Herbal Medicine for Rare Diseases

Many rare diseases are genetic and lack effective cures. Herbal medicine, developed by ancient healers without the benefit of modern cell biology knowledge, focuses on alleviating symptoms associated with uncommon conditions. *Herbal Medicine for Rare Diseases: Alleviating Symptoms by GMP Herbal Formulations* adopts an herbal medicine approach to addressing signs and symptoms of rare diseases.

Each herb possesses a multitude of compounds that allow it to treat various conditions, while a single condition can often be addressed by several different herbs, illustrating complex relationships that artificial intelligence (AI) excels at deciphering. The herbal prescriptions in this book are generated using AI models, trained on a decade's worth of medical insurance data from Taiwan, featuring the use of Good Manufacturing Practice (GMP)-certified traditional Chinese medicine (TCM) products. The connection between deep learning and big data ensures that the trained AI model represents the collective wisdom of ~5,000 herbal medical doctors in Taiwan who contributed to the training data.

Features

- Prescribes granulated herbal products sourced from GMP-certified manufacturers to ensure quality and safety
- Provides precise dosage information for the GMP herbal products in every prescription
- Includes a wealth of common and alternative herbal prescriptions tailored for specific conditions or combinations thereof
- Cites evidence from preclinical and clinical studies of the herb and formula to offer insights into their efficacy and mechanisms

In each section of *Herbal Medicine for Rare Diseases: Alleviating Symptoms by GMP Herbal Formulations*, AI-generated prescriptions are meticulously annotated with evidence from modern pharmacological and phytochemical studies of the herbs and multi-herb formulas included in the prescriptions. This book is beneficial for health professionals and practitioners, particularly those who specialize in complementary, alternative, and herbal medicine.

Herbal Medicine for Rare Diseases

Alleviating Symptoms by GMP Herbal Formulations

Sun-Chong Wang and Meng Hua Chen

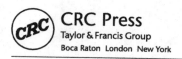

CRC Press
Taylor & Francis Group
Boca Raton   London   New York

CRC Press is an imprint of the
Taylor & Francis Group, an **informa** business

Designed cover image: Shutterstock

First edition published 2025
by CRC Press
2385 NW Executive Center Drive, Suite 320, Boca Raton FL 33431

and by CRC Press
4 Park Square, Milton Park, Abingdon, Oxon, OX14 4RN

CRC Press is an imprint of Taylor & Francis Group, LLC

© 2025 Taylor & Francis Group, LLC

ISBN: 978-1-032-72661-8 (hbk)
ISBN: 978-1-032-72223-8 (pbk)
ISBN: 978-1-032-72662-5 (ebk)

DOI: 10.1201/9781032726625

Typeset in Times
by KnowledgeWorks Global Ltd.

Contents

Preface

Ancient herbalists in China had no knowledge of genes and cells, but they utilized various parts of plants to alleviate patients' symptoms such as pain, fever, diarrhea, and insomnia. Over time, different herbs were combined into formulas and processed into decoctions to treat combinations of symptoms. Today, these decoctions are concentrated and dried into granules by Good Manufacturing Practice (GMP)-certified manufacturers, similar to how fresh milk is processed into instant milk powder. This book presents prescriptions made from the granular herbal products to relieve the symptoms of the 365 most common rare diseases, whose prevalences, estimated from the Orphanet database (https://www.orpha.net), are less than 1 in 2,000 and greater than 1 in 100,000.

ChatGPT has demonstrated to generate interesting texts with useful information. The texts and stories generated by ChatGPT appear to be genuine; however, some parts of the text may be fabricated and the text as a whole links factual information with nonfactual information. The reason for this behavior has to do with how ChatGPT was defined and trained. It was designed as a conditional probability model where, given user's input and model's generated words so far, it outputs the most probable next word. To achieve this, a window was randomly drawn from the training corpus that includes Wikipedia and webpages, and the model's parameters were adjusted so that the model correctly predicted the last word in the window given the preceding words. Our artificial intelligence (AI) model for herbal prescription generation is similar except that, with a training corpus consisting of pairs of disease diagnoses and herbal prescriptions, the model predicts herbal prescriptions based on the corresponding disease diagnoses. As the training data is structured and the task is specific, there is no room for our model to fabricate.

Taiwan is known for its semiconductor manufacturing and also its health insurance program, which is run by the government and covers all its residents. The health insurance program has reimbursed GMP granular herbal prescriptions since the program's establishment in 1995. The prescriptions shown throughout the book are based on the AI model trained on the health insurance reimbursement big data collected between 2004 and 2013, during which there were ~5,000 practicing herbal medical doctors in Taiwan. The prescriptions in this book represent the collective wisdom of 5,000 herbal medical doctors in Taiwan, not a single herbal medical doctor specializing in a specific field as in most other similar books. The diversity of the herbal medical doctors matches the heterogeneity of the rare diseases.

The health insurance reimbursement data recorded diseases in ICD-9 codes. As over two-thirds of the rare diseases are genetic and currently have no cures, symptomatic treatment of rare diseases by GMP herbal products is the approach adopted in the book. Diseases and symptoms (in MeSH; https://www.nlm.nih.gov/mesh/meshhome.html) are associated whenever they appeared in an article indexed in the PubMed database of the National Library of Medicine and National Institute of Health in the United States. Symptoms are ordered and treated as a sentence in one language; similarly, diseases and GMP granular herbal prescriptions are respectively ordered and treated as a sentence in a second and third language. Symptoms are translated to diseases, which in turn are translated to GMP granular herbal prescriptions by the AI Transformer model with a method called Multilingual Neural Machine Translation, which is a state-of-the-art and mature AI method underlying Google Translate.

The most common 365 rare diseases are grouped into chapters according to the affected organs/systems. Each section in a chapter starts with an introduction to the disease, followed by a table showing the symptoms of the diseases and the corresponding GMP herbal prescriptions. At the end of the section, the authors annotate the herbs/formulas appearing in the table, citing results of the latest peer-reviewed pharmacologic studies on the constituent herbs/formulas. The structure of the tables is detailed below.

Name of rare disease (Orphanet ID)
Disease prevalence
Disease-causing gene 1 (if any)
Disease-causing gene 2 (if any)
.
.
Mode of inheritance
Obligate phenotypes (if any)
Very frequent phenotypes
Frequent phenotypes
Occasional phenotypes
Disease onset

Obligate symptoms (ICD-9 code or MeSH descriptor ID) (if any):

| Common prescription 1. | Common prescription 1. |
| Common prescription 2. | Common prescription 2. |

Very frequent symptoms (ICD-9 code or MeSH descriptor ID):

| Common prescription 1. | Common prescription 1. |
| Common prescription 2. | Common prescription 2. |

Frequent symptoms (ICD-9 code or MeSH descriptor ID):

| Common prescription 1. | Common prescription 1. |
| Common prescription 2. | Common prescription 2. |

Occasional symptoms (ICD-9 code or MeSH descriptor ID) (if any):

| Common prescription 1. | Common prescription 1. |
| Common prescription 2. | Common prescription 2. |

The disease prevalence, genes, phenotypes, inheritance mode, and onset in the tables are based on the data downloaded from the Orphanet (https://www.orpha.net) in June 2023. The GMP herbal prescriptions, generated by the AI model, in the left table column are made up of classical multi-herb formulas and single herbs, while those in the right column of the table are made up of single herbs only. In herbal medicine, it is customary to prescribe multiple treatments for a single condition and to recommend a single treatment for multiple conditions. This versatile approach stems from the fact that herbs (and formulas) consist of various compounds, enabling them to target multiple pathways and functions within cells. This complexity results in many-to-many relationships between prescriptions and conditions, which are also best-suited for learning by AI models. An herbal prescription is generally taken three times a day. Moreover, the herbal medical doctor will give further instructions to pediatric patients and patients who are also taking conventional medicines.

About the Authors

Sun-Chong Wang, Ph.D., professor in the Department of Biomedical Sciences and Engineering, National Central University, Taiwan. Dr. Wang earned his PhD in physics from New York University, turned to bioinformatics, and specialized in epigenomics, herbalism, and deep learning. He has peer-reviewed publications in prestigious journals including *Nature Genetics, Nature Chemical Biology, Nature Structural and Molecular Biology, Nature Communications, Biological Psychiatry, Genome Biology,* and *Physical Review Letters.* He has contributed packages to R archive and Bioconductor. He is the author of six books on Amazon.com and two Android apps in Google Play.

Meng Hua Chen, member of Australia Acupuncture and Chinese Medicine Association (https://www.acupuncture.org.au). Dr. Chen is a dedicated and highly accomplished Chinese medicine practitioner with over three decades of experience. He possesses a bachelor of medical science in Chinese medicine from Guangzhou University of Chinese Medicine, China, and a PhD in complementary medicine from RMIT University, Australia. He demonstrates expertise in Chinese herbal medicine, acupuncture and holistic health consultation, providing integrative care to patients. He also publishes research works to esteemed international scientific journals, contributing to the advancement of complementary medicine.

1 GMP Herbal Medicine for Rare Developmental Defects During Embryogenesis

Human embryonic development begins with a single-celled fertilized egg and concludes around the eighth week after fertilization when the fetus takes form. During the eight weeks of pregnancy, a series of cell divisions and differentiations take place. For example, at about the third week, three primary germ layers—ectoderm, mesoderm, and endoderm—differentiate. Each layer eventually gives rise to specific tissues and organs. Specifically, the ectoderm later forms the eye, ear, tooth, mouth, anus, skin, hair, and the entire nervous system. The mesoderm develops into muscles, bones, lymph vessels, blood cells, spleen, kidneys, genital organs, and the circulatory system. The endoderm forms thyroid and parathyroid glands, urinary bladder, urethra, and the digestive and respiratory systems. Errors occurring in any stage of the embryonic development cause the conditions of this chapter, manifesting a wide range of signs and symptoms dependent on the affected parts or systems of the body. Over half of the errors involve mutated genes which can be inherited or acquired.

The single herbs that are frequently discussed in this chapter are Rhubarb Root and Rhizome (Dàhuáng), Licorice Root (Gāncǎo), Cardamon Seed (Shārén), Dahurian Angelica Root (Báizhǐ), Rehmannia Root (Dìhuáng), Scutellaria Root (Huángqín), Magnolia Bark (Hòupò), Figwort Root (Xuánshēn), Ophiopogon Tuber (Màiméndōng), Sweetflag Rhizome (Shíchāngpú), Immature Bitter Orange (Zhǐshí), and Chinese Senega Root (Yuǎnzhì). The multi-herb formulas that are commonly used in this chapter include Ginseng, Poria, and Atractylodes Powder (Shēnlíngbáizhúsǎn); Lycium, Chrysanthemum, and Rehmannia Pill (Qǐjúdìhuángwán); Aucklandia, Cardamon, and the Six Gentlemen Decoction (Xiāngshāliùjūnzǐtāng); Free and Easy Wanderer Plus (Augmented Rambling Powder; Jiāwèixiāoyáosǎn); Magnolia Flower and Gypsum Combination (Xīnyíqīngfèitāng); Tonify the Middle and Augment the Qi Decoction (Bǔzhōngyìqìtāng); Sweet Dew Decoction (Gānlùyǐn); Five Ingredient Formula with Poria (Wǔlíngsǎn); Minor Construct the Middle Decoction (Xiǎojiànzhōngtāng); Six Ingredient Pill with Rehmannia (Liùwèidìhuángwán); Achyranthes and Plantago Formula (Jìshēngshènqìwán); and Poria, Cinnamon, Atractylodis, and Licorice Decoction (Línggùishùgāntāng). Note that the herbal medicines in this book are in the form of concentrated extract granules manufactured by Good Manufacturing Practice (GMP)-certified pharmaceutical companies and that the safety and efficacy of the dispensing granules were found to be similar to those of traditional decoctions (Luo et al., 2012). Although the symptoms vary, many of the herbal regimens aim to improve the digestion of the affected newborns. For example, Shēnlíngbáizhúsǎn is known to relieve intestinal malabsorption and chronic diarrhea (Ji et al., 2019).

1.1 TRISOMY X

Trisomy X, also known as triple X syndrome or 47,XXX syndrome, is a form of chromosome number anomaly where females have three, rather than two, X chromosomes in their body cells. In most cases, the extra X came from an egg cell which failed to segregate the duplicated X chromosomes in concluding the egg-cell making process, called meiosis, in the ovary before ovulation. Therefore, although trisomy X is a genetic condition, it is not inherited and affected women can have normal children. The frequent symptoms of trisomy X include hypotonia and some patients may occasionally experience seizure and tremor.

DOI: 10.1201/9781032726625-1

TABLE 1.1

GMP Herbal Medicines for a One-Year-Old Girl with Trisomy X

Trisomy X (OrphaCode: 3375)

A malformation syndrome with a prevalence of ~4 in 10,000

Not applicable

Abnormality of chromosome segregation

Tall stature, Epicanthus, Hypotonia, Global developmental delay, Specific learning disability, Clinodactyly of the 5th finger, Cognitive impairment

Multicystic kidney dysplasia, Hypertelorism, Upslanted palpebral fissure, Depression, Anxiety, Pectus excavatum, Secondary amenorrhea, Seizure, Tremor, Hip dysplasia, Joint hyperflexibility, Attention deficit hyperactivity disorder, Renal hypoplasia/aplasia

Infancy, Childhood

Hypotonia (D009123):

Xiǎojiànzhōngtāng 5g + yùpíngfēngsǎn 5g.

Xiǎojiànzhōngtāng 5g + bǔzhōngyìqìtāng 5g.

Xiǎojiànzhōngtāng 5g + shēnlíngbáizhúsǎn 5-0g + shānzhā 1-0g + shénqū 1-0g + màiyá 1-0g + jīnèijīn 1-0g.

Sìjūnzǐtāng 5g + yùpíngfēngsǎn 5-0g + shānzhā 0g + shénqū 0g + màiyá 0g + jīnèijīn 0g.

Xìngsūyǐnyòukē 5g + xīnyíqīngfèitāng 5g.

Gāncǎo 5g + báizhǐ 5g + shārén 5g + dàhuáng 1-0g.

Zhǐqiào 5g + jílí 5-0g + chántuì 5-0g + júhóng 5-0g.

Jílí 5g + chántuì 5g + zhǐqiào 4-3g.

Huángqí 5g + chìsháo 1g + fángfēng 1g.

Seizure (345.9), Tremor (D014202):

Yìgānsǎn 5g + gāncǎoxiǎomàidàzǎotāng 5-2g.

Yìgānsǎn 5g + cháihújiālónggǔmǔlìtāng 5-0g + tiānmá 1-0g + gōuténg 1-0g.

Guìzhījiālónggǔmǔlìtāng 5-0g + yìgānsǎn 5-0g + tiānmá 1-0g + shíchāngpú 1-0g + yuǎnzhì 1-0g.

Wēndǎntāng 5g + shíchāngpú 1g + yuǎnzhì 1g + gōuténg 1g.

Tiānwángbǔxīndān 5g + shēnlíngbáizhúsǎn 5g + shíchāngpú 1g + yuǎnzhì 1g.

Xuánshēn 5g + dìhuáng 5g + màiméndōng 5g + yùzhú 5-0g + shāshēn 5-0g + hòupò 5-0g + zhǐshí 5-0g + dàhuáng 1-0g.

Gāncǎo 5g + báizhǐ 5g + shārén 4g + dàhuáng 0g.

The table first displays herbal medicines for trisomy X infants exhibiting hypotonia, followed by those for trisomy X infants with seizure and tremor. The prescriptions on the left column of the table comprise multi-herb formulas and also single herbs, while those on the right consist of single herbs only. Zero grams in a prescription in the table indicates that the weight of the medicinal granules is less than 0.5 grams, while *x*-*y*g indicates that the weight of the medicinal granules is anything between *x* and *y* grams. Xiǎojiànzhōngtāng has traditionally been used to improve the digestion of the patients and to strengthen the physique of children. Gāncǎo, i.e., Radix et Rhizoma Glycyrrhizae or licorice, a component herb in Xiǎojiànzhōngtāng, is believed to help energetics and digestion in traditional Chinese medicine (TCM). It is known today to be anti-inflammatory, antioxidative, antiallergenic, and antimicrobial through its corticosteroid-like activities; however, its habitual use can lead to hypokalemia and hypertension (Kwon et al., 2020). Yìgānsǎn was initially formulated for children experiencing panic, epilepsy, and convulsions by TCM physician Yang Shiying (1208–1274 AD) in the Southern Song Dynasty.

1.2　FETAL CYTOMEGALOVIRUS SYNDROME

A pregnant woman infected with cytomegalovirus can transmit the virus to the fetus, causing congenital cytomegalovirus infection in the newborn. Healthy adults infected with cytomegalovirus show no signs and symptoms. However, infants with antenatal cytomegalovirus infection can have long-term health conditions, including hearing loss and vision loss. Table 1.2 shows the herbal prescriptions for children with antenatal cytomegalovirus infection.

Xiǎocháihútāng has long been used for hearing problems, while Hángjú (Flos Chrysanthemi from Hangzhou/Zhejiang China) and Gǒuqǐzǐ (Fructus Lycii) have been known for their benefits to the

TABLE 1.2
GMP Herbal Medicines for a Two-Year-Old Toddler with Fetal Cytomegalovirus Syndrome

Fetal cytomegalovirus syndrome (OrphaCode: 294)

A disease with a prevalence of ~4 in 10,000

Not applicable

Sensorineural hearing impairment, Abnormality of the eye, Abnormality of vision

Splenomegaly, Anemia, Abnormality of coagulation, Hepatomegaly

Antenatal, Neonatal

Sensorineural hearing impairment (389.1), Abnormality of the eye (379.90):

Qǐjúdìhuángwán 5g + xiāngshāliùjūnzǐtāng 5-0g + shānzhā 1-0g + shíchāngpú 1-0g + yuǎnzhì 1-0g + gāncǎo 1-0g.

Qǐjúdìhuángwán 5g + zīshènmíngmùtāng 4-0g + mùzéicǎo 1-0g + xiàkūcǎo 1-0g + mìménghuā 1-0g + gāncǎo 1-0g.

Yùpíngfēngsǎn 5g + gāncǎo 2g.

Xiǎocháihútāng 5g + zhúyèshígāotāng 5g + mùzéicǎo 2g + juémíngzǐ 2g + gǔjīngcǎo 2g.

Xìngsūyǐnyòukē 5g + xǐgānmíngmùtāng 5g + cāngěrsǎn 5g + gāncǎo 1g.

Hángjú 5g + gǒuqǐzǐ 5g + shíchāngpú 4-2g + yuǎnzhì 4-2g + báizhú 2-0g + gāncǎo 2-0g.

Sīguāluò 5g + júhuā 5-4g + chántuì 4-0g + jílí 3-0g + júhóng 2-0g.

Shíchāngpú 5g + gǒuqǐzǐ 5g + yuǎnzhì 5g + hángjú 5-4g.

Anemia (285.9), Abnormality of coagulation (287.9):

Xiōngguījiāoàitāng 5g + guīpítāng 5-0g + shēnlíngbáizhúsǎn 3-0g + xiānhècǎo 2-0g + báimáogēn 2-0g + huángqí 1-0g.

Guīpítāng 5g + sìwùtāng 5-0g + bǔzhōngyìqìtāng 5-0g + xiānhècǎo 2-0g + báimáogēn 2-0g + ǒujiē 2-0g.

Shēnlíngbáizhúsǎn 5g + guīpítāng 5g + xiānhècǎo 2-0g + báimáogēn 2-0g + ējiāo 2-0g + dìhuáng 2-0g.

Xiānhècǎo 5g + xuánshēn 5-0g + báihuāshéshécǎo 5-0g + màiméndōng 5-0g + báimáogēn 5-0g + dìhuáng 5-0g + mǔdānpí 5-0g + chìsháo 5-0g + ǒujiē 5-0g + gāncǎo 2-0g.

Xuánshēn 5g + dìhuáng 5g + màiméndōng 5g + hòupò 3-0g + zhǐshí 3-0g + shānzhā 2-0g + shénqū 2-0g + dàhuáng 1-0g.

Gāncǎo 5g + shārén 5g + dàhuáng 0g.

eye. On the other hand, Xiānhècǎo (Herba Agrimoniae) has traditionally been used to stop bleeding. Moreover, the concurrent use of Xiānhècǎo and Guīpítāng was found to be associated with a reduced risk of anemia-related mortalities in patients with aplastic anemia (Chiu et al., 2021), where the potential hematopoietic effect of Xiānhècǎo and Guīpítāng was underscored. Other hematopoietic medicines in Table 1.2 will be elucidated when they appear again later in the book. Qǐjúdìhuángwán contains Gǒuqǐzǐ and Júhuā (Flos Chrysanthemi). The regimens in the table are composed to improve the visual, hearing, and anemia symptoms of children with fetal cytomegalovirus syndrome.

1.3 FRAGILE X SYNDROME

Fragile X syndrome (FXS) is caused by a repeat expansion and then silencing of the *FMR1* gene, whose products help develop connections and communications between the neurons in the brain. Affected individuals are thus intellectually disabled. Also, as one mutated allele of *FMR1* is enough to cause FXS, male FXS usually exhibits more severe learning disabilities than female FXS. Table 1.3 shows the herbal prescriptions for a two-year-old FXS toddler presenting various symptoms.

Xuánshēn (Radix Scrophulariae) has been used for sore and swollen throats (Lee et al., 2021; Wang, 2020). A modern study showed that compounds in Xuánshēn attenuate focal cerebral ischemia-reperfusion injury in rats (Chen et al., 2019). Gānlùxiāodúdān's modern use is for chronic liver disease (Wang, 2019), and in severe liver disease patients, toxins can build up and travel to the brain to cause neurocognitive impairment including language impairment (López-Franco et al., 2021). Xiǎocháihútāng (cf. Section 1.2) is known to address Shaoyang pattern, i.e., the "lesser yang syndrome" in TCM. As both foot-Shaoyang meridian and hand-Shaoyang meridian travel to the ear, Xiǎocháihútāng and Xiǎocháihútāngqùrénshēn are believed to heal hearing problems. Júhóng (Exocarpium Citri Rubrum) "regulates Qi, widens the

TABLE 1.3

GMP Herbal Medicines for a Two-Year-Old Child with Fragile X Syndrome

Fragile X syndrome (OrphaCode: 908)

A malformation syndrome with a prevalence of ~3 in 10,000

Disease-causing germline mutation(s) (loss of function): fragile X messenger ribonucleoprotein 1 (*FMR1* / Entrez: 2332) at Xq27.3

X-linked dominant

Macroorchidism, Chronic otitis media, Joint laxity, Pes planus, Neurological speech impairment, Intellectual disability–moderate, Folate-dependent fragile site at Xq28

Sinusitis, Macrocephaly, Narrow face, Long face, Mandibular prognathia, Otitis media, Protruding ear, Hypotonia, Large forehead, Frontal bossing, Gastroesophageal reflux, Attention deficit hyperactivity disorder

Strabismus, Autism, Anxiety, Seizure, Mitral valve prolapse, Cerebral cortical atrophy, Dilatation of the ascending aorta, Self-injurious behavior

Neonatal, Infancy, Childhood

Neurological speech impairment (D013064):

Gānlùxiāodúdān 5g + jīngfángbàidúsǎn 5-0g + xīnyíqīngfèitāng 5-0g + gāncǎo 0g.

Xìngsūyǐnyòukē 5g + xīnyíqīngfèitāng 5g + cāngěrsǎn 5g.

Xìngsūyǐnyòukē 5g + máxìnggānshítāng 5-2g + xīnyíqīngfèitāng 5-0g + bèimǔ 1-0g + yúxīngcǎo 1-0g.

Xiǎojiànzhōngtāng 5g.

Bǎohéwán 5g + gānlùxiāodúdān 5-0g + xiāngshāliùjūnzǐtāng 5-0g + gāncǎo 1-0g + jīnèijīn 1-0g.

Otitis media (382.9), Hypotonia (D009123), Gastroesophageal reflux (530.81):

Xiǎocháihútāngqùrénshēn 5g + qínjiāobiējiǎsǎn 3-2g + wūméi 1g + bǎihégùjīntāng 1-0g.

Xiǎocháihútāngqùrénshēn 5g + shēnsūyǐn 2-0g + bǎihégùjīntāng 2-0g + wūméi 1-0g.

Pǔjìxiāodúyǐn 5g + xiǎocháihútāngqùrénshēn 3g + wūméi 1g.

Strabismus (378.7, 378.6, 378.31), Autism (299.0), Seizure (345.9):

Gāncǎoxiǎomàidàzǎotāng 5g + yìgānsǎn 5-0g + cháihújiālónggǔmǔlìtāng 5-0g + tiānmá 2-0g + gōuténg 2-0g + acupuncture.

Gāncǎoxiǎomàidàzǎotāng 5g + báijiāngcán 1g + shíchāngpú 1g + yuǎnzhì 1g.

Xiǎocháihútāng 5g + báijiāngcán 1g + shíchāngpú 1g + yuǎnzhì 1g + gōuténg 1g.

Cháihújiālónggǔmǔlìtāng 5g + shíchāngpú 1g + yuǎnzhì 1g + chántuì 1g.

Guìzhījiālónggǔmǔlìtāng 5g + báijiāngcán 1g + shíchāngpú 1g + yuǎnzhì 1g + chántuì 1g + gōuténg 1g.

Sāngjúyǐn 5g + chántuì 1g + zhǐqiào 1g.

Xuánshēn 5g + dìhuáng 5g + hòupò 5g + zhǐshí 5g + màiméndōng 5g + yùzhú 5-0g + shāshēn 5-0g + dàhuáng 1-0g.

Báizhú 5g + gāncǎo 5-4g + shārén 5-4g + dàhuáng 1-0g.

Júhóng 5g + shānyào 2-0g.

Júhuā 5g + chántuì 5-0g + júhóng 2-0g.

Jílí 5g + júhuā 5-0g + júhóng 5-0g.

Zhǐqiào 5g + júhóng 5g + jílí 5-1g.

Jílí 5g + chántuì 5-0g + júhóng 2-0g + zhǐqiào 1-0g + sīguāluò 1-0g.

Chántuì 5g + júhóng 1-0g.

Gāncǎo 5g + jílí 5-0g + zhǐqiào 2-0g + sīguāluò 0g.

interior" and is used today for cough, chest pain, and dyspepsia (Wang, 2020). Qi is a form of energy responsible for life in many traditional medicines including TCM. Gāncǎoxiǎomàidàzǎotāng "cultivates the mind, calms the spirit" and is used nowadays for anxiety (Wang, 2019). Jílí, i.e., Fructus Tribuli, "brightens the eye" and was shown to ameliorate oxidant induced cell injury in human retinal pigment epithelial cells (Yuan et al., 2020). Note that expressions enclosed in double quotes represent the author's translations of Chinese phrases from classic TCM texts.

1.4   TURNER SYNDROME

Turner syndrome, or 45,X syndrome, is a chromosome abnormality affecting development in females. Girls and women with Turner syndrome have a complete or partial loss of one of the X chromosomes in all or some of their body cells. The functional X chromosome usually comes from

TABLE 1.4

GMP Herbal Medicines for a Four-Year-Old Girl with Turner Syndrome

Turner syndrome (OrphaCode: 881)

A malformation syndrome with a prevalence of ~3 in 10,000

Not applicable, Unknown

Abnormality of the ovary, Short neck, Delayed puberty, Increased circulating gonadotropin level, Short sternum, Osteopenia, Osteoporosis, Growth delay, Intrauterine growth retardation, Delayed skeletal maturation, Cubitus valgus, High urinary gonadotropins (primary hypogonadism), Short stature, Wide intermamillary distance, Aplasia/Hypoplasia of the nipples, Premature ovarian insufficiency, Female infertility, Postnatal growth retardation, Increased upper to lower segment ratio, Abnormal morphology of forearm bone, Enlarged thorax, Precocious menopause

High palate, Retrognathia, Micrognathia, Hearing impairment, Low-set ears, Recurrent otitis media, Webbed neck, Thickened nuchal skin fold, Broad neck, Behavioral abnormality, Anxiety, Impaired use of nonverbal behaviors, Primary amenorrhea, Hypertension, Glucose intolerance, Secondary amenorrhea, Hashimoto thyroiditis, Shield chest, Specific learning disability, Hepatic steatosis, Obesity, Failure to thrive in infancy, Hypoplastic toenails, Low posterior hairline, High and narrow palate, Kyphosis, Genu valgum, Elevated hepatic transaminase, Dilatation of the aortic arch, Dermatoglyphic ridges abnormal, Enlargement of the distal femoral epiphysis, Irregular proximal tibial epiphyses, Abnormal dermatoglyphics, Neck pterygia, Short 4th metacarpal, Short 5th metacarpal, Hypermobility of toe joints

Horseshoe kidney, Ectopic kidney, Abnormality of the dentition, Epicanthus, Cystic hygroma, Strabismus, Ptosis, Myopia, Depression, Pectus excavatum, Hyperinsulinemia, Atypical scarring of skin, Melanocytic nevus, Lymphedema, Vitiligo, Abnormal fingernail morphology, Hip dysplasia, Hepatic fibrosis, Alopecia, Atrial septal defect, Bicuspid aortic valve, Prolonged QT interval, Myocardial infarction, Coarctation of aorta, Pes planus, Hyperconvex fingernails, Short toe, Celiac disease, Cholestatic liver disease, Scoliosis, Autoimmunity, Madelung deformity, Inverted nipples, Nevus, Reduced bone mineral density, Numerous congenital melanocytic nevi, Type II diabetes mellitus, Attention deficit hyperactivity disorder, Combined hyperlipidemia, External ear malformation, Aplasia/Hypoplasia of the mandible, Splayed toes, Delayed social development, Thyroiditis

Antenatal, Neonatal, Infancy, Childhood

Osteoporosis (733.0), Premature ovarian insufficiency (256.31):

Guìzhījiālónggǔmǔlìtāng 5g + shānyào 2-0g + wǔwèizǐ 2-0g + fùpénzǐ 2-0g + dùzhòng 1-0g + bǔgǔzhī 1-0g + xùduàn 1-0g + shānzhā 1-0g + wūméi 1-0g.

Wūméi 5g + cāngzhú 5-2g + huáihuā 5-0g + wǔwèizǐ 5-0g.

Zhīmǔ 5g + gégēn 5g + mǔdānpí 2g + dìgǔpí 2-0g.

Dùzhòng 5g + xùduàn 5g.

Shānyào 5g + zhīmǔ 5-0g + gégēn 5-0g + dùzhòng 2-0g.

Hearing impairment (D034381), Hypertension (401-405.99), Hepatic steatosis (571.0), Obesity (278.00), Elevated hepatic transaminase (573.9):

Fángfēngtōngshèngsǎn 5g + dàcháihútāng 4-0g + shānzhā 1-0g + chēqiánzǐ 1-0g + héyè 1-0g + chénpí 1-0g + yìyǐrén 1-0g.

Fángfēngtōngshèngsǎn 5g + mázǐrénwán 5-0g.

Tiānmágōuténgyǐn 5g + fángfēngtōngshèngsǎn 3g + shānzhā 1g + gāncǎo 1g.

Tiānmágōuténgyǐn 5g + zhībódìhuángwán 5g + lóngdǎnxiègāntāng 5-0g.

Zhībódìhuángwán 5g + lóngdǎnxiègāntāng 5g + xiāngshāliùjūnzǐtāng 3g + shānzhā 1g + shénqū 1g + màiyá 1g.

Jiāwèixiāoyáosǎn 5g + zhībódìhuángwán 5g + shānzhā 1g + dānshēn 1g + héshǒuwū 1g + yīnchén 1g + chénpí 1g.

Gāncǎo 5g + bèimǔ 5-0g + zhīmǔ 5-0g + huángqín 5-0g + bǎihé 5-0g + dàhuáng 1-0g + huánglián 0g.

Shígāo 5g + zhīmǔ 5g + dàhuáng 0g.

Shānzhīzǐ 5g + gāncǎo 5g + zhīmǔ 5g + dàhuáng 0g + huánglián 0g.

Cháihú 5g + tiānhuā 4g + guìzhī 4g + huángqín 4g + gāncǎo 2g + mǔlì 2g + gānjiāng 2g.

Cháihú 5g + báisháo 5-2g + zhǐshí 5-2g + huángqín 5-2g + bànxià 2-1g + shēngjiāng 2-1g + dàzǎo 2-0g + dàhuáng 1-0g.

Strabismus (378.7, 378.6, 378.31), Ptosis (374.3), Myopia (367.1), Vitiligo (709.01), Alopecia (704.0), Celiac disease (579.0), Thyroiditis (245):

Jiāwèixiāoyáosǎn 5g + qǐjúdìhuángwán 5g + nǚzhēnzǐ 1-0g + héshǒuwū 1-0g + hànliáncǎo 1-0g + tùsīzǐ 1-0g.

Liùwèidìhuángwán 5-4g + xiāoyáosǎn 5-0g + gǒuqǐzǐ 1g + jílí 1g + nǚzhēnzǐ 1-0g + hànliáncǎo 1-0g + hónghuā 1-0g + táorén 1-0g + bǔgǔzhī 1-0g + tùsīzǐ 1-0g + héshǒuwū 1-0g.

Jílí 5g + chántuì 5-0g.

Báizhǐ 5g + shārén 5-2g + huángqín 3-0g + gāncǎo 2g + tiānhuā 1-0g + dàhuáng 0g.

Báizhǐ 5g + zhìgāncǎo 5g + shārén 5g + huángqín 3g + dàhuáng 0g.

the mother, indicating that Turner syndrome is often due to an error in chromosome separation that occurs when germ cells divide in the father.

Wūméi (Fructus Mume) aids digestion (Wang, 2020) and was shown to be antiosteoporosis in murine monocyte/macrophage-like cells (Yan et al., 2015). Dùzhòng (Cortex Eucommiae) was shown to prevent osteoporosis in ovariectomized rats (Zhang et al., 2009). Guìzhījiālónggǔmǔlìtāng has been used for individuals with "deficiency in both yin and yang." Fángfēngtōngshèngsǎn and Tiānmágōuténgyǐn are used nowadays for functional digestive disorders and essential hypertension, respectively (Wang, 2019). Lóngdǎnxiègāntāng "quenches fires of the Liver and Gallbladder" and is used today for chronic liver disease and cirrhosis (Wang, 2019). The bioactivities of Báizhǐ (Radix Angelicae Dahuricae), including its effects on the skin, were recently summarized (Zhao, Feng, et al., 2022). Jiāwèixiāoyáosǎn was the most commonly prescribed formula for hyperthyroidism, followed by Zhībódìhuángwán (Chang et al., 2022), which was derived from Liùwèidìhuángwán by adding two herbs to enhance the "heat-quenching" effect. The prescriptions in the table are seen to address various manifestations of Turner syndrome.

1.5 DOWN SYNDROME

Down syndrome, i.e., trisomy 21, is a chromosome condition where affected individuals have three copies of chromosome 21, instead of the normal two copies, in their body cells. In most cases, the extra copy comes from the mother when chromosome 21 fails to separate in cell division during egg cell making. In few cases, nonseparation of chromosomes occurs in early development of the embryo, resulting in trisomy 21 in only some, but not all, of the baby's body cells. Characteristics and symptoms of such mosaic Down syndrome patients are typically fewer and milder.

Huángqíwǔwùtāng "strengthens Qi and Blood" and is used today for paralytic syndromes (Wang, 2019); Shēnlíngbáizhúsǎn "enhances Qi and the Spleen" and is used today for disorders of function of stomach (Wang, 2019); Qǐjúdìhuángwán (cf. Section 1.2) "nourishes the Liver and the

TABLE 1.5

GMP Herbal Medicines for a One-Year-Old Baby with Down Syndrome

Down syndrome (OrphaCode: 870)

A malformation syndrome with a prevalence of ~3 in 10,000

Not applicable

Brachycephaly, Epicanthus, Short neck, Thickened nuchal skin fold, Upslanted palpebral fissure, Brachydactyly, Intellectual disability, Hypotonia, Joint laxity, Depressed nasal bridge, Flat face, Round ear

Decreased fertility, Macroglossia, Narrow mouth, Abnormality of the dentition, Thick lower lip vermilion, Narrow palate, Open mouth, Abnormality of the fontanelles or cranial sutures, Depressed nasal ridge, Microdontia, Obesity, Umbilical hernia, Sandal gap, Developmental regression, Malformation of the heart and great vessels, Downturned corners of mouth, Short nose, Clinodactyly of the 5th finger, Prematurely aged appearance, Bilateral single transverse palmar creases, Protruding tongue, Abnormality of immune system physiology, Abnormality of the lymphatic system

Conductive hearing impairment, Strabismus, Cataract, Myopia, Hypothyroidism, Hypotrichosis, Gait disturbance, Anal atresia, Aganglionic megacolon, Type II diabetes mellitus, Acute megakaryocytic leukemia, Impaired pain sensation, Renal hypoplasia/aplasia

Antenatal, Neonatal

Intellectual disability (D008607), Hypotonia (D009123):

Huángqíwǔwùtāng 5g + sháoyàogāncǎotāng 2-0g + dānshēn 2-0g + zhúrú 2-0g + yánhúsuǒ 2-0g + sāngzhī 2-0g + jiānghuáng 2-0g + gōuténg 2-0g + dāngguī 1-0g + acupuncture.
Bǔzhōngyìqìtāng 5g.

Gāncǎo 5g + shārén 5g + báizhǐ 5-0g + dàhuáng 0g.
Huángqí 5g + chìsháo 2-0g + fángfēng 2-0g + xìxīn 0g + huánglián 0g + dàhuáng 0g.
Běishāshēn 5g + yùzhú 5g + hòupò 5g + zhǐshí 5g + xuánshēn 5-0g + dìhuáng 5-0g + màiméndōng 5-0g + dàhuáng 1g.

(Continued)

TABLE 1.5 *(Continued)*
GMP Herbal Medicines for a One-Year-Old Baby with Down Syndrome

Obesity (278.00):

Shēnlíngbáizhúsǎn 5g + shānzhā 1-0g + shénqū 1-0g + màiyá 1-0g + jīnèijīn 1-0g + gāncǎo 1-0g.

Xiǎojiànzhōngtāng 5g + yùpíngfēngsǎn 2-0g + shānzhā 1-0g + shénqū 1-0g + màiyá 1-0g + gāncǎo 1-0g + jīnèijīn 0g.

Gāncǎo 5g + jīnyínhuā 4-0g + dàhuáng 1-0g + huánglián 0g.

Shānzhīzǐ 5g + gāncǎo 5g + huángqín 5-0g + zhīmǔ 5-0g + dàhuáng 0g + huánglián 0g.

Conductive hearing impairment (D006314), Strabismus (378.7, 378.6, 378.31), Cataract (366.8), Myopia (367.1), Hypothyroidism (244.9), Acute megakaryocytic leukemia (205.0):

Qǐjúdìhuángwán 5g + xiāngshāliùjūnzǐtāng 5g + jiāwèixiāoyáosǎn 5-3g + nǚzhēnzǐ 1-0g + hànliáncǎo 1-0g + juémíngzǐ 1-0g + acupuncture.

Xiǎocháihútāng 5g + zhúyèshígāotāng 5g + gǒuqǐzǐ 2g + júhuā 2g + xìxīn 0g + huánglián 0g + dàhuáng 0g.

Yùpíngfēngsǎn 5g + qǐjúdìhuángwán 5g + dānshēn 1g + shíchāngpú 1g + yuǎnzhì 1g + acupuncture.

Yùpíngfēngsǎn 5g + xìngsūyǐnyòukē 5g + cāngěrsǎn 5g + gāncǎo 1g.

Xìngsūyǐnyòukē 5g + xīnyíqīngfèitāng 4g + bèimǔ 1g + qiánhú 1g + yúxīngcǎo 1g + cāngěrzǐ 1g.

Hángjú 5g + gǒuqǐzǐ 5g + liánqiáo 5-0g + shíchāngpú 3-2g + yuǎnzhì 3-2g + gāncǎo 2-0g.

Yùzhú 5g + shāshēn 5g + màiméndōng 5-0g + hòupò 5-0g + zhǐshí 5-0g + xuánshēn 2-0g + dìhuáng 2-0g.

Gǒuqǐzǐ 5g + hángjú 4-2g + gāncǎo 2-1g + shíchāngpú 1g + yuǎnzhì 1g + báizhú 1-0g.

Kidney to improve eyesight" and is used today for disorders of lacrimal system (Wang, 2019). Yùzhú (Rhizoma Polygonati Odorati) "nourishes yin" and was demonstrated to ameliorate metabolic disorders in high-fat diet induced obese mice (Gu et al., 2013). Xìngsūyǐnyòukē, Xīnyíqīngfèitāng and Yùpíngfēngsǎn all benefit the respiratory system (Wang, 2019), infection of which can block the Eustachian tube to cause hearing loss.

1.6   22q11.2 DELETION SYNDROME

22q11.2 deletion syndrome, also known as DiGeorge syndrome or velocardiofacial syndrome, is a genetic condition marked by a deletion in a section of chromosome 22 at 22q11.2, where there are around 40 genes. The deletion is usually *de novo*, occurring during early development of the embryo. The remaining cases are inherited in an autosomal dominant pattern from a parent's, usually the mother's, germ cells with the deletion.

TABLE 1.6
GMP Herbal Medicines for a Three-Year-Old Child with 22q11.2 Deletion Syndrome

22q11.2 deletion syndrome (OrphaCode: 567)

A malformation syndrome with a prevalence of ~3 in 10,000

Disease-causing germline mutation(s): T-box transcription factor 1 (*TBX1* / Entrez: 6899) at 22q11.21

Role: the phenotype of T-box transcription factor 1 (*TBX1* / Entrez: 6899) at 22q11.21

Role: the phenotype of ARVCF delta catenin family member (*ARVCF* / Entrez: 421) at 22q11.21

Role: the phenotype of glycoprotein Ib platelet subunit beta (*GP1BB* / Entrez: 2812) at 22q11.21

Role: the phenotype of ubiquitin recognition factor in ER associated degradation 1 (*UFD1* / Entrez: 7353) at 22q11.21

Role: the phenotype of histone cell cycle regulator (*HIRA* / Entrez: 7290) at 22q11.21

Role: the phenotype of catechol-O-methyltransferase (*COMT* / Entrez: 1312) at 22q11.21

Modifying germline mutation: jumonji domain containing 1C (*JMJD1C* / Entrez: 221037) at 10q21.3

Modifying germline mutation: ras responsive element binding protein 1 (*RREB1* / Entrez: 6239) at 6p24.3

Modifying germline mutation: SEC24 homolog C, COPII coat complex component (*SEC24C* / Entrez: 9632) at 10q22.2

Autosomal dominant

(Continued)

TABLE 1.6 *(Continued)*

GMP Herbal Medicines for a Three-Year-Old Child with 22q11.2 Deletion Syndrome

Epicanthus, Low-set ears, Prominent nasal bridge, Wide nasal bridge, Upslanted palpebral fissure, Hypoplasia of the thymus, Atrial septal defect, Tetralogy of Fallot, Abnormal pulmonary valve morphology, Cleft palate, Conductive hearing impairment, Bulbous nose, Telecanthus, Abnormality of the pharynx, Hypotonia, Nasal speech, Ventricular septal defect, Truncus arteriosus, Abnormal facial shape, Dysphasia, Malformation of the heart and great vessels, Platybasia, Immunodeficiency, Abnormal aortic arch morphology

Malar flattening, Long philtrum, Small earlobe, Overfolded helix, Short neck, Ptosis, Posterior embryotoxon, Abnormal skull morphology, Tetany, Renal hypoplasia, Abnormality of the dentition, Long face, Hearing impairment, Chronic otitis media, Abnormal eyelid morphology, Carious teeth, Hypoparathyroidism, Seborrheic dermatitis, Acne, Arachnodactyly, Intellectual disability–mild, Global developmental delay, Specific learning disability, Constipation, Meningocele, Hypocalcemia, Myalgia, Short stature, Impaired T cell function, Attention deficit hyperactivity disorder, Occipital myelomeningocele, Corneal neovascularization, Anorectal anomaly, Abnormality of the tonsils

Vesicoureteral reflux, Polycystic kidney dysplasia, Abnormality of the uterus, Narrow mouth, Hydrocephalus, Microcephaly, Micrognathia, Strabismus, Downslanted palpebral fissures, Cataract, Microphthalmia, Abnormality of dental enamel, Behavioral abnormality, Autism, Anxiety, Hypopigmented skin patches, Retinal arteriolar tortuosity, Seizure, Polyhydramnios, Patent ductus arteriosus, Abnormal aortic valve morphology, Inguinal hernia, Cryptorchidism, Hypospadias, Turricephaly, Hypertelorism, Short philtrum, Choanal atresia, Glaucoma, Optic atrophy, Depression, Abnormality of the thorax, Hypothyroidism, Hyperthyroidism, Purpura, Cholelithiasis, Hand polydactyly, Intellectual disability, Arthritis, Failure to thrive, Intrauterine growth retardation, Obesity, Umbilical hernia, Laryngomalacia, Splenomegaly, Talipes equinovarus, Foot polydactyly, Abnormality of thrombocytes, Thrombocytopenia, Gastroesophageal reflux, Anal atresia, Asthma, Arrhinencephaly, Gastrointestinal hemorrhage, Aganglionic megacolon, Spina bifida, Intestinal malrotation, Bowel incontinence, Varicose veins, Scoliosis, Autoimmunity, Patellar dislocation, Multiple renal cysts, Joint hyperflexibility, Chronic obstructive pulmonary disease, Lung segmentation defects, Bipolar affective disorder, Feeding difficulties in infancy, Multiple suture craniosynostosis, Tricuspid atresia, Hypertensive crisis, Atelectasis, Schizophrenia

All ages

Tetralogy of Fallot (745.2), Cleft palate (749.0), Conductive hearing impairment (D006314), Hypotonia (D009123), Ventricular septal defect (745.4), Immunodeficiency (279.3):

Xīnyíqīngfèitāng 5g + shēnlíngbáizhúsǎn 5g + xiāngshāliùjūnzǐtāng 5-0g + shānzhā 1g + shénqū 1g + màiyá 1g + cāngěrzǐ 1-0g + jīnèijīn 1-0g.

Xiāngshāliùjūnzǐtāng 5g + bǎohéwán 4g + shānzhā 1g + shénqū 1g + màiyá 1g + jīnèijīn 1g.

Shēnlíngbáizhúsǎn 5g + xiǎoqīnglóngtāng 2-0g + shānzhā 1g + shénqū 1g + màiyá 1g + jīnèijīn 1-0g + wūméi 1-0g + huángqí 1-0g.

Huángqín 5g + báizhǐ 4g + zhìgāncǎo 3g + shārén 3g + dàhuáng 0g.

Gāncǎo 5g + báizhǐ 5g + shārén 5g + huángqín 5-0g + dàhuáng 1-0g.

Dìhuáng 5g + màiméndōng 5g + xuánshēn 3g + yùzhú 3g + shāshēn 3g.

Xuánshēn 5g + yùzhú 5g + dìhuáng 5g + shāshēn 5g + hòupò 5g + zhǐshí 5g + màiméndōng 5g + dàhuáng 1g.

Běishāshēn 5g + yùzhú 5g + xuánshēn 3g + dìhuáng 3g + màiméndōng 3g + dàhuáng 0g.

Báizhú 5g + fùzǐ 5g + cháihú 5g + báisháo 3g + fúlíng 3g + tiānhuā 2g + dǎngshēn 2g + guìzhī 2g + huángqín 2g + gāncǎo 1g + mǔlì 1g + gānjiāng 1g.

Ptosis (374.3), Tetany (D013746), Hearing impairment (D034381), Carious teeth (521.0, 521.07), Hypoparathyroidism (252.1), Seborrheic dermatitis (690.1), Constipation (564.0), Myalgia (D063806), Corneal neovascularization (370.6):

Jiāwèixiāoyáosǎn 5g + qǐjúdìhuángwán 5g + juémíngzǐ 1g + xiàkūcǎo 1g + mìménghuā 1-0g + jílí 1-0g + liánqiáo 1-0g.

Máxìnggānshítāng 5g + língguìshùgāntāng 5-0g + dàzǎo 1-0g + tínglìzǐ 1-0g.

Xǐgānmíngmùtāng 5g + qǐjúdìhuángwán 3g + xiāngshāliùjūnzǐtāng 2g.

Qǐjúdìhuángwán 5g + mázǐrénwán 5g + juémíngzǐ 2g + mìménghuā 2g + gǔjīngcǎo 2g + gāncǎo 1g.

Liùwèidìhuángwán 5g + hángjú 1g + xiàkūcǎo 1g + mìménghuā 1g + gāncǎo 1g + mázǐrénwán 0g.

Xuánshēn 5g + dìhuáng 5g + màiméndōng 5g + hòupò 5-1g + zhǐshí 5-1g + yùzhú 5-0g + dàhuáng 1-0g.

Huángqín 5g + gāncǎo 2g + báizhǐ 2g + shārén 2g + dàhuáng 0g.

Gāncǎo 5g + báizhǐ 5g + shārén 5g + huángqín 5-2g + dàhuáng 1g.

TABLE 1.6 *(Continued)*

GMP Herbal Medicines for a Three-Year-Old Child with 22q11.2 Deletion Syndrome

Vesicoureteral reflux (593.7), Polycystic kidney dysplasia (753.12), Hydrocephalus (331.4, 331.3), Microphthalmia (743.1), Autism (299.0), Seizure (345.9), Patent ductus arteriosus (747.0), Inguinal hernia (550), Cryptorchidism (752.51), Choanal atresia (748.0), Glaucoma (365), Optic atrophy (377.1), Hypothyroidism (244.9), Purpura (D011693), Intellectual disability (D008607), Obesity (278.00), Thrombocytopenia (287.5), Gastroesophageal reflux (530.81), Asthma (493):

Dìngchuǎntāng 5g + xīnyíqīngfèitāng 4-2g + xiāngshāliùjūnzǐtāng 2g + lóngdǎnxiègāntāng 2-0g + báijí 1-0g + hǎipiāoxiāo 1-0g.

Xiǎoqīnglóngtāng 5g + dìngchuǎntāng 5g + xīnyísǎn 2g + xiāngshāliùjūnzǐtāng 2g.

Dìngchuǎntāng 5g + xīnyísǎn 4g + xiāngshāliùjūnzǐtāng 4g + bǔzhōngyìqìtāng 2g.

Xiàkūcǎo 5g + shígāo 3g + hángjú 3g + ējiāo 3g + cháihú 3g + huángqín 3g + dāngguī 3g + shúdìhuáng 3g + dǎngshēn 3g.

Xiàkūcǎo 5g + cháihú 5g + yínyánghuò 5g + tùsīzǐ 5g + huángqín 5g + dāngguī 5g + shúdìhuáng 5g + dǎngshēn 5g + gāncǎo 2g + bànxià 2-0g + báizhú 2-0g + éshù 2-0g.

Huángqí 5g + shānzhūyú 2g + shānyào 2g + gāncǎo 2g + báizhú 2g + báisháo 2g + báizhǐ 2g + ējiāo 2g + cháihú 2g + huángqín 2g + dāngguī 2g + shúdìhuáng 2g + dǎngshēn 2g.

Xuánshēn 5g + shígāo 5g + màiméndōng 5g + gāncǎo 2g + báijí 2g + dìhuáng 2g + xīnyí 2g + jīnyínhuā 2g + cháihú 2g + huángqín 2g + dāngguī 2g.

Suānzǎorén 5g + bànxià 2g + xiàkūcǎo 2g + cháihú 2g + huángqín 2g + yuǎnzhì 2g.

Dìhuáng 5g + dāngguī 5g + nǚzhēnzǐ 4g + báisháo 4g + xiàkūcǎo 4g + huángqín 4g + cháihú 1g.

Huángqín (Radix Scutellariae) was shown to exert cardioprotection by stimulating the activity of catalase, an antioxidant enzyme, and improving vascular elasticity in rats with myocardial ischemia-reperfusion injury (Chan et al., 2011). Xīnyíqīngfèitāng contains Xīnyí (Flos Magnoliae) and Huángqín; a major bioactive compound in the former was shown to protect against myocardial ischemia/reperfusion injury in rats through inhibiting oxidative stress and myocardial apoptosis (Wang et al., 2015). Běishāshēn (Radix Glehniae) "nourishes yin, cleanses the Lung" and was reviewed to be immunoregulatory (Yang et al., 2019). Máxìnggānshítāng has been used for skin diseases (Fan & Xiong, 2018). Xiàkūcǎo (Spica Prunellae) "clears Liver fire, dissolves gall/scrofula" and is used today for hypertensive heart and chronic kidney disease (Wang, 2020). Dìngchuǎntāng translates into "antiasthma decoction." The prescriptions in the table target the varied manifestations of 22q11.2 deletion syndrome.

1.7 NOONAN SYNDROME

Noonan syndrome is characterized by distinctive physical features of the face, head and neck, chest and spine, heart defects, and bleeding problems. Noonan syndrome is caused by mutations in a number of genes critical for mediating cellular responses, including cellular growth, division and differentiation, to hormones and cytokines.

Báizhǐ (cf. Section 1.4) "releases exterior, dispels Wind, opens orifices, stops pain, eliminates dampness, arrests leukorrhea, reduces swelling, and drains pus." It was summarized to have anti-inflammatory, antitumor, antioxidant, analgesic, antiviral, antimicrobial, cardiovascular system protective, neuroprotective, hepatoprotective, skin protective, lipid metabolism regulatory, anti-diabetic, and immunoregulatory activities (Zhao, Feng, et al., 2022). Together with the GMP herb use data from medical insurance claims (Wang, 2020), we conclude that GMP Báizhǐ extract granules benefit patients with skin disease, upper respiratory infection, diseases of sebaceous glands, diseases of the oral soft tissues, heart disease, facial nerve disorders, symptoms involving head and neck, and disorders of joints; and the symptoms and anatomies it improves and affects

TABLE 1.7
GMP Herbal Medicines for a Two-Year-Old Child with Noonan Syndrome

Noonan syndrome (OrphaCode: 648)

A malformation syndrome with a prevalence of ~3 in 10,000

Candidate gene tested: RAS related (*RRAS* / Entrez: 6237) at 19q13.33

Disease-causing germline mutation(s): muscle RAS oncogene homolog (*MRAS* / Entrez: 22808) at 3q22.3

Disease-causing germline mutation(s): sprouty related EVH1 domain containing 2 (*SPRED2* / Entrez: 200734) at 2p14

Disease-causing germline mutation(s): RAS related 2 (*RRAS2* / Entrez: 22800) at 11p15.2

Disease-causing germline mutation(s): protein tyrosine phosphatase non-receptor type 11 (*PTPN11* / Entrez: 5781) at 12q24.13

Disease-causing germline mutation(s): Cbl proto-oncogene (*CBL* / Entrez: 867) at 11q23.3

Disease-causing germline mutation(s) (gain of function): SOS Ras/Rac guanine nucleotide exchange factor 1 (*SOS1* / Entrez: 6654) at 2p22.1

Disease-causing germline mutation(s): KRAS proto-oncogene, GTPase (*KRAS* / Entrez: 3845) at 12p12.1

Disease-causing germline mutation(s) (gain of function): Raf-1 proto-oncogene, serine/threonine kinase (*RAF1* / Entrez: 5894) at 3p25.2

Disease-causing germline mutation(s): NRAS proto-oncogene, GTPase (*NRAS* / Entrez: 4893) at 1p13.2

Disease-causing germline mutation(s) (gain of function): Ras like without CAAX 1 (*RIT1* / Entrez: 6016) at 1q22

Disease-causing germline mutation(s): leucine zipper like transcription regulator 1 (*LZTR1* / Entrez: 8216) at 22q11.21

Disease-causing germline mutation(s) (loss of function): RAS p21 protein activator 2 (*RASA2* / Entrez: 5922) at 3q23

Disease-causing germline mutation(s): SOS Ras/Rho guanine nucleotide exchange factor 2 (*SOS2* / Entrez: 6655) at 14q21.3

Autosomal dominant, Autosomal recessive

Hypogonadotrophic hypogonadism, Thick lower lip vermilion, High palate, Hypertelorism, Triangular face, Micrognathia, High forehead, Low-set and posteriorly rotated ears, Thickened helices, Webbed neck, Thickened nuchal skin fold, Cystic hygroma, Downslanted palpebral fissures, Ptosis, Proptosis, Pectus excavatum, Pectus carinatum, Dysarthria, Muscle weakness, Neurological speech impairment, Malformation of the heart and great vessels, Short stature, Pulmonary artery stenosis, Joint hyperflexibility, Wide intermamillary distance, Aplasia/Hypoplasia of the abdominal wall musculature, Midface retrusion, Enlarged thorax

Cryptorchidism, Abnormality of the genital system, Strabismus, Hypotonia, Abnormal pulmonary valve morphology, Abnormality of the spleen, Abnormal bleeding, Abnormality of coagulation, Low posterior hairline, Coarse hair, Hepatomegaly, Scoliosis, Delayed skeletal maturation, Abnormal dermatoglyphics, Feeding difficulties in infancy, Abnormal hair quantity, Arrhythmia, Abnormal platelet function, Abnormality of the lymphatic system

Sensorineural hearing impairment, Nystagmus, Melanocytic nevus, Lymphedema, Brachydactyly, Radioulnar synostosis, Clinodactyly of the 5th finger, Aplasia of the semicircular canal

Antenatal, Neonatal, Infancy, Childhood

Ptosis (374.3), Proptosis (376.30), Dysarthria (D004401), Muscle weakness (D018908), Neurological speech impairment (D013064):

Qǐjúdìhuángwán 5g + xiāngshāliùjūnzǐtāng 5g.	Báizhǐ 5g + gāncǎo 5-2g + shārén 5-2g + huángqín 5-0g + zhīzǐ 2-0g + liánqiáo 2-0g + dàhuáng 1-0g.
Xǐgānmíngmùtāng 5g + xiàkūcǎo 1g.	
Xǐgānmíngmùtāng 5g + xiāngshāliùjūnzǐtāng 5g.	
Xǐgānmíngmùtāng 5g + shēnlíngbáizhúsǎn 5g.	Báizhǐ 5g + zhìgāncǎo 5-3g + shārén 5-3g + huángqín 5-0g + guālóugēn 2-0g + xìxīn 1-0g + dàhuáng 1-0g.
Xiǎocháihútāng 5g + zhúyèshígāotāng 5g + mùzéicǎo 2g + juémíngzǐ 2g + chōngwèizǐ 2g + mìmēnghuā 2g + gǔjīngcǎo 2g.	Dìhuáng 5g + fángfēng 5g + gǒuqǐzǐ 5g + júhuā 5g + dāngguī 5g + xìxīn 1g + huánglián 1g.

Cryptorchidism (752.51), Strabismus (378.7, 378.6, 378.31), Hypotonia (D009123), Abnormality of coagulation (287.9):

Xìngsūyǐnyòukē 5g + bǎohéwán 5g.	Jílí 5g + chántuì 5g.
Xìngsūyǐnyòukē 5g + xīnyíqīngfèitāng 5g + bǎohéwán 5-0g.	Gāncǎo 5g + zhīmǔ 5g + huángqín 5g + dàhuáng 0g + huánglián 0g.
Gānlùyǐn 5g + zhǐqiào 3-2g + chántuì 2-0g.	Gāncǎo 5g + shārén 5g + báizhǐ 5-4g + huángqín 5-1g + tiānhuā 3-0g + dàhuáng 0g.

(Continued)

TABLE 1.7 *(Continued)*
GMP Herbal Medicines for a Two-Year-Old Child with Noonan Syndrome

Sensorineural hearing impairment (389.1), Nystagmus (379.53, 379.55, 379.50), Radioulnar synostosis (755.53):

Qǐjúdìhuángwán 5g + yìqìcōngmíngtāng 5g + shíchāngpú 1-0g + yuǎnzhì 1-0g.

Liùwèidìhuángwán 5g + yìqìcōngmíngtāng 5g + shíchāngpú 1g + gǒuqǐzǐ 1g + yuǎnzhì 1g.

Qǐjúdìhuángwán 5g + língguìshùgāntāng 5g + shíchāngpú 1g + yuǎnzhì 1g.

Yìqìcōngmíngtāng 5g + bǔzhōngyìqìtāng 5g + shíchāngpú 1g + yuǎnzhì 1g.

Yùzhú 5g + gǒuqǐzǐ 5g + shénqū 5g + màiyá 5g + huángqí 5-0g + júhuā 5-0g.

Gǒuqǐzǐ 5g + tùsīzǐ 5-0g + shíchāngpú 2g + hángjú 2g + yuǎnzhì 2g.

Shíchāngpú 5g + hángjú 5g + gǒuqǐzǐ 5g + yuǎnzhì 3g.

include fatigue, edema, headache, brain, hypoxia, fever, body weight, facial paralysis, back pain, and diarrhea.

1.8 BECKWITH-WIEDEMANN SYNDROME

Beckwith-Wiedemann syndrome, also known as exomphalos-macroglossia-gigantism syndrome, is an overgrowth of the newborn characterized by a large body size, an enlarged tongue, and abdominal wall defect. Children with Beckwith-Wiedemann syndrome are susceptible to childhood cancers, including kidney tumor and liver tumor, before age 4. The cause of Beckwith-Wiedemann syndrome is complex, including genetic and epigenetic changes in a region of chromosome 11 that controls growth.

Huángqín is mainly used for disorders of the intestine as we will see in Chapter 13 on rare gastroenterologic diseases. Èrchéntāng "dries dampness, eliminates phlegm, passes Qi, and

TABLE 1.8
GMP Herbal Medicines for a Three-Year-Old Child with Beckwith-Wiedemann Syndrome

Beckwith-Wiedemann syndrome (OrphaCode: 116)

A malformation syndrome with a prevalence of ~3 in 10,000

Disease-causing germline mutation(s) (loss of function): cyclin dependent kinase inhibitor 1C (*CDKN1C* / Entrez: 1028) at 11p15.4

Role: the phenotype of H19 imprinted maternally expressed transcript (*H19* / Entrez: 283120) at 11p15.5

Role: the phenotype of KCNQ1 opposite strand/antisense transcript 1 (*KCNQ1OT1* / Entrez: 10984) at 11p15.5

Role: the phenotype of insulin like growth factor 2 (*IGF2* / Entrez: 3481) at 11p15.5

Disease-causing germline mutation(s): nuclear receptor binding SET domain protein 1 (*NSD1* / Entrez: 64324) at 5q35.3

Autosomal dominant, Unknown

Tall stature, Large for gestational age, Neoplasm

Enlarged kidney, Nephropathy, Wide mouth, Macroglossia, Prominent occiput, Coarse facial features, Mandibular prognathia, Abnormality of earlobe, Proptosis, Congenital diaphragmatic hernia, Melanocytic nevus, Nevus flammeus, Choroideremia, Obesity, Hemihypertrophy, Umbilical hernia, Omphalocele, Polyhydramnios, Redundant skin, Premature birth, Exocrine pancreatic insufficiency, Hypoglycemia, Neonatal hypoglycemia, Hypercalciuria, Visceromegaly, Accelerated skeletal maturation, Large placenta, Posterior helix pit, Anterior creases of earlobe, Midface retrusion, Subchorionic septal cyst, Asymmetric growth, Infra-orbital crease, Abnormality of the shape of the midface

Inguinal hernia, Cryptorchidism, Ureteral duplication, Vesicoureteral reflux, Gonadoblastoma, Cleft palate, Large fontanelles, Wide anterior fontanel, Facial hemangioma, Otosclerosis, Nephrolithiasis, Hypothyroidism, Diastasis recti, Hypertrophic cardiomyopathy, Cardiomegaly, Splenomegaly, Polycythemia, Neurological speech impairment, Hepatomegaly, Malformation of the heart and great vessels, Nephroblastoma, Rhabdomyosarcoma, Hepatoblastoma, Neuroblastoma, Prominent metopic ridge, Multiple renal cysts, Elevated alpha-fetoprotein, Adrenocortical carcinoma, Adrenocortical cytomegaly, Congenital megaureter, Feeding difficulties in infancy, Sleep apnea, Abnormal pancreas morphology, Neurodevelopmental delay, Large intestinal polyposis, Leiomyosarcoma, Urogenital fistula

Antenatal, Neonatal

(Continued)

TABLE 1.8 *(Continued)*

GMP Herbal Medicines for a Three-Year-Old Child with Beckwith-Wiedemann Syndrome

Proptosis (376.30), Choroideremia (363.55), Obesity (278.00), Omphalocele (756.72), Hypoglycemia (251.2), Hypercalciuria (D053565):

Èrchéntāng 5g + bèimǔ 2g + xiàkūcǎo 2g + liánqiáo 2-0g.	Huángqín 5g + gāncǎo 2g + báizhǐ 2g +
Sǎnzhǒngkuìjiāntāng 5g + èrchéntāng 3-0g.	shārén 2g + jīnyínhuā 2-0g + dàhuáng 1-0g.
Jiāwèixiāoyáosǎn 5g + xiàkūcǎo 2g + xuánshēn 1g + bèimǔ 1g +	Xuánshēn 5g + dìhuáng 5g + hòupò 5g +
mǔlì 1g + acupuncture.	zhǐshí 5g + màiméndōng 5g + shāshēn 5-0g +
	dàhuáng 1g.
	Bǎihé 5g + gāncǎo 3g + dàhuáng 0g.

Inguinal hernia (550), Cryptorchidism (752.51), Vesicoureteral reflux (593.7), Cleft palate (749.0), Otosclerosis (387.8), Nephrolithiasis (592), Hypothyroidism (244.9), Hypertrophic cardiomyopathy (425.1), Neurological speech impairment (D013064), Sleep apnea (780.57):

Wǔlíngsǎn 5g + bǔzhōngyìqìtāng 5g + jìshēngshènqìwán 5-0g +	Xiǎohuíxiāng 5g + chuānliànzǐ 5g + mùxiāng 5g +
chuānliànzǐ 2g + yánhúsuǒ 2g + wūyào 2g + lìzhīhé 2g.	wúzhūyú 5g + wūyào 5g + lìzhīhé 5g + júhé 5g +
Júhéwán 5g + wǔlíngsǎn 5-0g + bǔzhōngyìqìtāng 3-0g + chuānliànzǐ	qīngpí 5-0g.
2-1g + mùxiāng 2-0g + lìzhīhé 2-0g + júhé 2-0g + xiǎohuíxiāng	Chuānliànzǐ 5g + wúzhūyú 5g + mùxiāng 2g +
1-0g + wúzhūyú 1-0g + yánhúsuǒ 1-0g + wūyào 1-0g.	wūyào 2g + lìzhīhé 2g + júhé 2g.
Sìnìtāng 5g + chuānliànzǐ 1g + yánhúsuǒ 1g + wūyào 1g + lìzhīhé 1g.	

harmonizes interior." In TCM, "phlegm-damp" can accumulate to block orifices including the eye. Co-application of Èrchéntāng and eyesight-improving herbs is said to "reduce opaqueness and brighten eyes." Xiǎohuíxiāng (Fructus Foeniculi) "disperses coldness, stops pain, regulates Qi, harmonizes interior" and is used for inguinal hernia and chronic glomerulonephritis (Wang, 2020). Chuānliànzǐ (Fructus Toosendan) "moves Qi, stops pain, kills worms, heals tinea" and is used for atherosclerosis, gastric ulcer, hernia, and so on (Wang, 2020). Lìzhīhé (Semen Litchi) has traditionally been used for hernia and was shown to decrease the tumor size in human prostate cancer xenograft mice (Guo et al., 2017).

1.9   47,XYY SYNDROME

47, XYY syndrome, also called double Y syndrome or Y disomy, results from an extra copy of the Y chromosome in a male's body cells. Y disomy is not inherited; it is caused by a random event during the father's sperm development. Y disomy usually presents with no symptoms except for a tall stature.

The term *yìqì* in Yìqìcōngmíngtāng and Bǔzhōngyìqìtāng means to "benefit Qi" and the term *cōngmíng* in Yìqìcōngmíngtāng is translated to "smartness," while the term *bǔzhōng* in Bǔzhōngyìqìtāng means to "strengthen interior." Therefore, based on traditional annotations of the formulas, the strategy of TCM for delayed speech and language development looks to promote growth and development of the affected boy. On the other hand, Bǔzhōngyìqìtāng was shown to elevate certain monoamines in the brain cortical tissues of mice to exert antiaging effects (Shih et al., 2000). Bǔzhōngyìqìtāng does have effects on the brain, in addition to the digestive tract. Huángqí, i.e., Radix Astragali, "replenishes Qi, raises yang, benefits defense, fortifies exterior, helps draining, reduces swelling, discharges pus, and regenerates tissues." Its use for immune-related diseases through improved innate and acquired immunities (Chen et al., 2020) links Qi (or "defense") to immunity. Based on the classical medical texts, modern phytochemical/pharmacological studies and health insurance claims data, we summarize the use of GMP Huángqí extract granules for heart disease, dermatoses, disorders of intestine, myoneural disorders, endocrine disorders, disorders of the nervous system, diabetes mellitus, liver disease, peripheral vascular disease, and diseases of upper respiratory tract; the symptoms and

TABLE 1.9

GMP Herbal Medicines for a Ten-Year-Old Boy with 47,XYY Syndrome

47,XYY syndrome (OrphaCode: 8)

A malformation syndrome with a prevalence of ~3 in 10,000

Not applicable, Unknown

Tall stature, Malar flattening, Low-set ears, Delayed speech and language development, Motor delay

Macrocephaly, Hypertelorism, Behavioral abnormality, Impaired social interactions, Hyperactivity, Intellectual disability, Neonatal hypotonia, Specific learning disability, Asthma, Attention deficit hyperactivity disorder, Congenital stationary night blindness, Finger clinodactyly, Impulsivity

Azoospermia, Cryptorchidism, Hypospadias, Macroorchidism, Micropenis, Hydrocephalus, Autistic behavior, Oligospermia, Increased circulating gonadotropin level, Seizure, Dysgenesis of the cerebellar vermis, Abnormal brainstem morphology, Male infertility, Cerebellar dysplasia, Increased serum testosterone level, Varicocele

All ages

Delayed speech and language development (D007805):

Bǔzhōngyìqìtāng 5g + yìqìcōngmíngtāng 5-0g.

Bǔzhōngyìqìtāng 5g + qǐjúdìhuángwán 5-0g + shíchāngpú 1-0g + yuǎnzhì 1-0g.

Bǔzhōngyìqìtāng 5g + liùwèidìhuángwán 4-0g.

Guìzhītāng 5g + cāngěrsǎn 1g + xìngrén 1g + hòupò 1g.

Língguìshùgāntāng 5g + gégēntāng 5g + jīngjiè 1g + liánqiáo 1g + cāngěrzǐ 1g.

Báizhǐ 5g + huángqín 5-0g + zhìgāncǎo 4-3g + shārén 4-3g + tiānhuā 2-0g + xìxīn 1-0g + dàhuáng 0g.

Huángqí 5g + chìsháo 1-0g + fángfēng 1-0g + xìxīn 0g + huánglián 0g + dàhuáng 0g.

Hyperactivity (D006948), Intellectual disability (D008607), Neonatal hypotonia (D009123), Asthma (493), Congenital stationary night blindness (368.61):

Xiǎoqīnglóngtāng 5g + xiāngshāliùjūnzǐtāng 3g + shānzhā 1g + shénqū 1g + màiyá 1g + jīnèijīn 1g.

Xiǎoqīnglóngtāng 5g + yùpíngfēngsǎn 5g + bǔzhōngyìqìtāng 5-0g.

Xiǎoqīnglóngtāng 5g + yùpíngfēngsǎn 5g + cāngěrsǎn 5-0g.

Máxìnggānshítāng 5g + cāngěrsǎn 5-0g + dìlóng 2-0g + jiégěng 2-0g + liánqiáo 2-0g + yúxīngcǎo 2-0g + gāncǎo 2-0g + dàhuáng 0g.

Huángqí 5g + zhìgāncǎo 3g + dāngguī 1g + wǔwèizǐ 0g.

Huángqí 5g + chìsháo 1g + fángfēng 1g + xìxīn 1g + huánglián 1g + dàhuáng 0g.

Azoospermia (606.0), Cryptorchidism (752.51), Hydrocephalus (331.4, 331.3), Seizure (345.9), Varicocele (456.4):

Yòuguīwán 5g + jìshēngshènqìwán 5g + ròucōngróng 2g + yínyánghuò 2g + tùsīzǐ 2g + bǔgǔzhǐ 2g.

Yòuguīwán 5g + zuǒguīwán 5g + ròucōngróng 1g + yínyánghuò 1g + bājǐtiān 1-0g + tùsīzǐ 1-0g.

Liùwèidìhuángwán 5g + xiāngshāliùjūnzǐtāng 5g + bājǐtiān 1g + ròucōngróng 1g + tùsīzǐ 1g.

Bǔyánghuánwǔtāng 5g + yòuguīwán 3g + bājǐtiān 1g + ròucōngróng 1g + yínyánghuò 1g + tùsīzǐ 1g.

Báizhú 5g + fùzǐ 5g + cháihú 5g + báisháo 4g + fúlíng 4g + tiānhuā 2g + zhǐshí 2g + guìzhī 2g + huángqín 2g + dǎngshēn 2g + gāncǎo 1g + mǔlì 1g + gānjiāng 1g.

Báizhú 5g + zhǐshí 5g + táorén 5g + gānjiāng 5g.

Bànxià 5g + ējiāo 5g + zǐcǎo 5g + dǎngshēn 5g + fùzǐ 3g + gānjiāng 3g + acupuncture.

anatomies on which Huángqí has an effect include body weight, brain, hypoxia, ataxia, fever, diarrhea, intellectual disability, edema, dizziness, adrenal glands, headache, pain, and back pain. Use of Yòuguīwán and Zuǒguīwán for male infertility is discussed in Section 12.1.

1.10 OMPHALOCELE

Omphalocele is the sticking out of abdominal organs such as intestines and liver through a hole in the abdominal wall near the belly button, with the protruding organs covered by a thin and transparent membrane. Omphalocele is an abdominal wall defect during the fetus's development in the womb and can accompany other signs and symptoms associated with chromosome number abnormality in the baby's cells.

TABLE 1.10

GMP Herbal Medicines for a One-Year-Old Infant with Omphalocele

Omphalocele (OrphaCode: 660)

A morphological anomaly with a prevalence of ~3 in 10,000

Not applicable

Omphalocele, Premature birthAntenatal

Omphalocele (756.72):

Xiǎojiànzhōngtāng 5g + shēnlíngbáizhúsǎn 5-0g + báizhú 1-0g + fángfēng 1-0g + huángqí 1-0g + acupuncture.	Zhìgāncǎo 5g + dàhuáng 0g.
Sìjūnzǐtāng 5g + yùpíngfēngsǎn 5g + gāncǎo 0g.	Xuánshēn 5g + dìhuáng 5g + màiméndōng 5g + hòupò 5-1g + zhǐshí 5-1g + dàhuáng 1-0g.
Shēnlíngbáizhúsǎn 5g + shānzhā 2g + shénqū 2g + màiyá 2g.	Gāncǎo 5g + hòupò 5g + zhǐshí 5g + dàhuáng 0g.

Dìhuáng (Radix Rehmanniae) "clears heat, cools blood, nourishes yin and generates saliva." It was reviewed and summarized to be effective for patients with various inflammatory and metabolic diseases such as diabetes (Kim et al., 2017); GMP Dìhuáng extract granule is used for functional disorder of intestine, diabetes, and pruritic disorder (Wang, 2020). Both Xiǎojiànzhōngtāng and Shēnlíngbáizhúsǎn are frequently prescribed to children with functional digestive disorders (Wang, 2019).

1.11 GASTROSCHISIS

Gastroschisis, or laparoschisis, is the sticking out of abdominal organs such as intestines and stomach through an opening in the abdominal wall next to the belly button, without a membrane covering the herniated organs. Unlike omphalocele, gastroschisis is usually an isolated condition without other birth defects. The cause of gastroschisis is not known, but it is associated with young maternal age and alcohol/tobacco use of the mother during pregnancy.

Zhìgāncǎo (Radix et Rhizoma Glycyrrhizae Praeparata cum Melle) is honey-roasted Gāncǎo (cf. Section 1.1). In comparison, Zhìgāncǎo is considered more tonifying and Gāncǎo is more "cooling." Changes in the pharmacokinetics of the active compounds in processed Gāncǎo explain the difference (Zhang et al., 2018). Guìzhītāng "dispels pathogenic wind from exterior, modulates both nutrition and defense." The formula therefore not only protects against infection but also aids in digestion.

TABLE 1.11

GMP Herbal Medicines for a One-Year-Old Infant with Gastroschisis

Gastroschisis (OrphaCode: 2368)

A morphological anomaly with a prevalence of ~3 in 10,000

Not applicable

Gastroschisis

Intestinal atresia

Abnormality of mesentery morphology

Antenatal

Gastroschisis (756.73):

Xiǎojiànzhōngtāng 5g + shēnlíngbáizhúsǎn 5-0g.	Zhìgāncǎo 5g + shārén 5-0g + xuánshēn 3-0g + dìhuáng 3-0g + màiméndōng 3-0g + dàhuáng 1-0g.
Xiǎojiànzhōngtāng 5g + yùpíngfēngsǎn 5-0g.	
Guìzhītāng 5g + báisháo 1-0g + gāncǎo 1-0g + dàhuáng 0g.	Gāncǎo 5g + báizhǐ 5g + shārén 5g + dàhuáng 0g.
	Xuánshēn 5g + dìhuáng 5g + màiméndōng 5g + hòupò 1g + zhǐshí 1g + dàhuáng 0g.

1.12 ESOPHAGEAL ATRESIA

Esophageal atresia is a congenital anatomic defect in which the esophagus does not connect correctly to the stomach. In most cases of esophageal atresia, the upper esophagus ends in a closed pouch without continuing to the lower esophagus or the stomach. The cause of esophageal atresia is not known; however, advanced paternal age and assisted reproductive technology increase the risk for the condition.

TABLE 1.12
GMP Herbal Medicines for a One-Year-Old Infant with Esophageal Atresia

Esophageal atresia (OrphaCode: 1199)

A morphological anomaly with a prevalence of ~3 in 10,000

Not applicable

Tracheoesophageal fistula

Failure to thrive in infancy, Vomiting, Dysphagia, Restrictive ventilatory defect, Recurrent respiratory infections, Gastrointestinal dysmotility, Excessive salivation, Chronic obstructive pulmonary disease, Feeding difficulties in infancy, Absence of stomach bubble on fetal sonography, Bronchitis, Oral aversion, Immunologic hypersensitivity, Esophagitis

Abnormality of the urinary system, Abnormality of the genitourinary system, Cyanosis, Pallor, Growth delay, Small for gestational age, Polyhydramnios, Vocal cord paresis, Subglottic stenosis, Gastroesophageal reflux, Pyloric stenosis, Respiratory distress, Aspiration, Abnormal vertebral morphology, Episodic respiratory distress, Laryngotracheomalacia, Abnormal respiratory system morphology, Morphological abnormality of the gastrointestinal tract, Anorectal anomaly, Clinodactyly, Abnormality of cardiovascular system morphology, Abnormality of limbs, Abnormality of skeletal muscles

Neonatal

Vomiting (D014839), Bronchitis (466.0, 490, 491), Esophagitis (530.1):

Bànxiàxièxīntāng 5g + gāncǎo 2-1g + xìngrén 1-0g + fúlíng 1-0g.

Sūzǐjiàngqìtāng 5g + báisháo 2-1g + shēngjiāng 1g.

Gāncǎo 5g + xìngrén 5-0g + bèimǔ 5-0g + qiánhú 5-0g + jiégěng 5-0g + sāngbáipí 5-0g + guālóurén 5-0g + fúlíng 5-0g + chénpí 5-0g + zǐsūyè 5-0g + júhóng 5-0g.

Gāncǎo 5g + hòupò 5-0g + zhǐshí 5-0g + dàhuáng 1-0g + huánglián 1-0g.

Cyanosis (D003490), Pallor (D010167), Vocal cord paresis (D014826), Gastroesophageal reflux (530.81), Respiratory distress (D004417):

Wǔlíngsǎn 5g + gāncǎo 1g + báisháo 1g + tiáowèichéngqìtāng 1-0g + dàhuáng 0g.

Lǐzhōngtāng 5g + gāncǎo 1g + báisháo 1g + fùzǐ 1-0g + dàhuáng 0g.

Guìzhītāng 5g + xìngrén 1g + hòupò 1g + dàhuáng 0g.

Gāncǎo 5g + hòupò 5g + zhǐshí 5g + dàhuáng 0g.

Gāncǎo 5g + báizhǐ 5g + shārén 5g + huángqín 5-0g + dàhuáng 1-0g.

Xìngrén (Semen Armeniacae Amarum) "stops cough, quells asthma, moistens bowels, passes stools." It was reviewed to have such pharmacological effects as antitussive, antiasthmatic, anti-inflammatory, analgesic, antioxidant, antitumor, cardioprotective, antifibrotic, immune regulatory, bowel relaxing, insecticidal, and so on (Wei et al., 2023) and is used today for chest pain and cough (Wang, 2020). Bànxiàxièxīntāng "harmonizes the Stomach, lowers ascent, removes lumps, and eliminates fullness." Sūzǐjiàngqìtāng "lowers Qi, quells asthma, dispels phlegm, stops coughing" and is used today for asthma (Wang, 2019).

1.13 ISOLATED CLEFT LIP

Isolated cleft lip is a fissure extending from the upper lip to the nasal base without other birth defects. An isolated cleft lip is usually unilateral on the left side of the lip. The mother's genetic predispositions and exposures to medications and smoking during pregnancy are believed to increase the risk for isolated cleft lip.

Jílí (Section 1.3) was shown to be anti-inflammatory in monocyte/macrophage-like cells derived from mice (Tian et al., 2020). So was Júhuā (Tian et al., 2020). Yínqiàosǎn was shown to relieve

TABLE 1.13
GMP Herbal Medicines for a One-Year-Old Infant with Isolated Cleft Lip

Isolated cleft lip (OrphaCode: 199302)

A morphological anomaly with a prevalence of ~3 in 10,000

Major susceptibility factor: tumor protein p63 (*TP63* / Entrez: 8626) at 3q28

Major susceptibility factor: interferon regulatory factor 6 (*IRF6* / Entrez: 3664) at 1q32.2

Major susceptibility factor: nectin cell adhesion molecule 1 (*NECTIN1* / Entrez: 5818) at 11q23.3

Major susceptibility factor: msh homeobox 1 (*MSX1* / Entrez: 4487) at 4p16.2

Multigenic/multifactorial

Chronic otitis media, Non-midline cleft lip

Velopharyngeal insufficiency, Behavioral abnormality, Small for gestational age, Macrodontia, Supernumerary maxillary incisor, Speech articulation difficulties, Maternal teratogenic exposure, Low self-esteem, Abnormality of the Eustachian tube, Bilateral cleft lip

Neonatal, Infancy

Unspecified otitis media (382.9):	
Yínqiàosǎn 5g.	Jílí 5g.
Sāngjúyǐn 5g + zhǐqiào 1-0g + chántuì 1-0g + sāngbáipí 0g.	Gāncǎo 5g.
	Júhuā 5g + júhóng 2g.
	Zhǐqiào 5-0g + chántuì 5-0g + jílí 2g.

the fever of children who are hypersensitive to conventional anti-inflammatory medicines such as paracetamol and ibuprofen (Liew et al., 2015).

1.14   CLEFT LIP/PALATE

Cleft lip/palate, also called cleft lip-alveolus-palate syndrome, is a split across the upper lip, upper gum ridge, and mouth roof, as a result of developmental abnormality of the fetus in the womb. An interaction of genetic factors and environmental factors is believed to contribute to the formation of cleft lip/palate.

Shārén (Fructus Amomi) "removes dampness, moves Qi, warms interior, stops vomiting, stops diarrhea, and prevents miscarriage." It was shown to attenuate nasal inflammation in mice with allergic rhinitis (Fan et al., 2022) and is used for gastric ulcer and allergic rhinitis (Wang, 2020). Note that Shārén is edible. Yìqìcōngmíngtāng is a formula that benefits both hearing and vision as we will see its applications again in Chapter 6 on ophthalmic disorders and other chapters of the book.

TABLE 1.14
GMP Herbal Medicines for a One-Year-Old Infant with Cleft lip/palate

Cleft lip/palate (OrphaCode: 199306)

A morphological anomaly with a prevalence of ~3 in 10,000

Major susceptibility factor: Rho GTPase activating protein 29 (*ARHGAP29* / Entrez: 9411) at 1p22.1

Major susceptibility factor: tumor protein p63 (*TP63* / Entrez: 8626) at 3q28

Major susceptibility factor: bone morphogenetic protein 4 (*BMP4* / Entrez: 652) at 14q22.2

Major susceptibility factor: nectin cell adhesion molecule 1 (*NECTIN1* / Entrez: 5818) at 11q23.3

Major susceptibility factor: cadherin 1 (*CDH1* / Entrez: 999) at 16q22.1

Major susceptibility factor: interferon regulatory factor 6 (*IRF6* / Entrez: 3664) at 1q32.2

Major susceptibility factor: platelet derived growth factor receptor alpha (*PDGFRA* / Entrez: 5156) at 4q12

Major susceptibility factor: msh homeobox 1 (*MSX1* / Entrez: 4487) at 4p16.2

Major susceptibility factor: discs large MAGUK scaffold protein 1 (*DLG1* / Entrez: 1739) at 3q29

Disease-causing germline mutation(s): distal-less homeobox 4 (*DLX4* / Entrez: 1748) at 17q21.33

Multigenic/multifactorial

(Continued)

TABLE 1.14 *(Continued)*
GMP Herbal Medicines for a One-Year-Old Infant with Cleft lip/palate

Abnormality of dental eruption

Cleft palate, Oral cleft, Velopharyngeal insufficiency, Recurrent otitis media, Delayed speech and language development, Poor suck, Feeding difficulties in infancy, Speech articulation difficulties, Unilateral cleft palate, Oral-pharyngeal dysphagia

Conductive hearing impairment, Dental malocclusion, Nasal speech, Malnutrition, Peg-shaped maxillary lateral incisors, Palate fistula, Abnormal number of permanent teeth, Bilateral cleft palate, Agenesis of lateral incisor

Neonatal, Infancy

Cleft palate (749.0), Delayed speech and language development (D007805):

Xìngsūyǐnyòukē 5g + xīnyíqīngfèitāng 5g.

Sìjūnzǐtāng 5g + shānzhā 1-0g + shénqū 1-0g + màiyá 1-0g.

Gānlùyǐn 5g + bǎohéwán 3-0g + gāncǎo 0g.

Shēnlíngbáizhúsǎn 5g + shénqū 0g + màiyá 0g.

Gāncǎo 5g + shārén 5g + báizhǐ 5-0g + dàhuáng 1-0g.

Shénqū 5g + màiyá 5g.

Xuánshēn 5g + dìhuáng 5g + màiméndōng 5g + hòupò 1-0g + zhǐshí 1-0g + dàhuáng 0g.

Conductive hearing impairment (D006314):

Yìqìcōngmíngtāng 5g + shíchāngpú 1-0g + yuǎnzhì 1-0g.

Guìzhītāng 5g + màiyá 2g + huángqín 1g + xiāngfù 1g + dàhuáng 0g.

Guìzhītāng 5g + xìngrén 2g + hòupò 2g + dàhuáng 0g.

Shārén 5g + gāncǎo 4-3g + báizhǐ 4-3g + huángqín 4-0g + tiānhuā 2-0g + dàhuáng 0g.

1.15 DOUBLE OUTLET RIGHT VENTRICLE

In a normal heart structure, the aorta, the main and largest artery in the body, connects to the left ventricle. Infants with double outlet right ventricle (DORV) have their aorta connected to the right ventricle. The cause of DORV is unknown although chromosomal abnormalities are suggested.

Gānjiāng (Rhizoma Zingiberis) extract was shown to reduce heart structural abnormalities in diabetic rats (Ilkhanizadeh et al., 2016). Wǔlíngsǎn was concluded to be safe and effective for the treatment of chronic heart failure in a systematic review and meta-analysis of randomized controlled trials (Li et al., 2022). Moreover, Wǔlíngsǎn, Sìnìtāng, Shēnlíngbáizhúsǎn, and Xiǎojiànzhōngtāng all improve digestion. In addition to digestion, Wǔlíngsǎn relieves symptoms involving the skin, urinary system, and heart; Sìnìtāng relieves heart diseases, endocrine disorders, symptoms involving

TABLE 1.15
GMP Herbal Medicines for a One-Year-Old Infant with Double Outlet Right Ventricle

Double outlet right ventricle (OrphaCode: 3426)

A morphological anomaly with a prevalence of ~3 in 10,000

Multigenic/multifactorial

Double outlet right ventricle

Cyanosis

Narrow mouth, Cleft palate, Submucous cleft hard palate, Hypertelorism, Intellectual disability–mild, Failure to thrive, Ventricular septal defect, Pulmonic stenosis, Tachycardia, Tachypnea, Short stature, Hypoplastic left heart, Depressed nasal bridge, Feeding difficulties, Heart murmur, Narrow palpebral fissure, Abnormality of cartilage of external ear

Hypoparathyroidism, Tetralogy of Fallot, Truncus arteriosus, Coarctation of aorta, Intestinal malrotation, Hypocalcemia, Pulmonary artery atresia, Aplasia/Hypoplasia of the thymus, Heterotaxy

Neonatal, Infancy

Cyanosis (D003490):

Wǔlíngsǎn 5g + píngwèisǎn 5-0g.

Sìnìtāng 5g + píngwèisǎn 5-0g + guìzhī 1-0g + máhuáng 1-0g + xìxīn 1-0g + bànxià 1-0g + hòupò 1-0g + fúlíng 1-0g + dàhuáng 0g.

Gānjiāng 5g + huángqín 5g + huánglián 5g + dǎngshēn 5g + dàhuáng 1g.

Gānjiāng 5g + rénshēn 3-2g + bànxià 3-2g + dàhuáng 0g.

(Continued)

TABLE 1.15 *(Continued)*
GMP Herbal Medicines for a One-Year-Old Infant with Double Outlet Right Ventricle

Cleft palate (749.0), Ventricular septal defect (745.4), Tachypnea (D059246), Hypoplastic left heart (746.7), Heart murmur (D006337):

Shēnlíngbáizhúsǎn 5g + sháoyàogāncǎotāng 2g + shānzhā 1g + shénqū 1g + màiyá 1g + jīnèijīn 1-0g.	Běishāshēn 5g + yùzhú 5g + báizhú 5g + shíhú 5g + màiyá 5g + màiméndōng 5-0g + huángqín 5-0g.
Shēnlíngbáizhúsǎn 5g + xīnyíqīngfèitāng 4g + gāncǎo 1g + fángfēng 1g + jīngjiè 1g + cāngěrzǐ 1g.	Xuánshēn 5g + dìhuáng 5g + màiméndōng 5g + hòupò 5-1g + zhǐshí 5-1g + yùzhú 5-0g + dàhuáng 1-0g.
Gānlùyǐn 5g + yínqiàosǎn 5g + gāncǎo 1g + wūméi 1g.	
Xiǎoqīnglóngtāng 5g + xiāngshāliùjūnzǐtāng 3g + shānzhā 1g + shénqū 1g + màiyá 1g + jīnèijīn 1g.	Gāncǎo 5g + báizhǐ 4g + shārén 4g + huángqín 3g + dàhuáng 0g.

Hypoparathyroidism (252.1), Tetralogy of Fallot (745.2):

Xiǎojiànzhōngtāng 5g + gāncǎo 1-0g.	Yùzhú 5g + shāshēn 5g + màiméndōng 5-3g + xuánshēn 3-2g + dìhuáng 3-2g + hòupò 3-0g + zhǐshí 3-0g + dàhuáng 0g.
Gāncǎoxiǎomàidàzǎotāng 5g + gāncǎo 0g.	
Xiǎocháihútāng 5g + xuánshēn 1-0g + mǔlì 1-0g + bèimǔ 1-0g + xiàkūcǎo 1-0g.	Zhìgāncǎo 5g + báizhǐ 4g + shārén 4g + dàhuáng 0g.
	Gāncǎo 5g + júhuā 5g + júhóng 5g.

the respiratory system, and disorders of the nervous system; Xiǎojiànzhōngtāng relieves diseases of upper respiratory tract such as allergic rhinitis, and complications of heart disease such as cardiac dysrhythmias. Shēnlíngbáizhúsǎn contains Rénshēn (Radix Ginseng), whose cardiovascular benefits and mechanisms were reviewed (Kim, 2012).

1.16   PARTIAL ATRIOVENTRICULAR SEPTAL DEFECT

Partial atrioventricular septal defect (partial AVSD) is a condition where there is a hole in the wall separating the two upper chambers near the center of the heart of the newborn. The left heart valve may also be leaky. Symptoms may not appear until early adulthood. The exact cause of partial AVSD is unknown but may involve a combination of genetic and environmental factors during baby's heart development in the womb.

Fùzǐ (Radix Aconiti Lateralis Preparata) "restores dying yang, dispels coldness, and kills pain." It was shown to protect against myocardial infarction in rats by improving myocardial energy metabolism abnormalities and changing phospholipids levels and distribution patterns to stabilize the cardiomyocyte membrane structure (Wu et al., 2019). Furthermore, Gāncǎo (cf. Section 1.1) was shown to reduce the toxicity and increase the efficacy of Fùzǐ on heart failure in mice (Yan et al.,

TABLE 1.16
GMP Herbal Medicines for a 19-Year-Old Adult with Partial Atrioventricular Septal Defect

Partial atrioventricular septal defect (OrphaCode: 1330)

A morphological anomaly with a prevalence of ~3 in 10,000

Not applicable

Partial atrioventricular canal defect

Mitral regurgitation, Palpitations, Recurrent respiratory infections, Exertional dyspnea, Exercise-induced muscle fatigue, Heart murmur

Syncope, Tetralogy of Fallot, Patent ductus arteriosus, Bicuspid aortic valve, Aortic valve stenosis, Coarctation of aorta, Angina pectoris, Atrial arrhythmia, Abnormal tricuspid valve morphology, Double outlet right ventricle, Transient ischemic attack, Hypoplastic left heart, Atrial flutter, Bacterial endocarditis, Anomalous pulmonary venous return, Common atrium, Heterotaxy, Coronary sinus enlargement

All ages

(Continued)

TABLE 1.16 *(Continued)*

GMP Herbal Medicines for a 19-Year-Old Adult with Partial Atrioventricular Septal Defect

Mitral regurgitation (396.3, 746.6), Heart murmur (D006337):

Zhēnwǔtāng 5g + fùzǐ 1g + gānjiāng 1-0g + tiáowèichéngqìtāng 1-0g + dàhuáng 0g.

Zhēnwǔtāng 5g + fùzǐ 1g + xìxīn 1g + dǐdāngtāng 0g + dàhuáng 0g.

Zhìgāncǎotāng 5g + xuèfǔzhúyūtāng 5-3g + dānshēn 1g + yùjīn 1g + yánhúsuǒ 1-0g.

Fùzǐ 5g + gāncǎo 4-3g + gānjiāng 4-3g + fúlíng 4-0g + suānzǎorén 4-0g + dǎngshēn 3-0g.

Dānshēn 5g + gāncǎo 5g + báisháo 5g + shíhú 5g + bǎihé 5g + chēqiánzǐ 5g + fúlíng 5g + màiméndōng 5g.

Dānshēn 5g + niúxī 5g + gāncǎo 5g + báisháo 5g + xìngrén 5g + sāngjìshēng 5g + chénpí 5g + màiméndōng 5g + xùduàn 5g.

Syncope (D013575), Tetralogy of Fallot (745.2), Patent ductus arteriosus (747.0), Aortic valve stenosis (395.0, 746.3), Angina pectoris (D000787), Double outlet right ventricle (745.11), Hypoplastic left heart (746.7):

Shēngmàiyǐn 5g + xuèfǔzhúyūtāng 5-4g + xiāngshāliùjūnzǐtāng 4-0g + dānshēn 1g + sānqī 1-0g + bèimǔ 1-0g + guālóurén 1-0g + yùjīn 1-0g.

Shēngmàiyǐn 5g + bǔzhōngyìqìtāng 5-4g + zhìgāncǎotāng 5-0g + dānshēn 1g + bèimǔ 1-0g + xiàkūcǎo 1-0g + gǔsuìbǔ 1-0g + yùjīn 1-0g + sānqī 1-0g + chìsháo 1-0g + xiōngqióng 1-0g.

Báizhú 5g + fùzǐ 5g + cháihú 5g + báisháo 4g + fúlíng 4g + tiānhuā 2g + dǎngshēn 2g + guìzhī 2g + huángqín 2g + xìxīn 2-0g + wǔwèizǐ 2-0g + shēngjiāng 2-0g + gāncǎo 1g + mǔlì 1g + gānjiāng 1g.

Huángqín 5g + báizhǐ 4g + gāncǎo 2g + jīnyínhuā 2g + shārén 2g + dàhuáng 1g.

2020). Zhēnwǔtāng was shown to reduce the weight and volume of the heart, improve the cardiac function, inhibit hyperplasia of collagen, and reverse myocardial hypertrophy in rats with left ventricular hypertrophy (Xie et al., 2010).

1.17 MICROTIA

Microtia refers to underdevelopment or absence of one or both external ears, which is present at birth. The ear canal may be narrow or missing. The cause of microtia is unknown for the most part, although some cases are associated with mutations in the *HOXA2* gene which is a transcription

TABLE 1.17

GMP Herbal Medicines for a Two-Year-Old Child with Microtia

Microtia (OrphaCode: 83463)

A morphological anomaly with a prevalence of ~3 in 10,000

Disease-causing germline mutation(s): homeobox A2 (*HOXA2* / Entrez: 3199) at 7p15.2

Autosomal dominant, Autosomal recessive, Not applicable

Microtia

Abnormality of the pinna, Atresia of the external auditory canal, Delayed speech and language development, Hypoplastic helices, Anotia

Holoprosencephaly, Attention deficit hyperactivity disorder

Neonatal, Infancy

Delayed speech and language development (D007805):

Sìjūnzǐtāng 5g + yùpíngfēngsǎn 5-0g + guìzhītāng 5-0g + shānzhā 2-0g + shénqū 2-0g + màiyá 2-0g.

Xiǎoxùmìngtāng 5g + gégēntāng 5g.

Bǔzhōngyìqìtāng 5g + shānzhā 1g + shénqū 1g + màiyá 1g.

Báizhǐ 5g + zhìgāncǎo 4g + shārén 4g + dàhuáng 0g.

Huángqí 5g + chìsháo 1g + fángfēng 1g + xìxīn 1-0g + huánglián 1-0g.

Tiānmá 5g + báisháo 5g + dìhuáng 5g + mànjīngzǐ 5g + gōuténg 5g + niúxī 3g + bànxià 3g + báizhǐ 3g + hángjú 3g + màiméndōng 3g + dānguī 3g + gǎoběn 3g + xìxīn 2g.

factor that is temporally and spatially expressed during embryonic development for the positional identities in hindbrain development.

Sìjūnzǐtāng "tastes sweet and warm, benefits Qi, strengthens the Spleen, and nourishes the Stomach." The formula consists of four herbs, each of which improves the function of the Spleen which governs digestion. Sìjūnzǐtāng was shown to rescue brain neurons and improve neurobehavioral function in rats following cerebral ischemia-reperfusion (Yang et al., 2019); it is commonly prescribed to pediatric patients with chronic sinusitis (Wang, 2019). Xiǎoxùmìngtāng "warms meridians, activates yang, strengthens the body, dispels Wind" and is used today for cerebrovascular disease, and late effects of cerebrovascular disease (Wang, 2019).

1.18   CONGENITAL PRIMARY APHAKIA

Congenital primary aphakia is a condition present at birth where the lens is missing. Congenital primary aphakia is caused by mutations in the *FOXE3* gene which is a lens-specific transcription factor that is important for lens formation in vertebrates.

TABLE 1.18

GMP Herbal Medicines for a One-Year-Old Infant with Congenital Primary Aphakia

Congenital primary aphakia (OrphaCode: 83461)

A malformation syndrome with a prevalence of ~3 in 10,000

Disease-causing germline mutation(s): forkhead box E3 (*FOXE3* / Entrez: 2301) at 1p33

Autosomal recessive

Microphthalmia, Congenital aphakia, Aplasia/Hypoplasia affecting the anterior segment of the eye

Abnormality of vision, Sclerocornea, Retinal dysplasiaNeonatal, Infancy

Microphthalmia (743.1):

Shēnlíngbáizhúsǎn 5g + shānzhā 1-0g + shénqū 1-0g + màiyá 1-0g.	Yùzhú 5g + shāshēn 5g + màiméndōng 5-0g + hòupò 5-0g + zhǐshí 5-0g + dàhuáng 1-0g.
Xìngsūyǐnyòukē 5g + xīnyíqīngfèitāng 5g.	Báizhǐ 5g + shārén 4g + gāncǎo 2g + dàhuáng 0g.
Xiǎojiànzhōngtāng 5g + shānzhā 1g + shénqū 1g + màiyá 1g.	Báizhǐ 5g + zhìgāncǎo 5g + shārén 5g + huángqín 2g + dàhuáng 0g.
Guìzhītāng 5g + gāncǎo 1g + xìngrén 1g + hòupò 1g + dàhuáng 0g.	Xuánshēn 5g + dìhuáng 5g + màiméndōng 5g + hòupò 2g + zhǐshí 2g + dàhuáng 1g.

The edible and yin-nourishing properties of Yùzhú (cf. Section 1.5) may explain its prescription to infants with microphthalmia in the table. Báizhǐ, being edible too, is annotated in Section 1.7 to "open orifices," which in TCM includes eyes, ears, and mouth (cf. Table 1.17). Xìngsūyǐnyòukē, Xiǎojiànzhōngtāng, and Guìzhītāng all treat allergic rhinitis (Wang, 2019). Moreover, they all contain Shēngjiāng (Rhizoma Zingiberis Recens), which was shown to improve ocular blood flow in rats (Takahashi et al., 2023) and lower increased intraocular pressure in rabbits (Akpalaba et al., 2009).

1.19   CLEFT VELUM

The back of the roof of the mouth is called the soft palate or velum. Exposure to alcohol, tobacco, or drugs during pregnancy of a genetically susceptible mother is implicated to induce an error in the palatine fusion process of the baby in utero, causing cleft velum in the newborn.

Gāncǎo is introduced in Section 1.1 to be anti-inflammatory. Línguìshùgāntāng "warms yang, strengthens the Spleen, promotes urination, eliminates dampness" and is used for vertiginous syndromes and other disorders of vestibular system, and for general symptoms (Wang, 2019). In

TABLE 1.19

GMP Herbal Medicines for a One-Year-Old Infant with Cleft Velum

Cleft velum (OrphaCode: 99772)

A morphological anomaly with a prevalence of ~3 in 10,000

Major susceptibility factor: grainyhead like transcription factor 3 (*GRHL3* / Entrez: 57822) at 1p36.11

Candidate gene tested: ubiquitin B (*UBB* / Entrez: 7314) at 17p11.2

Multigenic/multifactorial, Not applicable

Cleft soft palate, Velopharyngeal insufficiency, Poor suck, Receptive language delay, Nasal regurgitation, Oral-pharyngeal dysphagia

Hypoplasia of the maxilla, Recurrent otitis media, Conductive hearing impairment, Nasal speech, Speech articulation difficulties, Short face, Aspiration pneumonia

Neonatal, Infancy

Recurrent otitis media [Unspecified otitis media 382.9)], Conductive hearing impairment (D006314):

Xiǎocháihútāng 5g + yínqiàosǎn 5g + shíchāngpú 1g + yuǎnzhì 1g.

Xiǎocháihútāng 5g + língguìshùgāntāng 5g + liánqiáo 2-1g + shíchāngpú 2-0g + jiégěng 2-0g + shénqū 2-0g + yuǎnzhì 2-0g + jiégěng 1-0g + jīngjiè 1-0g.

Sāngjúyǐn 5g + chántuì 2g.

Gāncǎo 5g + shārén 5g + báizhǐ 5-0g + huángqín 5-0g + tiānhuā 2-0g + dàhuáng 0g.

Jílí 5g + zhǐqiào 5-0g.

addition, Língguìshùgāntāng was shown to alleviate non-alcoholic fatty liver disease in rats (Dang et al., 2019). The liver is associated with the ear through the TCM meridian system where Qi flows.

1.20 NEUROFIBROMATOSIS TYPE 1

Neurofibromatosis type 1, also known as nonmosaic neurofibromatosis type 1 or von Recklinghausen disease, is characterized by formation of multiple noncancerous or cancerous tumors on the nerves and skin. Neurofibromatosis type 1 is caused by mutations in the *NF1* gene whose products function in cells of and around the nerve as tumor suppressor proteins.

TABLE 1.20

GMP Herbal Medicines for a Two-Year-Old Child with Neurofibromatosis Type 1

Neurofibromatosis type 1 (OrphaCode: 636)

A disease with a prevalence of ~2 in 10,000

Disease-causing germline mutation(s) (loss of function): neurofibromin 1 (*NF1* / Entrez: 4763) at 17q11.2

Autosomal dominant

Abnormality of the nervous system, Delayed puberty, Melanocytic nevus, Multiple lipomas, Intellectual disability–mild, Specific learning disability, Subcutaneous nodule, Meningioma, Generalized hyperpigmentation, Multiple cafe-au-lait spots, Neoplasm of the skin, Astrocytoma, Plexiform neurofibroma, Lisch nodules, Macule

Cryptorchidism, Tall stature, Hearing abnormality, Hearing impairment, Abnormality of the eye, Abnormality of vision, Proptosis, Heterochromia iridis, Ataxia, Freckling, Neurological speech impairment, Headache, Memory impairment, Skeletal dysplasia, Recurrent fractures, Genu valgum, Slender long bone, Paresthesia, Attention deficit hyperactivity disorder

Kyphosis, Hydrocephalus, Macrocephaly, Abnormal eyelid morphology, Glaucoma, Visual impairment, Abnormal electroretinogram, Cataract, Myopia, Chorioretinal coloboma, Abnormality of the endocrine system, Hypertension, Precocious puberty, Abnormality of the skeletal system, Hypopigmented skin patches, Seizure, Joint stiffness, Leukemia, Abnormality of the respiratory system, Scoliosis, Neoplasm, Pheochromocytoma, Genu varum, Abnormality of the hip bone, Short stature, Chronic myelogenous leukemia, Neoplasm of the gastrointestinal tract, Abnormality of retinal pigmentation, Corneal opacity, Spinal neurofibromas, Urinary tract neoplasm, Abnormality of the upper urinary tract, Abnormal hair quantity, Sarcoma, Arterial stenosis

Neonatal, Infancy

(Continued)

TABLE 1.20 *(Continued)*

GMP Herbal Medicines for a Two-Year-Old Child with Neurofibromatosis Type 1

Multiple lipomas (214):

Shíliùwèiliúqìyǐn 5g + sǎnzhǒngkuìjiāntāng 5g.
Èrchéntāng 5g + guìzhīfúlíngwán 5g.
Èrchéntāng 5g + sǎnzhǒngkuìjiāntāng 5-0g + zhēnrénhuómìngyǐn 5-0g + xuánshēn 2-0g + mǔlì 2-0g + bèimǔ 2-0g + xiàkūcǎo 2-0g + sānléng 1-0g + éshù 1-0g.

Báijièzǐ 5g + kūnbù 5g + xiàkūcǎo 5-0g + bèimǔ 2g + hǎipiāoxiāo 2-0g + gāncǎo 0g.
Xiàkūcǎo 5g + bèimǔ 2g + gāncǎo 0g.
Tiānhuā 5g + gāncǎo 5g + báizhǐ 5g + shārén 5g + huángqín 5g + dàhuáng 1g.

Cryptorchidism (752.51), Hearing impairment (D003638), Abnormality of the eye (379.90), Proptosis (376.30), Ataxia (D002524), Neurological speech impairment (D013064), Headache (D006261), Memory impairment (D008569), Skeletal dysplasia (756.56, 756.4), Paresthesia (D010292):

Wǔlíngsǎn 5g + zīshènmíngmùtāng 5-0g + gǒuqǐzǐ 2-1g + tùsīzǐ 2-1g + chēqiánzǐ 1g + wǔwèizǐ 1g + fùpénzǐ 1-0g.
Zīshènmíngmùtāng 5g + qǐjúdìhuángwán 5-0g + gǒuqǐzǐ 2-0g + júhuā 2-0g.

Gāncǎo 5g + huángqín 5g + huánglián 5-1g + dàhuáng 0g.
Gāncǎo 5g + gǒuqǐzǐ 5g + júhuā 5g + gānjiāng 5-0g.

Hydrocephalus (331.4, 331.3), Glaucoma (365), Visual impairment (D014786), Cataract (366.8), Myopia (367.1), Abnormality of the endocrine system (259.9), Hypertension (401-405.99), Seizure (345.9), Leukemia (208), Neoplasm (199), Neoplasm of the gastrointestinal tract (239.0):

Yìqìcōngmíngtāng 5g + qǐjúdìhuángwán 5-0g + liùwèidìhuángwán 5-0g + shíchāngpú 1g + tiānmá 1-0g + yuǎnzhì 1-0g + acupuncture.
Jiāwèixiāoyáosǎn 5g + qǐjúdìhuángwán 5g + tiānmá 1g + shíchāngpú 1g + xiàkūcǎo 1g + cǎojuémíng 1g + yuǎnzhì 1g.
Jiāwèixiāoyáosǎn 5g + língguìshùgāntāng 5g + tiānmá 1g + báijiāngcán 1g + shíchāngpú 1g + yuǎnzhì 1g.

Nǚzhēnzǐ 5g + tiānméndōng 5g + dìhuáng 5g + gǒuqǐzǐ 5g + màiméndōng 5g + júhuā 5g + huángqín 5g + dāngguī 5-0g + chuānxiōng 4-0g.
Gǒuqǐzǐ 5-3g + júhuā 5-0g + huángqí 5-0g + dìhuáng 3-0g + fángfēng 3-0g + dāngguī 3-0g + xìxīn 1-0g + huánglián 1-0g + dàhuáng 1-0g.

Báijièzǐ (Semen Sinapis) "warms the Lung, transforms phlegm, moves Qi, and dissolves congelation (i.e., nodule)." It was shown to reduce formation of colon adenomas in mice (Yuan et al., 2011) and is used for cough, lipoma, and so on (Wang, 2020). Tiānhuā (Radix Trichosanthis) is anti-cancer and the mechanisms in the treatment of lung cancer were investigated in silico (Cui et al., 2024). Shíliùwèiliúqìyǐn "rectifies Qi, activates circulation, benefits Qi, opens collaterals, reduces swelling, drains pus" and is used today for simple and unspecified goiter (Wang, 2019). Nǚzhēnzǐ (Fructus Ligustri Lucidi) "nourishes yin of the Liver and Kidney, strengthens the waist and knees, darkens the hair, and brightens the eye." It was reviewed to have such pharmacological effects as antitumor, liver protection, blood glucose/lipid-lowering, and immune regulation (Cao et al., 2023), and is used today for disease of pancreas, disorder of globe, lumbago, and so on (Wang, 2020).

1.21 PROXIMAL 16p11.2 MICRODELETION SYNDROME

Proximal 16p11.2 microdeletion syndrome, also called proximal monosomy 16p11.2, is characterized by impaired communications and socialization. Proximal 16p11.2 microdeletion syndrome is caused by deletion of a piece of chromosome 16 on p11.2, which includes about two dozen genes, one of which, i.e., *SH2B1*, encodes proteins that function in growth factor receptor signaling.

Báizhú, or Rhizoma Atractylodis Macrocephalae, was shown to have antihallucination-like effects in mice (Murayama et al., 2014). It was also demonstrated to ameliorate learning and memory impairment in rats (Zhao et al., 2015). Fúlíng, i.e., Poria cocos, was shown to retard ototoxicity of kanamycin in guinea pigs (Liu et al., 1995). Sìjūnzǐtāng, Yùpíngfēngsǎn, and Bǔzhōngyìqìtāng all contain Báizhú; Yùpíngfēngsǎn and Bǔzhōngyìqìtāng both contain Huángqí (cf. Section 1.9); and Sìjūnzǐtāng contains Fúlíng.

TABLE 1.21

GMP Herbal Medicines for a Three-Year-Old Child with Proximal 16p11.2 Microdeletion Syndrome

Proximal 16p11.2 microdeletion syndrome (OrphaCode: 261197)

A malformation syndrome with a prevalence of ~2 in 10,000

Role: the phenotype of SH2B adaptor protein 1 (*SH2B1* / Entrez: 25970) at 16p11.2

Autosomal dominant, Not applicable

Behavioral abnormality, Autistic behavior, Global developmental delay

Macrocephaly, Delayed speech and language development, Intellectual disability, Intellectual disability–mild, Motor delay, Specific learning disability, Severe expressive language delay, Attention deficit hyperactivity disorder, Speech articulation difficulties, Moderate receptive language delay, Brain imaging abnormality

Hypertelorism, Broad forehead, Micrognathia, Conductive hearing impairment, Sensorineural hearing impairment, Autism, Stereotypy, Impaired social interactions, Seizure, Choreoathetosis, Dystonia, Failure to thrive, Obesity, Abnormal heart morphology, Atrial septal defect, Abnormal aortic valve morphology, Abnormal facial shape, Gastroesophageal reflux, Ventriculomegaly, Enlarged cisterna magna, Scoliosis, Platybasia, Abnormal vertebral morphology, Chiari type I malformation, Paroxysmal dyskinesia, Speech apraxia, Midface retrusion, Feeding difficulties, Arachnoid cyst

Childhood

Delayed speech and language development (D007805), Intellectual disability (D008607):

Guìzhītāng 5g + yùpíngfēngsǎn 3-0g + xìngrén 1-0g + hòupò 1-0g + gāncǎo 1-0g + dàhuáng 0g + acupuncture.
Sìjūnzǐtāng 5g + bǔzhōngyìqìtāng 5g.

Huángqí 5g + chìsháo 1-0g + fángfēng 1-0g + xìxīn 0g + huánglián 0g + dàhuáng 0g.

Conductive hearing impairment (D006314), Sensorineural hearing impairment (389.1), Autism (299.0), Stereotypy (307.3), Seizure (345.9), Dystonia (D004421), Obesity (278.00), Abnormal heart morphology (746.9), Gastroesophageal reflux (530.81), Paroxysmal dyskinesia (D002819), Speech apraxia (D001072):

Xīnyíqīngfèitāng 5g + yìqìcōngmíngtāng 4g + báijiāngcán 1g + shíchāngpú 1g + dìlóng 1g + jīnchán 1g + acupuncture.
Xīnyíqīngfèitāng 5g + máxìnggānshítāng 5g + shíchāngpú 2g + yuǎnzhì 2g + gāncǎo 1g.
Xīnyíqīngfèitāng 5g + cháihújiālónggǔmǔlìtāng 5g + shíchāngpú 2g + yuǎnzhì 2g + chántuì 2-0g.
Xiǎocháihútāng 5g + báijiāngcán 1g + shíchāngpú 1g + héyè 1g + yuǎnzhì 1g.

Báizhú 5g + fúlíng 5g + shíchāngpú 4g + bèimǔ 4g + cháihú 4g + huángqín 4g + yuǎnzhì 4g + dǎngshēn 4g + zéxiè 4-0g + bànxià 2-0g.
Shārén 5-2g + guālóugēn 5-2g + huángqín 5-2g + gāncǎo 5-1g + cháihú 5-0g + báizhú 5-0g + huángbò 3-0g + guìzhī 2-0g + wūwèizǐ 1-0g + mǔlì 1-0g + gānjiāng 1-0g + xìxīn 1-0g + dāngguī 1-0g + dàhuáng 1-0g.
Tiānméndōng 5g + bèimǔ 5g + liánqiáo 5g + huángqín 5g + mǔdānpí 4g + hòupò 4g + zéxiè 4g.

1.22 HEREDITARY HEMORRHAGIC TELANGIECTASIA

Hereditary hemorrhagic telangiectasia (HHT), also known as Rendu-Osler-Weber disease, is a genetic condition where arteries connect directly to veins instead of through capillaries. High arterial pressure can rupture the veins, leading to bleeding such as nosebleeds. Mutations in the genes whose products are involved in blood vessel development cause HHT. Affected tissues and types of HHT depend on which gene(s) were mutated.

Huánglián (Rhizoma Coptidis) is best known for its "fire extinguishing" effect (Moon et al., 2017). In TCM, "yin deficiency and fire excess" forces a frenetic movement of blood, causing non-traumatic bleeding. Huánglián is believed to stop bleeding from the mouth and nose. Qīngzàojiùfèitāng "clears dryness, moistens the Lungs" and is used today for chronic bronchitis (Wang, 2019). Zàojiǎocì (Spina Gleditsiae) was shown to induce cancer cell apoptosis in rats transplanted with rat hepatocellular carcinoma cells (Cai et al., 2019). Dàcháihútāng was demonstrated to protect against acute intrahepatic cholestasis in mice (Xu et al., 2022). Tiānmá (Rhizoma Gastrodiae) was shown to suppress acute seizures in mice with temporal lobe epilepsy (Yip et al., 2020). Dìlóng (Pheretima) reduced the cerebral infarction areas in rats with middle cerebral artery occlusion (Liu et al., 2012). Bǔyánghuánwǔtāng contains Dìlóng.

TABLE 1.22

GMP Herbal Medicines for an 11-Year-Old Child with Hereditary Hemorrhagic Telangiectasia

Hereditary hemorrhagic telangiectasia (OrphaCode: 774)

A disease with a prevalence of ~2 in 10,000

Disease-causing germline mutation(s): activin A receptor like type 1 (*ACVRL1* / Entrez: 94) at 12q13.13

Disease-causing germline mutation(s): SMAD family member 4 (*SMAD4* / Entrez: 4089) at 18q21.2

Disease-causing germline mutation(s): endoglin (*ENG* / Entrez: 2022) at 9q34.11

Disease-causing germline mutation(s): growth differentiation factor 2 (*GDF2* / Entrez: 2658) at 10q11.22

Autosomal dominant

Epistaxis, Mucosal telangiectasiae, Telangiectasia of the skin

Cavernous hemangioma, Spontaneous hematomas, Visceral angiomatosis, Cholecystitis, Portal hypertension, Microcytic anemia, Migraine, Abnormality of cardiovascular system physiology, Arteriovenous malformation

Cholelithiasis, Seizure, Cirrhosis, Hepatic failure, Congestive heart failure, Pulmonary arterial hypertension, Subarachnoid hemorrhage, Pulmonary embolism, Transient ischemic attack, Abnormality of the cerebral vasculature, Intestinal polyposis, Conjunctival telangiectasia, Amblyopia, Nephrolithiasis, Hematuria, Cerebral hemorrhage, Esophageal varix, Hemoptysis, Gastrointestinal hemorrhage, Venous thrombosis, Retinal telangiectasia, Peripheral arteriovenous fistula

All ages

Epistaxis (D004844) [Epistaxis (784.7)]:

Qīngzàojiùfèitāng 5g + xīnyíqīngfèitāng 5-0g + xiānhècǎo 1g + báimáogēn 1g + ǒujiē 1g + dìhuáng 1-0g.	Huángqín 5-4g + huánglián 5-3g + dàhuáng 1-0g.
Qīngzàojiùfèitāng 5g + gānlùyǐn 5g + xiānhècǎo 1g + ǒujiē 1g + báimáogēn 1-0g + dìhuáng 1-0g.	
Qīngzàojiùfèitāng 5g + máxìnggānshítāng 5g + bèimǔ 1g + jiégěng 1g + sāngbáipí 1g + yúxīngcǎo 1g.	

Cholecystitis (575.10), Portal hypertension (572.3), Migraine (346):

Dàcháihútāng 5g + yùjīn 1g + chuānliànzǐ 1-0g + jīnqiáncǎo 1-0g + chìsháo 1-0g + huǒmárén 0g.	Zàojiǎocì 5g + rǔxiāng 5g + gǒujǐ 5g + púhuáng 5-0g + fùzǐ 4-3g + dàhuáng 2g.
	Bànxià 5g + fúlíng 5g + fùzǐ 4g + xìxīn 4g + dàhuáng 2g.

Seizure (345.9), Cirrhosis (D008103) [Cirrhosis of liver without mention of alcohol (571.5)], Congestive heart failure (428, 428.0), Subarachnoid hemorrhage (D013345), Amblyopia (368.01, 368.00), Nephrolithiasis (592), Hematuria (D006417), Cerebral hemorrhage (D002543) [Intracerebral hemorrhage (431)], Hemoptysis (D006469), Gastrointestinal hemorrhage (D006471):

Bǔyánghuánwǔtāng 5g + wēndǎntāng 5-4g + tiānmá 1g + shíchāngpú 1g + yuǎnzhì 1g + acupuncture.	Tiānmá 5g + dìlóng 5g + zhǐshí 5g + shénqū 5g + huángqí 5g + shíchāngpú 4g + yuǎnzhì 4g + dàhuáng 2-1g + acupuncture.
Bǔyánghuánwǔtāng 5g + cháihújiālónggǔmǔlìtāng 4-0g + sānqī 1g + dānshēn 1g + shíchāngpú 1g + yuǎnzhì 1g + tiānmá 1-0g + acupuncture.	Huángqín 5g + báizhǐ 4g + gāncǎo 3-2g + shārén 3-2g + guālóugēn 2-1g + dàhuáng 1g + acupuncture.

1.23 FAMILIAL CEREBRAL CAVERNOUS MALFORMATION

Familial cerebral cavernous malformation, or hereditary brain cavernous angioma, is characterized by multiple collections of abnormal capillaries in the brain or spinal cord. These capillaries have thin walls and thus prone to leak. Familial cerebral cavernous malformation is caused by mutations in the genes such as *KRIT1* whose protein products play roles in cell-cell interactions to prevent blood vessel leakage.

Sānléng (Rhizoma Sparganii) "breaks blood clots, moves Qi, dissipates stagnation, stops pain" and was reviewed and summarized to have antitumor, antithrombotic, estrogen antagonistic, anti-inflammatory, analgesic, antioxidant, and anti-organ fibrosis activities (Jia et al., 2021). Zhēnrénhuómìngyǐn "clears heat, detoxifies, de-swells, destroys hardening, activates circulation, stops pain" and is used for eczema and hemorrhoids (Wang, 2019). Oral Xiāofēngsǎn was shown

TABLE 1.23

GMP Herbal Medicines for a 25-Year-Old Adult with Familial Cerebral Cavernous Malformation

Familial cerebral cavernous malformation (OrphaCode: 221061)

A malformation syndrome with a prevalence of ~1 in 10,000

Disease-causing germline mutation(s) (loss of function): CCM2 scaffold protein (*CCM2* / Entrez: 83605) at 7p13

Disease-causing germline mutation(s) (loss of function): KRIT1 ankyrin repeat containing (*KRIT1* / Entrez: 889) at 7q21.2

Disease-causing germline mutation(s): programmed cell death 10 (*PDCD10* / Entrez: 11235) at 3q26.1

Autosomal dominant

Seizure, Cerebral hemorrhage, Headache

Hemangioma, Increased intracranial pressure, Scoliosis, Meningioma, Focal T2 hyperintense brainstem lesion, Focal T2 hypointense brainstem lesion, Neuroma

Episodic vomiting, Choroidal hemangioma, Vascular skin abnormality, Retinal cavernous angioma, Venous malformation, Cognitive impairment, Spinal cord lesion

All ages

Seizure (345.9), Cerebral hemorrhage (D002543) [Intracerebral hemorrhage (431)], Headache (D006261):

Cháihújiālónggǔmǔlìtāng 5g + wēndǎntāng 5-2g + shíchāngpú 1g + yuǎnzhì 1g + tiānmá 1-0g + dānshēn 1-0g + gōuténg 1-0g + acupuncture.

Tiānmágōuténgyǐn 5g + bǔyánghuánwǔtāng 4g + dānshēn 1g + shíchāngpú 1g + yuǎnzhì 1g.

Gāncǎoxiǎomàidàzǎotāng 5g + cháihújiālónggǔmǔlìtāng 5g + shíchāngpú 1g + yuǎnzhì 1g.

Huángqí 5g + chìsháo 1g + fángfēng 1g + xìxīn 1-0g + huánglián 1-0g + dàhuáng 0g.

Hemangioma (228.00):

Shíliùwèiliúqìyǐn 5g + sǎnzhǒngkuìjiāntāng 5g + sānléng 1-0g + éshù 1-0g.

Xuèfǔzhúyūtāng 5g + cháihúshūgāntāng 5g + dānshēn 1g + yùjīn 1g.

Zhēnrénhuómìngyǐn 5g + sǎnzhǒngkuìjiāntāng 5g + tiānhuā 1g + xuánshēn 1g + bèimǔ 1g + xiàkūcǎo 1g + púgōngyīng 1g.

Sǎnzhǒngkuìjiāntāng 5g + dānshēn 1g + xuánshēn 1g + mǔlì 1g + bèimǔ 1g + xiàkūcǎo 1g + biējiǎ 1g.

Báijièzǐ 5g + zàojiǎocì 5g + bèimǔ 5g + fángfēng 5g + jiégěng 5g + jīngjiè 5g + fúlíng 5g + dǎngshēn 5g + gāncǎo 4g + dìhuáng 4g + báizhú 4-0g + dāngguī 4-0g.

Sānléng 5g + tiānhuā 5g + gāncǎo 5g + chìsháo 5g + cháihú 5g + huángbò 5g + dāngguīwěi 5g + púgōngyīng 5g + hónghuā 3g + táorén 3g.

Dānshēn 5g + dìhuáng 5g + héshǒuwū 5g + fúlíng 5g + dǎngshēn 5g + kuǎndōnghuā 5g + báizhú 3g + báisháo 3g + qiàncǎo 3g + dāngguī 3g.

Zàojiǎocì 5g + rǔxiāng 5g + gǒujǐ 5g + púhuáng 5g + fùzǐ 3g + dàhuáng 2g.

Vascular skin abnormality (709.1):

Xiāoyáosǎn 5g + dāngguīyǐnzǐ 5-0g + nǚzhēnzǐ 1-0g + hànliáncǎo 1-0g + tùsīzǐ 1-0g + jīxuèténg 1-0g + dānshēn 1-0g + mǔdānpí 1-0g + chìsháo 1-0g.

Huángliánjiědútāng 5g + xiāofēngsǎn 3g + dāngguīyǐnzǐ 3g + yèjiāoténg 2g + báixiānpí 1g + dìfūzǐ 1g.

Jiědúsìwùtāng 5g + xiāofēngsǎn 5-4g.

Huángqín 5g + báizhǐ 4g + zhìgāncǎo 3g + shārén 3g + tiānhuā 2g + dàhuáng 1g.

Báizhǐ 5-4g + huángqín 5-4g + gāncǎo 4-2g + shārén 4-2g + tiānhuā 2g + dàhuáng 1-0g.

to be effective and safe for severe, refractory, extensive, and nonexudative atopic dermatitis by a randomized, double-blinded, placebo-controlled trial (Cheng et al., 2011).

1.24 SUPRAVALVULAR AORTIC STENOSIS

Supravalvular aortic stenosis is obstructive narrowing of the section of the aorta just above the aortic valve, which controls blood flow from the left ventricle into the aorta. Supravalvular aortic stenosis is caused by mutations in the *ELN* gene whose products form structures providing resilience and flexibility to tissues and organs including the blood vessels and heart.

TABLE 1.24

GMP Herbal Medicines for a 13-Year-Old Adolescent with Supravalvular Aortic Stenosis

Supravalvular aortic stenosis (OrphaCode: 3193)

A morphological anomaly with a prevalence of ~1 in 10,000

Disease-causing germline mutation(s) (loss of function): elastin (*ELN* / Entrez: 2006) at 7q11.23

Autosomal dominant

Supravalvular aortic stenosis, ArrhythmiaAll ages

Arrhythmia (D001145) [Cardiac dysrhythmia, unspecified (427.9)]:

Zhìgāncǎotāng 5g + dānshēn 0g + bèimǔ 0g + fúlíng 0g + zǐsū 0g.	Zhìgāncǎo 5g + gānjiāng 5g + fùzǐ 3g + gǒuqǐzǐ 3-0g + júhuā 3-0g.
Shēngjiāng 5g + zhìgāncǎo 5g + ròuguì 4g + fùzǐ 4g + hǎigé 4g.	Huángqí 5g + zhīmǔ 2g + shēngmá 1g + gāncǎo 1g + jiégěng 1g + cháihú 1g.
	Zhìgāncǎo 5g + guìzhī 5g + táorén 5g + dàhuáng 0g.

Huángqí and Zhìgāncǎotāng, which contains Zhìgāncǎo, were found to be among the most commonly used herbs and formulas to reduce the mortality risk for ischemic heart disease in patients with type 2 diabetes in Taiwan (Tsai et al., 2017). Shēngjiāng (cf. Section 1.18) was shown to protects heart by suppressing myocardial ischemia/reperfusion induced inflammation in rats (Xu et al., 2019).

1.25 NON-SYNDROMIC METOPIC CRANIOSYNOSTOSIS

Non-syndromic metopic craniosynostosis, also known as isolated trigonocephaly, is premature closure of a growth seam such as the median frontal suture in the skull of the newborn, without other related anomalies. Some of the cases of non-syndromic metopic craniosynostosis are associated with mutations in the *FGFR1* gene whose products are receptors on cell membrane to set off reactions inside the cell for cell differentiation in response to growth factors outside of the cell. *FGFR1* is shown to be important for the development and growth of bones including the craniofacial bones.

Zhìgāncǎo (cf. Section 1.11) "nourishes the Spleen, harmonizes the Stomach, benefits Qi, and restores pulse." Xuánshēn (cf. Section 1.3) "clears heat, cools Blood, nourishes yin, and removes toxins." Both Xiǎojiànzhōngtāng (cf. Sections 1.1 and 1.15) and Guìzhītāng (cf. Section 1.11) help digestion as well as immunity. It was reported that pre-surgical acupuncture reduces anxiety and stress;

TABLE 1.25

GMP Herbal Medicines for a One-Year-Old Infant with Non-Syndromic Metopic Craniosynostosis

Non-syndromic metopic craniosynostosis (OrphaCode: 3366)

A morphological anomaly with a prevalence of ~1 in 10,000

Disease-causing germline mutation(s): fibroblast growth factor receptor 1 (*FGFR1* / Entrez: 2260) at 8p11.23

Disease-causing germline mutation(s): FRAS1 related extracellular matrix 1 (*FREM1* / Entrez: 158326) at 9p22.3

Autosomal dominant, Not applicable

Trigonocephaly

Prominent supraorbital ridges, Wide nasal bridge, Hypotelorism, Synophrys

Omphalocele

Neonatal, Infancy

Omphalocele (756.72):

Xiǎojiànzhōngtāng5g + shēnlíngbáizhúsǎn 5-0g + báizhú 1-0g + báisháo 1-0g + fángfēng 1-0g + chénpí 1-0g + acupuncture.	Zhìgāncǎo 5g + dàhuáng 0g.
	Gāncǎo 5g + shārén 5g + dàhuáng 0g.
Guìzhītāng 5g + gāncǎo 1-0g + acupuncture.	Xuánshēn 5g + dìhuáng 5g + màiméndōng 5g + hòupò 5-1g + zhǐshí 5-1g + yùzhú 5-0g + shāshēn 5-0g + dàhuáng 1-0g.

acupuncture during surgery reduces narcotics use and maintains respiratory stability; and post-surgical acupuncture alleviates post-operative discomforts and enhances recovery (Yuan & Wang, 2019).

1.26 CHARGE SYNDROME

CHARGE syndrome, also known as Hall-Hittner syndrome, is a fetal development condition affecting multiple organs. The letters in CHARGE stand for: Coloboma–Heart defects–Atresia choanae–Retardation of growth and development–Genitourinary problems–Ear abnormalities, although these manifestations no longer make the diagnosis. CHARGE syndrome is associated with new mutations in the *CHD7* gene whose products regulate activities of other genes through packaging DNA into loose or tight configurations of chromatin inside the nucleus.

TABLE 1.26

GMP Herbal Medicines for a One-Year-Old Infant with CHARGE Syndrome

CHARGE syndrome (OrphaCode: 138)

A malformation syndrome with a prevalence of ~9 in 100,000

Candidate gene tested: semaphorin 3E (*SEMA3E* / Entrez: 9723) at 7q21.11

Disease-causing germline mutation(s): chromodomain helicase DNA binding protein 7 (*CHD7* / Entrez: 55636) at 8q12.2

Autosomal dominant, Unknown

Cryptorchidism, Hypogonadotrophic hypogonadism, Micropenis, Abnormality of the inner ear, Hearing impairment, Overfolded helix, Anosmia, Iris coloboma, Delayed puberty, Global developmental delay, Abnormal cranial nerve morphology, External ear malformation, Feeding difficulties in infancy, Aplasia/Hypoplasia of the earlobes, Hypoplasia of the semicircular canal

Abnormal morphology of female internal genitalia, Bifid scrotum, Labial hypoplasia, Narrow mouth, Cleft palate, Cleft upper lip, Narrow face, Facial asymmetry, Low-set and posteriorly rotated ears, Choanal atresia, Strabismus, Ptosis, Anophthalmia, Chorioretinal coloboma, Microphthalmia, Nystagmus, Optic atrophy, Delayed eruption of teeth, Autism, Obsessive-compulsive behavior, Anterior hypopituitarism, Intellectual disability, Hypotonia, Polyhydramnios, Tetralogy of Fallot, Patent ductus arteriosus, Abnormal aortic valve morphology, Abnormal cardiac septum morphology, Gastroesophageal reflux, Malformation of the heart and great vessels, Short stature, Dilatation of the aortic arch, Depressed nasal bridge, Attention deficit hyperactivity disorder, Postnatal growth retardation, Facial palsy, Chin dimple, Interrupted aortic arch, Abnormality of the soft palate

Vesicoureteral reflux, Horseshoe kidney, Hydronephrosis, Microcephaly, Epicanthus, Hypertelorism, Preauricular skin tag, Abnormality of the eye, Abnormality of vision, Eyelid coloboma, Lacrimation abnormality, Abnormality of the ribs, Abnormality of the adrenal glands, Brachydactyly, Dandy-Walker malformation, Holoprosencephaly, Intrauterine growth retardation, Laryngomalacia, Talipes, Respiratory insufficiency, Aqueductal stenosis, Highly arched eyebrow, Tracheoesophageal fistula, Scoliosis, Hemivertebrae, Abnormality of tibia morphology, Clinodactyly of the 5th finger, Abnormality of bone mineral density, Cranial nerve paralysis, Aplasia/Hypoplasia of the cerebellum, Microtia, Bifid femur, Hypoplasia of the zygomatic bone, Abnormality of immune system physiology

Neonatal

Cryptorchidism (752.51), Hearing impairment (D034381), Anosmia (D000857):

Wǔlíngsǎn 5g + píngwèisǎn 5-0g + gāncǎo 0g.

Sìjūnzǐtāng 5g.

Bāwèidìhuángwán 5g.

Júhóng 5g + jílí 3g.

Chántuì 5g + júhóng 5-0g.

Cleft palate (749.0), Optic atrophy (377.1), Obsessive-compulsive behavior (300.3), Intellectual disability (D008607), Hypotonia (D009123), Tetralogy of Fallot (745.2), Gastroesophageal reflux (530.81), Facial palsy (351.0):

Bànxiàxièxīntāng 5g + gāncǎoxiǎomàidàzǎotāng 5g + xiāngshāliùjūnzǐtāng 5g + mǔlì 2g + hǎipiāoxiāo 2g + mǔlì 2-0g + mázǐrénwán 2-0g.

Guìzhītāng 5g + xìngrén 2g + hòupò 2g + dàhuáng 0g.

Tiānmágōuténgyǐn 5g + qǐjúdìhuángwán 5g + dānshēn 1g + shíchāngpú 1g + yuǎnzhì 1g.

Jiāwèixiāoyáosǎn 5g + zhǐqiào 2g + jílí 1g + chántuì 0g.

Chuānxiōng 5g + tiānméndōng 5g + báizhú 5g + báisháo 5g + dìhuáng 5g + héshǒuwū 5g + fúlíng 5g + dāngguī 5g + júhuā 5-0g + màiyá 5-0g + suānzǎorén 5-0g.

Gǒuqǐzǐ 5g + júhuā 5g + dìhuáng 4-3g + dāngguī 4-3g + fángfēng 4-3g + xìxīn 2-1g + huánglián 2-1g + dàhuáng 2-0g.

(Continued)

TABLE 1.26 *(Continued)*

GMP Herbal Medicines for a One-Year-Old Infant with CHARGE Syndrome

Vesicoureteral reflux (593.7), Hydronephrosis (591), Abnormality of the eye (379.90), Abnormality of the adrenal glands
(255.9), Aqueductal stenosis (331.4, 331.3), Cranial nerve paralysis (352.9):

Sāngpiāoxiāosǎn 5g + qǐjúdìhuángwán 5-4g + jìshēngshènqìwán 5-0g + bǔzhōngyìqìtāng 5-0g + xiāngshāliùjūnzǐtāng 4-0g.	Shénqū 5g + màiyá 5g.
Qǐjúdìhuángwán 5g + zhūlíngtāng 5g + jìshēngshènqìwán 5g.	Shānzhīzǐ 5g + gāncǎo 5g + huángbò 5g + dàhuáng 0g + huánglián 0g.
Sāngpiāoxiāosǎn 5g + bǔzhōngyìqìtāng 5g + fùpénzǐ 1g.	Gāncǎo 5g + zhīmǔ 5g.
Xiāngshāliùjūnzǐtāng 5g + shēnlíngbáizhúsǎn 5g + jìshēngshènqìwán 5g + shānzhā 2g + shénqū 2g + màiyá 2g.	Gāncǎo 5g + shénqū 2g + jīnèijīn 2g + dàhuáng 0g + huánglián 0g.

Chuānxiōng (Radix Chuanxiong) "enlivens Blood, moves Qi, dispels Wind, and stops pain."
Pretreatment with Chuānxiōng was shown to alleviate ischemic stroke in mice with middle cerebral
artery occlusion-induced ischemic stroke (Lim et al., 2024); Chuānxiōng was shown to promote angiogenesis in human umbilical vein endothelial cells and in quail embryo chorioallantoic membranes (Cheng
et al., 2023); Chuānxiōng is used for cardiovascular and cerebrovascular diseases including chest pain
and headache (Wang, 2020). Sāngpiāoxiāosǎn "modulates and replenishes the Heart/Kidney, astringes
semen, arrests spermatorrhea" and is used for symptoms involving the urinary system (Wang, 2019).

1.27   DUODENAL ATRESIA

Duodenal atresia is a congenital condition where the upper section of the small bowel, called the duodenum, is narrowed or blocked in the newborn. The underlying cause of duodenal atresia is unknown.

TABLE 1.27

GMP Herbal Medicines for a One-Year-Old Infant with Duodenal Atresia

Duodenal atresia (OrphaCode: 1203)

A morphological anomaly with a prevalence of ~9 in 100,000

Unknown

Polyhydramnios, Duodenal atresia

Abnormality of the pancreas, Annular pancreas, Abnormality of the pulmonary artery

Antenatal, Neonatal, Infancy, Childhood

Atresia and stenosis of small intestine (751.1):

Shēnlíngbáizhúsǎn 5g + bǎohéwán 2-0g + shānzhā 1-0g + shénqū 1-0g + màiyá 1-0g + jīnèijīn 1-0g.	Gāncǎo 5g + hòupò 5-0g + zhǐshí 5-0g + dàhuáng 1-0g.
Xiāngshāliùjūnzǐtāng 5g + shānzhā 1g + màiyá 1g.	Xuánshēn 5g + dìhuáng 5g + màiméndōng 5g + hòupò 3-2g + zhǐshí 3-2g + dàhuáng 0g.

Màiméndōng (Radix Ophiopogonis) "nourishes yin, moistens the Lung and skin" and is used
today for cough, bronchitis, chest pain, pruritic disorder, and dyspepsia, including constipation
(Wang, 2020). Xiāngshāliùjūnzǐtāng "benefits the Stomach, replenishes interior, rectifies Qi, harmonizes the Stomach" and is used for disorders of function of stomach, and functional digestive
disorders (Wang, 2019).

1.28   CLASSIC CONGENITAL ADRENAL HYPERPLASIA
DUE TO 21-HYDROXYLASE DEFICIENCY

Classic congenital adrenal hyperplasia due to 21-hydroxylase deficiency, also known as classic
21-OHD CAH, simple virilizing form, is characterized by excessive production of androgens.
Classic congenital adrenal hyperplasia due to 21-hydroxylase deficiency is caused by mutations in

TABLE 1.28

GMP Herbal Medicines for a One-Year-Old Infant with Classic Congenital Adrenal Hyperplasia Due to 21-hydroxylase Deficiency

Classic congenital adrenal hyperplasia due to 21-hydroxylase deficiency (OrphaCode: 90794)

A disease with a prevalence of ~7 in 100,000

Disease-causing germline mutation(s): cytochrome P450 family 21 subfamily A member 2 (*CYP21A2* / Entrez: 1589) at 6p21.33

Autosomal recessive

Decreased circulating cortisol level, Increased circulating androgen concentration, Abnormal response to ACTH stimulation test, Elevated circulating 17-hydroxyprogesterone, Increased circulating progesterone

Renal salt wasting, Abnormality of the menstrual cycle, Decreased fertility, Abnormal external genitalia, Hyperactive renin-angiotensin system, Oligomenorrhea, Hirsutism, Acne, Growth abnormality, Failure to thrive, Weight loss, Dehydration, Neonatal hypoglycemia, Vomiting, Hyperkalemia, Hypotension, Hyponatremia, Hypochloremia, Increased circulating ACTH level, Elevated urinary epinephrine, Premature fusion of the radial epiphyseal plates, Decreased circulating aldosterone level, Short stature, Accelerated skeletal maturation, Hyperkalemic metabolic acidosis, Primary adrenal insufficiency, Clitoral hypertrophy, Hypovolemia, Feeding difficulties, Premature pubarche, Hypocapnia, Hypernatriuria, Increased serum androstenedione, Increased serum testosterone level, Abnormal ovarian physiology, Abnormal serum dehydroepiandrosterone level

Long penis, Hypogonadotrophic hypogonadism, Ambiguous genitalia, female, Ambiguous genitalia, Tall stature, Aplasia of the uterus, Frontal balding, Spontaneous abortion, Decreased testicular size, Precocious puberty in females, Premature adrenarche, Testicular adrenal rest tumor, Fused labia majora, Shock, Urogenital sinus anomaly

Antenatal, Neonatal, Infancy, Childhood, Adolescent, Adult

Hirsutism (D006628), Weight loss (D015431), Vomiting (D014839), Hypovolemia (D020896), Hypocapnia (D016857):

Zhēnrénhuómìngyǐn 5g + gāncǎo 1-0g.

Jiāwèixiāoyáosǎn 5g + bǎohéwán 5g + gāncǎo 0g.

Zhēnrénhuómìngyǐnqùchuānshānjiǎ 5g + púgōngyīng 2-1g + jīnyínhuā 1g + liánqiáo 1-0g + yìyǐrén 1-0g + gāncǎo 1-0g.

Gāncǎo 5g + báizhǐ 5g + shārén 5g + huángqín 5-0g + dàhuáng 1-0g.

Ambiguous genitalia (752.7), Frontal balding (704.0):

Jiāwèixiāoyáosǎn 5g + zhǐqiào 2-1g + jílí 2-0g.

Zhībódìhuángwán 5g + zhǐqiào 1g.

Zhǐqiào 5g + jílí 5-0g.

Chántuì 5g.

---

the *CYP21A2* gene whose products, i.e., 21-hydroxylase, catalyze production of cortisol and aldosterone in the adrenal glands. Deficiency in 21-hydroxylase decreases cortisol and aldosterone production, resulting in androgen overproduction.

Liánqiáo (Fructus Forsythiae) "clears heat, detoxifies, reduces carbuncle, dissolves scrofula" and is used today mainly for skin conditions such as dermatitis, eczema, pruritis, urticaria, and acne (Wang, 2020). Zhēnrénhuómìngyǐn (cf. Section 1.23) along with Liánqiáo was found to be the most commonly used GMP concentrated herbal extract granule combination for the treatment of acne (H. Chen et al., 2016), which is caused by increased, androgen-induced sebum production at the sebaceous follicle.

1.29 HYPOHIDROTIC ECTODERMAL DYSPLASIA

Hypohidrotic ectodermal dysplasia, or anhidrotic ectodermal dysplasia, is abnormal development of the tissues deriving from the outermost layer of the embryo called the ectoderm, including the skin, sweat glands, hair, nails, and teeth. Many cases of hypohidrotic ectodermal dysplasia are caused by mutations in the *EDA* gene whose products work with other proteins in signaling pathways between different embryonic layers which are required for normal formation of the sweat glands, teeth, and so on.

Zīshènmíngmùtāng "replenishes Qi and Blood, clears heat, cleans eyes" and is used today for disorders of the lacrimal system (Wang, 2019). Yùpíngfēngsǎn was shown to be safe for the treatment of idiopathic sweating in end-stage cancer patients (Chiu et al., 2009). In addition, Yùpíngfēngsǎn

TABLE 1.29

GMP Herbal Medicines for a One-Year-Old Infant with Hypohidrotic Ectodermal Dysplasia

Hypohidrotic ectodermal dysplasia (OrphaCode: 238468)

A disease with a prevalence of ~7 in 100,000

Disease-causing germline mutation(s): ectodysplasin A (*EDA* / Entrez: 1896) at Xq13.1

Disease-causing germline mutation(s): ectodysplasin A2 receptor (*EDA2R* / Entrez: 60401) at Xq12

Disease-causing germline mutation(s): ectodysplasin A receptor (*EDAR* / Entrez: 10913) at 2q13

Disease-causing germline mutation(s): EDAR associated via death domain (*EDARADD* / Entrez: 128178) at 1q42.3-q43

Disease-causing germline mutation(s): Wnt family member 10A (*WNT10A* / Entrez: 80326) at 2q35

Disease-causing germline mutation(s): cystatin B (*CSTB* / Entrez: 1476) at 21q22.3

Disease-causing germline mutation(s): TNF receptor associated factor 6 (*TRAF6* / Entrez: 7189) at 11p12

Disease-causing germline mutation(s): keratinocyte differentiation factor 1 (*KDF1* / Entrez: 126695) at 1p36.11

Autosomal dominant, Autosomal recessive, X-linked recessive

Abnormality of the dentition, Hypoplasia of the maxilla, Dry skin, Thin skin, Keratoconjunctivitis sicca, Abnormal facial shape, Abnormality of dental morphology, Irregular hyperpigmentation, Reduced number of teeth, Abnormality of immune system physiology, Thick vermilion border

Nephrotic syndrome, Xerostomia, Sinusitis, Anteverted nares, Hyperkeratosis, Eczema, Hypohidrosis, Frontal bossing, Slow-growing hair, Abnormality of the abdominal wall, Trichorrhexis nodosa, Generalized hypopigmentation of hair, Cough, Inflammatory abnormality of the eye, Aplasia/Hypoplasia of the eyebrow

Failure to thrive, Abnormality of the nail, Abnormal hair quantity, Cognitive impairment, Breast aplasia

Neonatal, Infancy

Keratoconjunctivitis sicca (375.15):

Zīshènmíngmùtāng 5g + qǐjúdìhuángwán 5-0g + gǒuqǐzǐ 1-0g + júhuā 1-0g.	Gǒuqǐzǐ 5g + júhuā 5g + niúbàngzǐ 3g + shègān 3g + xìxīn 1g + huánglián 1g.
Gānlùyǐn 5g + júhuā 2-1g + chántuì 2-1g + jiāwèixiāoyáosǎn 2-0g + jílí 1g + zhǐqiào 1-0g.	Gǒuqǐzǐ 5g + shíchāngpú 2g + hángjú 2g + yuǎnzhì 2g.
	Zhǐqiào 5-4g + jílí 5-0g + chántuì 5-0g + júhóng 2-0g.

Nephrotic syndrome (581), Hypohidrosis (705.0), Cough (D003371):

Yùpíngfēngsǎn 5g + bǔzhōngyìqìtāng 5-0g + fúxiǎomài 2-0g + máhuánggēn 2-0g + huángqí 1-0g.	Huángqí 5g + báizhú 2g + fángfēng 2g.
Liùwèidìhuángwán 5g + wǔwèizǐ 1g + huángqí 1g.	Báimáogēn 5g + dìhuáng 5g + huángqí 5g + yìyǐrén 5-0g.
	Fúlíng 5g + gāncǎo 3g + wǔwèizǐ 2g + xìxīn 1g + gānjiāng 0g.
	Gāncǎo 5g + báizhǐ 5g + shārén 5-3g + dàhuáng 0g.

as a feed additive was reviewed to promote growth and enhance immunity of the animals in the farming industry (Chu et al., 2023).

1.30 PRADER-WILLI SYNDROME

Prader-Willi syndrome, also known as Prader-Labhart-Willi syndrome, is a complex genetic disorder characterized by muscle weakness, obesity and low testosterone. Prader-Willi syndrome is caused by loss of function of the genes at the 15q11-13 region of chromosome 15. This region of the human genome expresses gene copies from only one of the parents through a process called genomic imprinting. If only genes from the father (mother) are to be expressed in a zygote, but these genes are somehow missing during spermatogenesis (oogenesis), then Prader-Willi syndrome (Angelman syndrome) results.

Huánshǎodān is translated to "youth restoring elixir." It was formulated to "replenish deficiency in the Heart, Kidney, Spleen and Stomach," in particular in the Kidney yang, which in TCM concerns the functions and activities of the body's development and reproduction. Sīguāluò (Retinervus Luffae Fructus) was shown to lower blood glucose in diabetic rats (El-Fiky et al., 1996). Dàhuáng (Radix et Rhizoma Rhei) and Cháihújiālónggǔmǔlìtāng are among the most commonly used GMP herbal products for non-motor symptoms of Parkinson's disease in Taiwan (Lin et al., 2021).

TABLE 1.30

GMP Herbal Medicines for a One-Year-Old Infant with Prader-Willi Syndrome

Prader-Willi syndrome (OrphaCode: 739)

A disease with a prevalence of ~5 in 100,000

Role: the phenotype of small nucleolar RNA, C/D box 115 cluster (*SNORD115* / HGNC: 32780) at 15q11.2

Role: the phenotype of small nuclear ribonucleoprotein polypeptide N (*SNRPN* / Entrez: 6638) at 15q11.2

Role: the phenotype of MAGE family member L2 (*MAGEL2* / Entrez: 54551) at 15q11.2

Role: the phenotype of necdin, MAGE family member (*NDN* / Entrez: 4692) at 15q11.2

Role: the phenotype of OCA2 melanosomal transmembrane protein (*OCA2* / Entrez: 4948) at 15q12-q13.1

Role: the phenotype of small nucleolar RNA, C/D box 116 cluster (*SNORD116* / HGNC: 32781) at 15q11.2

Autosomal dominant, Not applicable

Cryptorchidism, Infertility, Motor delay, Short stature, Central hypotonia

Scrotal hypoplasia, Hypoplastic labia majora, Clitoral hypoplasia, Hypoplastic labia minora, Hypogonadism, Abnormality of the dentition, Strabismus, Periodontitis, Behavioral abnormality, Delayed speech and language development, Primary amenorrhea, Diabetes mellitus, Growth hormone deficiency, Osteopenia, Osteoporosis, Edema, Hypopigmentation of the skin, Erysipelas, Intellectual disability–mild, Hyporeflexia, Specific learning disability, Failure to thrive, Decreased fetal movement, Weak cry, Short foot, Abnormal facial shape, Poor suck, Ventriculomegaly, Recurrent respiratory infections, Abnormal rapid eye movement sleep, Gastroparesis, Polyphagia, Scoliosis, Increased susceptibility to fractures, Obstructive sleep apnea, External genital hypoplasia, Hypopigmentation of hair, Intellectual disability–borderline, Attention deficit hyperactivity disorder, Decreased testicular size, Central sleep apnea, Impaired temperature sensation, Central adrenal insufficiency, Small pituitary gland, Perisylvian polymicrogyria, Abdominal obesity, Decreased circulating gonadotropin level, Small hand, Brain imaging abnormality

Xerostomia, Narrow nasal bridge, Psychosis, Autistic behavior, Hypertension, Seizure, Stroke, Hip dysplasia, Vomiting, Excessive daytime sleepiness, Intellectual disability–moderate, Abnormal cerebral white matter morphology, Downturned corners of mouth, Almond-shaped palpebral fissure, Nasogastric tube feeding in infancy, Central hypothyroidism, Premature pubarche, Premature adrenarche, Decreased inhibin B level

Antenatal, Neonatal

Cryptorchidism (752.51):

Huánshǎodān 5g + píngwèisǎn 2-0g + gāncǎo 0g.
Huánshǎodān 5g + bǎohéwán 2-0g.
Wǔlíngsǎn 5g.

Chántuì 5g + zhǐqiào 4-0g + jílí 3-0g.
Jílí 5-1g + chántuì 5-0g + zhǐqiào 5-0g.

Strabismus (378.7, 378.6, 378.31), Delayed speech and language development (D007805), Diabetes mellitus (250), Osteoporosis (733.0), Edema (D004487), Erysipelas (035), Gastroparesis (536.3), Polyphagia (D006963), Obstructive sleep apnea (327.23), Abdominal obesity (D056128):

Xiāofēngsǎn 5g + jīnyínhuā 2g + cāngzhú 2-0g + púgōngyīng 2-0g.
Yīnchénwǔlíngsǎn 5g + dàqīngyè 2-0g + jīnyínhuā 2-0g + púgōngyīng 2-0g + jīxuèténg 2-0g + dàqīngyè 1-0g + báijí 1-0g + cāngzhú 1-0g + dàhuáng 0g.

Sīguāluò 5g + júhuā 5g + jílí 5g + chántuì 5-0g + zéxiè 5-0g.
Jílí 5g + huángqí 4g + shānyào 4-0g + chántuì 3-0g.

Psychosis (295.4, 295.7), Hypertension (401-405.99), Seizure (345.9), Vomiting (D014839):

Gāncǎoxiǎomàidàzǎotāng 5g + cháihújiālónggǔmǔlìtāng 5g + wēndǎntāng 5-0g.
Liùwèidìhuángwán 5g + shēnlíngbáizhúsǎn 5g.
Èrchéntāng 5g + shíchāngpú 1g + yuǎnzhì 1g.
Wēndǎntāng 5g + shíchāngpú 1g + fúshén 1g + yuǎnzhì 1g.

Dàhuáng 5g + gāncǎo 5g.
Gāncǎo 5g + hòupò 5-0g + zhǐshí 5-0g + dàhuáng 2-0g.
Yùzhú 5g + shāshēn 5g + hòupò 2g + zhǐshí 2g + dàhuáng 0g.

1.31 WOLF-HIRSCHHORN SYNDROME

Wolf-Hirschhorn syndrome, also known as distal deletion 4p or telomeric deletion 4p, is characterized by distinctive facial features, delayed growth, intellectual disability, and seizures. Wolf-Hirschhorn syndrome is caused by deletion of the genetic material at the end of the short arm of chromosome 4. Severity of the symptoms correlates with the size of the deletion. The chromosomal

TABLE 1.31
GMP Herbal Medicines for a One-Year-Old Infant with Wolf-Hirschhorn Syndrome

Wolf-Hirschhorn syndrome (OrphaCode: 280)

A malformation syndrome with a prevalence of ~5 in 100,000

Role: the phenotype of phosphatidylinositol glycan anchor biosynthesis class G (*PIGG* / Entrez: 54872) at 4p16.3

Role: the phenotype of complexin 1 (*CPLX1* / Entrez: 10815) at 4p16.3

Role: the phenotype of C-terminal binding protein 1 (*CTBP1* / Entrez: 1487) at 4p16.3

Role: the phenotype of nuclear receptor binding SET domain protein 2 (*NSD2* / Entrez: 7468) at 4p16.3

Candidate gene tested: negative elongation factor complex member A (*NELFA* / Entrez: 7469) at 4p16.3

Role: the phenotype of leucine zipper and EF-hand containing transmembrane protein 1 (*LETM1* / Entrez: 3954) at 4p16.3

Multigenic/multifactorial, Not applicable

Hypospadias, Abnormality of the mouth, Abnormal lip morphology, Microcephaly, Dolichocephaly, Epicanthus, Abnormality of the philtrum, Hypertelorism, Short philtrum, Micrognathia, High forehead, Low-set and posteriorly rotated ears, Wide nasal bridge, Downslanted palpebral fissures, Hypodontia, Seizure, Ataxia, Hypotonia, Global developmental delay, Failure to thrive, Intrauterine growth retardation, Decreased fetal movement, Frontal bossing, Low posterior hairline, Highly arched eyebrow, Downturned corners of mouth, Microtia, High anterior hairline, Intellectual disability–severe

Cryptorchidism, Abnormality of the kidney, Cleft upper lip, Hearing impairment, Ptosis, Iris coloboma, Optic atrophy, Abnormality of the thorax, Congenital diaphragmatic hernia, Rib fusion, Abnormality of the vertebral column, Sacral dimple, Hemangioma, Arachnodactyly, Split hand, Preaxial hand polydactyly, Skull defect, Atrial septal defect, Abnormal heart valve morphology, Abnormal cardiac septum morphology, Abnormality of the foot, Talipes equinovarus, Tethered cord, Malformation of the heart and great vessels, Scoliosis, Delayed skeletal maturation, Kyphosis, Abnormal form of the vertebral bodies, Abnormal vertebral morphology, Rib segmentation abnormalities, Aplasia/Hypoplasia of the lungs, Aplasia cutis congenita of scalp, Hypoplastic pubic rami, Short thumb, Short hallux

Abnormality of the genital system, Abnormality of the urinary system, Cleft palate, Chronic otitis media, Megalocornea, Strabismus, Retinopathy, Proptosis, Nystagmus, Sclerocornea, Osteoporosis, Agenesis of corpus callosum, Disproportionate tall stature, Recurrent respiratory infections, Abnormality of the immune system, Abdominal situs inversus, Abnormality of the gallbladder, Aplasia/Hypoplasia of the nipples, Aplasia/Hypoplasia of the cerebellum, Abnormality of movement, Hernia

Antenatal, Neonatal

Hypodontia (520.0), Seizure (345.9), Ataxia (D002524), Hypotonia (D009123):

Gānlùxiāodúdān 5g + zhǐqiào 5-1g + jílí 5-0g + chántuì 5-0g.

Gānlùyǐn 5g + zhǐqiào 5g + jílí 5g + chántuì 5g + júhuā 5-0g.

Yínqiàosǎn 5g + zhǐqiào 1g + jílí 1-0g + chántuì 1-0g.

Zhǐqiào 5g + júhóng 5-0g.

Zhǐqiào 5g + júhuā 5-0g + chántuì 5-0g.

Zhǐqiào 5g + jílí 5-0g + chántuì 4-0g.

Cryptorchidism (752.51), Cleft upper lip (749.1, 749.11), Hearing impairment (D003638), Ptosis (374.3), Optic atrophy (377.1), Hemangioma (228.00), Talipes equinovarus (754.51):

Jiāwèixiāoyáosǎn 5g + qǐjúdìhuángwán 5g + xiāngshāliùjūnzǐtāng 5g + xìngsūyǐnyòukē 2-0g.

Qǐjúdìhuángwán 5g + zīshènmíngmùtāng 5-4g + jiāwèixiāoyáosǎn 5-0g + juémíngzǐ 1-0g + mùzéicǎo 1-0g + cǎojuémíng 1-0g + mìménghuā 1-0g + gǔjīngcǎo 1-0g.

Huángqín 5g + fúlíng 5g + chénpí 5g + báizhú 5-3g + báisháo 5-3g + dāngguī 5-3g + chuānxiōng 3g + bànxià 3-0g + shārén 3-0g + cháihú 3-0g + zhīzǐ 3-0g.

Gǒuqǐzǐ 5g + júhuā 5g + fángfēng 4g + dāngguī 4g + xìxīn 2g + huánglián 2g.

Gāncǎo 5g + jīnyínhuā 5g + huánglián 5g.

Cleft palate (749.0), Retinopathy (362.9), Proptosis (376.30), Nystagmus (379.53, 379.55, 379.50), Osteoporosis (733.0), Abdominal situs inversus (759.3), Hernia (618.6):

Qǐjúdìhuángwán 5g + zīshènmíngmùtāng 5-0g + dānshēn 1-0g + shíchāngpú 1-0g + yuǎnzhì 1-0g.

Qǐjúdìhuángwán 5g + xiāngshāliùjūnzǐtāng 5-0g + nǚzhēnzǐ 2-0g + hànliáncǎo 2-0g.

Gānlùyǐn 5g + qǐjúdìhuángwán 4g + gāncǎo 1g + gǔsuìbǔ 1g.

Xuánshēn 5g + gāncǎo 5g + dìhuáng 5g + jīnyínhuā 5g + liánqiáo 5g.

Shānzhīzǐ 5g + gāncǎo 5-2g + huángqín 5-0g + zhīmǔ 5-0g + huángbò 2-0g + dàhuáng 2-0g + huánglián 1-0g.

deletion occurs at random during reproductive cell production or during early embryonic development. Wolf-Hirschhorn syndrome is not inherited.

Zhǐqiào (Fructus Aurantii) has traditionally been used to "rectify Qi, displace phlegm and decumulate foods." It, together with stir-fried wheat bran, was shown to increase gastrointestinal motility and gastrointestinal hormone levels in rats with functional dyspepsia (Zhu et al., 2020); it is used today for flatulence, eructation, gas pain, chest pain, and functional disorder of the intestine (Wang, 2020). Gānlùxiāodúdān was shown in vitro to be effective against enterovirus 71 infection (Hsieh et al., 2016), which can cause meningoencephalitis with such neurologic sequelae as seizures. Furthermore, Gānlùxiāodúdān was reported to treat viral oral ulcers (herpangina and herpetic gingivostomatitis) in children (Lee et al., 2017).

1.32 RUBINSTEIN-TAYBI SYNDROME

Rubinstein-Taybi syndrome, also known as broad thumb-hallux syndrome, is characterized as broad thumbs and first toes, short stature, distinctive facial features, and intellectual disability. Many cases of Rubinstein-Taybi syndrome are caused by mutations or deletion in the *CREBBP* gene whose products are a histone acetyltransferase that promotes gene expression by uncompacting chromosomes.

TABLE 1.32

GMP Herbal Medicines for a One-Year-Old Infant with Rubinstein-Taybi Syndrome

Rubinstein-Taybi syndrome (OrphaCode: 783)

A malformation syndrome with a prevalence of ~5 in 100,000

Disease-causing germline mutation(s): CREB binding protein (*CREBBP* / Entrez: 1387) at 16p13.3

Role: the phenotype of CREB binding protein (*CREBBP* / Entrez: 1387) at 16p13.3

Disease-causing germline mutation(s) (loss of function): E1A binding protein p300 (*EP300* / Entrez: 2033) at 22q13.2

Autosomal dominant, Unknown

High palate, Hypertelorism, Low-set ears, Convex nasal ridge, Downslanted palpebral fissures, Telecanthus, Brachydactyly, Intellectual disability, Global developmental delay, Failure to thrive in infancy, Short stature, Joint hyperflexibility, Feeding difficulties in infancy, Broad hallux phalanx, Broad thumb

Cryptorchidism, Abnormality of the dentition, Microcephaly, Epicanthus, Micrognathia, Wide nasal bridge, Strabismus, Glaucoma, Nasolacrimal duct obstruction, Carious teeth, Irritability, Anxiety, Constipation, Respiratory insufficiency, Generalized hirsutism, Highly arched eyebrow, Malformation of the heart and great vessels, Clinodactyly of the 5th finger, Attention deficit hyperactivity disorder, Abnormal distal phalanx morphology of finger, Clubbing of toes

Hearing impairment, Ptosis, Atypical scarring of skin, Seizure, Hip dysplasia, Polyhydramnios, Capillary hemangioma, Finger syndactyly, Keloids

Antenatal, Neonatal

Intellectual disability (D008607):

Xiǎojiànzhōngtāng 5g + shānzhā 1g + shénqū 1g + màiyá 1-0g + jīnèijīn 1-0g.

Shēnlíngbáizhúsǎn 5g + shānzhā 0g + shénqū 0g + màiyá 0g.

Yùpíngfēngsǎn 5g + guìzhītāng 5g + gāncǎo 0g.

Xuánshēn 5g + dìhuáng 5g + màiméndōng 5g + hòupò 5-1g + zhǐshí 5-1g + gāncǎo 1-0g + dàhuáng 1-0g.

Cryptorchidism (752.51), Strabismus (378.7, 378.6, 378.31), Glaucoma (365), Carious teeth (521.0, 521.07), Constipation (564.0), Clubbing of toes (754.51):

Jiāwèixiāoyáosǎn 5g + qǐjúdìhuángwán 5g + mázǐrénwán 5-2g + xuánshēn 2g + dìhuáng 2g + màiméndōng 2g + cǎojuémíng 2-0g + huǒmárén 2-0g.

Mázǐrénwán 5g + dàcháihútāng 3g.

Xiāngshāliùjūnzǐtāng 5g + mùxiāngbīnglángwán 1g + mázǐrénwán 1g + shānzhā 1g + shénqū 1g + màiyá 1g.

Gāncǎo 5g + dàhuáng 5-2g + zhīmǔ 5-0g.

Gāncǎo 5g + zhīmǔ 5g + huángqín 5g + dàhuáng 0g + huánglián 0g.

Běishāshēn 5g + yùzhú 5-0g + hòupò 5-0g + zhǐshí 5-0g + xuánshēn 5-0g + dìhuáng 5-0g + màiméndōng 5-0g + dàhuáng 1g.

(Continued)

TABLE 1.32 *(Continued)*
GMP Herbal Medicines for a One-Year-Old Infant with Rubinstein-Taybi Syndrome

Hearing impairment (D034381), Ptosis (374.3), Seizure (345.9), Keloids (D007627):

Línngguìshùgāntāng 5g + xiǎocháihútāng 5-0g + tiānmá 2-0g + shíchāngpú 2-0g + yuǎnzhì 2-0g + gōuténg 1-0g.
Shēnlíngbáizhúsǎn 5g + xiāngshāliùjūnzǐtāng 5-0g + tiānmá 1g + shíchāngpú 1-0g + yuǎnzhì 1-0g + gōuténg 1-0g.

Gāncǎo 5g + báizhǐ 5-4g + shārén 5-2g + dàhuáng 1-0g.

Xuánshēn (cf. Sections 1.3 and 1.25) has neuroprotective effects on the central nervous system as it was shown to protect focal cerebral ischemia and reperfusion injury in mice (Meng et al., 2018) and to increase the viability of human neuroblastoma cells under oxidative stress (Lee et al., 2019). Dìhuáng (cf. Section 1.10) was shown to have a significant neuroprotective effect against neuronal impairment and memory dysfunction caused by scopolamine in rats (Lee et al., 2011). Yùpíngfēngsǎn contains Huángqí and Báizhú as the Monarch and Minister herbs, both of which benefit the brain (cf. Sections 1.9 and 1.21).

1.33 SAETHRE-CHOTZEN SYNDROME

Saethre-Chotzen syndrome, also known as acrocephalosyndactyly type 3, is due to premature fusion of some skull bones, e.g., the frontal and parietal bones, before or after birth, resulting in an abnormally shaped head and/or asymmetric face. Saethre-Chotzen syndrome is caused by mutations in the *TWIST1* gene whose products are a transcription factor important for bone and muscle formation in the head and face during embryonic development.

The flavones in Huángqín (cf. Section 1.6) were reviewed and summarized to be beneficial for such ocular diseases as cataracts, glaucoma, and age-related macular degeneration (Xiao et al., 2014). Xiǎoqīnglóngtāng "relieves exterior, removes abnormal water distributions, stops coughing, and calms asthma." Xiǎoqīnglóngtāng, Xīnyíqīngfèitāng, and Xīnyísǎn are used today for allergic

TABLE 1.33
GMP Herbal Medicines for a One-Year-Old Infant with Saethre-Chotzen Syndrome

Saethre-Chotzen syndrome (OrphaCode: 794)

A malformation syndrome with a prevalence of ~5 in 100,000

Candidate gene tested: fibroblast growth factor receptor 3 (*FGFR3* / Entrez: 2261) at 4p16.3

Candidate gene tested: fibroblast growth factor receptor 2 (*FGFR2* / Entrez: 2263) at 10q26.13

Disease-causing germline mutation(s) (loss of function): twist family bHLH transcription factor 1 (*TWIST1* / Entrez: 7291) at 7p21.1

Autosomal dominant

Facial asymmetry, Abnormal skull morphology, Craniosynostosis, Clinodactyly of the 5th finger, High forehead, Finger syndactyly

Narrow palate, Brachycephaly, Delayed cranial suture closure, Low anterior hairline, Hypertelorism, Prominent nasal bridge, Strabismus, Plagiocephaly, Microtia, Open bite, Narrow internal auditory canal, Convex nasal ridge, Ptosis, Blepharospasm, Brachydactyly, Hyperlordosis, Depressed nasal bridge, Bilateral single transverse palmar creases, External ear malformation, Abnormality of the antihelix, Prominent crus of helix

Cryptorchidism, Cleft palate, Epicanthus, Hypoplasia of the maxilla, Hearing impairment, Low-set ears, Conductive hearing impairment, Hypotelorism, Hallux valgus, Increased intracranial pressure, Malformation of the heart and great vessels, Abnormal form of the vertebral bodies, Short stature, Sleep apnea, Sensorineural hearing impairment, Amblyopia, Optic atrophy, Triphalangeal thumb, Seizure, Migraine, Intellectual disability–moderate, Scoliosis, Proximal radio-ulnar synostosis, Abnormal hair pattern, Broad thumb

Antenatal, Neonatal

(Continued)

TABLE 1.33 *(Continued)*
GMP Herbal Medicines for a One-Year-Old Infant with Saethre-Chotzen Syndrome

Strabismus (378.7, 378.6, 378.31), Ptosis (374.3), Blepharospasm (333.81):

Yìgānsǎn 5g + gāncǎoxiǎomàidàzǎotāng 2g + báijiāngcán 1g + mǔlì 1g + chántuì 1-0g + gōuténg 1-0g.

Liùwèidìhuángwán 5g + shēnlíngbáizhúsǎn 4g + tiānmá 1g + báijiāngcán 1g + mǔlì 1g + xiàkūcǎo 1g + gōuténg 1g.

Gāncǎoxiǎomàidàzǎotāng 5g + cháihújiālónggǔmǔlìtāng 5-0g + báijiāngcán 1-0g + chántuì 1-0g + gōuténg 1-0g + gāncǎo 1-0g + shíchāngpú 0g + yuǎnzhì 0g + jílí 0g.

Báizhú 5g + fúlíng 5g.

Huángqín 5g + báizhǐ 5-4g + gāncǎo 4-2g + shārén 4-2g + tiānhuā 1-0g + dàhuáng 0g.

Báizhǐ 5g + shārén 4g + zhìgāncǎo 3g + huángqín 2g + dàhuáng 0g.

Cryptorchidism (752.51), Cleft palate (749.0), Hearing impairment (D034381), Sleep apnea (780.57), Amblyopia (368.01, 368.00), Optic atrophy (377.1), Seizure (345.9), Migraine (346):

Xiǎoqīnglóngtāng 5g + bǔzhōngyìqìtāng 5g + xiāngshāliùjūnzǐtāng 5-0g.

Xīnyísǎn 5g + xiǎoqīnglóngtāng 2g + xiāngshāliùjūnzǐtāng 2g + báizhǐ 1g + zàojiǎocì 1g + lùlùtōng 1g.

Bǔzhōngyìqìtāng 5g + xiǎoqīnglóngtāng 5-4g + xīnyíqīngfèitāng 5-0g + báizhǐ 2-0g + shíchāngpú 2-0g + xīnyí 2-0g + gāncǎo 1-0g + xiōngqióng 1-0g + yúxīngcǎo 1-0g + cāngěrzǐ 1-0g.

Gǒuqǐzǐ 5g + júhuā 5g + dìhuáng 3g + dāngguī 3g + niúbàngzǐ 2g + xuánshēn 2g + fángfēng 2g + xìxīn 1g + huánglián 1g.

Gǒuqǐzǐ 5g + yuǎnzhì 5-2g + huángqí 5-0g + shíchāngpú 3-2g + hángjú 3-0g + bǎihé 3-0g + gāncǎo 2-0g + acupuncture.

rhinitis (Wang, 2019), which can affect the middle and inner ear, leading to conductive and sensorineural hearing loss (Sahni et al., 2022). Note that Báizhú "clarifies the eye" according to the Materia Medica in the Ming and Qing dynasties; however, modern pharmacological studies on its eye-benefiting effects are lacking (Zhang et al., 2021).

1.34 ALAGILLE SYNDROME

Alagille syndrome, also known as arteriohepatic dysplasia or syndromic bile duct paucity, is a genetic condition where the bile ducts are narrow or blocked. Alagille syndrome is caused by mutations or deletion in the *JAG1* gene whose products are involved in a signaling pathway, called Notch

TABLE 1.34
GMP Herbal Medicines for a One-Year-Old Infant with Alagille Syndrome

Alagille syndrome (OrphaCode: 52)

A malformation syndrome with a prevalence of ~5 in 100,000

Role: the phenotype of jagged canonical Notch ligand 1 (*JAG1* / Entrez: 182) at 20p12.2

Disease-causing germline mutation(s): jagged canonical Notch ligand 1 (*JAG1* / Entrez: 182) at 20p12.2

Disease-causing germline mutation(s): notch receptor 2 (*NOTCH2* / Entrez: 4853) at 1p12

Autosomal dominant

Corneal dystrophy, Cholestasis, Failure to thrive, Ventricular septal defect, Hepatomegaly, Reduced number of intrahepatic bile ducts

Coarse facial features, Pointed chin, Round face, Protruding ear, Intrauterine growth retardation, Frontal bossing, Long nose, Spina bifida occulta, Abnormal form of the vertebral bodies, Vertebral segmentation defect, Butterfly vertebral arch, Telangiectasia of the skin

Cryptorchidism, Abnormality of the ureter, Nephrotic syndrome, Brachycephaly, Hypertelorism, Short philtrum, Micrognathia, Strabismus, Deeply set eye, Downslanted palpebral fissures, Keratoconus, Abnormal pupil morphology, Abnormality of the ribs, Hypertension, Delayed puberty, Intellectual disability–mild, Specific learning disability, Atrial septal defect, Delayed skeletal maturation, Hypoplasia of the ulna, Clinodactyly of the 5th finger, Peripheral pulmonary artery stenosis, Renal hypoplasia/aplasia, Short distal phalanx of finger, Flat face

All ages

(Continued)

TABLE 1.34 *(Continued)*

GMP Herbal Medicines for a One-Year-Old Infant with Alagille Syndrome

Cholestasis (576.2), Ventricular septal defect (745.4):

Xiǎocháihútāng 5g + shānzhā 2-0g + gāncǎo 1-0g.	Gāncǎo 5g + jílí 5-0g + chántuì 5-0g.
Xiǎocháihútāng 5g + sìjūnzǐtāng 5-0g.	Júhuā 5g + zhǐqiào 5g.
Xiǎocháihútāng 5g + píngwèisǎn 5-0g.	

Cryptorchidism (752.51), Nephrotic syndrome (581), Strabismus (378.7, 378.6, 378.31), Deeply set eye (376.5), Keratoconus (371.6), Hypertension (401-405.99):

Bǔzhōngyìqìtāng 5g + jìshēngshènqìwán 5-0g + xiāngshāliùjūnzǐtāng 5-0g + guīpítāng 5-0g.	Jílí 5g + zhǐqiào 5-0g.
Shēnlíngbáizhúsǎn 5-2g + bǔzhōngyìqìtāng 5-0g + mázǐrénwán 2-0g + shānzhā 1-0g + shénqū 1-0g + màiyá 1-0g.	Júhuā 5g + chántuì 5g.
	Zhǐqiào 5g + júhóng 5g.
	Dàhuáng 5g + gāncǎo 5g + báizhǐ 5g + shārén 5g + huángqín 5g.

signaling, important for the development of the liver, heart, eye, and spinal column in early embryonic development.

Xiǎocháihútāng was reviewed to treat liver diseases, including chronic hepatitis, hepatic fibrosis, cirrhosis, and hepatocarcinoma (Shimizu, 2000; Zheng et al., 2013). Júhuā (cf. Section 1.2) "evacuates wind-heat, normalizes the Liver, brightens the eye" and was shown to protect rats from liver injury through antioxidant and antiapoptotic pathways (Zhou et al., 2021) and to lessen visual fatigue in rats through multiple components, multiple targets, and multiple pathways (Qiu et al., 2022). Bǔzhōngyìqìtāng "benefits Qi, raises yang, lifts collapsing, and adjusts and replenishes the Spleen and Stomach."

1.35 CAT-EYE SYNDROME

Cat-eye syndrome is a chromosomal anomaly characterized by a hole in the quadrant of the iris inferior to the horizontal meridian and medial to the vertical meridian, making the pupil look oval or comet shaped. Cat-eye syndrome is caused by four or three copies of the short arm and a small

TABLE 1.35

GMP Herbal Medicines for a One-Year-Old Infant with Cat-Eye Syndrome

Cat-eye syndrome (OrphaCode: 195)

A malformation syndrome with a prevalence of ~5 in 100,000

Not applicable

Preauricular skin tag, Anal atresia, Preauricular pit

Hydronephrosis, Hypertelorism, Downslanted palpebral fissures, Chorioretinal coloboma, Iris coloboma, Abnormality of the ribs, Hypotonia, Intellectual disability–mild, Hip dysplasia, Intrauterine growth retardation, Malformation of the heart and great vessels, Short stature, Renal hypoplasia/aplasia, Abnormal localization of kidney

Abnormality of the genital system, Hearing impairment, Microphthalmia

Antenatal, Neonatal

Hydronephrosis (591), Hypotonia (D009123):

Wǔlíngsǎn 5g + píngwèisǎn 5-0g + gāncǎo 1-0g.	Zhǐqiào 5g + jílí 5-3g.
Wǔlíngsǎn 5g + shēnlíngbáizhúsǎn 5-0g + chēqiánzǐ 1-0g + zéxiè 1-0g.	Chántuì 5g.
	Júhóng 5g + jílí 5-0g + zhǐqiào 4-0g.

Hearing impairment (D034381), Microphthalmia (743.1):

Wǔlíngsǎn 5g + gāncǎo 1g + dàhuáng 0g.	Gāncǎo 5g + báizhǐ 5-4g + shārén 5-4g + dàhuáng 1-0g.
Língguìshùgāntāng 5g + gāncǎo 1-0g + mázǐrénwán 1-0g + dàhuáng 0g.	

section of the long arm of chromosome 22, instead of the normal two copies. The extra chromosomes result from a random event during formation of reproductive cells in the parent and are not inherited.

Jílí (cf. Sections 1.3) was shown to elicit a positive diuresis in rats, evoke a contractile activity on guinea pig ileum, and therefore proposed as a therapeutic agent for urinary stones (Al-Ali et al., 2003). Wǔlíngsǎn (cf. Section 1.15), in combination with an oral steroid, was shown to treat aged patients with acute low-tone sensorineural hearing loss (Okada et al., 2012). Língguìshùgāntāng was shown to be effective in the treatment of patients with dizziness caused by orthostatic dysregulation (Sakata & Egami, 2021).

1.36 APERT SYNDROME

Apert syndrome, also known as acrocephalosyndactyly type 1, is characterized by distinctive malformations of the skull, face, hands, and feet due to premature fusion of the bones during early fetal development. Apert syndrome is caused by *de novo* or germline mutations in the *FGFR2* gene, whose products are receptors on a cell surface receiving growth factors from outside the cell to trigger cell division or differentiation into bone cells for the head, hands, and feet during embryonic development.

TABLE 1.36

GMP Herbal Medicines for a One-Year-Old Infant with Apert Syndrome

Apert syndrome (OrphaCode: 87)

A malformation syndrome with a prevalence of ~5 in 100,000

Disease-causing germline mutation(s) (gain of function): fibroblast growth factor receptor 2 (*FGFR2* / Entrez: 2263) at 10q26.13

Autosomal dominant

Brachyturricephaly, Hypoplasia of the maxilla, Broad forehead, Conductive hearing impairment, Proptosis, Toe syndactyly, Frontal bossing, Acrobrachycephaly, Depressed nasal bridge, Finger syndactyly, Flat face

Narrow palate, Large fontanelles, Mandibular prognathia, Hypertelorism, Facial asymmetry, Convex nasal ridge, Strabismus, Downslanted palpebral fissures, Delayed eruption of teeth, Hypertension, Intellectual disability, Agenesis of corpus callosum, Absent septum pellucidum, Vertebral segmentation defect, Cervical vertebrae fusion (C5/C6), Feeding difficulties in infancy, Aplasia/Hypoplasia of the thumb, Broad thumb, Morphological abnormality of the semicircular canal, Midface retrusion

Cleft palate, Bifid uvula, Hydrocephalus, Sensorineural hearing impairment, Choanal atresia, Visual impairment, Optic atrophy, Esophageal atresia, Respiratory insufficiency, Ventriculomegaly, Arnold-Chiari malformation, Malformation of the heart and great vessels, Cloverleaf skull, Micromelia, Ectopic anus, Ovarian neoplasm, Corneal erosion

Antenatal, Neonatal

Conductive hearing impairment (D006314), Proptosis (376.30):

Língguìshùgāntāng 5g + xiǎocháihútāng 5-0g + gāncǎo 2-0g + xìngrén 1-0g + hòupò 1-0g + tiáowèichéngqìtāng 1-0g.

Guìzhītāng 5g + báisháo 1g + dàhuáng 0g.

Gāncǎo 5g + shārén 5g + báizhǐ 5-0g + dàhuáng 1-0g.

Strabismus (378.7, 378.6, 378.31), Hypertension (401-405.99), Intellectual disability (D008607):

Yùpíngfēngsǎn 5g + guìzhītāng 5-0g + xiǎojiànzhōngtāng 5-0g.

Xìngsūyǐnyòukē 5g + xīnyíqīngfèitāng 5g.

Sāngjúyǐn 5g + zhǐqiào 3g + chántuì 3g.

Bǔzhōngyìqìtāng 5g + bǎohéwán 4g + gāncǎo 0g.

Báizhú 5g + fúlíng 5g + gāncǎo 5-0g + dǎngshēn 5-0g.

Gāncǎo 5g + hòupò 5g + zhǐshí 5g + dàhuáng 1g.

Báizhǐ 5g + gāncǎo 5-3g + shārén 4-3g + dàhuáng 0g.

Cleft palate (749.0), Hydrocephalus (331.4, 331.3), Sensorineural hearing impairment (389.1), Choanal atresia (748.0), Visual impairment (D015354), Optic atrophy (377.1):

Liùwèidìhuángwán 5g + shíchāngpú 1g + yuǎnzhì 1g + acupuncture.

Bǔyánghuánwǔtāng 5g + shíchāngpú 1g + yuǎnzhì 1g.

Xīnyíqīngfèitāng 5g + yínqiàosǎn 5g + xìngrén 1-0g + bèimǔ 1-0g + bǎnlángēn 1-0g + jiégěng 1-0g + acupuncture.

Shíchāngpú 5g + yuǎnzhì 5g + dǎngshēn 5g + huángqí 5-0g + fúlíng 5-0g + shēngmá 2-0g + cháihú 2-0g.

Shíchāngpú 5g + yuǎnzhì 5g + guībǎn 5-0g.

Huángqín 5g + báizhǐ 4g + dàhuáng 2g + tiānhuā 2g + gāncǎo 2g + shārén 2g.

A case was reported that Xiǎocháihútāng as adjuvant therapy relieves the hearing difficulty, tinnitus, and dizziness of a patient with relapsing polychondritis (Kimura et al., 1996). Yùpíngfēngsǎn is translated to "jade windscreen powder" and was elucidated to treat allergic rhinitis by regulating immunological functions, diminishing inflammation, and improving immunity through different pathways (Yang et al., 2021). Note that Yùpíngfēngsǎn contains Huángqí (cf. Section 1.9) as the Monarch herb and Báizhú (cf. Section 1.33) as the Minister herb. Huángqí was shown to ameliorate dry eye injury in rabbits (Chu et al., 2021). Xìngsūyǐnyòukē contains Xìngrén (cf. Section 1.12), which was shown to be anti-cholinesterase and neuroprotective in electric eels and in rat pheochromocytoma cells, respectively (Vahedi-Mazdabadi et al., 2020). Shíchāngpú (Rhizoma Acori Tatarinowii) "opens orifices, calms the mind, transforms dampness, and harmonizes the Stomach." There are nine orifices in TCM, including eyes, ears, nostrils, mouth, tongue, and throat (cf. *Nan Jing: The Classic of Difficult Issues*).

1.37 TREACHER-COLLINS SYNDROME

Treacher-Collins syndrome, also known as Franceschetti-Klein syndrome or mandibulofacial dysostosis without limb anomalies, is deformities of the cheekbones, chin, eyes, and ears due to underdevelopment of the facial bones. Treacher-Collins syndrome is most often caused by mutations in the *TCOF1* gene, whose protein products compose structures in early embryonic development that become bones of the face.

Guìzhīsháoyàozhīmǔtāng "dispels Wind, removes dampness, warms meridians, disperses coldness, nourishes yin, and clears heat." It was concluded by systematic review and meta-analysis of randomized controlled trials to be effective in the treatment of rheumatoid arthritis (Feng et al., 2021)

TABLE 1.37

GMP Herbal Medicines for a One-Year-Old Infant with Treacher-Collins Syndrome

Treacher-Collins syndrome (OrphaCode: 861)

A malformation syndrome with a prevalence of ~5 in 100,000

Disease-causing germline mutation(s): RNA polymerase I subunit B (*POLR1B* / Entrez: 84172) at 2q14.1

Disease-causing germline mutation(s): treacle ribosome biogenesis factor 1 (*TCOF1* / Entrez: 6949) at 5q32-q33.1

Disease-causing germline mutation(s): RNA polymerase I and III subunit D (*POLR1D* / Entrez: 51082) at 13q12.2

Disease-causing germline mutation(s): RNA polymerase I and III subunit C (*POLR1C* / Entrez: 9533) at 6p21.1

Autosomal dominant, Autosomal recessive

Malar flattening, Retrognathia, Hypoplasia of the maxilla, Micrognathia, Downslanted palpebral fissures, Abnormal facial shape, Abnormality of bone mineral density, Open bite, Short face, Midface retrusion, Skeletal dysplasia, Hypoplasia of the zygomatic bone

Abnormality of the dentition, Low anterior hairline, Abnormality of the middle ear, Conductive hearing impairment, Wide nasal bridge, Strabismus, Visual impairment, Absent eyelashes, Iris coloboma, Eyelid coloboma, Frontal bossing, Microtia, Reduced number of teeth, Narrow internal auditory canal

Cryptorchidism, Scrotal hypoplasia, Rectovaginal fistula, Wide mouth, Narrow mouth, Glossoptosis, Cleft palate, Cleft upper lip, High palate, Brachycephaly, Hypertelorism, Preauricular skin tag, Choanal atresia, Cataract, Microphthalmia, Blepharospasm, Abnormality of dental enamel, Hypoplasia of the thymus, Abnormality of the adrenal glands, Abnormality of the vertebral column, Global developmental delay, Failure to thrive, Abnormality of the hair, Patent ductus arteriosus, Facial cleft, Encephalocele, Respiratory insufficiency, Malformation of the heart and great vessels, Tracheoesophageal fistula, Multiple enchondromatosis, Thyroid hypoplasia, Abnormality of dental morphology, Hypoplasia of penis, Branchial fistula, Dysphasia

Neonatal

Skeletal dysplasia (756.56, 756.4):

Guìzhīsháoyàozhīmǔtāng 5g + gāncǎo 0g.

Shēnlíngbáizhúsǎn 5g + liùwèidìhuángwán 5-0g + acupuncture.

Dúhuójìshēngtāng 5g + gāncǎo 0g.

Xuánshēn 5g + dìhuáng 5g + màiméndōng 5g + hòupò 5-0g + zhǐshí 5-0g + dàhuáng 1-0g.

Gāncǎo 5g + báizhǐ 5g + shārén 5g + dàhuáng 0g.

(Continued)

TABLE 1.37 *(Continued)*
GMP Herbal Medicines for a One-Year-Old Infant with Treacher-Collins Syndrome

Conductive hearing impairment (D006314), Strabismus (378.7, 378.6, 378.31), Visual impairment (D015354):

Xiǎojiànzhōngtāng 5g + yùpíngfēngsǎn 5-0g + gāncǎo 1-0g. Gāncǎo 5g + bǎohéwán 5g.

Jīngfángbàidúsǎn 5g + gāncǎo 1g + jīnyínhuā 1g + liánqiáo 1g.

Báizhǐ 5g + gāncǎo 5-4g + shārén 4g + huángqín 4-0g + tiānhuā 2-0g + dàhuáng 0g.

Cryptorchidism (752.51), Cleft palate (749.0), Choanal atresia (748.0), Cataract (366.8), Microphthalmia (743.1), Blepharospasm (333.81), Abnormality of the adrenal glands (255.9), Patent ductus arteriosus (747.0):

Jiāwèixiāoyáosǎn 5g + qǐjúdìhuángwán 5g + zīshènmíngmùtāng 5-0g + nǔzhēnzǐ 1g + hànliáncǎo 1g + xiàkūcǎo 1-0g + dānshēn 1-0g + mǔlì 1-0g + bèimǔ 1-0g + hángjú 1-0g + gǒuqǐzǐ 1-0g.

Jiāwèixiāoyáosǎn 5g + xiāngshāliùjūnzǐtāng 4g + qīngxīnliánzǐyǐn 4g + yúxīngcǎo 1g + yánhúsuǒ 1g + ròudòukòu 0g.

Jiāwèixiāoyáosǎn 5g + zuǒguīwán 3g + gǒuqǐzǐ 1g + xiàkūcǎo 1g + cǎojuémíng 1g + mìmēnghuā 1g + júhuā 1g.

Gǒuqǐzǐ 5g + júhuā 5g + zhìgāncǎo 3g + dǎngshēn 3g + fùzǐ 2g + gānjiāng 2g.

Gǒuqǐzǐ 5g + júhuā 5g + niúbàngzǐ 3g + xuánshēn 3g + shègān 3g + xìxīn 1g + huánglián 1g.

Gǒuqǐzǐ 5g + júhuā 5g + dìhuáng 4-3g + dāngguī 4-3g + fángfēng 4-2g + xìxīn 2-1g + huánglián 2-1g + dàhuáng 0g.

Gǒuqǐzǐ 5g + júhuā 5g + dāngguī 5g + shúdìhuáng 5g + fángfēng 4-2g + xìxīn 2g + huánglián 2g.

---

and gout (Zhang et al., 2020) and is used today for rheumatoid arthritis (Wang, 2019). Gǒuqǐzǐ (cf. Section 1.2) was shown to protect retinal pigment epithelial cells against oxidative stress in age-related macular degeneration mice (Xu et al., 2013).

1.38 MONOSOMY 18p

Monosomy 18p, also known as De Grouchy syndrome, results in developmental delays and facial/body deformities, such as droopy eyelids, large ears, cleft lip, and small hands, due to deletion of the whole or part of the short arm of chromosome 18. The chromosomal error occurs spontaneously during early embryonic development and is not inherited.

Gānlùyǐn "nourishes yin, moisturizes dryness, clears heat, detoxifies" and was shown to alleviate periodontitis in rats through inhibiting osteoclast differentiation and suppressing bone resorption (Inagaki et al., 2021). Gégēntāng "induces sweating, resolves exterior, generates saliva, and relaxes meridians." It was concluded to reduce symptoms of patients with cervical spondylotic radiculopathy in a systematic review and meta-analysis of randomized controlled trials (Lee & Hyun, 2018) and is used today for symptoms involving head and neck (Wang, 2019). Note that orofacial clefts are associated with oral and respiratory tract infections in children (Sato et al., 2022; Zhou et al., 2022).

TABLE 1.38
GMP Herbal Medicines for a One-Year-Old Infant with Monosomy 18p

Monosomy 18p (OrphaCode: 1598)

A disease with a prevalence of ~5 in 100,000

Not applicable, Unknown

Short philtrum, Protruding ear, Hypodontia, Delayed speech and language development, Brachydactyly, Intellectual disability, Global developmental delay, Short stature, Abnormality of the antihelix

Macrotia, Cleft palate, Brachycephaly, Microcephaly, Epicanthus, Micrognathia, Wide nasal bridge, Webbed neck, Short neck, Ptosis, Carious teeth, Misalignment of teeth, Pectus excavatum, Hypertension, Hypotonia, Low posterior hairline, Downturned corners of mouth, Kyphoscoliosis, Wide intermamillary distance, Enlarged thorax

Microphthalmia, Behavioral abnormality, Hypothyroidism, Lymphedema, Holoprosencephaly, Alopecia, Malformation of the heart and great vessels, Autoimmunity, Generalized dystonia

Neonatal

(Continued)

TABLE 1.38 *(Continued)*
GMP Herbal Medicines for a One-Year-Old Infant with Monosomy 18p

Hypodontia (520.0), Delayed speech and language development (D007805), Intellectual disability (D008607):

Gānlùyǐn 5g + zhúyèshígāotāng 5g + zhǐqiào 2-0g + chántuì 2-0g.	Gāncǎo 5g + báizhǐ 5g + shārén 5g + dàhuáng 1-0g.
Gānlùyǐn 5g + bǎohéwán 5g.	Xuánshēn 5g + yùzhú 5g + dìhuáng 5g + shāshēn 5g + hòupò 5g + zhǐshí 5g + màiméndōng 5g + dàhuáng 0g.
Qīngwèisǎn 5g.	Báizhǐ 5g + zhìgāncǎo 5g + shārén 5g + dàhuáng 1g.

Cleft palate (749.0), Ptosis (374.3), Carious teeth (521.0, 521.07), Hypertension (401-405.99), Hypotonia (D009123):

Xīnyíqīngfèitāng 5g + gégēntāng 5g + yínqiàosǎn 5g + lóngdǎnxiègāntāng 5-0g.	Gāncǎo 5g + báizhǐ 5g + shārén 5g + jīnyínhuā 5-0g + huángqín 5-0g + tiānhuā 2-0g + dàhuáng 1g.
Xīnyísǎn 5g + xiǎoqīnglóngtāng 3-2g + xiāngshāliùjūnzǐtāng 3-1g + yínqiàosǎn 2-0g + lóngdǎnxiègāntāng 2-0g + mázǐrénwán 1-0g.	Báizhǐ 5g + gāncǎo 4g + shārén 4g + xìxīn 1g + dàhuáng 0g.
	Báizhǐ 5g + zhìgāncǎo 5g + shārén 5g + huángqín 5g + dàhuáng 0g.
	Hángjú 5g + gǒuqǐzǐ 5g + dìhuáng 4g + fángfēng 4g + dāngguī 4g + xìxīn 2g + huánglián 1g.

Microphthalmia (743.1), Hypothyroidism (244.9), Alopecia (704.0):

Liùwèidìhuángwán 5g + xiāngshāliùjūnzǐtāng 5g + shēnlíngbáizhúsǎn 5g.	Báizhǐ 5g + gāncǎo 5-2g + shārén 5-2g + huángqín 5-0g + tiānhuā 2-0g + dàhuáng 1-0g.
Zhǐbódìhuángwán 5g + xiāngshāliùjūnzǐtāng 5g + shānzhā 1g + shénqū 1g + màiyá 1g.	Báizhǐ 5g + zhìgāncǎo 4g + shārén 4g + dàhuáng 0g.
Xiāngshāliùjūnzǐtāng 5g + bǎohéwán 2g.	
Jiāwèixiāoyáosǎn 5g + shēnlíngbáizhúsǎn 5g + gāncǎo 1g + báizhú 1g + báisháo 1g + fángfēng 1g + chénpí 1g.	

1.39 NAIL-PATELLA SYNDROME

Nail-patella syndrome, also known as onychoosteodysplasia or Turner-Kieser syndrome, is characterized by underdevelopment or abnormality of the nails and kneecaps. Nail-patella syndrome is caused by mutations in the *LMX1B* gene which is a transcription factor important for limb development in early embryonic development.

Bǎohéwán is translated to "harmony preserving pill" and was shown to improve the intestinal contents and intestinal mucosal microbial activity of mice fed with a high-fat and high-protein diet (Guo et al., 2022). Shānzhīzǐ (Fructus Gardeniae) was shown to be anti-hyperuricemic in mice with renal dysfunction (Hu et al., 2013). However, long-term or high-dose administration of Shānzhīzǐ was found to damage the liver and kidney functions in rats (Li et al., 2021). Attention should therefore be paid to its dosing. Zhūlíngtāng "improves urination, soaks dampness, clears heat, nourishes yin" and is used for symptoms involving the urinary system, contact dermatitis, and other eczema (Wang, 2019).

TABLE 1.39
GMP Herbal Medicines for a Three-Year-Old Child with Nail-Patella Syndrome

Nail-patella syndrome (OrphaCode: 2614)

A malformation syndrome with a prevalence of ~5 in 100,000

Disease-causing germline mutation(s): LIM homeobox transcription factor 1 beta (*LMX1B* / Entrez: 4010) at 9q33.3

Autosomal dominant

Abnormality of the nail, Abnormal digit morphology

Abnormality of the kidney, Arthritis, Flexion contracture, Pes planus, Constipation, Abnormality of the knee, Elbow flexion contracture, Decreased muscle mass, Back pain, Abnormal iris pigmentation, Equinovarus deformity, Iliac horns, Abnormality of the elbow, Morphological abnormality of the gastrointestinal tract, Fingernail dysplasia

(Continued)

TABLE 1.39 *(Continued)*
GMP Herbal Medicines for a Three-Year-Old Child with Nail-Patella Syndrome

Renal insufficiency, Proteinuria, Nephrotic syndrome, Nephritis, High forehead, Abnormality of the eye, Pectus excavatum, Hematuria, Osteoporosis, Seizure, Limited elbow extension, Talipes equinovarus, Achilles tendon contracture, Talipes equinovalgus, Talipes calcaneovalgus, Scoliosis, Abnormality of femur morphology, Lumbar hyperlordosis, Cubitus valgus, Abnormality of tibia morphology, Patellar dislocation, Abnormal patella morphology, Patellar hypoplasia, Dislocated radial head, Spondylolisthesis, Spondylolysis, Stage 5 chronic kidney disease, Clinodactyly of the 5th finger, Reduced bone mineral density, Thickening of the glomerular basement membrane, Proximal finger joint hyperextensibility, Hypoplasia of dental enamel, Knee flexion contracture, Limited pronation/supination of forearm, Patellar aplasia, Impaired pain sensation, Ocular hypertension, Primary congenital glaucoma, Talipes calcaneovarus, Contracture of the distal interphalangeal joint of the fingers, Antecubital pterygium, Lester's sign, High anterior hairline, Impaired temperature sensation, Osteochondritis Dissecans, Open angle glaucoma, Knee pain, Acroparesthesia, Abnormal cranial nerve physiology, Toe walking, Knee joint hypermobility, Toenail dysplasia

Neonatal, Infancy, Childhood

Constipation (564.0), Back pain (D001416), Equinovarus deformity (754.51):

Bǎohéwán 5g + mázǐrénwán 5-2g + xiāngshāliùjūnzǐtāng 5-0g + gāncǎo 1-0g.

Bǎohéwán 5g + xiāngshāliùjūnzǐtāng 5g + rùnchángwán 5g.

Xiǎojiànzhōngtāng 5-0g + shēnlíngbáizhúsǎn 5-0g + mázǐrénwán 1g + shānzhā 1g + shénqū 1g + màiyá 1g + ròucōngróng 1-0g + jīnèijīn 1-0g.

Xuánshēn 5g + dìhuáng 5g + màiméndōng 5g + hòupò 5-1g + zhǐshí 5-1g + yùzhú 5-0g + shāshēn 5-0g + dàhuáng 1-0g.

Renal insufficiency (586), Proteinuria (791.0), Nephrotic syndrome (581), Abnormality of the eye (379.90), Osteoporosis (733.0), Seizure (345.9), Talipes equinovarus (754.51), Osteochondritis Dissecans (732.7):

Zhūlíngtāng 5g + liùwèidìhuángwán 3g + huángqí 1g.

Zhūlíngtāng 5g + jìshēngshènqìwán 5g + dānshēn 2g + báimáogēn 2g + chēqiánzǐ 2g + yìmǔcǎo 2g + zélán 2-0g + bìxiè 2g.

Bìxièfēnqīngyǐn 5g + jìshēngshènqìwán 4g + yìmǔcǎo 2g + huángqí 1g + dàhuáng 0g.

Shēnlíngbáizhúsǎn 5g + jìshēngshènqìwán 4g + dīngshùxiū 2g + dānshēn 1g + dàhuáng 0g.

Shānzhīzǐ 5-3g + zhīmǔ 5-3g + dàzǎo 2-1g + huánglián 1-0g + dàhuáng 0g.

Zhīmǔ 5g + gāncǎo 3g + huángqín 3g + huángbò 2g + dàhuáng 0g + huánglián 0g.

1.40 ISOLATED PIERRE ROBIN SYNDROME

Isolated Pierre Robin syndrome is characterized by underdevelopment of the lower jaw, retraction of the tongue, and obstruction of the upper airways. The three anomalies take place sequentially before birth with one anomaly giving rise to the next. Isolated Pierre Robin syndrome is caused by mutations in the enhancer of the *SOX9* gene, which is a transcription factor regulating other genes important for the development of the lower jaw.

TABLE 1.40
GMP Herbal Medicines for a One-Year-Old Infant with Isolated Pierre Robin Syndrome

Isolated Pierre Robin syndrome (OrphaCode: 718)

A malformation syndrome with a prevalence of ~5 in 100,000

Disease-causing germline mutation(s): SRY-box transcription factor 9 (*SOX9* / Entrez: 6662) at 17q24.3

Autosomal dominant, Multigenic/multifactorial, Not applicable, Unknown

Glossoptosis, Cleft palate, Micrognathia

Abnormality of the pharynx, Neonatal respiratory distress, Upper airway obstructionAntenatal, Neonatal

Cleft palate (749.0):

Gānlùyǐn 5g + bǎohéwán 5-0g + gāncǎo 1-0g.

Sāngjúyǐn 5g + zhǐqiào 2-0g + chántuì 2-0g.

Báizhǐ 5g + gāncǎo 5-4g + shārén 5-4g + dàhuáng 1-0g.

Shénqū 5g + màiyá 5g.

Xuánshēn 5g + dìhuáng 5g + màiméndōng 5g + dàhuáng 0g + hòupò 0g + zhǐshí 0g.

Shénqū (Massa Medicata Fermentata) was shown to alleviate disturbance in the intestinal micro-flora and metabolites in rats with functional dyspepsia (Bai et al., 2023). Sāngjúyǐn "scatters Wind, clears heat, widens the Lung, stops coughing" and is used for upper respiratory tract infections (Nabil et al., 2015). The prescriptions are believed to enhance the immunity and digestion of the affected baby.

1.41 SOTOS SYNDROME

Sotos syndrome, also known as cerebral gigantism, is characterized by overgrowth in the first few years of life, learning disabilities, and a large and narrow head with a slightly protrusive fore-head and pointed chin. Sotos syndrome is caused by mutations in the *NSD1* gene, which encodes

---

TABLE 1.41

GMP Herbal Medicines for a One-Year-Old Infant with Sotos Syndrome

Sotos syndrome (OrphaCode: 821)

A disease with a prevalence of ~5 in 100,000

Disease-causing germline mutation(s) (loss of function): nuclear receptor binding SET domain protein 1 (*NSD1* / Entrez: 64324) at 5q35.3

Disease-causing germline mutation(s) (loss of function): SET domain containing 2, histone lysine methyltransferase (*SETD2* / Entrez: 29072) at 3p21.31

Disease-causing germline mutation(s) (loss of function): APC regulator of WNT signaling pathway 2 (*APC2* / Entrez: 10297) at 19p13.3

Autosomal dominant, Autosomal recessive

Tall stature, Coarse facial features, Increased arm span

Dolichocephaly, Narrow face, Long face, Hearing impairment, Chronic otitis media, Astigmatism, Downslanted palpebral fissures, Behavioral abnormality, Seizure, Hypotonia, Intellectual disability–mild, Global developmental delay, Joint laxity, Constipation, Scoliosis, Sparse anterior scalp hair, Accelerated skeletal maturation, Prolonged neonatal jaundice, Prominent forehead, Feeding difficulties, Flushing, Increased head circumference, Tall chin, Brain imaging abnormality

Vesicoureteral reflux, Abnormality of the kidney, Renal insufficiency, Abnormality of the dentition, Macrocephaly, Aggressive behavior, Autistic behavior, Anxiety, Large hands, Cerebellar vermis hypoplasia, Tremor, Flexion contracture, Abnormal heart morphology, Ventricular septal defect, Atrial septal defect, Patent ductus arteriosus, Pes planus, Gastroesophageal reflux, Cerebral atrophy, Bilateral tonic-clonic seizure, Ventriculomegaly, Generalized non-motor (absence) seizure, Generalized myoclonic seizures, Enlarged cisterna magna, Intellectual disability–moderate, Poor coordination, Focal impaired awareness seizure, Cavum septum pellucidum, Dyscalculia, Kyphosis, Aortic aneurysm, Aplasia/Hypoplasia of the corpus callosum, Pedal edema, Intellectual disability–severe

Antenatal, Neonatal

Hearing impairment (D034381), Astigmatism (367.2), Seizure (345.9), Hypotonia (D009123), Constipation (564.0):

Sāngjúyǐn 5g + zhǐqiào 2-0g + jílí 2-0g + chántuì 1-0g.	Shíchāngpú 5g + yuǎnzhì 5g + chántuì 5-0g.
	Jílí 5g + zhǐqiào 5-0g + júhóng 5-0g.

Vesicoureteral reflux (593.7), Renal insufficiency (586), Tremor (D014202), Abnormal heart morphology (746.9), Ventricular septal defect (745.4), Patent ductus arteriosus (747.0), Gastroesophageal reflux (530.81), Bilateral tonic-clonic seizure (D012640), Aortic aneurysm (441.1, 441.3, 441.5, 441.6):

Xiāngshāliùjūnzǐtāng 5g + shēnlíngbáizhúsǎn 5g + jìshēngshènqìwán 5g + báijí 2g + bèimǔ 2g + hǎipiāoxiāo 2g + jīnèijīn 2-0g.	Shānzhīzǐ 5g + gāncǎo 3g + huángbò 3g + huánglián 0g.
Shēnlíngbáizhúsǎn 5g + mázǐrénwán 5g + mùxiāngbīnglángwán 2g + shānzhā 1g + shénqū 1g + màiyá 1g + jīnèijīn 1g.	Shúdìhuáng 5g + guībǎn 5g + zhīmǔ 3g + huángbò 3g + ējiāo 2g + huángqín 2g + huánglián 2g.
	Shānzhīzǐ 5g + dìhuáng 5g + chēqiánzǐ 5g + huángqín 5g + zéxiè 5g + dùzhòng 5-0g + chuānxiōng 4-3g + niúxī 4-3g + báisháo 3-0g + dāngguī 3-0g + fùzǐ 2-0g.
Shēnlíngbáizhúsǎn 5-4g + xīnyíqīngfèitāng 5-0g + xiǎoqīnglóngtāng 2g + xiāngshāliùjūnzǐtāng 2g + hǎipiāoxiāo 1g + báijí 1-0g + huángqí 1-0g + bèimǔ 1-0g + mázǐrénwán 0g.	Dìhuáng 5g + chēqiánzǐ 5g + fúlíng 5g + huángqín 5g + zéxiè 5g + dǎngshēn 5g + niúxī 3g + fùzǐ 3g + dāngguī 3g.

---

a histone methyltransferase that regulates the activities of other genes important for growth and development through histone modifications.

Yuǎnzhì (Radix Polygalae) "quiets the mind, calms the spirit, removes phlegm, opens orifices, resolves carbuncle/swelling" and is used for hypertension, sleep disturbances, absence of menstruation, tinnitus, palpitations, intracerebral hemorrhage, and so on (Wang, 2020). Shēnlíngbáizhúsǎn was shown to reduce serum uric acid levels and increase uric acid excretion in quails with hyperuricemia (Wang, Lin, et al., 2022), which causes such kidney diseases as nephrolithiasis.

1.42   STURGE-WEBER SYNDROME

Sturge-Weber syndrome, also known as encephalofacial angiomatosis, Sturge-Weber-Dimitri syndrome, or Sturge-Weber-Krabbe syndrome, is characterized by port-wine birthmarks on one side of the face, growths of blood vessels in the two innermost layers covering the brain and spinal cord, and high pressure inside the eye. Sturge-Weber syndrome is caused by spontaneous mutations in the *GNAQ* gene in a cell of the embryo whose products are involved in the signaling pathway for the development and function of blood vessels.

TABLE 1.42

GMP Herbal Medicines for a One-Year-Old Infant with Sturge-Weber Syndrome

Sturge-Weber syndrome (OrphaCode: 3205)

A malformation syndrome with a prevalence of ~5 in 100,000

Disease-causing somatic mutation(s): G protein subunit alpha q (*GNAQ* / Entrez: 2776) at 9q21.2

Not applicable

Seizure, Capillary hemangioma

Strabismus, Glaucoma, Optic atrophy, Behavioral abnormality, Intellectual disability, Stroke, Hyperreflexia, Attention deficit hyperactivity disorder, Abnormality of the cerebral vasculature

Gingival overgrowth, Hydrocephalus, Macrocephaly, Hearing abnormality, Abnormality of the eye, Abnormality of eye movement, Abnormality of vision, Conjunctival telangiectasia, Retinal detachment, Abnormal choroid morphology, Iris coloboma, Blindness, Autistic behavior, Heterochromia iridis, Corneal dystrophy, Dysphagia, Cerebral cortical atrophy, Neurological speech impairment, Pulmonary embolism, Arnold-Chiari malformation, Cerebral calcification, Venous thrombosis, Abnormal retinal vascular morphology, Hemianopia, Visceral angiomatosis, Hyperostosis

Neonatal

Seizure (345.9):

Gāncǎoxiǎomàidàzǎotāng 5g + cháihújiālónggǔmǔlìtāng 5g + wēndǎntāng 5-0g.

Tiānmágōuténgyǐn 5g + yìgānsǎn 5g.

Shēnlíngbáizhúsǎn 5g + shānzhā 1g + màiyá 1g + jīnèijīn 1g.

Xuánshēn 5g + dìhuáng 5g + màiméndōng 5g + hòupò 5-0g + zhǐshí 5-0g + dàhuáng 1-0g.

Strabismus (378.7, 378.6, 378.31), Glaucoma (365), Optic atrophy (377.1), Intellectual disability (D008607), Hyperreflexia (D012021):

Qǐjúdìhuángwán 5g + yìqìcōngmíngtāng 5g + shíchāngpú 1-0g + yuǎnzhì 1-0g + acupuncture.

Sāngjúyǐn 5g + zhǐqiào 2g + jílí 2-1g + chántuì 2-0g.

Zhǐqiào 5g + jílí 5-4g + chántuì 5-0g.

Jílí 5g + zhǐqiào 4-3g + chántuì 4-0g.

Hydrocephalus (331.4, 331.3), Abnormality of the eye (379.90), Retinal detachment (361.9), Neurological speech impairment (D013064), Hemianopia (D006423):

Qǐjúdìhuángwán 5g + yìqìcōngmíngtāng 5g + shíchāngpú 1g + yuǎnzhì 1g + chántuì 1g + acupuncture.

Qǐjúdìhuángwán 5g + zīshènmíngmùtāng 5g + yìqìcōngmíngtāng 5-0g + juémíngzǐ 1-0g.

Liùwèidìhuángwán 5g + yìqìcōngmíngtāng 5g + shíchāngpú 1g + gǒuqǐzǐ 1g + yuǎnzhì 1g.

Júhuā 5g + gāncǎo 5-0g + júhóng 5-0g + chántuì 5-0g.

Zhǐqiào 5g + jílí 5g.

Xuánshēn 5g + dìhuáng 5g + màiméndōng 5g + hòupò 5-2g + zhǐshí 5-2g + yùzhú 4-0g + shāshēn 4-0g + dàhuáng 1g.

Xuánshēn and Dìhuáng, introduced in Section 1.32, were neuroprotective on the central nervous system in murine models. Gāncǎoxiǎomàidàzǎotāng was shown to possess anxiolytic-like effects in mice (Chen et al., 2019). Wēndǎntāng was concluded to be more effective than conventional therapy for both ischemic stroke and hemorrhagic stroke in a systematic review and meta-analysis of randomized controlled trials (Xu et al., 2015). Note that acupuncture was demonstrated to be effective in clinical treatment of dry eye by a randomized, double-blinded, sham-acupuncture-controlled study (Dhaliwal et al., 2019).

1.43 TUBEROUS SCLEROSIS COMPLEX

Tuberous sclerosis complex, also known as Bourneville syndrome, is characterized by benign tumors in many parts of the body, including the cerebral cortex of the brain, kidneys, skin, retina, and lungs. Tuberous sclerosis complex is caused by mutations in the *TSC1* or *TSC2* genes, whose products work together as tumor suppressors.

The antidepressant effect of Gāncǎo and its molecular mechanisms were expounded in a recent review (Wang et al., 2023). In addition, GMP Shēnlíngbáizhúsǎn (cf. Table 1.42), Cháihújiālónggǔmǔlìtāng, Shíchāngpú, Dàhuáng, Tiānmá, Yuǎnzhì, and Gāncǎo concentrated extract granules were found to be among the most commonly used TCM products in children with cerebral palsy in Taiwan (Liao et al., 2017). Yìgānsǎn (cf. Section 1.1) was shown to significantly improve low mood,

---

TABLE 1.43

GMP Herbal Medicines for a One-Year-Old Infant with Tuberous Sclerosis Complex

Tuberous sclerosis complex (OrphaCode: 805)

A disease with a prevalence of ~5 in 100,000

Modifying germline mutation: interferon gamma (*IFNG* / Entrez: 3458) at 12q15

Disease-causing germline mutation(s): TSC complex subunit 1 (*TSC1* / HGNC:12362) at 9q34

Disease-causing germline mutation(s): TSC complex subunit 2 (*TSC2* / Entrez: 7249) at 16p13.3

Autosomal dominant

Abnormality of the kidney, Behavioral abnormality, Seizure, Cortical dysplasia, Subependymal nodules, Cortical tubers, Hypomelanotic macule, Generalized abnormality of skin

Renal cyst, Depression, Autism, Aggressive behavior, Autistic behavior, Hyperactivity, Intellectual disability, Specific learning disability, Status epilepticus, Sleep disturbance, Focal-onset seizure, Confetti-like hypopigmented macules, Repetitive compulsive behavior, Retinal hamartoma, Shagreen patch, Cardiac rhabdomyoma, Angiofibromas, Epileptic spasm, Abnormal social behavior, Infantile spasms, Chronic kidney disease, Neurodevelopmental delay, Pulmonary lymphangiomyomatosis, Chorioretinal hypopigmentation, Impulsivity, Self-injurious behavior, Skin plaque

Renal insufficiency, Anxiety, Hypertension, Hepatic cysts, Respiratory distress, Hemoptysis, Poor speech, Renal angiomyolipoma, Attention deficit hyperactivity disorder, Subependymal giant-cell astrocytoma, Noncommunicating hydrocephalus, Respiratory tract infection, Ungual fibroma, Epidermoid cyst

All ages

Seizure (345.9):

Gāncǎoxiǎomàidàzǎotāng 5g + cháihújiālónggǔmǔlìtāng 5-0g + wēndǎntāng 5-0g + tiānmá 1-0g + gōuténg 1-0g.

Wēndǎntāng 5g + gāncǎoxiǎomàidàzǎotāng 3-0g + shíchāngpú 2-1g + yuǎnzhì 2-1g.

Xuánshēn 5g + dìhuáng 5g + màiméndōng 5g + hòupò 2-0g + zhǐshí 2-0g + dàhuáng 1-0g.

Gāncǎo 5g + báizhǐ 5g + shārén 5g + dàhuáng 0g.

Autism (299.0), Hyperactivity (D006948), Intellectual disability (D008607), Focal-onset seizure (D012640), Chronic kidney disease (D051436):

Gāncǎoxiǎomàidàzǎotāng 5g + cháihújiālónggǔmǔlìtāng 5g + tiānmá 2g + shíchāngpú 2-0g + yuǎnzhì 2-0g + gōuténg 2-0g.

Cháihújiālónggǔmǔlìtāng 5g + shēnlíngbáizhúsǎn 5g + shíchāngpú 1g + yuǎnzhì 1g.

Yìgānsǎn 5g + wēndǎntāng 5-0g + shēnlíngbáizhúsǎn 5-0g + shíchāngpú 2-1g + yuǎnzhì 2-1g.

Gāncǎo 5g + báizhǐ 5-0g + shārén 5-0g + huángqín 5-0g + dàhuáng 1-0g.

(Continued)

TABLE 1.43 *(Continued)*
GMP Herbal Medicines for a One-Year-Old Infant with Tuberous Sclerosis Complex

Renal insufficiency (586), Hypertension (401-405.99), Respiratory distress (D004417), Hemoptysis (D006469), Noncommunicating hydrocephalus (331.4, 331.3):

Wǔlíngsǎn 5g + shēnlíngbáizhúsǎn 5-0g + jìshēngshènqìwán 5-0g + huángqí 2-0g + dǎngshēn 2-0g + dàhuáng 0g.

Yùpíngfēngsǎn 5g + shēnsūyǐn 5-0g + shēnlíngbáizhúsǎn 5-0g + shénqū 1-0g + màiyá 1-0g + jīnèijīn 1-0g.

Xìngrén 5g + bèimǔ 5g + qiánhú 5g + jiégěng 5g + sāngbáipí 5g + guālóurén 5g + fúlíng 5g + chénpí 5g + zǐsūyè 5g + huángqín 5-0g.

Gāncǎo 5g + hòupò 5g + zhǐshí 5g + dàhuáng 1g.

Dàzǎo 5g + gāncǎo 2g + xìngrén 2g + hòupò 2g + máhuáng 2g + tínglìzǐ 2g + dàhuáng 1-0g.

impulsivity, and aggression in patients with borderline personality disorder (Miyaoka et al., 2008) and decrease visual hallucinations in patients with Charles Bonnet syndrome (Miyaoka et al., 2011). Yìgānsǎn was also shown to restore the brain glutathione content and ameliorate the pathological symptoms of schizophrenia in mice (Makinodan et al., 2009). Shēnsūyǐn "benefits Qi, resolves exterior, widens the Lung, dissolves phlegm" and is used today for chronic bronchitis (Wang, 2019).

1.44 USHER SYNDROME

Usher syndrome, also known as retinitis pigmentosa-deafness syndrome, is characterized by impairment of the inner ear and retina leading to loss of hearing and peripheral vision. Most cases of Usher syndrome are caused by mutations in the *MYO7A* gene, whose products constitute the hair-like protrusions on the surface of the hair cells in the inner ear, as well as sites of melanin production and storage inside the retinal pigment epithelial cells.

Qǐjúdìhuángwán (cf. Sections 1.2 and 1.5) was shown to protect rats against retinal ischemia (Cheng et al., 2016) and was reviewed to effectively alleviate dry eye symptoms in patients with dry

TABLE 1.44
GMP Herbal Medicines for a Ten-Year-Old Child with Usher Syndrome

Usher syndrome (OrphaCode: 886)

A disease with a prevalence of ~5 in 100,000

Disease-causing germline mutation(s): Usher syndrome 1K (autosomal recessive) (*USH1K* / HGNC:43724) at 10p11.21-q21.1

Disease-causing germline mutation(s) (loss of function): cadherin related 23 (*CDH23* / Entrez: 64072) at 10q22.1

Disease-causing germline mutation(s) (loss of function): USH1 protein network component harmonin (*USH1C* / Entrez: 10083) at 11p15.1

Disease-causing germline mutation(s) (loss of function): USH1 protein network component sans (*USH1G* / Entrez: 124590) at 17q25.1

Disease-causing germline mutation(s) (loss of function): myosin VIIA (*MYO7A* / Entrez: 4647) at 11q13.5

Disease-causing germline mutation(s) (loss of function): protocadherin related 15 (*PCDH15* / Entrez: 65217) at 10q21.1

Disease-causing germline mutation(s): Usher syndrome 1E (autosomal recessive, severe) (*USH1E* / HGNC:12599) at 21q21

Disease-causing germline mutation(s): Usher syndrome 1H (autosomal recessive) (*USH1H* / HGNC:22433) at 15q22-q23

Disease-causing germline mutation(s): calcium and integrin binding family member 2 (*CIB2* / Entrez: 10518) at 15q25.1

Disease-causing germline mutation(s): espin (*ESPN* / Entrez: 83715) at 1p36.31

Disease-causing germline mutation(s): usherin (*USH2A* / Entrez: 7399) at 1q41

Disease-causing germline mutation(s): adhesion G protein-coupled receptor V1 (*ADGRV1* / Entrez: 84059) at 5q14.3

Disease-causing germline mutation(s): myosin VIIA (*MYO7A* / Entrez: 4647) at 11q13.5

Disease-causing germline mutation(s): whirlin (*WHRN* / Entrez: 25861) at 9q32

Modifying germline mutation: PDZ domain containing 7 (*PDZD7* / Entrez: 79955) at 10q24.31

(Continued)

TABLE 1.44 *(Continued)*

GMP Herbal Medicines for a Ten-Year-Old Child with Usher Syndrome

Disease-causing germline mutation(s): centrosomal protein 78 (*CEP78* / Entrez: 84131) at 9q21.2

Disease-causing germline mutation(s): arylsulfatase G (*ARSG* / Entrez: 22901) at 17q24.2

Disease-causing germline mutation(s): clarin 1 (*CLRN1* / Entrez: 7401) at 3q25.1

Disease-causing germline mutation(s): mitochondrially encoded tRNA-Ser (AGU/C) 2 (*MT-TS2* / Entrez: 4575) at mitochondria

Disease-causing germline mutation(s): histidyl-tRNA synthetase 1 (*HARS1* / Entrez: 3035) at 5q31.3

Autosomal recessive

Sensorineural hearing impairment, Visual impairment, Abnormal electroretinogram, Progressive visual loss, Blindness, Nyctalopia, Visual field defect, Vestibular dysfunction, Abnormality of retinal pigmentation, Vestibular areflexia

Cataract, Myopia, Ataxia, High hypermetropia, Cognitive impairment

Decreased fertility, Tinnitus, Astigmatism, Nystagmus, Carious teeth, Abnormality of dental enamel, Microdontia, Psychosis, Depression, Hallucinations, Anxiety, Hypertrophic cardiomyopathy, Cerebral cortical atrophy, Myopathy, EMG abnormality, Aplasia/Hypoplasia of the cerebellum, Hyperacusis, Abnormality of cardiovascular system physiology, Abnormality of dental color

Neonatal, Infancy, Childhood

Sensorineural hearing impairment (389.1), Blindness (D001766), Nyctalopia (368.6):

Qǐjúdìhuángwán 5g + yìqìcōngmíngtāng 5g + shíchāngpú 2-0g + yuǎnzhì 2-0g + acupuncture.	Shíchāngpú 5g + júhuā 5-2g + jílí 5-2g + chántuì 5-2g.
Zīshènmíngmùtāng 5g + qǐjúdìhuángwán 5-0g + yìqìcōngmíngtāng 4-0g + shíchāngpú 1-0g + yuǎnzhì 1-0g + acupuncture.	Shíchāngpú 5g + hángjú 5g + gǒuqǐzǐ 5g + yuǎnzhì 5g + dǎngshēn 5g + fúlíng 5-0g.
	Huángqín 5g + báizhǐ 4g + zhìgāncǎo 3g + shārén 3g + tiānhuā 2g + dàhuáng 1g.

Cataract (366.8), Myopia (367.1), Ataxia (D002524):

Jiāwèixiāoyáosǎn 5g + zhǐqiào 1g + chántuì 1g + jílí 1-0g + júhuā 1-0g.	Jílí 5g + zhǐqiào 5-4g + chántuì 5-0g.
Qǐjúdìhuángwán 5g + zīshènmíngmùtāng 5g + jiāwèixiāoyáosǎn 5-0g + juémíngzǐ 1-0g.	Júhuā 5g + jílí 5g + chántuì 5g.

Tinnitus (D014012), Astigmatism (367.2), Nystagmus (379.53, 379.55, 379.50), Carious teeth (521.0, 521.07), Psychosis (295.4, 295.7), Hallucinations (D006212), Hypertrophic cardiomyopathy (425.1), Myopathy (359.9), Hyperacusis (D012001):

Qǐjúdìhuángwán 5g + zīshènmíngmùtāng 5-0g + língguìshùgāntāng 5-0g + chēqiánzǐ 2-0g + chōngwèizǐ 2-0g + shénqū 2-0g + yuǎnzhì 2-0g + acupuncture.	Gǒuqǐzǐ 5g + hángjú 5-4g + shíchāngpú 4-2g + yuǎnzhì 4-2g + nǚzhēnzǐ 2-0g + huángqí 2-0g + gāncǎo 2-0g.
Liùwèidìhuángwán 5g + língguìshùgāntāng 5-0g + shíchāngpú 2-1g + gǒuqǐzǐ 2-1g + yuǎnzhì 2-1g + xīnyí 2-0g + júhuā 1-0g.	Hángjú 5g + gǒuqǐzǐ 5g + fángfēng 2g + dìhuáng 2g + dāngguī 1g + xìxīn 1g + huánglián 1g + gāncǎo 0g.

eye disease (Su et al., 2021). Adjunctive use of GMP Jiāwèixiāoyáosǎn (cf. Section 1.4) or Huángqín (cf. Sections 1.6 and 1.33) extract granules was found to be associated with a lower occurrence of diabetic retinopathy in female patients with type 2 diabetes (Tsai, Li, et al., 2017).

1.45 WAARDENBURG SYNDROME

Waardenburg syndrome is characterized by varying degrees of congenital hearing loss and diminished coloration of the iris, hair, and skin. Waardenburg syndrome can be caused by mutations in the *PAX3* gene, which regulates the *MITF* gene whose products play a role in the development of melanocytes that produce pigment, i.e., melanin.

Gāncǎo was introduced in Section 1.1 to be anti-inflammatory. Drops of topical solutions of Gāncǎo extract were shown in rabbits to inhibit inflammation-associated corneal neovascularization (Shah et al., 2018), the development of which reduces corneal transparency and deteriorates visual

TABLE 1.45
GMP Herbal Medicines for a One-Year-Old Infant with Waardenburg Syndrome

Waardenburg syndrome (OrphaCode: 3440)

A disease with a prevalence of ~5 in 100,000

Disease-causing germline mutation(s): paired box 3 (*PAX3* / Entrez: 5077) at 2q36.1

Disease-causing germline mutation(s): KIT ligand (*KITLG* / Entrez: 4254) at 12q21.32

Modifying germline mutation: tyrosinase (*TYR* / Entrez: 7299) at 11q14.3

Disease-causing germline mutation(s): snail family transcriptional repressor 2 (*SNAI2* / Entrez: 6591) at 8q11.21

Disease-causing germline mutation(s): SRY-box transcription factor 10 (*SOX10* / Entrez: 6663) at 22q13.1

Disease-causing germline mutation(s): melanocyte inducing transcription factor (*MITF* / Entrez: 4286) at 3p13

Disease-causing germline mutation(s) (loss of function): endothelin receptor type B (*EDNRB* / Entrez: 1910) at 13q22.3

Disease-causing germline mutation(s): endothelin 3 (*EDN3* / Entrez: 1908) at 20q13.32

Disease-causing germline mutation(s): endothelin receptor type B (*EDNRB* / Entrez: 1910) at 13q22.3

Autosomal dominant, Autosomal recessive

Hearing impairment, Conductive hearing impairment, Prominent nasal bridge, Abnormality of vision, Synophrys, Abnormality of skin pigmentation, Hypopigmented skin patches, Heterochromia iridis, Abnormal facial shape, Premature graying of hair, Hypopigmentation of hair

Abnormality of the mouth, Abnormal lip morphology, Abnormality of the face, Underdeveloped nasal alae, Wide nasal bridge, Abnormality of the eye, Telecanthus, Abnormal eyebrow morphology, Lacrimation abnormality, White forelock

Abnormality of the uterus, Abnormality of the vagina, Oral cleft, Ptosis, Aganglionic megacolon, Myelomeningocele, Intestinal obstruction, Abnormality of the gastrointestinal tract, Aplasia/Hypoplasia of the colon

Neonatal, Infancy

Hearing impairment (D034381):

Jiāwèixiāoyáosǎn 5g + língguìshùgāntāng 5g + xiǎoqīnglóngtāng 2g + shānzhā 1g + shārén 1g.	Gāncǎo 5g + báizhǐ 5g + shārén 5-4g + dàhuáng 1-0g.
Jiāwèixiāoyáosǎn 5g + língguìshùgāntāng 5g + chuānxiōngchádiàosǎn 2g + shārén 1g + fùzǐ 1-0g + shānzhā 1-0g + liánqiáo 1-0g.	Shārén 5g + gāncǎo 4-2g + báizhǐ 3-2g + huángqín 3-0g + cāngěrzǐ 2-0g + tiānhuā 2-0g + dàhuáng 1-0g.
Língguìshùgāntāng 5g + báisháo 1-0g + mázǐrénwán 1-0g + bànxià 1-0g + dàhuáng 0g.	

Abnormality of the eye (379.90):

Xiǎocháihútāng 5g + zhúyèshígāotāng 5g + mùzéicǎo 2g + juémíngzǐ 2g + gǔjīngcǎo 2g + júhóng 2-0g.	Gāncǎo 5g + báizhǐ 5-0g + shārén 4-0g + dàhuáng 0g.
Xìngsūyǐnyòukē 5g + xǐgānmíngmùtāng 5g + mùzéicǎo 1g + chántuì 1g.	Gāncǎo 5g + shārén 5-0g + huángqín 3-0g + dàhuáng 0g.
Yùpíngfēngsǎn 5g + qǐjúdìhuángwán 5g + gāncǎo 1g.	Jílí 5g + chántuì 5g.
Sāngjúyǐn 5g + cāngěrsǎn 5g + gāncǎo 0g.	

Ptosis (374.3), Intestinal obstruction (560.9), Abnormality of the gastrointestinal tract (520-579.99):

Xìngsūyǐnyòukē 5g + xīnyíqīngfèitāng 5g + xiāngshāliùjūnzǐtāng 5-0g + bǎohéwán 5-0g.	Gāncǎo 5g + huángqín 5-0g + dàhuáng 1-0g + huánglián 0g.
Shēnlíngbáizhúsǎn 5g + xìngsūyǐnyòukē 4-0g + shānzhā 1-0g + shénqū 1-0g + màiyá 1-0g + jīnèijīn 1-0g.	

acuity. Xiǎocháihútāng is a reconciling formula for the Shaoyang meridians (cf. Section 1.36), stagnation of Qi flow over which degrades the orifices, leading to hearing loss, red eyes, fullness in the chest, and irritability. Xìngsūyǐnyòukē and Xīnyíqīngfèitāng are used for respiratory tract infections with such viruses as adenoviruses, which can also infect the eye to cause viral conjunctivitis.

1.46 TRICUSPID ATRESIA

Tricuspid atresia is a heart defect present at birth where the valve between the two right chambers of the heart, called the tricuspid valve, is missing. The exact cause of tricuspid atresia is unknown; however, alcohol, smoking, viral illness, and certain medications of the mother before or during pregnancy increase the risk for the underdevelopment of the fetus's heart.

TABLE 1.46

GMP Herbal Medicines for a One-Year-Old Infant with Tricuspid Atresia

Tricuspid atresia (OrphaCode: 1209)

A morphological anomaly with a prevalence of ~5 in 100,000

Not applicable

Tricuspid atresia

Cyanosis, Ventricular septal defect

Atrial septal defect, Patent foramen ovale, Transposition of the great arteries, Hypoplasia of right ventricle, Persistent left superior vena cava

Coarctation of aorta, Pulmonary artery atresia

Antenatal, Neonatal

Cyanosis (D003490), Ventricular septal defect (745.4):

Sìnìtāng 5g + bànxià 1-0g + gāncǎo 1-0g.	Gāncǎo 5g + báizhǐ 5-0g + shārén 5-0g + dàhuáng 1-0g.
Zhēnwǔtāng 5g + gāncǎo 1g.	Gānjiāng 5g + gāncǎo 2g.

Some compounds in Gānjiāng (cf. Section 1.15) were found to be hemostatic, while others promote blood circulation in an in vitro study (Li et al., 2023). Sìnìtāng, containing Gānjiāng and Gāncǎo, was shown to improve early ventricular remodeling and cardiac function in rats after myocardial infarction (Liu et al., 2014). Zhēnwǔtāng was introduced in Section 1.16 to protect the heart of rats. Sìnìtāng "activates the heart" and Zhēnwǔtāng "reduces the burden of the heart by eliminating excessive body fluid." In other words, Zhēnwǔtāng is used for chronic heart diseases while Sìnìtāng for acute heart conditions.

1.47 CONGENITAL LOBAR EMPHYSEMA

Congenital lobar emphysema, also known as infantile lobar hyperinflation, is a respiratory distress condition where the air can enter but cannot escape the lungs due to unusual structures inside or outside the airways, resulting in overinflation of the lobes of the lung. The cause of most cases of congenital lobar emphysema is unknown.

Xìngrén (cf. Section 1.12) was shown to protect against acute lung injury in rats through its anti-inflammatory and antioxidant effects (Zhao, Zhang, et al., 2022). Xiǎoqīnglóngtāng (cf. Section 1.33) was shown to exhibit anti-airway inflammatory, anti-airway remodeling, and specific

TABLE 1.47

GMP Herbal Medicines for a One-Year-Old Infant with Congenital Lobar Emphysema

Congenital lobar emphysema (OrphaCode: 1928)

A morphological anomaly with a prevalence of ~5 in 100,000

Not applicable

Emphysema, Respiratory distress

Abnormality of immune system physiology

Neonatal, Infancy, Childhood, Adult

Emphysema (492.8), Respiratory distress (D004417):

Xiǎoqīnglóngtāng 5g + yùpíngfēngsǎn 5-0g + gāncǎo 1-0g.	Xìngrén 5g + máhuáng 5g + chénpí 5-3g + gāncǎo 5-2g + bànxià 3-0g.
Xìngsūyǐnyòukē 5g + xīnyíqīngfèitāng 5-0g.	
Máxìnggānshítāng 5g + gāncǎo 2-0g + dàzǎo 1-0g + tínglìzǐ 1-0g + dàhuáng 0g.	Gāncǎo 5g + xìngrén 5g + bèimǔ 5g + qiánhú 5g + jiégěng 5g + chénpí 5g + sāngbáipí 5-0g + guālóurén 5-0g + fúlíng 5-0g.

immunoregulatory effects in chronic asthmatic mice (Wang et al., 2012). Máxìnggānshítāng was demonstrated in rats to prevent bleomycin-induced lung fibrosis (Chang et al., 2011) and protect PM2.5 induced acute lung injury (Fei et al., 2019). Note that Máxìnggānshítāng, cooler than Xiǎoqīnglóngtāng, is prescribed to patients manifesting also hyperthermia and thirst.

1.48 46,XX GONADAL DYSGENESIS

46,XX gonadal dysgenesis—also called 46,XX complete gonadal dysgenesis; 46,XX pure gonadal dysgenesis; and XX female gonadal dysgenesis—refers to the absence of puberty and menstruation due to a primary ovarian defect in an otherwise phenotypic female. 46,XX gonadal dysgenesis can be caused by mutations in the *FSHR* gene, which encodes follicle stimulating hormone receptors important for ovary development.

Tiānméndōng (Radix Asparagi) was shown to enhance the expression of estrogen receptors in the frontal cortex and hippocampus of ovariectomized rats (Lalert et al., 2018), and was also shown to ameliorate menopausal depression in ovariectomized rats (Kim et al., 2020). Liùwèidìhuángwán

---

TABLE 1.48

GMP Herbal Medicines for a 12-Year-Old Girl with 46,XX Gonadal Dysgenesis

46,XX gonadal dysgenesis (OrphaCode: 243)

A malformation syndrome with a prevalence of ~5 in 100,000

Disease-causing germline mutation(s): nuclear receptor subfamily 5 group A member 1 (*NR5A1* / Entrez: 2516) at 9q33.3

Disease-causing germline mutation(s): mitochondrial ribosomal protein S22 (*MRPS22* / Entrez: 56945) at 3q23

Disease-causing germline mutation(s) (loss of function): follicle stimulating hormone receptor (*FSHR* / Entrez: 2492) at 2p16.3

Disease-causing germline mutation(s): bone morphogenetic protein 15 (*BMP15* / Entrez: 9210) at Xp11.22

Disease-causing germline mutation(s): PSMC3 interacting protein (*PSMC3IP* / Entrez: 29893) at 17q21.2

Disease-causing germline mutation(s): nucleoporin 107 (*NUP107* / Entrez: 57122) at 12q15

Disease-causing germline mutation(s): basonuclin 1 (*BNC1* / Entrez: 646) at 15q25.2

Disease-causing germline mutation(s): zinc finger SWIM-type containing 7 (*ZSWIM7* / Entrez: 125150) at 17p12

Disease-causing germline mutation(s) (loss of function): RNA polymerase III subunit H (*POLR3H* / Entrez: 171568) at 22q13.2

Disease-causing germline mutation(s) (loss of function): scaffold protein involved in DNA repair (*SPIDR* / Entrez: 23514) at 8q11.21

Autosomal dominant, Autosomal recessive, Not applicable, X-linked recessive

Gonadal dysgenesis, Premature ovarian insufficiency, Precocious menopause

Decreased fertility, Primary amenorrhea, Delayed puberty, Increased circulating gonadotropin level, Decreased serum estradiol, Abnormality of secondary sexual hair

Osteopenia, Sparse pubic hair, Delayed skeletal maturation, Reduced bone mineral density, Osteoporosis of vertebrae, Aplasia/hypoplasia of the uterus, Aplasia/Hypoplasia of the breasts, Streak ovary

Hearing impairment, Secondary amenorrhea, Abnormality of metabolism/homeostasis, Short stature

Adolescent, Adult

Gonadal dysgenesis (758.6), Premature ovarian insufficiency (256.31):

Liùwèidìhuángwán 5g + jiāwèixiāoyáosǎn 5g + nǚzhēnzǐ 1g + hànliáncǎo 1g + tùsīzǐ 1-0g.

Jiāwèixiāoyáosǎn 5g + zuǒguīwán 5g + nǚzhēnzǐ 1g + hànliáncǎo 1g.

Jiāwèixiāoyáosǎn 5g + dāngguīsháoyàosǎn 5g + xiāngfù 1g + yìmǔcǎo 1g.

Guìzhījiālónggǔmǔlìtāng 5g + yìgānsǎn 4g + wǔwèizǐ 1g.

Dāngguīsháoyàosǎn 5g + shānyào 1g + dùzhòng 1g + xùduàn 1g.

Tiānméndōng 5g + yùzhú 5g + dìhuáng 5g + mǔdānpí 5g + jīnyínhuā 5g + huángqín 5g + yīnchén 5-0g + liánqiáo 5-0g.

Huángqí 5g + chuānxiōng 4g + tiānméndōng 4g + niúxī 4g + báisháo 4g + huángqín 4g + gǔsuìbǔ 2g + xùduàn 2g.

Báizhú 5g + dìhuáng 5g + huángqí 5g + dǎngshēn 5g + chuānxiōng 4g + guìzhī 4g + huángqín 2g.

Běishāshēn 5g + dìhuáng 5g + mǔdānpí 5g + zhǐqiào 5g + sāngzhī 5g + huángqín 5g + chuānxiōng 2g.

was shown to regulate proliferation and migration of rat vascular smooth muscle cells via modulation of estrogen receptors (Zhang, Qian, et al., 2018). A modified GMP concentrated Zuǒguīwán extract was shown to restore the ovarian function effectively and promptly in a woman with premature ovarian failure (Chao et al., 2003).

1.49   VAN DER WOUDE SYNDROME

Van der Woude syndrome (VWS), also called lip-pit syndrome, is characterized by the presence of cleft lip/palate and pits in the center of the lower lip in the newborn. Most VWS cases are caused by mutations in the *IRF6* gene whose products are a transcription factor activating other genes important for the early development and maturation of tissues in the head and face.

TABLE 1.49

GMP Herbal Medicines for a One-Year-Old Infant with van der Woude Syndrome

Van der Woude syndrome (OrphaCode: 888)

A malformation syndrome with a prevalence of ~5 in 100,000

Disease-causing germline mutation(s): interferon regulatory factor 6 (*IRF6* / Entrez: 3664) at 1q32.2

Disease-causing germline mutation(s): grainyhead like transcription factor 3 (*GRHL3* / Entrez: 57822) at 1p36.11

Autosomal dominant, Not applicable

Lip pit

Cleft palate, Lower lip pit

Cleft upper lip, Hypodontia, Abnormal salivary gland morphology

Neonatal

Cleft palate (749.0):	
Gānlùyǐn 5g + bǎohéwán 5-0g + gāncǎo 1-0g.	Gāncǎo 5-4g + shārén 5-3g + báizhǐ 5-0g + dàhuáng 1-0g.
Sāngjúyǐn 5g + zhǐqiào 2-1g + júhuā 1-0g + chántuì 1-0g.	Shénqū 5g + màiyá 5g.
Cleft upper lip (749.1, 749.11), Hypodontia (520.0):	
Sāngjúyǐn 5g + zhǐqiào 1g.	Báizhǐ 5g + gāncǎo 4g + shārén 4g + dàhuáng 0g.
Yínqiàosǎn 5g + zhǐqiào 1g + jílí 1g + chántuì 1g.	Xuánshēn 5g + dìhuáng 5g + màiméndōng 5g + hòupò 5-1g +
Gānlùyǐn 5g + zhǐqiào 0g + chántuì 0g.	zhǐshí 5-1g + yùzhú 5-0g + shāshēn 5-0g + dàhuáng 1-0g.

Drinking Gāncǎo extract solution was found to lower orofacial cleft occurrence in mouse fetuses in an observational study (Chimedtseren et al., 2023). Gānlùyǐn, Sāngjúyǐn, and Yínqiàosǎn all contain Gāncǎo. Furthermore, babies with a cleft lip sometimes experience dry lips and dry gums. Gānlùyǐn and Sāngjúyǐn were combined in a prescription to relieve the dry mouth and dry eye symptoms of Sjögren's syndrome (Lee et al., 2021).

1.50   CHOANAL ATRESIA

Choanal atresia refers to narrowing or blockage of the two openings in the back of the nasal passage joining the nasal cavity and nasopharynx. Choanal atresia results from problems with prenatal development and is associated with exposure to endocrine disrupters, secondhand smoke, caffeine, and medications during pregnancy.

Aqueous Gāncǎo extract was shown to alleviate the severity of pulmonary fibrosis in mice (Ghorashi et al., 2017). Guìzhītāng was demonstrated to exhibit anti-inflammatory effects on airway inflammation in human bronchial epithelial cells (Kim et al., 2021). Guìzhītāng is listed as a formula drug in the KEGG database with the following efficacy: analgesic, anti-inflammatory, antipyretic, sedative, and cold remedy (https://www.genome.jp/entry/D06947).

TABLE 1.50
GMP Herbal Medicines for a Two-Year-Old Girl with Choanal Atresia

Choanal atresia (OrphaCode: 137914)

A morphological anomaly with a prevalence of ~5 in 100,000

Not applicable

Nasal obstruction, Chronic sinusitis, Abnormal nasal mucus secretion

Cyanosis, Craniosynostosis, Laryngomalacia, Subglottic stenosis, Respiratory distress, Recurrent respiratory infections, Tracheomalacia, Upper airway obstruction, Mandibulofacial dysostosis, Feeding difficulties, Inappropriate crying, Choking episodes

Neonatal, Infancy, Childhood

Cyanosis (D003490), Respiratory distress (D004417):

Guìzhītāng 5g + xìngrén 1g + hòupò 1g + dàhuáng 0g. Wǔlíngsǎn 5g.	Gāncǎo 5g + báizhǐ 5g + shārén 5-3g + huángqín 5-0g + tiānhuā 2-0g + dàhuáng 1-0g.
Máxìnggānshítāng 5g + cāngěrsǎn 5g + dōngguāzǐ 2g + jiégěng 2g + liánqiáo 2g + yúxīngcǎo 2g.	Zhìgāncǎo 5g + hòupò 5g + zhǐshí 5g + dàhuáng 1g.

1.51 EEC SYNDROME

EEC syndrome stands for ectrodactyly-ectodermal dysplasia-cleft lip/palate syndrome, and is characterized by missing or malformation of one or more central fingers or toes; abnormalities of the hair, teeth, nails, skin, and sweat glands; and cleft lip/palate. EEC syndrome is most often caused by mutations in the *TP63* gene whose products function as a transcription factor important for regulation of layering of the undifferentiated embryonic ectoderm.

A meta-analysis of randomized controlled trials concluded that combination of modified Yùnǔjiān with Western medicine improved the total effective rate, compared with Western medicine alone,

TABLE 1.51
GMP Herbal Medicines for a One-Year-Old Infant with EEC Syndrome

EEC syndrome (OrphaCode: 1896)

A malformation syndrome with a prevalence of ~5 in 100,000

Disease-causing germline mutation(s): tumor protein p63 (*TP63* / Entrez: 8626) at 3q28

Autosomal dominant

Sparse eyebrow, Thick eyebrow, Lacrimation abnormality, Carious teeth, Taurodontia, Abnormality of dental enamel, Microdontia, Dry skin, Hyperkeratosis, Split hand, Nail pits, Split foot, Coarse hair, Nail dystrophy, Reduced number of teeth, Ectrodactyly

Urethral atresia, Hydronephrosis, Oral cleft, Keratitis, Blepharitis, Photophobia, Slow-growing hair, Generalized hypopigmentation, Aplasia/Hypoplasia of the skin, Renal hypoplasia/aplasia, Corneal erosion, Inflammatory abnormality of the eye

Hypospadias, Vesicoureteral reflux, Cleft palate, Xerostomia, Abnormality of the inner ear, Abnormality of the middle ear, Sensorineural hearing impairment, Choanal atresia, Entropion, Hypoplasia of the thymus, Growth hormone deficiency, Anterior hypopituitarism, Intellectual disability, Toe syndactyly, Fine hair, Lymphoma, Nevus, Short stature, Finger syndactyly, Aplasia/Hypoplasia of the nipples, External ear malformation, Aplasia/Hypoplasia of the thumb, Proximal placement of thumb, Aplasia/Hypoplasia of the breasts, Hypohidrosis

Antenatal, Neonatal

Carious teeth (521.0, 521.07):

Yùnǔjiān 5g + gānlùyǐn 5-0g + xuánshēn 1-0g + dìhuáng 1-0g + màiméndōng 1-0g + jīnyínhuā 1-0g + liánqiáo 1-0g. Qīngwèisǎn 5g + yùnǔjiān 5-0g.	Báizhǐ 5g + gāncǎo 5-4g + shārén 5-4g + huángqín 5-0g + tiānhuā 2-0g + dàhuáng 1-0g.
	Báizhǐ 5g + zhìgāncǎo 4g + shārén 4g + huángqín 4g + dàhuáng 0g.

(Continued)

TABLE 1.51 *(Continued)*

GMP Herbal Medicines for a One-Year-Old Infant with EEC Syndrome

Hydronephrosis (591), Keratitis (370), Blepharitis (373.0, 373.4), Photophobia (D020795):

Yuèbìjiāshùtāng 5g + wǔlíngsǎn 4-0g + chēqiánzǐ 1-0g.	Gāncǎo 5g + júhuā 5g + jílí 5g + júhóng
Wǔlíngsǎn 5g + chēqiánzǐ 1-0g.	5-0g.
Sāngjúyǐn 5g + chántuì 0g.	Júhuā 5g + júhóng 2g.
Xǐgānmíngmùtāng 5g.	Chántuì 5g + jílí 5-2g.

Vesicoureteral reflux (593.7), Cleft palate (749.0), Sensorineural hearing impairment (389.1), Choanal atresia (748.0), Entropion (374.00), Intellectual disability (D008607), Hypohidrosis (705.0):

Xīnyíqīngfèitāng 5g + máxìnggānshítāng 5g + yínqiàosǎn 5g.	Gāncǎo 5g + báizhǐ 5g + shārén 5g +
Xīnyíqīngfèitāng 5g + xiǎoqīnglóngtāng 3g + gégēntāng 3g + xiāngshāliùjūnzǐtāng 1g.	huángqín 5g + guālóugēn 5-0g + dàhuáng 1g.
Xīnyíqīngfèitāng 5g + dìngchuǎntāng 4g + yínqiàosǎn 4g + bèimǔ 1g + bǎnlángēn 1g.	
Yuèbìjiāshùtāng 5g + báizhú 2g + fùzǐ 2g + fúlíng 2g + gānjiāng 1g + dǎngshēn 1g.	

in patients with periodontitis (Yue et al., 2021). Gāncǎo, introduced in Section 1.1 to be antioxidant, was demonstrated to ameliorate nephrotoxicity in rats with acute tubular necrosis through improving antioxidant defense (Aksoy et al., 2012). Yuèbìtāng was shown to regulate renal microvascular permeability, alleviate edema, and reduce renal function impairment in rats with nephrotic syndrome (Li et al., 2023). Yuèbìjiāshùtāng is Yuèbìtāng plus Báizhú.

1.52　STERNAL CLEFT

Sternal cleft, also called cleft sternum or sternum bifidum, is characterized by a cleft in the center of the chest due to a partial or complete failure of the breastbone fusion during early embryonic development. The cause of sternal cleft is unknown; however, a form of vitamin B12 deficiency and alcohol abuse during pregnancy were suggested to be associated with the condition.

Zhúyèshígāotāng "clears heat, generates saliva, benefits Qi, and harmonizes the Stomach." It was formulated to clear lingering heat and calm the spirit. For example, it is used for dengue fever for those experiencing fever, muscle ache, general weakness, poor appetite, and stomachache (Chen et al., 2020). Zàojiǎocì (cf. Section 1.22) was reviewed to have anticancer, anti-inflammatory, anti-atherogenic, antimicrobial, antiallergic, and antiviral activities (Gao et al., 2016).

TABLE 1.52

GMP Herbal Medicines for a One-Year-Old Infant with Sternal Cleft

Sternal cleft (OrphaCode: 2017)

A morphological anomaly with a prevalence of ~5 in 100,000

Not applicable

Abnormality of the neck, Webbed neck, Abnormality of the eye, Abnormality of vision

Antenatal, Neonatal

Webbed neck (744.5), Abnormality of the eye (379.90):

Zhúyèshígāotāng 5g + zàojiǎocì 2g + fángfēng 2g + jīngjiè 2g + júhóng 2g + xuánfùhuā 2-0g.	Gāncǎo 5g + júhuā 5g + jílí 5g + júhóng 5g + chántuì 5-0g.
Xǐgānmíngmùtāng 5g + bǎohéwán 2g + gāncǎo 1g.	Zhǐqiào 5-2g + jílí 5-0g + gāncǎo 5-0g + chántuì 2-0g.
Qǐjúdìhuángwán 5g + zīshènmíngmùtāng 5g.	
Jiāwèixiāoyáosǎn 5g + zhǐqiào 1g + jílí 1g.	

1.53 ISOLATED SPLIT HAND-SPLIT FOOT MALFORMATION

Isolated split hand-split foot malformation (SHFM), also called ectrodactyly, is absence of certain fingers and toes without congenital defects in other body parts. Mutations in many genes have been associated with split hand/foot malformation, giving different SHFM subtypes and inheritance patterns. SHFM type 1 is caused by mutations in the *DLX5* or *DLX6* gene whose products are transcription factors and play a role in bone development and fracture healing.

TABLE 1.53
GMP Herbal Medicines for a One-Year-Old Infant with Isolated Split Hand-Split Foot Malformation

Isolated split hand-split foot malformation (OrphaCode: 2440)

A malformation syndrome with a prevalence of ~5 in 100,000

Disease-causing germline mutation(s): distal-less homeobox 6 (*DLX6* / Entrez: 1750) at 7q21.3

Disease-causing germline mutation(s) (loss of function): epidermal growth factor receptor pathway substrate 15 like 1 (*EPS15L1* / Entrez: 58513) at 19p13.11

Disease-causing germline mutation(s): tumor protein p63 (*TP63* / Entrez: 8626) at 3q28

Candidate gene tested: SEM1 26S proteasome subunit (*SEM1* / Entrez: 7979) at 7q21.3

Disease-causing germline mutation(s): Wnt family member 10B (*WNT10B* / Entrez: 7480) at 12q13.12

Disease-causing germline mutation(s): distal-less homeobox 5 (*DLX5* / Entrez: 1749) at 7q21.3

Candidate gene tested: beta-transducin repeat containing E3 ubiquitin protein ligase (*BTRC* / Entrez: 8945) at 10q24.32

Role: the phenotype of F-box and WD repeat domain containing 4 (*FBXW4* / Entrez: 6468) at 10q24.32

Autosomal dominant, Autosomal recessive, X-linked recessive

Oligodactyly

Finger syndactyly

Sensorineural hearing impairment, Aniridia, Split hand, Absent hand

Neonatal, Infancy

Sensorineural hearing impairment (389.1), Aniridia (743.45):

Xìngsūyǐnyòukē 5g + xīnyíqīngfèitāng 5g + bèimǔ 1-0g + guālóurén 1-0g.	Shíchāngpú 5g + yuǎnzhì 5g.
	Júhuā 5g + júhóng 0g.
Shēnlíngbáizhúsǎn 5g + shānzhā 1g + shénqū 1g + màiyá 1g.	Gāncǎo 5g.
	Hángjú 5g.
Sāngjúyǐn 5g + jílí 2-0g + zhǐqiào 1-0g + chántuì 0g.	Chántuì 5g.
	Yùzhú 5g + shāshēn 5g + màiméndōng 5g + xuánshēn 4g + dìhuáng 4g + hòupò 4g + zhǐshí 4g + dàhuáng 1g.

Shíchāngpú, introduced in Section 1.36 to open orifices in TCM, was shown to significantly stimulate the expression and secretion of neurotrophic factors, i.e., nerve growth factor, brain derived neurotrophic factor and glial derived neurotrophic factor, in cultured rat astrocytes in dose-dependent manners (Lam et al., 2019). Xìngsūyǐnyòukē, Xīnyíqīngfèitāng, and Sāngjúyǐn are all used for upper respiratory infections. Many of the prescriptions in Table 1.53 aim to enhance the immunity of the newborn.

1.54 ISOLATED ANIRIDIA

Isolated aniridia is partial or complete absence of the iris, which controls the size of the pupil in the center of the eyeball. Most isolated aniridia cases are caused by mutations or deletions in the *PAX6* gene whose products are a transcription factor regulating other genes important for the eye development before birth and eye structures after birth.

Xiǎocháihútāng plus Wǔlíngsǎn, called Sairei-to in Kampo, was reviewed to treat uveitis in humans (Hayasaka et al., 2012). Zhǐqiào (cf. Section 1.31) is a component herb in a modern Chinse

TABLE 1.54

GMP Herbal Medicines for a One-Year-Old Infant with Isolated Aniridia

Isolated aniridia (OrphaCode: 250923)

A morphological anomaly with a prevalence of ~5 in 100,000

Disease-causing germline mutation(s) (loss of function): paired box 6 (*PAX6* / Entrez: 5080) at 11p13

Disease-causing germline mutation(s) (gain of function): tripartite motif containing 44 (*TRIM44* / Entrez: 54765) at 11p13

Disease-causing germline mutation(s): forkhead box C1 (*FOXC1* / Entrez: 2296) at 6p25.3

Autosomal dominant, Not applicable

Aniridia, Visual loss, Nystagmus, Aplasia/Hypoplasia of the macula

Glaucoma, Cataract, Peters anomalyNeonatal

Aniridia (743.45), Nystagmus (379.53, 379.55, 379.50):

Xiǎocháihútāng 5g + zhúyèshígāotāng 5g + mùzéicǎo 2-1g + juémíngzǐ 2-1g + chōngwèizǐ 2-1g + qīngxiāngzǐ 2-0g + gǔjīngcǎo 1-0g + mìmēnghuā 1-0g.	Hángjú 5g + gǒuqǐzǐ 5g + dìhuáng 3g + fángfēng 3g + dāngguī 3-0g + xìxīn 2-1g + huánglián 2-1g.
Xiāngshāliùjūnzǐtāng 5g.	Gāncǎo 5g + júhuā 5g + jílí 5g.
Qǐjúdìhuángwán 5g + bǎohéwán 2g + gāncǎo 0g.	Yùzhú 5g + shāshēn 5g + hòupò 3g + zhǐshí 3g + xuánshēn 2g + dìhuáng 2g + màiméndōng 2g + dàhuáng 1g.
	Gǒuqǐzǐ 5g + júhuā 5g + dìhuáng 2g + fángfēng 2g + xìxīn 1g + huánglián 1g + dāngguī 1g + dàhuáng 1g.

Glaucoma (365), Cataract (366.8):

Sāngjúyǐn 5g + zhǐqiào 2-0g + jílí 2-0g + chántuì 2-0g + júhuā 1-0g.	Jílí 5g + chántuì 5g.
	Zhǐqiào 5g + jílí 5-3g + chántuì 5-0g.

herbal formula that was shown to prevent diabetic retinopathy in rats (Chen et al., 2017). Chántuì (Periostracum Cicadae; cicada slough) was summarized to be mainly used for external wind heat, cold aversion, cough, measles and poor respiration, itchy skin, sore throat and hoarseness, red and swollen eyes, children's convulsions, and night crying (Xie et al., 2023). Sāngjúyǐn contains Júhuā, which benefits the eye (cf. Sections 1.2 and 1.34).

1.55 POLAND SYNDROME

Poland syndrome, also called Poland anomaly, is characterized by underdevelopment of the muscles, breast, and nipple on one side of the chest and a deformed hand on the same side. The cause of Poland syndrome is unknown; however, a prevailing theory says that disruptions of arterial blood flow to the tissues that later develop into the chest and hand during early embryogenesis cause Poland syndrome.

Dìhuáng (cf. Sections 1.10 and 1.32) was shown to alleviate symptoms of high-fat diet induced diabetic mice through its anti-inflammatory effect (Meng et al., 2021). Its combination with Xuánshēn (cf. Sections 1.25, 1.3, and 1.32) was also shown to protect the kidney in diabetic nephropathy rats through reduction in renal microinflammation (Zhang et al., 2022). Wēndǎntāng was concluded to

TABLE 1.55

GMP Herbal Medicines for a 12-Year-Old Boy with Poland Syndrome

Poland syndrome (OrphaCode: 2911)

A malformation syndrome with a prevalence of ~5 in 100,000

Autosomal dominant, Autosomal recessive, Multigenic/multifactorial, Not applicable

Asymmetry of the thorax, Aplasia/Hypoplasia of the nipples, Lack of subcutaneous fatty tissue, Aplasia of the pectoralis major muscle, Aplasia/Hypoplasia of the breasts

Renal hypoplasia, Abnormality of the hand, Unilateral brachydactyly, Finger symphalangism, Small hand

(Continued)

TABLE 1.55 *(Continued)*

GMP Herbal Medicines for a 12-Year-Old Boy with Poland Syndrome

Cryptorchidism, Hypospadias, Ureterocele, Vesicoureteral reflux, Duplicated collecting system, Microcephaly, Abnormality of the outer ear, Short neck, Myopia, Abnormality of the sternum, Pectus carinatum, Abnormality of the ribs, Short ribs, Congenital diaphragmatic hernia, Diabetes mellitus, Sprengel anomaly, Missing ribs, Brachydactyly, Hand polydactyly, Split hand, Abnormality of the liver, Atrial septal defect, Dextrocardia, Encephalocele, Low posterior hairline, Acute leukemia, Scoliosis, Kyphosis, Abnormality of the lower limb, Hemivertebrae, Abnormality of the ulna, Abnormality of the humerus, Spina bifida occulta, Vertebral segmentation defect, Absent hand, Reduced bone mineral density, Finger syndactyly, Aplasia/Hypoplasia of the radius, Aplasia/Hypoplasia of the sternum, Abnormal dermatoglyphics, Renal hypoplasia/aplasia, Retinal hamartoma, Aplasia/Hypoplasia of the thumb, Cone-shaped epiphysis, Neoplasm of the breast
Neonatal, Infancy

Cryptorchidism (752.51), Vesicoureteral reflux (593.7), Myopia (367.1), Diabetes mellitus (250), Abnormality of the liver (573.9):

Qǐjúdìhuángwán 5g + jiāwèixiāoyáosǎn 5-4g + nǚzhēnzǐ 1g + dānshēn 1g + gǒuqǐzǐ 1g + huángqí 1g + màiméndōng 1-0g + dìhuáng 0g.

Liùwèidìhuángwán 5g + jiāwèixiāoyáosǎn 4g + huángqí 1g + nǚzhēnzǐ 1g + gǒuqǐzǐ 1g + màiméndōng 1g.

Wēndāntāng 5g + qǐjúdìhuángwán 4g + shēnlíngbáizhúsǎn 3g + huángqí 1g + mùtōng 1g + fángfēng 1g + xìxīn 0g.

Gǒuqǐzǐ 5g + júhuā 5g + fángfēng 4-3g + dìhuáng 4-2g + dānggui 4-2g + xìxīn 1g + huánglián 1g.

Gǒuqǐzǐ 5g + júhuā 5g + niúbàngzǐ 4g + shègān 4g + xìxīn 1g + huánglián 1g.

Xuánshēn 5g + dìhuáng 5g + hòupò 5g + zhǐshí 5g + màiméndōng 5g + yùzhú 5-0g + shāshēn 5-0g + dàhuáng 0g.

be safe and effective for nonalcoholic fatty liver disease in a systematic review and meta-analysis of randomized controlled trials, improving the liver function as well as blood lipid and blood glucose-related indicators (Zhang, Liu, et al., 2022).

1.56 MICROFORM HOLOPROSENCEPHALY

Microform holoprosencephaly is also called holoprosencephaly-like or holoprosencephaly, minor form (HPE, minor form). HPE is a forehead malformation due to incomplete separation of the embryonic forehead into two cerebral hemispheres in early gestation, resulting in neurocognitive impairment and midline craniofacial anomalies. Depending on the extent of incomplete separation, symptoms of HPE can vary from benign to incompatible with life. Microform holoprosencephaly is the mildest of HPE, manifesting subtle midline defects, such as closely spaced eyes, a flat nose, cleft lip, narrow inner nostrils, and a single central incisor on the upper jaw, with normal intelligence. Microform holoprosencephaly can be caused by mutations in many genes, including the *SHH* gene, whose products are signaling proteins important for establishing the midline of the underside of the forebrain.

TABLE 1.56

GMP Herbal Medicines for a One-Year-Old Infant with Microform Holoprosencephaly

Microform holoprosencephaly (OrphaCode: 280200)

A malformation syndrome with a prevalence of ~5 in 100,000

Candidate gene tested: fibroblast growth factor receptor 1 (*FGFR1* / Entrez: 2260) at 8p11.23

Candidate gene tested: SUFU negative regulator of hedgehog signaling (*SUFU* / Entrez: 51684) at 10q24.32

Disease-causing germline mutation(s): patched 1 (*PTCH1* / Entrez: 5727) at 9q22.32

Disease-causing germline mutation(s): SIX homeobox 3 (*SIX3* / Entrez: 6496) at 2p21

Disease-causing germline mutation(s): TGFB induced factor homeobox 1 (*TGIF1* / Entrez: 7050) at 18p11.31

Disease-causing germline mutation(s): Zic family member 2 (*ZIC2* / Entrez: 7546) at 13q32.3

Disease-causing germline mutation(s): GLI family zinc finger 2 (*GLI2* / Entrez: 2736) at 2q14.2

Disease-causing germline mutation(s): teratocarcinoma-derived growth factor 1 (*TDGF1* / Entrez: 6997) at 3p21.31

Disease-causing germline mutation(s): forkhead box H1 (*FOXH1* / Entrez: 8928) at 8q24.3

(Continued)

TABLE 1.56 *(Continued)*

GMP Herbal Medicines for a One-Year-Old Infant with Microform Holoprosencephaly

Disease-causing germline mutation(s): fibroblast growth factor 8 (*FGF8* / Entrez: 2253) at 10q24.32

Disease-causing germline mutation(s): dispatched RND transporter family member 1 (*DISP1* / Entrez: 84976) at 1q41

Disease-causing germline mutation(s): cell adhesion associated, oncogene regulated (*CDON* / Entrez: 50937) at 11q24.2

Disease-causing germline mutation(s): nodal growth differentiation factor (*NODAL* / Entrez: 4838) at 10q22.1

Disease-causing germline mutation(s): delta like canonical Notch ligand 1 (*DLL1* / Entrez: 28514) at 6q27

Disease-causing germline mutation(s): growth arrest specific 1 (*GAS1* / Entrez: 2619) at 9q21.33

Disease-causing germline mutation(s): sonic hedgehog signaling molecule (*SHH* / Entrez: 6469) at 7q36.3

Multigenic/multifactorial

Choanal atresia, Single median maxillary incisor, Midnasal stenosis

Microcephaly, Short philtrum, Narrow nasal bridge, Hypotelorism, Intellectual disability, Intrauterine growth retardation, Premature birth, Short stature, Tented upper lip vermilion

Ambiguous genitalia, Renal agenesis, Cleft palate, Oral cleft, Anteverted nares, Strabismus, Iris coloboma, Hypothyroidism, Panhypopituitarism, Hemangioma, Seizure, Agenesis of corpus callosum, Holoprosencephaly, Tetralogy of Fallot, Asthma, Duodenal atresia, Malformation of the heart and great vessels, Scoliosis, Short nose, EMG: myopathic abnormalities, Hypoplasia of penis, Maternal diabetes, Cyclopia

Neonatal, Infancy, Childhood

Choanal atresia (748.0):	
Xiǎojiànzhōngtāng 5-0g + shēnlíngbáizhúsǎn 5-0g + shānzhā 1-0g + shénqū 1-0g + màiyá 1-0g + jīnèijīn 1-0g.	Júhuā 5g + zhǐqiào 3-0g.
Sìjūnzǐtāng 5g.	Zhǐqiào 5g + jílí 5-0g.
Sāngjúyǐn 5g + zhǐqiào 1g + jílí 1-0g.	Júhóng 5g.
Xìngsūyǐnyòukē 5g + xīnyíqīngfèitāng 5g.	
Intellectual disability (D008607):	
Xiǎojiànzhōngtāng 5g + shānzhā 2-1g + shénqū 2-1g + màiyá 2-0g.	Xuánshēn 5g + dìhuáng 5g + màiméndōng 5g + hòupò 5-1g + zhǐshí 5-1g + dàhuáng 1-0g.
Liùjūnzǐtāng 5g.	Zhǐqiào 5g + jílí 2g.
Xiǎocháihútāngqùrénshēn 5g + qínjiāobiējiǎsǎn 2g + bǎihégùjīntāng 1g.	Gāncǎo 5g + báizhǐ 5g + shārén 5g + dàhuáng 0g.
Ambiguous genitalia (752.7), Cleft palate (749.0), Strabismus (378.7, 378.6, 378.31), Hypothyroidism (244.9), Panhypopituitarism (253.2), Hemangioma (228.00), Seizure (345.9):	
Liùwèidìhuángwán 5g + shēnlíngbáizhúsǎn 5g + shānzhā 2-1g + shénqū 2-1g + màiyá 2-1g + jīnèijīn 1-0g.	Jílí 5g + zhǐqiào 2-0g.
Guìzhījiālónggǔmǔlìtāng 5g + màiyá 2g + púgōngyīng 2g.	
Shēnlíngbáizhúsǎn 5g + bǎohéwán 3g + shānzhā 2g + shénqū 2g + màiyá 2g + jīnèijīn 2g.	

Integrative therapy with Sìjūnzǐtāng, introduced in Section 1.17 for children with chronic sinusitis, was shown to be more effective than conventional therapy alone in the treatment of severe ventilator-associated pneumonia in children in a randomized controlled trial (Han & Wang, 2019). Moreover, Sìjūnzǐtāng was demonstrated to promote restoration of intestinal function in a rabbit model of intestinal obstruction by regulating intestinal homeostasis (Yu et al., 2014). Liùjūnzǐtāng was concluded in a meta-analysis of randomized controlled trials to be safe and effective for the treatment of functional dyspepsia (Xiao et al., 2012). Xiǎocháihútāngqùrénshēn is used today for neurotic disorders (Wang, 2019).

1.57   ISOLATED BILIARY ATRESIA

Isolated biliary atresia, also called non-syndromic biliary atresia, is progressive scarring or blockage of the bile ducts inside and outside the liver occurring in the time before and soon after birth, resulting in jaundice of the infant. Isolated biliary atresia is caused by the interaction of genetics, environment, immunity, and infections.

TABLE 1.57
GMP Herbal Medicines for a One-Year-Old Infant with Isolated Biliary Atresia

Isolated biliary atresia (OrphaCode: 30391)

A morphological anomaly with a prevalence of ~5 in 100,000

Multigenic/multifactorial

Jaundice, Cholestasis, Failure to thrive

Decreased liver function, Severe failure to thrive, Hepatomegaly, Fat malabsorption, Conjugated hyperbilirubinemia, Elevated hepatic transaminase, Elevated alkaline phosphatase, Prolonged neonatal jaundice, Prolonged prothrombin time, Atretic gallbladder, Acholic stools, Elevated gamma-glutamyltransferase activity, Dark yellow urine

Ophthalmoplegia, Hypothyroidism, Pruritus, Seizure, Cirrhosis, Periportal fibrosis, Bile duct proliferation, Small for gestational age, Splenomegaly, Abnormal facial shape, Hypopituitarism

Antenatal, Neonatal, Infancy

Jaundice (D007565), Cholestasis (576.2):

Xiǎocháihútāng 5g + wǔlíngsǎn 5–0g + píngwèisǎn 5–0g.

Yīnchénwǔlíngsǎn 5g + shānzhā 1–0g + shénqū 0g + màiyá 0g.

Xiǎojiànzhōngtāng 5g + shānzhā 1g + shénqū 1g + màiyá 1g.

Yīnchén 5g.

Zhǐqiào 5g + jílí 3–0g.

Gāncǎo 5g + báizhǐ 5–0g + shārén 5–0g + dàhuáng 0g.

Decreased liver function (573.9):

Xiǎocháihútāng 5g + sìjūnzǐtāng 5–0g + yīnchén 1–0g.

Xiǎocháihútāng 5g + liùjūnzǐtāng 5–0g + yīnchén 1–0g.

Cháihúshūgāntāng 5g + shānzhā 1g + shénqū 1g + màiyá 1g.

Júhuā 5g + júhóng 5g.

Júhuā 5g + zhǐqiào 3–2g.

Ophthalmoplegia (378.56), Hypothyroidism (244.9), Pruritus (D011537), Seizure (345.9):

Yìgānsǎn 5g + gāncǎoxiǎomàidàzǎotāng 2g + gāncǎo 1–0g.

Yùpíngfēngsǎn 5g + bǔzhōngyìqìtāng 5g + gāncǎo 1g.

Xiāofēngsǎn 5g.

Yínqiàosǎn 5g + gāncǎo 1g + dàhuáng 0g.

Huángqín 5g + báizhǐ 4–2g + zhìgāncǎo 4–2g + shārén 4–2g + tiānhuā 2–0g + dàhuáng 1–0g.

Yīnchén (Herba Artemisiae Scopariae) has long been used for a variety of liver diseases and the molecular mechanisms against chronic hepatitis B were explored (He et al., 2021). The flavonoids in Zhǐqiào (cf. Section 1.31), having antioxidative, anticytotoxic, anti-inflammatory, antifibrotic, and antitumor activities, were reviewed to be potential therapeutic agents for liver diseases (Wu et al., 2020). Xiǎocháihútāng and Júhuā were introduced in Section 1.34 for liver diseases. Yìgānsǎn (cf. Sections 1.1 and 1.43) was shown to inhibit seizures in planarians (Park et al., 2014), a type of flatworm possessing mammalian-like neurotransmitters for epilepsy research.

1.58   48,XXXY SYNDROME

48,XXXY syndrome manifests developmental delays and intellectual disability, including speech and language learning difficulties, in boys. Men with 48,XXXY are infertile. 48,XXXY is caused by fertilization of an egg with two extra Xs, i.e., XXX, by a normal sperm with a Y, or fertilization of a normal egg with an X by an abnormal sperm with two extra Xs, i.e., XXY. The abnormality, called nondisjunction, occurs at random during the reproductive cell production process and is not inherited.

Bājǐtiān (Radix Morindae Officinalis) was shown to enhance the sexual function of male mice and protect human sperm DNA from hydrogen peroxide damage; in other words, it is a potential androgen-like drug that modulates hormone levels without producing reproductive-organ lesions (Wu et al., 2015). Ròucōngróng (Herba Cistanches) was demonstrated to improve the cognitive and independent living ability of moderate Alzheimer's disease patients by slowing down volume changes of the hippocampus and reducing the levels of total tau, TNF-α, and IL-1β (Li et al., 2015). Bǔzhōngyìqìtāng, combined with biological mesh during rehabilitation after inguinal hernia repairment, was shown to have superior safety and benefit on post-operative rehabilitation, including reduced post-operative pain and hospital stay in a randomized controlled study (Zhu et al., 2022).

TABLE 1.58

GMP Herbal Medicines for a Two-Year-Old Boy with 48,XXXY Syndrome

48,XXXY syndrome (OrphaCode: 96263)

A malformation syndrome with a prevalence of ~5 in 100,000

Not applicable, Unknown

Azoospermia, Hypogonadism, Infertility, Intellectual disability–mild, Global developmental delay, Language impairment, Decreased testicular size

Cryptorchidism, Scrotal hypoplasia, Tall stature, Epicanthus, Hypertelorism, Chronic otitis media, Depressed nasal ridge, Strabismus, Upslanted palpebral fissure, Carious teeth, Taurodontia, Abnormality of dental enamel, Delayed eruption of teeth, Autism, Gynecomastia, Hypotonia, Pes planus, Constipation, Asthma, Recurrent respiratory infections, Radioulnar synostosis, Elbow dislocation, Clinodactyly of the 5th finger, Joint hyperflexibility, Abnormality of epiphysis morphology, Attention deficit hyperactivity disorder, Hypoplasia of penis, Open bite, Down-sloping shoulders

Inguinal hernia, Renal dysplasia, Cleft palate, Brachycephaly, Mandibular prognathia, Facial asymmetry, Short neck, Blepharophimosis, Irritability, Anxiety, Delayed speech and language development, Seizure, Tremor, Obesity, Talipes equinovarus, Gastroesophageal reflux, Pulmonary embolism, Malformation of the heart and great vessels, Scoliosis, Coxa valga, Hip dislocation, Venous thrombosis, Type II diabetes mellitus, Abnormal aggressive, impulsive, or violent behavior, Abnormal social behavior, Schizophrenia

Neonatal, Infancy

Azoospermia (606.0), Language impairment (D007806):

Liùwèidìhuángwán 5g + shēnlíngbáizhúsăn 5g.

Liùwèidìhuángwán 5g + bǔzhōngyìqìtāng 5g + shānyào 2-0g + gǒuqǐzǐ 2-0g + tùsīzǐ 2-0g.

Liùwèidìhuángwán 5g + ròucōngróng 1-0g + gǒuqǐzǐ 1-0g + tùsīzǐ 1-0g + fùpénzǐ 1-0g + yínyánghuò 0g + suǒyáng 0g.

Zuǒguīwán 5g + shēnlíngbáizhúsăn 5g.

Bājǐtiān 5g + ròucōngróng 5g + yínyánghuò 5g + tùsīzǐ 5g + fùpénzǐ 5-0g.

Gǒuqǐzǐ 5g + tùsīzǐ 5g + chēqiánzǐ 4-0g + yínyánghuò 2-0g + fùpénzǐ 2-0g + wǔwèizǐ 1-0g.

Ròucōngróng 5g + chēqiánzǐ 2g + gǒuqǐzǐ 2g + tùsīzǐ 2g + fùpénzǐ 2g + wǔwèizǐ 2g.

Cryptorchidism (752.51), Strabismus (378.7, 378.6, 378.31), Carious teeth (521.0, 521.07), Autism (299.0), Gynecomastia (778.7), Hypotonia (D009123), Constipation (564.0), Asthma (493), Radioulnar synostosis (755.53):

Máxìnggānshítāng 5g + xīnyíqīngfèitāng 5-0g + dàzǎo 1-0g + tínglìzǐ 1-0g + bèimǔ 1-0g + guālóurén 1-0g + yúxīngcǎo 1-0g + jiégěng 1-0g + sāngbáipí 1-0g.

Bǔzhōngyìqìtāng 5g + xuánshēn 1g + dìhuáng 1g + màiméndōng 1g.

Dìngchuǎntāng 5g + xīnyíqīngfèitāng 4g + mázǐrénwán 2g + bèimǔ 1g + guālóurén 1g.

Dàhuáng 5g + gāncǎo 5g + báizhǐ 5g + shārén 5g + huángqín 5-0g.

Xuánshēn 5g + dìhuáng 5g + màiméndōng 5g + dàhuáng 1g + hòupò 1g + zhǐshí 1g.

Gǒuqǐzǐ 5g + zhīmǔ 5-0g + júhuā 5-0g + dìhuáng 4-0g + dāngguī 4-0g + huángqín 4-0g + fángfēng 2-0g + dàhuáng 1g + huánglián 1g + xìxīn 1-0g.

Inguinal hernia (550), Cleft palate (749.0), Blepharophimosis (374.46), Delayed speech and language development (D007805), Seizure (345.9), Tremor (D014202), Obesity (278.00), Talipes equinovarus (754.51), Gastroesophageal reflux (530.81):

Bǔzhōngyìqìtāng 5g + zhībódìhuángwán 4-0g + dùzhòng 1-0g + xùduàn 1-0g.

Bǔzhōngyìqìtāng 5g + jìshēngshènqìwán 5-0g.

Bǔzhōngyìqìtāng 5g + dúhuójìshēngtāng 5-0g.

Bǔzhōngyìqìtāng 5g + xiāngshāliùjūnzǐtāng 5-0g + chuānliànzǐ 1-0g + yánhúsuǒ 1-0g + zhǐshí 1-0g.

Huángqí 5g + dǎngshēn 5g + shānyào 4g + báizhú 4g + báisháo 4g + dìhuáng 4g + dùzhòng 4g + gǒuqǐzǐ 4g + fúlíng 4g + dāngguī 4g + shúdìhuáng 4g + xùduàn 4g + yìyǐrén 4-0g.

Báizhú 5-4g + fúlíng 5-1g + huángqí 5-0g + zhǐshí 4-0g.

Dìhuáng 5g + ròucōngróng 5g + dùzhòng 5g + gǒuqǐzǐ 5g + yínyánghuò 5g + tùsīzǐ 5g + huángqí 5g + dāngguī 5g + xùduàn 5g.

1.59   SMITH-MAGENIS SYNDROME

Smith-Magenis syndrome, also known as 17p11.2 microdeletion syndrome, is characterized by difficulty sleeping, distinctive facial features, and behavioral problems. Smith-Magenis syndrome is caused by deletion in a region on chromosome 17 containing the *RAI1* gene, whose products are a transcription factor controlling other genes important for the regulation of circadian rhythm,

TABLE 1.59

GMP Herbal Medicines for a One-Year-Old Infant with Smith-Magenis Syndrome

Smith-Magenis syndrome (OrphaCode: 819)

A malformation syndrome with a prevalence of ~4 in 100,000

Candidate gene tested: DEAF1 transcription factor (*DEAF1* / Entrez: 10522) at 11p15.5

Disease-causing germline mutation(s): retinoic acid induced 1 (*RAI1* / Entrez: 10743) at 17p11.2

Candidate gene tested: FLII actin remodeling protein (*FLII* / Entrez: 2314) at 17p11.2

Candidate gene tested: IQ motif and Sec7 domain ArfGEF 2 (*IQSEC2* / Entrez: 23096) at Xp11.22

Autosomal dominant

Brachycephaly, Broad forehead, Wide nasal bridge, Deeply set eye, Upslanted palpebral fissure, Synophrys, Taurodontia, Delayed eruption of primary teeth, Stereotypy, Anxiety, Delayed speech and language development, Brachydactyly, Intellectual disability, Hypotonia, Global developmental delay, Hyporeflexia, Obesity, Hoarse voice, Frontal bossing, Neurological speech impairment, Sleep disturbance, Depressed nasal bridge, Abnormal tracheobronchial morphology, Corticospinal tract hypoplasia, Attention deficit hyperactivity disorder, Tented upper lip vermilion, Midface retrusion, Self-injurious behavior, Large face

Open mouth, Mandibular prognathia, Hypertelorism, Short philtrum, Micrognathia, Chronic otitis media, Conductive hearing impairment, Anteverted nares, Microcornea, Strabismus, Myopia, Gait disturbance, Failure to thrive in infancy, Decreased fetal movement, Pes planus, Toe syndactyly, Constipation, Gastroesophageal reflux, Ventriculomegaly, Hypertriglyceridemia, EEG abnormality, Malformation of the heart and great vessels, Scoliosis, Hypercholesterolemia, Short nose, Abnormal form of the vertebral bodies, Clinodactyly of the 5th finger, Short stature, Impaired pain sensation, Aplasia/Hypoplasia of the corpus callosum, Feeding difficulties in infancy, Peripheral neuropathy, Hyperacusis

Abnormality of the ureter, Cleft palate, Cleft upper lip, Microcephaly, Retinal detachment, Hypothyroidism, Delayed puberty, Precocious puberty, Hand polydactyly, Seizure, Joint stiffness, Renal hypoplasia/aplasia, Abnormal localization of kidney

Neonatal, Infancy, Childhood, Adolescent, Adult

Stereotypy (307.3), Delayed speech and language development (D007805), Intellectual disability (D008607), Hypotonia (D009123), Obesity (278.00), Hoarse voice (D006685), Neurological speech impairment (D013064):

Gāncǎoxiǎomàidàzǎotāng 5g + jiāwèixiāoyáosǎn 5-0g + mǔlì 2-0g + lónggǔ 2-0g + suānzǎorén 1-0g.

Gāncǎoxiǎomàidàzǎotāng 5g + cháihújiālónggǔmǔlìtāng 5-0g + suānzǎorén 3-0g + yèjiāoténg 2-0g + fúshén 2-0g + yuǎnzhì 2-0g.

Gāncǎo 5g + shānzhīzǐ 3-2g + zhīmǔ 3-2g + dàhuáng 0g + huánglián 0g.

Gāncǎo 5g + huángqín 5g + zhīmǔ 5-0g + dàzǎo 2-0g + dàhuáng 1-0g + huánglián 1-0g.

Conductive hearing impairment (D006314), Strabismus (378.7, 378.6, 378.31), Myopia (367.1), Constipation (564.0), Gastroesophageal reflux (530.81), Hyperacusis (D012001):

Xìngsūyǐnyòukē 5g + xīnyíqīngfèitāng 5g + yínqiàosǎn 5g + bèimǔ 1g + jiégěng 1g.

Sāngjúyǐn 5g + xīnyíqīngfèitāng 3g + bèimǔ 1g + xiàkūcǎo 1g + jiégěng 1g.

Língguìshùgāntāng 5g + shíchāngpú 1g + yuǎnzhì 1g + dàhuáng 0g.

Sāngjúyǐn 5g + cāngěrsǎn 4g + shíchāngpú 1g + yuǎnzhì 1g.

Júhuā 5g.

Zhǐqiào 5g.

Hángjú 5g.

Jílí 5g + chántuì 5g + zhǐqiào 4-0g.

Júhóng 5g

---

including the sleep-wake cycle. The chromosomal deletion occurs at random during reproductive cell formation or early embryonic development, and is not inherited.

Gāncǎo (cf. Section 1.1) was shown to ameliorate the cognitive impairment in a mouse model of inflammation-induced memory and cognitive deficit (Cho et al., 2018). Gāncǎoxiǎomàidàzǎotāng, Jiāwèixiāoyáosǎn, and Wēndǎntāng all contain Gāncǎo. Cāngěrsǎn "dispels Wind, opens nostrils, stops headache" and is used today for upper respiratory tract infections including rhinitis, sinusitis, and nasopharyngitis (Wang, 2019). Recall that the Eustachian tube links the nasopharynx to the middle ear.

1.60 KABUKI SYNDROME

Kabuki syndrome, also known as Niikawa-Kuroki syndrome, is characterized by growth delays, intellectual disability, and distinctive facial features resembling the stage makeup of Kabuki actors in traditional Japanese theater arts. Kabuki syndrome is caused by *de novo* mutations in the *KMT2D*

TABLE 1.60

GMP Herbal Medicines for a One-Year-Old Infant with Kabuki Syndrome

Kabuki syndrome (OrphaCode: 2322)

A malformation syndrome with a prevalence of ~3 in 100,000

Disease-causing germline mutation(s): lysine methyltransferase 2D (*KMT2D* / Entrez: 8085) at 12q13.12

Disease-causing germline mutation(s): lysine demethylase 6A (*KDM6A* / Entrez: 7403) at Xp11.3

Autosomal dominant, Not applicable

Macrotia, Protruding ear, Long eyelashes, Short columella, Highly arched eyebrow, Hemivertebrae, Abnormal form of the vertebral bodies, Butterfly vertebrae, Sparse lateral eyebrow, Short middle phalanx of finger, Abnormal dermatoglyphics, Eversion of lateral third of lower eyelids, Vertebral clefting, Short 5th finger

Abnormality of the dentition, Cleft palate, Oral cleft, High palate, Hydrocephalus, Microcephaly, Conductive hearing impairment, Sensorineural hearing impairment, Strabismus, Ptosis, Hypodontia, Widely spaced teeth, Microdontia, Hypotonia, Failure to thrive, Abnormal cardiac septum morphology, Coarctation of aorta, Ventriculomegaly, Cerebral cortical atrophy, Scoliosis, Recurrent infections, Short stature, Joint hyperflexibility, Abnormality of dental morphology, Abnormality of immune system physiology, Feeding difficulties

Cryptorchidism, Hypospadias, Ureteropelvic junction obstruction, Duplicated collecting system, Hydronephrosis, Mask-like facies, Preauricular skin tag, Microcornea, Coloboma, Blue sclerae, Nystagmus, Congenital diaphragmatic hernia, Precocious puberty, Seizure, Obesity, EEG abnormality, Hip dislocation, Crossed fused renal ectopia, Renal hypoplasia/aplasia, Hypoplasia of penis, Lip pit, Abnormal localization of kidney, Small hand

Antenatal, Neonatal, Infancy

Cleft palate (749.0), Hydrocephalus (331.4, 331.3), Conductive hearing impairment (D006314), Sensorineural hearing impairment (389.1), Strabismus (378.7, 378.6, 378.31), Ptosis (374.3), Hypodontia (520.0), Hypotonia (D009123):

Liùwèidìhuángwán 5g + shíchāngpú 1g + yuǎnzhì 1g.

Xīnyíqīngfèitāng 5g + língguìshùgāntāng 5-0g + shíchāngpú 1g + yuǎnzhì 1g.

Xīnyíqīngfèitāng 5g + yìqìcōngmíngtāng 5-0g + shíchāngpú 1g + yuǎnzhì 1g + chántuì 1-0g.

Shíchāngpú 5g + zhìgāncǎo 5g + shārén 5g + huángbò 5g + guībǎn 5g.

Shíchāngpú 5g + fúshén 5g + dǎngshēn 5-4g + yuǎnzhì 5-4g + huángqí 5-0g + báizhú 5-0g + fúlíng 5-0g + gǒuqǐzǐ 4-0g + júhuā 2-0g.

Cryptorchidism (752.51), Hydronephrosis (591), Nystagmus (379.53, 379.55, 379.50), Seizure (345.9), Obesity (278.00):

Wǔlíngsǎn 5g + jìshēngshènqìwán 5g + chēqiánzǐ 2g + gǒuqǐzǐ 2g + tùsīzǐ 2g + fùpénzǐ 2-0g.

Wēndǎntāng 5g + tiānmá 1g + shíchāngpú 1g + yuǎnzhì 1g + dàhuáng 0g.

Liùwèidìhuángwán 5g + wǔlíngsǎn 4g + shíchāngpú 1g + chēqiánzǐ 1g + gǒuqǐzǐ 1g + tùsīzǐ 1g + bǔgǔzhī 1g + yuǎnzhì 1g.

Jìshēngshènqìwán 5g + guīpítāng 4g + tiānmá 1g + shíchāngpú 1g + yuǎnzhì 1g + dàhuáng 0g.

Shānzhīzǐ 5g + gāncǎo 5g + zhīmǔ 5g + dàhuáng 1-0g + huánglián 1-0g.

Gāncǎo 5g + huángbò 5g + dàhuáng 0g.

Gāncǎo 5g + huángqín 5-4g + dàhuáng 1-0g + huánglián 1-0g.

---

or *KDM6A* gene, whose products control activities of genes important for early embryological development through modification of chromatin structures to allow or disallow access of genes to the transcriptional machinery in the nucleus.

Yuǎnzhì (cf. Section 1.41) has long been touted as a cognitive enhancer. As an example of its nootropic effects, it was shown to ameliorate behavioral defects in mice with Alzheimer's disease by promoting degradation of the amyloid precursor protein (Li et al., 2016). The other example showed that it prevents axonal degeneration and memory deficits in mice with Alzheimer's disease by inhibiting endocytosis (Kuboyama et al., 2017). Yìqìcōngmíngtāng (cf. Section 1.14) was demonstrated to prevent age-related hearing loss by modulating the apoptosis process in mouse auditory cells (Yang et al., 2022).

1.61 BOR SYNDROME

BOR syndrome, i.e., Branchiootorenal syndrome, is characterized by the formation of a neck mass called branchial cleft cysts and malformation of the ear and kidney. Many cases of BOR syndrome are caused by mutations in the *EYA1* gene whose products interact with other proteins, including

TABLE 1.61
GMP Herbal Medicines for a Three-Year-Old Child with BOR Syndrome

BOR syndrome (OrphaCode: 107)

A malformation syndrome with a prevalence of ~2 in 100,000

Disease-causing germline mutation(s): SIX homeobox 1 (*SIX1* / Entrez: 6495) at 14q23.1

Disease-causing germline mutation(s): EYA transcriptional coactivator and phosphatase 1 (*EYA1* / Entrez: 2138) at 8q13.3

Disease-causing germline mutation(s): SIX homeobox 5 (*SIX5* / Entrez: 147912) at 19q13.32

Autosomal dominant

Hearing impairment

Preauricular skin tag, External ear malformation, Renal hypoplasia/aplasia, Enlarged cochlear aqueduct, Stenosis of the external auditory canal, Atresia of the external auditory canal, Abnormality of the middle ear ossicles, Hypoplasia of the cochlea, Branchial cyst

Ureteropelvic junction obstruction, Renal insufficiency, Cleft palate, Retrognathia, Multicystic kidney dysplasia, Vesicoureteral reflux, Hydronephrosis, Facial palsy, Abnormal lacrimal duct morphology

Neonatal, Infancy, Childhood

Hearing impairment (D034381):

Jiāwèixiāoyáosǎn 5g + língguìshùgāntāng 5g + chuānxiōngchádiàosǎn 2g + bǎnlángēn 1-0g + jiégěng 1-0g + shānzhā 1-0g + shārén 1-0g + fùzǐ 1-0g.

Jiāwèixiāoyáosǎn 5g + língguìshùgāntāng 5g + xiǎoqīnglóngtāng 2g + shānzhā 1g + shārén 1g.

Jiāwèixiāoyáosǎn 5g + língguìshùgāntāng 5g + gégēntāng 2g + shānzhā 1g + qīngpí 1g.

Língguìshùgāntāng 5g + màiméndōngtāng 5g + bèimǔ 1g + jiégěng 1g.

Huángbò 5g + shārén 4g + gāncǎo 2g.

Shārén 5g + gāncǎo 5-3g + báizhǐ 5-3g + huángqín 2-0g + dàhuáng 0g.

Renal insufficiency (586), Cleft palate (749.0), Vesicoureteral reflux (593.7), Hydronephrosis (591), Facial palsy (351.0):

Zhūlíngtāng 5g + jìshēngshènqìwán 5g + báimáogēn 2-1g + dānshēn 2-0g + dōngguāzǐ 2-0g + chēqiánzǐ 2-0g + jīnqiáncǎo 2-0g + bìxiè 2-0g + chìsháo 1-0g + yìmǔcǎo 1-0g + dàhuáng 0g.

Qǐjúdìhuángwán 5g + zhūlíngtāng 5g + báimáogēn 2g + jīnqiáncǎo 2g + jīxuèténg 2g + dàhuáng 0g.

Shānyào 5g + báizhú 5g + fúlíng 5g + huángqí 5g + dǎngshēn 5g + gāncǎo 2-0g.

Dàzǎo 5g + shānyào 5g + gāncǎo 5g + báizhú 5g + báisháo 5g + ējiāo 5g + huángqí 5g + dāngguī 5g + shúdìhuáng 5g + dǎngshēn 5g.

Gāncǎo 5g + báizhú 5g + fúlíng 5g + chénpí 5g + zhūlíng 5g + zéxiè 5g.

Jílí 5g.

those encoded by the *SIX1* and *SIX5* genes, to regulate the development of tissues that later form the neck, ears, and kidneys during embryonic development.

Huángbò (Cortex Phellodendri Chinensis) is a component herb in Yìqìcōngmíngtāng of the last section. Màiméndōngtāng "cleans and nourishes the Lung/Stomach, lowers ascending Qi" and is used today for symptoms involving the respiratory system and other chest symptoms such as chronic bronchitis (Wang, 2019). Màiméndōngtāng contains Rénshēn (cf. Section 1.15) as the minister herb in the formula. Korean red ginseng was shown to attenuate noise-induced hearing loss in rats (Durankaya et al., 2021). Use of GMP concentrated Jìshēngshènqìwán and/or Dānshēn (Radix et Rhizoma Salviae Miltiorrhizae) extract granules was found to improve the long-term survival rate of patients with chronic kidney disease (Huang et al., 2018).

1.62 46,XX TESTICULAR DISORDER OF SEX DEVELOPMENT

46,XX testicular disorder of sex development is also known as de la Chapelle syndrome, or XX, male syndrome. 46,XX testicular disorder of sex development is a congenital intersex condition where an affected individual carries a 46,XX genotype in each of the body cells but shows a male phenotype, including male external genitalia. 46,XX testicular disorder of sex development is

TABLE 1.62

GMP Herbal Medicines for a 12-Year-Old Boy with 46,XX Testicular Disorder of Sex Development

46,XX testicular disorder of sex development (OrphaCode: 393)

A malformation syndrome with a prevalence of ~2 in 100,000

Disease-causing germline mutation(s): SRY-box transcription factor 9 (*SOX9* / Entrez: 6662) at 17q24.3

Disease-causing germline mutation(s): sex determining region Y (*SRY* / Entrez: 6736) at Yp11.2

Disease-causing germline mutation(s) (gain of function): SRY-box transcription factor 3 (*SOX3* / Entrez: 6658) at Xq27.1

Role: the phenotype of nuclear receptor subfamily 0 group B member 1 (*NR0B1* / Entrez: 190) at Xp21.2

Disease-causing germline mutation(s) (loss of function): nuclear receptor subfamily 5 group A member 1 (*NR5A1* / Entrez: 2516) at 9q33.3

Autosomal dominant

Male hypogonadism, Ambiguous genitalia, Polycystic ovaries, Decreased testicular size

Antenatal, Neonatal, Adolescent

Ambiguous genitalia (752.7), Polycystic ovaries (256.4):

Guìzhīfúlíngwán 5g + shānyào 3-2g + hónghuā 2-1g + táorén 2-1g + dàhuáng 0g. Guìzhījiālónggǔmǔlìtāng 5g + shānyào 2g + hónghuā 2g + táorén 2g.	Shānyào 5g + dùzhòng 5g + gǒuqǐzǐ 5g + tùsīzǐ 5g + shúdìhuáng 5g + gǔsuìbǔ 5-0g + xùduàn 5-0g + shānzhūyú 3-2g + dāngguī 3-0g. Dùzhòng 5g + chuānxiōng 2g + niúxī 2g + dìhuáng 2g + guìzhī 2g + gǔsuìbǔ 2g + huángqín 2g + xùduàn 2g. Dìhuáng 5g + dùzhòng 5g + guìzhī 5g + gǔsuìbǔ 5g + xùduàn 5g + jīxuèténg 5-0g + chuānxiōng 4g + àiyè 2-0g.

caused by an X chromosome from the father that contains of a section of the Y chromosome that contains the *SRY* gene whose products direct the fetus's development as a male. This misplacement of the *SRY* gene on X, called translocation, occurs as a random event during the sperm formation. As the affected individuals have a male appearance from birth, they are typically raised as boys and develop a male gender identity.

Shānyào (Rhizoma Dioscoreae; wild yam), an herbal food, is in "Kidney essence reinforcing" formulas for the treatment of infertility (Zhang & Liu, 2022). Shānyào was also shown to decrease the anxiety and IL-2 levels in the brain of ovariectomized rats (Ho et al., 2007). Dùzhòng (cf. Section 1.4) was demonstrated to improve the erectile function of diabetic rats by enhancing the hypothalamic-pituitary-gonadal axis (Fu et al., 2019). The efficacy of Guìzhīfúlíngwán for the treatment of ovarian cancer has been confirmed by a number of clinical studies (Wang et al., 2022).

1.63   NIJMEGEN BREAKAGE SYNDROME

Nijmegen breakage syndrome (NBS) is also known as ataxia-telangiectasia, variant 1; Berlin breakage syndrome; microcephaly-immunodeficiency-lymphoid malignancy syndrome; and Seemanova syndrome type 2. NBS is characterized by a smaller-than-normal head, compromised immunity, cancer of the lymphatic system, and distinctive facial features. NBS is caused by mutations in the *NBN* gene whose products repair DNA damage which can occur in cell replication and radiation exposure.

Báizhú (cf. Section 1.21) is recognized as an immune enhancer. For example, Báizhú was shown to boost the immune responses of mice immunized with a commercial FMDV (foot-and-mouth disease virus) vaccine (Li et al., 2009), and increase the cytokine levels and alleviate the decline in lymphocyte activation in mice treated with cyclophosphamide (Xiang et al., 2020), which is a medication to suppress immunity in chemotherapy. Guīpítāng, Shēnlíngbáizhúsǎn, Sìjūnzǐtāng, and Xiāngshāliùjūnzǐtāng all contain Báizhú. Běishāshēn, introduced in Section 1.6 to "clean the Lung," was shown to be anti-lung cancer in vitro (Li et al., 2017; Wang et al., 2017). Gānlùyǐn (cf. Section 1.38) was demonstrated to inhibit proliferation and migration of mouse leukemia cells and inhibit tumor growth in mice (Liu et al., 2013).

TABLE 1.63
GMP Herbal Medicines for a One-Year-Old Infant with Nijmegen Breakage Syndrome

Nijmegen breakage syndrome (OrphaCode: 647)

A malformation syndrome with a prevalence of ~2 in 100,000

Disease-causing germline mutation(s): nibrin (*NBN* / Entrez: 4683) at 8q21.3

Autosomal recessive

Microcephaly, Abnormality of the face, Retrognathia, Low anterior hairline, Sloping forehead, Hearing abnormality, Macrotia, Prominent nasal bridge, Convex nasal ridge, Prominent nose, Short neck, Upslanted palpebral fissure, Mental deterioration, Abnormality of the hair, Thrombocytopenia, Hemolytic anemia, Autoimmune hemolytic anemia, Deep philtrum, Anal atresia, Anal stenosis, Chronic diarrhea, Recurrent respiratory infections, Abnormality of chromosome stability, Short stature, Cachexia, Depressed nasal bridge, Recurrent sinopulmonary infections, Recurrent pneumonia, Attention deficit hyperactivity disorder, Abnormal hair quantity, Anorectal anomaly

Neoplasm, Pollakisuria

Cleft palate, Abnormal eyelid morphology, Cutaneous photosensitivity, Muscle weakness, Freckling, Abnormality of neuronal migration, Acute leukemia, Lymphoma, Rhabdomyosarcoma, Respiratory failure, Abnormality of the musculature, Skeletal muscle atrophy, Glioma, T-cell lymphoma, B-cell lymphoma, Non-midline cleft lip

Neonatal, Infancy

Thrombocytopenia (287.5), Autoimmune hemolytic anemia (283.0), Abnormality of chromosome stability (D019457) [Other conditions due to chromosome anomalies (758.89)], Cachexia (D002100):

Guīpítāng 5g + shēnlíngbáizhúsǎn 5-0g + sìjūnzǐtāng 2-0g + xiāngshāliùjūnzǐtāng 2-0g.	Báizhú 5g + huángqí 5g + dǎngshēn 5g + yùzhú 5-0g + màiyá 5-0g + shúdìhuáng 5-0g + gāncǎo 2-0g + dàzǎo 2-0g.
Sìjūnzǐtāng 5g + sìwùtāng 5g + huángqí 1g.	

Neoplasm (199):

Gānlùyǐn 5g + qīngwèisǎn 5g.	Běishāshēn 5g + xuánshēn 5g + yùzhú 5g + dìhuáng 5g + hòupò 5g + zhǐshí 5g + màiméndōng 5g + dàhuáng 1-0g.
Gānlùyǐn 5g + liánggésǎn 5g.	
Gānlùyǐn 5g + xiāngshāliùjūnzǐtāng 5g + shānzhā 1g + shénqū 1g + màiyá 1g + jīnèijīn 1g.	Xuánshēn 5g + dìhuáng 5g + màiméndōng 5g + hòupò 5-3g + zhǐshí 5-3g + yùzhú 5-0g + shāshēn 5-0g + dàhuáng 1-0g.
Gānlùyǐn 5g + zhúyèshígāotāng 5g + tiānhuā 1g + shíhú 1g.	

Cleft palate (749.0), Muscle weakness (D018908), Skeletal muscle atrophy (D009133):

Gānlùyǐn 5g + bǎohéwán 5-0g + gāncǎo 1-0g.	Gāncǎo 5g + báizhǐ 5g + shārén 5-3g + dàhuáng 1-0g.
Gānlùyǐn 5g + xīnyíqīngfèitāng 5-0g + gāncǎo 1g.	
Wǔlíngsǎn 5g + yùpíngfēngsǎn 5g + gāncǎo 0g.	
Gānlùxiāodúdān 5g + gāncǎo 0g.	

1.64 ISOLATED DANDY-WALKER MALFORMATION

Isolated Dandy-Walker malformation is a brain development condition characterized by underdevelopment of the middle cerebellum, enlargement of the space near the cerebellum and brainstem, including the fluid-filled cavity that drains brain fluid into the spinal cord. Isolated Dandy-Walker malformation can also affect the heart. Most cases of isolated Dandy-Walker malformation result sporadically from defects in early embryonic development of the cerebellum. The first identified gene variants associated with isolated Dandy-Walker malformation include *ZIC1* and *ZIC4,* whose products are transcription activators important for cerebellum maturation.

Gāncǎo (cf. Section 1.1) was shown to exert cardioprotection in rats with myocardial necrosis by reducing oxidative stress, augmenting endogenous antioxidants, and restoring functional parameters as well as maintaining structural integrity (Ojha et al., 2015). However, because of a correlation between Gāncǎo intake and blood pressure increase, a no-effect dose of 6 g licorice a day for a person with a body weight of 60 kg was recommended (Van Gelderen et al., 2000). On the other hand, the antihypertensive effect of Báizhǐ (cf. Section 1.7) was demonstrated through its vasorelaxant

TABLE 1.64
GMP Herbal Medicines for a One-Year-Old Infant with Isolated Dandy-Walker Malformation

Isolated Dandy-Walker malformation (OrphaCode: 217)

A morphological anomaly with a prevalence of ~2 in 100,000

Role: the phenotype of Zic family member 1 (*ZIC1* / Entrez: 7545) at 3q24

Role: the phenotype of Zic family member 4 (*ZIC4* / Entrez: 84107) at 3q24

Disease-causing germline mutation(s): nidogen 1 (*NID1* / Entrez: 4811) at 1q42.3

Multigenic/multifactorial

Prominent occiput, Dandy-Walker malformation, Platybasia

Frontal bossing

Cleft palate, Abnormality of the cardiovascular system, Tetralogy of Fallot, Encephalocele, Aplasia/Hypoplasia of the corpus callosum

Antenatal, Neonatal

Cleft palate (749.0), Abnormality of the cardiovascular system (429.2), Tetralogy of Fallot (745.2):

Gānlùyǐn 5g + màiméndōng 2-0g + gāncǎo 1-0g + jiégěng 1-0g.	Gāncǎo 5g + shārén 5g + huángbò 5g.
Gānlùyǐn 5g + xiāngshāliùjūnzǐtāng 5-0g + gāncǎo 2-0g.	Báizhǐ 5g + gāncǎo 5-3g + shārén 5-3g + huángqín 5-0g + dàhuáng 1-0g.

effect on the isolated rat aortic rings (Lee et al., 2015). Gānlùyǐn was shown to suppress vascular smooth muscle cell migration, and thus luminal scar tissue overgrowth, in rats receiving carotid artery balloon injury (Chien et al., 2012).

1.65   ISOLATED KLIPPEL-FEIL SYNDROME

Isolated Klippel-Feil syndrome, also known as congenital cervical vertebral fusion, is fusion of two or more cervical vertebrae due to faulty segmentation along the embryo's developing axis during early gestation. Most isolated Klippel-Feil syndrome cases occur randomly for unknown reasons. Others are found in families associated with mutations in the *GDF6* gene whose products are required for normal formation of bones and joints in the skull and axial skeleton.

Báisháo (Radix Paeoniae Alba) was suggested to down-regulate fetal Th1/Th2/Th17 cytokines and receptors to benefit embryonic survival and development in mice (Xu et al., 2017). Dǎngshēn

TABLE 1.65
GMP Herbal Medicines for a One-Year-Old Infant with Isolated Klippel-Feil Syndrome

Isolated Klippel-Feil syndrome (OrphaCode: 2345)

A malformation syndrome with a prevalence of ~2 in 100,000

Disease-causing germline mutation(s): growth differentiation factor 3 (*GDF3* / Entrez: 9573) at 12p13.31

Disease-causing germline mutation(s): mesenchyme homeobox 1 (*MEOX1* / Entrez: 4222) at 17q21.31

Disease-causing germline mutation(s): growth differentiation factor 6 (*GDF6* / Entrez: 392255) at 8q22.1

Autosomal dominant, Autosomal recessive, Not applicable

Facial asymmetry, Webbed neck, Short neck, Abnormality of the vertebral column, Low posterior hairline, Cervical C2/C3 vertebral fusion, Abnormal vertebral segmentation and fusion

Hearing impairment, Abnormality of the ribs, Sprengel anomaly, Scoliosis, Abnormality of the shoulder, Congenital muscular torticollis

Cleft palate, Abnormal cranial nerve morphology, Ventricular septal defect, Anal atresia, Spina bifida, Malformation of the heart and great vessels, Hemiplegia/hemiparesis, Ectopic anus, Abnormal sacrum morphology, Renal hypoplasia/aplasia, Cognitive impairment

Neonatal, Infancy

(Continued)

TABLE 1.65 (Continued)
GMP Herbal Medicines for a One-Year-Old Infant with Isolated Klippel-Feil Syndrome

Cervical C2/C3 vertebral fusion (756.16):

Xiǎojiànzhōngtāng 5g + língguìshùgāntāng 5-0g + báizhǐ 2g + shígāo 2g + yītiáogēn 2-0g + dàfùpí 2-0g + niúxī 2-0g + xìngrén 2-0g.

Shūjīnghuóxuètāng 5g + guìzhīsháoyàozhīmǔtāng 5-0g + báizhǐ 2g + yītiáogēn 2-0g.

Báisháo 5g + fúlíng 5g + dǎngshēn 5-2g + cháihú 5-0g + báizhú 2-1g + fùzǐ 2-1g.

Chántuì 5g + hónghuā 3g + báisháo 2g + fùzǐ 2g + dǎngshēn 2g + báizhú 1g.

Cleft palate (749.0), Ventricular septal defect (745.4), Spina bifida (741):

Xìngsūyǐnyòukē 5g + xīnyíqīngfèitāng 5g + yúxīngcǎo 2-0g + bèimǔ 1-0g + guālóurén 1-0g.

Xuánshēn 5g + dìhuáng 5g + màiméndōng 5g + yùzhú 5-0g + shāshēn 5-0g + hòupò 5-0g + zhǐshí 5-0g + dàhuáng 1-0g.

Shēnlíngbáizhúsǎn 5g + shānzhā 1-0g + màiyá 1-0g + wūméi 0g + shénqū 0g + jīnèijīn 0g.

Gāncǎo 5g + báizhǐ 5g + shārén 5g + dàhuáng 0g.

(Radix Codonopsis) is a component herb in an oral herbal formula for chronic neck pain with radicular signs or symptoms (Cui et al., 2010). Yītiáogēn (Flemingia prostrata Roxb. f. ex Roxb.) "dispels wind-dampness, relaxes muscles, activates circulation, clears heat, stops pain" and is used for neuralgia, neuritis, and radiculitis (Wang, 2020). Xuánshēn (cf. Section 1.3) was shown to attenuate ventricular remodeling in rats with coronary artery ligation (Huang et al., 2012). Furthermore, Xuánshēn was introduced in Section 1.32 for neuroprotection.

1.66 POSTERIOR URETHRAL VALVE

Posterior urethral valve (PUV) is a condition in which boys are born with an extra membranous tissue in the urethra close to the bladder, which can partially or completely block the urine outflow. The cause of PUV is unknown; however, some PUV cases are associated with mutations in the *BNC2* gene whose products are a transcription factor playing roles in early urinary tract development.

Fúlíng (cf. Section 1.21) was shown to ameliorate chronic kidney disease in rats by intervening in fatty acid metabolism, phospholipid metabolism, purine metabolism, and tryptophan metabolism (Zhao et al., 2013). Liùwèidìhuángwán was demonstrated to be antidiabetic in diabetic mice

---

TABLE 1.66
GMP Herbal Medicines for a Ten-Year-Old Boy with Posterior Urethral Valve

Posterior urethral valve (OrphaCode: 93110)

A morphological anomaly with a prevalence of ~2 in 100,000

Disease-causing germline mutation(s): basonuclin 2 (*BNC2* / Entrez: 54796) at 9p22.3-p22.2

Autosomal recessive, Not applicable, X-linked recessive

Recurrent urinary tract infections, Congenital posterior urethral valve, Chronic kidney disease

Vesicoureteral reflux, Hydronephrosis

Urinary incontinence, Renal insufficiency, Hypertension, Stage 5 chronic kidney disease, Unilateral renal dysplasia, Postnatal growth retardation, Enuresis nocturna, Fetal pyelectasis, Pyelonephritis

All ages

Chronic kidney disease (D051436):

Liùwèidìhuángwán 5g + shēnlíngbáizhúsǎn 5-3g + dānshēn 1-0g + huángqí 1-0g + shānzhā 1-0g + shénqū 1-0g + màiyá 1-0g.

Liùwèidìhuángwán 5g + xiāngshāliùjūnzǐtāng 5g + shānzhā 1g + shénqū 1g + màiyá 1g.

Jìshēngshènqìwán 5g + shēnlíngbáizhúsǎn 5-0g + wǔlíngsǎn 5-0g + chēqiánzǐ 1-0g.

Fúlíng 5g + gāncǎo 2g + fùzǐ 2g + dǎngshēn 2g + gānjiāng 1g.

Fúlíng 5g + báisháo 4-3g + fùzǐ 4-3g + dǎngshēn 4-3g + báizhú 2-1g.

Xuánshēn 5g + dìhuáng 5g + màiméndōng 5g + hòupò 5-1g + zhǐshí 5-1g + dàhuáng 0g.

(Continued)

TABLE 1.66 *(Continued)*

GMP Herbal Medicines for a Ten-Year-Old Boy with Posterior Urethral Valve

Vesicoureteral reflux (593.7), Hydronephrosis (591):

Liùwèidìhuángwán 5g + sāngpiāoxiāosǎn 5g + bǔzhōngyìqìtāng 5-0g.

Bìxièfēnqīngyǐn 5g + jìshēngshènqìwán 5g + shānyào 1g + wūyào 1g + yìzhìrén 1g.

Shēnlíngbáizhúsǎn 5g + bǔzhōngyìqìtāng 5g + shānyào 1g + qiànshí 1g.

Zhūlíngtāng 5g + jìshēngshènqìwán 5g + báimáogēn 1g + chēqiánzǐ 1g + jīnqiáncǎo 1g.

Liùwèidìhuángwán 5g + zhūlíngtāng 5g + báimáogēn 1g + jīnqiáncǎo 1g.

Báimáogēn 5g + chēqiánzǐ 5-2g + jīnqiáncǎo 5-2g + niúxī 2g.

Chìxiǎodòu 5g + chēqiánzǐ 5g + yìmǔcǎo 5g + dāngguī 2g.

Chìxiǎodòu 5g + báimáogēn 5-3g + chēqiánzǐ 5-3g + huáshí 3-0g + dāngguī 2g + púhuáng 2-0g.

Urinary incontinence (D014549), Renal insufficiency (586), Hypertension (401-405.99), Pyelonephritis (590.80):

Zhūlíngtāng 5g + jìshēngshènqìwán 5g + báimáogēn 2-0g + chēqiánzǐ 2-0g + jīnqiáncǎo 2-0g.

Wǔlíngsǎn 5g + jìshēngshènqìwán 5g.

Sāngpiāoxiāosǎn 5g + liùwèidìhuángwán 2g + yìzhìrén 1g + fùpénzǐ 1g.

Dàhuáng 5g + dānshēn 5g + chēqiánzǐ 5g + wūyào 5g + wǔlíngsǎn 5g + zhībódìhuángwán 5g + sāngpiāoxiāosǎn 5g.

Chìxiǎodòu 5g + dāngguī 5g + chēqiánzǐ 3g + niúxī 2-0g.

Bànxià 5g + fùzǐ 5g + fúlíng 5g + dàhuáng 2g + xìxīn 2g.

Báimáogēn 5g + chìxiǎodòu 5g + chēqiánzǐ 5g + yìmǔcǎo 5g + dāngguī 2g + dàhuáng 0g. Gāncǎo 5g + dàhuáng 2g.

(Wang et al., 2018). Note that Liùwèidìhuángwán, Shēnlíngbáizhúsǎn, Xiāngshāliùjūnzǐtāng, Jìshēngshènqìwán, Wǔlíngsǎn, Zhūlíngtāng, and Zhībódìhuángwán all contain Fúlíng. Báimáogēn (Rhizoma Imperatae) was shown to ameliorate pathological changes of the renal tissue in rats with nephrosis (Chen et al., 2015). Chìxiǎodòu (Semen Phaseoli) herbal-acupuncture at Yingu (KI10) was shown to relieve acute nephritis in rats (Kwak et al., 2013).

1.67 FIBULAR HEMIMELIA

Fibular hemimelia—also called congenital longitudinal deficiency of the fibula; fibular longitudinal meromelia—is a shortening (or missing completely) of the calf bone and toes in one of the feet at birth. Fibular hemimelia results from disruptions during limb development of the fetus in utero with unknown reasons.

Xiāngshāliùjūnzǐtāng, Shēnlíngbáizhúsǎn, Liùjūnzǐtāng, Xiǎojiànzhōngtāng, and Sìjūnzǐtāng were introduced in previous sections to improve digestion. On the other hand, Yùpíngfēngsǎn and Xīnyíqīngfèitāng were introduced earlier for respiratory tract infections. The prescriptions were

TABLE 1.67

GMP Herbal Medicines for a One-Year-Old Boy with Fibular Hemimelia

Fibular hemimelia (OrphaCode: 93323)

A morphological anomaly with a prevalence of ~2 in 100,000

Not applicable

Difficulty walking, Abnormality of fibula morphology

Talipes equinovarus, Genu valgum, Tibial bowing, Shortening of the tibia, Disproportionate prominence of the femoral medial condyle, Limb undergrowth, Abnormal morphology of bones of the lower limbs, Lower limb asymmetry

Proximal femoral focal deficiency, Impairment of activities of daily living, Knee joint hypermobility, Limitation of joint mobility, Joint stiffness, Joint laxity, Toe syndactyly, Talipes equinovalgus, Short toe, Bowing of the legs, Fibular hypoplasia, Short femur, Decreased hip abduction, Arthralgia of the hip, Limited knee flexion/extension, Finger syndactyly, Increased laxity of ankles, Structural foot deformity, Abnormal bone ossification, Oligodactyly, Pain, Hip subluxation

Antenatal

(Continued)

TABLE 1.67 *(Continued)*
GMP Herbal Medicines for a One-Year-Old Boy with Fibular Hemimelia

Difficulty walking (D051346):

Xiāngshāliùjūnzǐtāng 5g + shēnlíngbáizhúsǎn 5-0g + shānzhā 0g + shénqū 0g + màiyá 0g.

Liùjūnzǐtāng 5g + xìngsūyǐnyòukē 5-0g.

Liùjūnzǐtāng 5g + yùpíngfēngsǎn 5-0g.

Shūjīnghuóxuètāng 5g.

Gāncǎo 5g + báizhǐ 5g + shārén 5-3g + huángqín 5-0g + tiānhuā 2-0g + dàhuáng 1-0g.

Talipes equinovarus (754.51):

Xiǎojiànzhōngtāng 5g + shēnlíngbáizhúsǎn 5-0g + shānzhā 1-0g + shénqū 1-0g + màiyá 1-0g.

Xiǎojiànzhōngtāng 5g + yùpíngfēngsǎn 5-0g + shānzhā 1-0g + shénqū 1-0g + màiyá 1-0g.

Xìngsūyǐnyòukē 5g + xīnyíqīngfèitāng 5g.

Sìjūnzǐtāng 5g + shēnlíngbáizhúsǎn 5g + acupuncture.

Yùpíngfēngsǎn 5g + xiāngshāliùjūnzǐtāng 5g + shānzhā 2g + shénqū 2g + màiyá 2g + jīnèijīn 2g.

Báizhǐ 5g + zhìgāncǎo 5g + shārén 5g + dàhuáng 1-0g.

Pain (D010146):

Shēnlíngbáizhúsǎn 5g + xiǎojiànzhōngtāng 5-0g + shānzhā 1g + shénqū 1g + màiyá 1g + jīnèijīn 1-0g.

Xiǎojiànzhōngtāng 5g + shānzhā 1g + shénqū 1g + màiyá 1-0g + jīnèijīn 1-0g.

Xuánshēn 5g + dìhuáng 5g + màiméndōng 5g + hòupò 5-2g + zhǐshí 5-2g + dàhuáng 1-0g.

therefore seen to promote smooth growth of the affected newborns. Xuánshēn (cf. Section 1.3) was found to be one of the six core herbs in TCM for the management of cancer pain in cancer patients (Jo et al., 2022).

1.68 8p23.1 DUPLICATION SYNDROME

8p23.1 duplication syndrome, also called trisomy 8p23.1, is characterized by developmental delay, learning difficulty, facial dysmorphisms, and congenital heart defect. 8p23.1 duplication syndrome is due to duplication of a 4 Mbp interval at p23.1 of chromosome 8 containing five genes. The cause of the chromosome rearrangement resulting in this chromosome structure abnormality is unknown.

TABLE 1.68
GMP Herbal Medicines for a One-Year-Old Infant with 8p23.1 Duplication Syndrome

8p23.1 duplication syndrome (OrphaCode: 251076)

A malformation syndrome with a prevalence of ~2 in 100,000

Not applicable, Unknown

Intellectual disability, Global developmental delay, Language impairment, Highly arched eyebrow, Malformation of the heart and great vessels

Hydronephrosis, Hypertelorism, Long philtrum, Hearing impairment, Wide nose, Deeply set eye, Adrenal insufficiency, Ventricular septal defect, Tetralogy of Fallot, Pulmonic stenosis, Toe syndactyly, Thick vermilion border, Exostoses

Neonatal, Infancy

Intellectual disability (D008607), Language impairment (D007806):

Huángqíwǔwùtāng 5g + shānzhā 1-0g + shénqū 1-0g + màiyá 1-0g + gāncǎo 0g.

Bǔzhōngyìqìtāng 5g + huángqíwǔwùtāng 5-0g.

Huángqí 5g + gāncǎo 4g + báizhǐ 4g + shārén 4g + dàhuáng 0g.

Huángqí 5g + chìsháo 1g + fángfēng 1g + xìxīn 1-0g + huánglián 1-0g + dàhuáng 0g.

Huángqí 5g + báizhú 2g + fángfēng 2g + fúlíng 2-0g.

(Continued)

TABLE 1.68 *(Continued)*

GMP Herbal Medicines for a One-Year-Old Infant with 8p23.1 Duplication Syndrome

Hydronephrosis (591), Hearing impairment (D034381), Deeply set eye (376.5), Ventricular septal defect (745.4), Tetralogy of Fallot (745.2), Exostoses (726.91):

Wǔlíngsǎn 5g + yuèbìjiāshùtāng 5-0g.	Zhìgāncǎo 5g + dàhuáng 1-0g.
Wǔlíngsǎn 5g + jìshēngshènqìwán 5-0g.	Gāncǎo 5g + báizhú 5g + fúlíng 5g + dǎngshēn 5g.
Wǔlíngsǎn 5g + bǔzhōngyìqìtāng 5-0g.	Gāncǎo 5g + huángqín 5g + huánglián 0g.
Zhìgāncǎotāng 5g + zhūlíngtāng 5g.	
Língguìshùgāntāng 5g.	

Huángqíwǔwùtāng was shown to ameliorate neuronal injury in rats after ischemic stroke through modulating M2 microglia polarization and synaptic plasticity (Ou et al., 2023). Huángqí (cf. Section 1.9) was found to significantly recover the clinical symptoms of cerebral infarction patients in a randomized, double-blind, placebo-controlled clinical trial (Li et al., 2023). Use of GMP-concentrated Zhìgāncǎotāng, Jìshēngshènqìwán, Bǔzhōngyìqìtāng, Huángqí, or Dǎngshēn extract granules, together with conventional medicine, was shown to improve the survival of heart failure patients in a retrospective population-based cohort study in Taiwan (Tsai et al., 2017).

1.69 COFFIN-LOWRY SYNDROME

Coffin-Lowry syndrome (CLS) is characterized by intellectual disability, craniofacial abnormalities, and skeletal abnormalities, including a curved spine and prominent breast bone. CLS is caused by mutations in the *RPS6KA3* gene whose products are protein kinases for signaling within cells and regulate other genes important for cell proliferation, differentiation, and apoptosis, i.e., self-destruction.

Qīngwèisǎn was shown to facilitate healing of oral ulcer, ameliorate pathological morphologies of gastric and oral mucosa, and decrease the levels of pro-inflammatory cytokines in diabetic

TABLE 1.69

GMP Herbal Medicines for a Two-Year-Old Child with Coffin-Lowry Syndrome

Coffin-Lowry syndrome (OrphaCode: 192)

A malformation syndrome with a prevalence of ~2 in 100,000

Disease-causing germline mutation(s): ribosomal protein S6 kinase A3 (*RPS6KA3* / Entrez: 6197) at Xp22.12

X-linked dominant

Thick lower lip vermilion, Open mouth, Everted lower lip vermilion, Coarse facial features, Epicanthus, Hypertelorism, Anteverted nares, Downslanted palpebral fissures, Hypodontia, Widely spaced teeth, Pectus excavatum, Pectus carinatum, Abnormal diaphysis morphology, Brachydactyly, Large hands, Tapered finger, Intellectual disability, Hypotonia, Broad finger, Frontal bossing, Neurological speech impairment, Scoliosis, Delayed skeletal maturation, Kyphosis, Abnormal form of the vertebral bodies, Short stature, Craniofacial hyperostosis, Depressed nasal bridge, Joint hyperflexibility, Abnormality of dental morphology, Thick nasal alae, Severe global developmental delay

Wide mouth, Narrow palate, High palate, Microcephaly, Hypoplasia of the maxilla, Protruding ear, Wide nose, Hypertonia, Gait disturbance, Redundant skin, Pes planus, Hypoplastic fingernail, Hyperconvex fingernails, Ventriculomegaly, Progressive spasticity, Narrow iliac wings, Feeding difficulties in infancy, Pseudoepiphyses of the metacarpals, Short distal phalanx of finger, Short metacarpal

Sensorineural hearing impairment, Strabismus, Cataract, Optic atrophy, Delayed eruption of teeth, Seizure, Muscle weakness, Abnormal mitral valve morphology, Abnormal aortic valve morphology, Abnormal tricuspid valve morphology, Cerebral cortical atrophy, Abnormality of neuronal migration, Skeletal muscle atrophy, Advanced eruption of teeth, Aplasia/Hypoplasia of the cerebellum, Aplasia/Hypoplasia of the corpus callosum, Abnormality of retinal pigmentation, Sleep apnea, Death in early adulthood, Self-injurious behavior

Neonatal, Infancy, Childhood

(Continued)

TABLE 1.69 *(Continued)*

GMP Herbal Medicines for a Two-Year-Old Child with Coffin-Lowry Syndrome

Hypodontia (520.0), Intellectual disability (D008607), Neurological speech impairment (D013064):

Yùnǚjiān 5g + gānlùyǐn 5g.

Gānlùyǐn 5g + bǎohéwán 5g.

Qīngwèisǎn 5g + gānlùyǐn 5-0g + gāncǎo 0g.

Yùnǚjiān 5g + qīngwèisǎn 5g + gāncǎo 0g.

Gānlùyǐn 5g + huòxiāngzhèngqìsǎn 5g + yèjiāoténg 3g + hǎipiāoxiāo 3g + chántuì 3g + bózǐrén 2g.

Báizhǐ 5g + gāncǎo 5-4g + shārén 5-3g + tiānhuā 4-0g + dàhuáng 1-0g.

Xuánshēn 5g + yùzhú 5g + dìhuáng 5g + shāshēn 5g + hòupò 5g + zhǐshí 5g + màiméndōng 5g + dàhuáng 1g.

Hypertonia (D009122):

Xiǎohuóluòdān 5g + shūjīnghuóxuètāng 5g + dúhuójìshēngtāng 5-0g + dāngguīniántòngtāng 5-0g.

Xiǎohuóluòdān 5g + shūjīnghuóxuètāng 5g + báisháo 1-0g + yánhúsuǒ 1-0g + acupuncture.

Wūyàoshùnqìsǎn 5g + shūjīnghuóxuètāng 5g + acupuncture.

Tiānnánxīng 5g + bànxià 5g + zhúrú 5g + zhǐqiào 5g.

Tiānnánxīng 5g + bànxià 5g + shíchāngpú 5g + fúlíng 5g + gānjiāng 5-0g.

Dìlóng 5g + táorén 5g + huángbò 5g + dānguī 5g + gāncǎo 2g + guìzhī 2g + máhuáng 2g + sūmù 2g + chuānwū 1g.

Jílí 5g + chántuì 3g.

Sensorineural hearing impairment (389.1), Strabismus (378.7, 378.6, 378.31), Cataract (366.8), Optic atrophy (377.1), Seizure (345.9), Muscle weakness (D018908), Sleep apnea (780.57):

Yìqìcōngmíngtāng 5g + shíchāngpú 1g + yuǎnzhì 1g + xiōngqióng 1-0g + acupuncture.

Xìngsūyǐnyòukē 5g + xīnyíqīngfèitāng 5g + gégēntāng 5g + acupuncture.

Xìngsūyǐnyòukē 5g + xīnyíqīngfèitāng 5g + yínqiàosǎn 5g + acupuncture.

Huángbò 5g + shārén 4-3g + gāncǎo 2g + shānzhīzǐ 2-0g + dìhuáng 2-0g + bǎihé 2-0g + dàndòuchǐ 2-0g + chìsháo 2-0g + ējiāo 2-0g + huángqín 2-0g + jiānghuáng 2-0g + jiāngcán 2-0g + chántuì 2-0g + dàhuáng 0g.

Shíchāngpú 5g + chìsháo 5g + hòupò 5g + jiégěng 5g + táorén 5g + qiàncǎo 5g + zǐcǎogēn 5g + yuǎnzhì 5g + jiānghuáng 5g + jiāngcán 5g + chántuì 5g + dàhuáng 3g.

Huángbò 5g + zhìgāncǎo 3g + shārén 3g + shíchāngpú 2g + yuǎnzhì 2g.

mice subjected to stomach heat syndrome (Shi et al., 2022). Tiānnánxīng (Rhizoma Arisaematis Praeparata) was shown to have a protective effect on febrile seizures in rats through regulating neurotransmitters and suppressing neuroinflammation (Su et al., 2022). The therapeutic effects of Dìlóng (cf. Section 1.22) on neuropathies were reviewed and summarized (Moon & Kim, 2018). Xiǎohuóluòdān "dispels wind, removes dampness, dissolves phlegm, opens collaterals, activates blood, stops pain" and is used for nerve root and plexus disorders, peripheral enthesopathies and allied syndromes, and intervertebral disc disorders (Wang, 2019). Note that Xiǎohuóluòdān contains Dìlóng.

1.70 EBSTEIN MALFORMATION OF THE TRICUSPID VALVE

Ebstein malformation of the tricuspid valve is a congenital heart defect where the valve separating the right upper and lower heart chamber is misplaced or abnormal in such a way that blood goes the wrong way back to the upper chamber while the heart pumps. The cause of most cases of Ebstein malformation of the tricuspid valve is unknown, although maternal ingestion of lithium was associated. Other cases are linked to mutations in the *MYH7* gene whose protein products are found in the heart and skeletal muscles.

Xuèfǔzhúyūtāng was concluded to be effective for the treatment of post-stroke depression, hyperlipidemia, and stable angina pectoris by meta-analysis of randomized controlled trials (Shao et al., 2020; Wang & Qiu, 2019; Yi et al., 2014). Shēngmàiyǐn injection was concluded to be a safe and effective adjuvant treatment of chronic heart failure in a systematic review and meta-analysis of randomized controlled trials (Wang et al., 2020). Sìnìtāng was shown to improve left ventricular

TABLE 1.70

GMP Herbal Medicines for a 13-Year-Old Adolescent with Ebstein Malformation of the Tricuspid Valve

Ebstein malformation of the tricuspid valve (OrphaCode: 1880)

A morphological anomaly with a prevalence of ~1 in 100,000

Disease-causing germline mutation(s): myosin heavy chain 7 (*MYH7* / Entrez: 4625) at 14q11.2

Autosomal dominant, Not applicable

Premature birth, Atrial septal defect, Respiratory insufficiency, Malformation of the heart and great vessels, Ebstein anomaly of the tricuspid valve, Imperforate tricuspid valve, Fatigue

Patent ductus arteriosus, Abnormal cardiac septum morphology, Atrial fibrillation, Arrhythmia, Right bundle branch block, Chest pain

Congestive heart failure, Sudden cardiac death, Cerebral ischemia, Abnormality of the endocardium, Arterial thrombosis

All ages

Ebstein anomaly of the tricuspid valve (746.2), Fatigue (D005221):

Xuèfǔzhúyūtāng 5g + zhìgāncǎotāng 5g + sānqī 1-0g + dānshēn 1-0g.	Zhìgāncǎo 5g + shēngjiāng 2g + fùzǐ 2g + guìzhī 2g + gānjiāng 2g.
Shēngmàiyǐn 5g + xuèfǔzhúyūtāng 5g + chuānqī 1g + dānshēn 1g.	Zhìgāncǎo 5g + gānjiāng 5g + fùzǐ 3g + wúzhūyú 2-0g.
Sìnìtāng 5g + shēngmàiyǐn 5g + zhìgāncǎotāng 5g + dānshēn 2-0g.	Gāncǎo 5g + báizhǐ 5g + shārén 4g + tiānhuā 2g + dàhuáng 0g.
	Huángqí 5g + zhìgāncǎo 3g + wǔwèizǐ 1g + dāngguī 1g.

Patent ductus arteriosus (747.0), Atrial fibrillation (427.31), Right bundle branch block (D002037), Chest pain (D002637):

Shēngmàiyǐn 5g + zhìgāncǎotāng 5-0g + bǔzhōngyìqìtāng 5-0g + sānqī 1-0g + dānshēn 1-0g + yùjīn 1-0g + gāncǎo 1-0g.	Huángqí 5-4g + běishāshēn 5-2g + yùzhú 5-2g + gǔsuìbǔ 5-2g + guìzhī 5-1g + báizhú 5-0g + xùduàn 2g + chuānxiōng 2-0g.
Xuèfǔzhúyūtāng 5g + sānqī 1g + dānshēn 1g + mùxiāng 1g + yùjīn 1g.	Huángqí 5g + dǎngshēn 5g + chuānxiōng 4-2g + guìzhī 4-2g + gǔsuìbǔ 4-2g + xùduàn 4-2g + tiānméndōng 3-0g + báizhú 3-0g + dùzhòng 2-0g.

Congestive heart failure (428, 428.0):

Shēngmàiyǐn 5g + xuèfǔzhúyūtāng 5g + jìshēngshènqìwán 5g + bànxiàxièxīntāng 2-0g + dānshēn 1g + yùjīn 1-0g.	Zhìgāncǎo 5g + guìzhī 5g + táorén 5g + zhǐqiào 3-0g + dàhuáng 1-0g + hónghuā 0g.
Xuèfǔzhúyūtāng 5g + bǔzhōngyìqìtāng 5-0g + zhēnwǔtāng 5-0g + dānshēn 1g + chuānqī 1-0g + yùjīn 1-0g.	Dānshēn 5g + báisháo 5g + dìhuáng 5g + fúlíng 5g + huángjīng 5g + kuǎndōnghuā 3g + báibiǎndòu 3g + qiàncǎo 3g + dāngguī 3g.
Sìnìtāng 5g + gānlùyǐn 5g + shēngmàiyǐn 2g.	

---

systolic function in heart failure after myocardial infarction in rats by inhibiting the excessive activation of Renin-Angiotensin-Aldosterone system (Zhu et al., 2018).

1.71 GORLIN SYNDROME

Gorlin syndrome, also known as basal cell nevus syndrome or nevoid basal cell carcinoma syndrome, is characterized by a predisposition to the development of jaw cysts and multiple basal cell carcinomas, a type of skin cancer that rarely spreads to other parts of the body, on the face, back, and chest. Gorlin syndrome is caused by mutations in the *PTCH1* gene, which is a tumor suppressor gene.

Tiānméndōng (cf. Section 1.48) is yin-nourishing in TCM and has been prescribed to patients with Lung yin or Kidney yin deficiency, manifesting dry cough or tidal fever/spermatorrhea. Báisháo (cf. Section 1.65) was demonstrated to lessen the behavioral loss in mice with Parkinson's disease (Zheng et al., 2019). Shúdìhuáng (Radix Rehmanniae Praeparata) was shown in mice to inhibit renal fibrosis progression (Liu et al., 2022), which, prevalent in end-stage renal diseases, causes renal failure. Both Jìshēngshènqìwán and Liùwèidìhuángwán contain Shúdìhuáng, while

TABLE 1.71

GMP Herbal Medicines for a 25-Year-Old Adult with Gorlin Syndrome

Gorlin syndrome (OrphaCode: 377)

A malformation syndrome with a prevalence of ~1 in 100,000

Disease-causing germline mutation(s) (loss of function): patched 1 (*PTCH1* / Entrez: 5727) at 9q22.32

Disease-causing germline mutation(s) (loss of function): SUFU negative regulator of hedgehog signaling (*SUFU* / Entrez: 51684) at 10q24.32

Disease-causing germline mutation(s): patched 2 (*PTCH2* / Entrez: 8643) at 1p34.1

Autosomal dominant

Melanocytic nevus, Cerebral calcification, Neoplasm, Palmar pits, Plantar pits

Wide nasal bridge, Abnormality of the neck, Brachydactyly, Scoliosis, Vertebral fusion, Vertebral wedging

Cryptorchidism, Hypogonadotrophic hypogonadism, Hydrocephalus, Brachycephaly, Epicanthus, Mandibular prognathia, Hypertelorism, Strabismus, Glaucoma, Telecanthus, Cataract, Iris coloboma, Carious teeth, Arachnodactyly, Intellectual disability, Frontal bossing, Hemivertebrae, Abnormality of the sense of smell

Adolescent, Adult

Cryptorchidism (752.51), Hydrocephalus (331.4, 331.3), Strabismus (378.7, 378.6, 378.31), Glaucoma (365), Cataract (366.8), Carious teeth (521.0, 521.07), Intellectual disability (D008607):

Bǔzhōngyìqìtāng 5g + jìshēngshènqìwán 5g + ròucōngróng 2g + gǒuqǐzǐ 2g + yínyánghuò 2g + tùsīzǐ 2g + fùpénzǐ 2-0g + bǔgǔzhǐ 2-0g.

Liùwèidìhuángwán 5g + bǔzhōngyìqìtāng 5g + mázǐrénwán 2g + bājǐtiān 1g + ròucōngróng 1g + héshǒuwū 1g + acupuncture.

Bǔyánghuánwǔtāng 5g + liùwèidìhuángwán 4g + mázǐrénwán 2-0g + ròucōngróng 1g + gǒuqǐzǐ 1g + bājǐtiān 1-0g + tùsīzǐ 1-0g + fùpénzǐ 1-0g + huángqí 1-0g + nǚzhēnzǐ 1-0g + hǎipiāoxiāo 1-0g.

Tiānméndōng 5g + běishāshēn 5g + dìhuáng 5g + huángqín 5g + huángqí 5-4g + chuānxiōng 4g + yuǎnzhì 4g + dāngguī 4-0g.

Báisháo 5g + dìhuáng 4g + màiméndōng 4g + huǒmárén 2g + mǔlì 2g + zhìgāncǎo 2g + ējiāo 2g + guībǎn 2g + biējiǎ 2g.

Shúdìhuáng 5g + báizhú 4g + fùzǐ 4g + báisháo 3g + fúlíng 3g + báijièzǐ 2g + dǎngshēn 2g + dàhuáng 1g + shēngjiāng 1g + máhuáng 1g + huánglián 0g.

Báizhú 5g + fùzǐ 5g + cháihú 5g + báisháo 4g + fúlíng 4g + tiānhuā 2g + dǎngshēn 2g + dàhuáng 2g + guìzhī 2g + huángqín 2g + gāncǎo 1g + mǔlì 1g + gānjiāng 1g.

Mázǐrénwán contains Báisháo. Bǔzhōngyìqìtāng was demonstrated to reverse chemotherapy-induced renal injury in mice (Xiong et al., 2016). Use of Bǔyánghuánwǔtāng for rehabilitation of ischemic stroke patients was supported in a systematic review and meta-analysis of randomized controlled trials (Gao et al., 2021).

REFERENCES

Akpalaba, R., Agu, C., Adeleke, O. O., & Asonye, C. (2009). Effect of orally administered *Zingiber officinale* on the intra ocular pressure of experimental rabbits. *International Journal of Health Research*, 2(3). https://doi.org/10.4314/ijhr.v2i3.47911

Aksoy, N., Doğan, Y., İriadam, M., Bıtıren, M., Uzer, E., Özgönül, A., & Aksoy, Ş (2012). Protective and therapeutic effects of licorice in rats with acute tubular necrosis. *Journal of Renal Nutrition*, 22(3), 336–343. https://doi.org/10.1053/j.jrn.2011.07.002

Al-Ali, M., Wahbi, S., Twaij, H. A., & Al-Badr, A. (2003). *Tribulus terrestris*: Preliminary study of its diuretic and contractile effects and comparison with *Zea mays*. *Journal of Ethnopharmacology*, 85(2–3), 257–260. https://doi.org/10.1016/s0378-8741(03)00014-x

Bai, Y., Zheng, M., Fu, R., Du, J., Wang, J., Zhang, M., Fan, Y., Huang, X., & Li, Z. (2023). Effect of Massa Medicata Fermentata on the intestinal flora of rats with functional dyspepsia, *Microbial Pathogenesis*, 174, 105927. https://doi.org/10.1016/j.micpath.2022.105927

Cai, Y., Zhang, C., Zhan, L., Cheng, L., Lu, D., Wang, X., Xu, H., Wang, S., Wu, D. C., & Ruan, L. (2019). Anticancer effects of *Gleditsia sinensis* extract in rats transplanted with hepatocellular carcinoma cells. *Oncology Research*, 27(8), 889–899. https://doi.org/10.3727/096504018x15482423944678

Cao, M., Wu, J., Peng, Y., Dong, B., Jiang, Y., Hu, C., Yu, L., & Chen, Z. (2023). Ligustri Lucidi Fructus, a traditional Chinese medicine: Comprehensive review of botany, traditional uses, chemical composition, pharmacology, and toxicity. *Journal of Ethnopharmacology, 301*, 115789. https://doi.org/10.1016/j.jep.2022.115789

Chan, E., Liu, X. X., Guo, D. J., Kwan, Y. W., Leung, G. P., Lee, S. M., & Chan, S. W. (2011). Extract of *Scutellaria baicalensis* Georgi root exerts protection against myocardial ischemia-reperfusion injury in rats. *American Journal of Chinese Medicine, 39*(4), 693–704. https://doi.org/10.1142/s0192415x11009135

Chang, C., Lin, C., Lien, H., Lin, Y., Chen, Y., Chang, F., & Li, Z. (2011). Effects of Ma-Xing-Shi-Gan-Tang on bleomycin-induced lung fibrosis in rats. *Journal of Food and Drug Analysis, 19*(2), 13. https://doi.org/10.38212/2224-6614.2259

Chang, C. T., Wu, S., Lai, Y., Hung, Y., Hsu, C. Y., Chen, H., Chu, C., Cheng, J., Hu, W., & Kuo, C. (2022). The utilization of Chinese herbal products for hyperthyroidism in National Health Insurance System (NHIRD) of Taiwan: A population-based study. *Evidence-Based Complementary and Alternative Medicine, 2022*, 1–11. https://doi.org/10.1155/2022/5500604

Chao, S., Huang, L., & Yen, H. (2003). Pregnancy in premature ovarian failure after therapy using Chinese herbal medicine. *Chang Gung Medical Journal, 26*(6), 449–452. https://pubmed.ncbi.nlm.nih.gov/12956293

Chen, L., Chen, Z., Wang, C., Luo, Y., Luo, Y., Duan, M. Y., & Liu, R. (2015). Protective effects of different extracts of imperatae rhizoma in rats with adriamycin nephrosis and influence on expression of TGF-β1, and NF-κB p65]. *Zhong Yao Cai, 38*(11), 2342–2347. [Article in Chinese] https://pubmed.ncbi.nlm.nih.gov/27356389

Chen, H., Gu, L., Yang, Y., & Guo, J. (2019). GABA and 5-HT systems are involved in the anxiolytic effect of Gan-Mai-Da-Zao decoction. *Frontiers in Neuroscience, 12*. https://doi.org/10.3389/fnins.2018.01043

Chen, H., Lin, Y., & Chen, Y. C. (2016). Identifying Chinese herbal medicine network for treating acne: Implications from a nationwide database. *Journal of Ethnopharmacology, 179*, 1–8. https://doi.org/10.1016/j.jep.2015.12.032

Chen, W., Yao, X., Zhou, C., Zhang, Z., Gui, G., & Lin, B. (2017). Danhong Huayu Koufuye prevents diabetic retinopathy in Streptozotocin-induced diabetic rats via antioxidation and anti-inflammation. *Mediators of Inflammation, 2017*, 1–8. https://doi.org/10.1155/2017/3059763

Chen, Y., Ho, T. S., Lee, P. C., Chang, H. H., Shieh, G. S., Lee, C. I., Hu, W. L., & Hung, Y. C. (2020). Effects of Chinese and Western medicine on patients with dengue fever. *American Journal of Chinese Medicine, 48*(02), 329–340. https://doi.org/10.1142/s0192415x20500160

Chen, Y., Zhang, L., Gong, X., Gong, H., Cheng, R., Qiu, F., Zhong, X., & Huang, Z. (2019). Iridoid glycosides from Radix Scrophulariae attenuates focal cerebral ischemia-reperfusion injury via inhibiting endoplasmic reticulum stress-mediated neuronal apoptosis in rats. *Molecular Medicine Reports*. https://doi.org/10.3892/mmr.2019.10833

Chen, Z., Liu, L., Gao, C., Chen, W., Vong, C. T., Yao, P., Yang, Y., Li, X., Tang, X., Wang, S., & Wang, Y. (2020). Astragali Radix (Huangqi): A promising edible immunomodulatory herbal medicine. *Journal of Ethnopharmacology, 258*, 112895. https://doi.org/10.1016/j.jep.2020.112895

Cheng, H., Chiang, L. C., Jan, Y. M., Chen, G. W., & Li, T. (2011). The efficacy and safety of a Chinese herbal product (Xiao-Feng-San) for the treatment of refractory atopic dermatitis: A randomized, double-blind, placebo-controlled trial. *International Archives of Allergy and Immunology, 155*(2), 141–148. https://doi.org/10.1159/000318861

Cheng, J.-M., Liu, X.-Q., Liu, J.-H., Pan, W., Zhang, X.-M., Hu, L., & Chao, H.-M. (2016). Chi-Ju-Di-Huang-Wan protects rats against retinal ischemia by downregulating matrix metalloproteinase-9 and inhibiting p38 mitogen-activated protein kinase. *Chinese Medicine, 11*(1). https://doi.org/10.1186/s13020-016-0109-6

Cheng, X., Yang, X. R., Cui, H., Zhang, B., Chen, K., Yang, X., Jiao, J., Du, Y., Zhang, Q., Zheng, J., Xie, W., Li, F., & Lei, H. (2023). Chuanxiong improves angiogenesis via the PI3K/AKT/Ras/MAPK pathway based on network pharmacology and DESI-MSI metabolomics. *Frontiers in Pharmacology, 14*. https://doi.org/10.3389/fphar.2023.1135264

Chien, Y. C., Sheu, M. J., Wu, C. H., Lin, W., Chen, Y. Y., Cheng, P. L., & Cheng, H. (2012). A Chinese herbal formula "Gan-Lu-Yin" suppresses vascular smooth muscle cell migration by inhibiting matrix metalloproteinase-2/9 through the PI3K/AKT and ERK signaling pathways. *BMC Complementary and Alternative Medicine, 12*(1). https://doi.org/10.1186/1472-6882-12-137

Chimedtseren, I., Niimi, T., Inoue, M., Furukawa, H., Imura, H., Minami, K., Garidkhuu, A., Gantugs, A., & Natsume, N. (2023). Prevention of cleft lip and/or palate in A/J mice by licorice solution. *Congenital Anomalies, 63*(5), 141–146. https://doi.org/10.1111/cga.12527

Chiu, M., Hsu, Y., Chen, C., Li, T., Chiou, J., Tsai, F., Lin, T., Liao, C., Huang, S., Chou, C., Liang, W., & Lin, Y. (2021). Chinese herbal medicine therapy reduces the risks of overall and Anemia-related mortalities in patients with aplastic anemia: A nationwide retrospective study in Taiwan. *Frontiers in Pharmacology, 12*. https://doi.org/10.3389/fphar.2021.730776

Chiu, S., Lai, Y., Chang, H., Chang, K., Chen, S., Liao, H., Chen, Y., & Chen, Y. (2009). The therapeutic effect of modified Yu Ping Feng San on idiopathic sweating in end-stage cancer patients during hospice care. *Phytotherapy Research*, *23*(3), 363–366. https://doi.org/10.1002/ptr.2633

Cho, M. J., Kim, J. H., Park, C. H., Lee, A. Y., Shin, Y. S., Lee, J. H., Park, C. G., & Cho, E. J. (2018). Comparison of the effect of three licorice varieties on cognitive improvement via an amelioration of neuroinflammation in lipopolysaccharide-induced mice. *Nutrition Research and Practice*, *12*(3), 191. https://doi.org/10.4162/nrp.2018.12.3.191

Chu, H., Zong, Y., Yang, H., Chen, S., Ma, Z., & Li, H. (2023). Effects of Yu-Ping-Feng polysaccharides on animal growth performance and immune function: A review. *Frontiers in Veterinary Science*, *10*. https://doi.org/10.3389/fvets.2023.1260208

Chu, L., Ma, S., Chen, Z., & Cao, W. (2021). Astragalus IV ameliorates the dry eye injury in rabbit model via MUC1-ErbB1 pathway. *European Journal of Histochemistry*, *65*(2). https://doi.org/10.4081/ejh.2021.3198

Cui, Q., Sun, S., Lu, M., Huang, Y., & Lyu, W. (2024). Mechanism of radix trichosanthis in the treatment of lung cancer based on network pharmacology and molecular docking. *International Medicine and Health Guidance News*, *30*(6), 881–889. http://www.imhgn.com/EN/10.3760/cma.j.issn.1007-1245.2024.06.001

Cui, X., Trinh, K., & Wang, Y. (2010). Chinese herbal medicine for chronic neck pain due to cervical degenerative disc disease. *Cochrane Library*. https://doi.org/10.1002/14651858.cd006556.pub2

Dang, Y., Hao, S., Zhou, W., Zhang, L., & Ji, G. (2019). The traditional Chinese formulae Ling-gui-zhu-gan decoction alleviated non-alcoholic fatty liver disease via inhibiting PPP1R3C mediated molecules. *BMC Complementary and Alternative Medicine*, *19*(1). https://doi.org/10.1186/s12906-018-2424-1

Dhaliwal, D. K., Zhou, S. P., Samudre, S. S., Lo, N. J., & Rhee, M. K. (2019). Acupuncture and dry eye: Current perspectives. A double-blinded randomized controlled trial and review of the literature. *Clinical Ophthalmology*, *13*, 731–740. https://doi.org/10.2147/opth.s175321

Durankaya, S. M., Olgun, Y., Aktaş, S., Eskicioğlu, H. E., Gürkan, S., Altun, Z., Mutlu, B., Kolatan, E., Doğan, E., Yılmaz, O., & Kırkım, G. (2021). Effect of Korean red ginseng on noise-induced hearing loss. *Turk Arch Otorhinolaryngol*, *59*(2), 111–117. https://doi.org/10.4274/tao.2021.2021-1-5

El-Fiky, F. K., Abou-Karam, M. A., & Afify, E. A. (1996). Effect of *Luffa aegyptiaca* (seeds) and *Carissa edulis* (leaves) extracts on blood glucose level of normal and streptozotocin diabetic rats. *Journal of Ethnopharmacology*, *50*(1), 43–47. https://doi.org/10.1016/0378-8741(95)01324-5

Fan, Y., Nguyen, T., Piao, C. H., Shin, H. S., Song, C. H., & Chai, O. H. (2022). Fructus Amomi extract attenuates nasal inflammation by restoring Th1/Th2 balance and down-regulation of NF-κB phosphorylation in OVA-induced allergic rhinitis. *Bioscience Reports*, *42*(3). https://doi.org/10.1042/bsr20212681

Fan, Y., & Xiong, X. (2018). Chinese classical formulas Ephedra associated prescriptions for treatment of skin diseases]. *Zhongguo Zhong Yao Za Zhi*, *43*(12), 2431–2434. [Article in Chinese] https://doi.org/10.19540/j.cnki.cjcmm.2018.0074

Fei, Y., Zhao, B., Yin, Q., Qiu, Y., Ren, G., Wang, B., Wang, Y., Fang, W., & Li, Y. (2019). Ma Xing Shi Gan decoction attenuates PM2.5 induced lung injury via inhibiting HMGB1/TLR4/NFKB signal pathway in RAT. *Frontiers in Pharmacology*, *10*. https://doi.org/10.3389/fphar.2019.01361

Feng, C., Chen, R., Wang, K., Wen, C., & Xu, Z. (2021). Chinese traditional medicine (GuiZhi-ShaoYao-ZhiMu decoction) as an add-on medication to methotrexate for rheumatoid arthritis: A meta-analysis of randomized clinical trials. *Therapeutic Advances in Chronic Disease*, *12*, 204062232199343. https://doi.org/10.1177/2040622321993438

Fu, H., Bai, X., Le, L., Tian, D., Gao, H., Qi, L., & Hu, K. (2019). *Eucommia ulmoides* Oliv. leaf extract improves erectile dysfunction in Streptozotocin-induced diabetic rats by protecting endothelial function and ameliorating hypothalamic-pituitary-gonadal axis function. *Evidence-based Complementary and Alternative Medicine*, *2019*, 1–12. https://doi.org/10.1155/2019/1782953

Gao, J., Yang, X., & Yin, W. (2016). From Traditional usage to pharmacological evidence: A systematic mini-review of Spina Gleditsiae. *Evidence-based Complementary and Alternative Medicine*, *2016*, 1–6. https://doi.org/10.1155/2016/3898957

Gao, L., Xiao, Z., Jia, C., & Wang, W. (2021). Effect of Buyang Huanwu decoction for the rehabilitation of ischemic stroke patients: A meta-analysis of randomized controlled trials. *Health and Quality of Life Outcomes*, *19*(1). https://doi.org/10.1186/s12955-021-01728-6

Ghorashi, M., Rezaee, M. A., Rezaie, M. J., Mohammadi, M., Jalili, A., & Rahmani, M. (2017). The attenuating effect of aqueous extract of licorice on bleomycin-induced pulmonary fibrosis in mice. *Food and Agricultural Immunology*, *28*(1), 67–77. https://doi.org/10.1080/09540105.2016.1203294

Gu, M., Zhang, Y., Fan, S., Ding, X., & Ji, G. (2013). Extracts of rhizoma polygonati odorati prevent high-fat diet-induced metabolic disorders in C57BL/6 mice. *PloS One*, *8*(11), e81724. https://doi.org/10.1371/journal.pone.0081724

Guo, H., Luo, H., Yuan, H., Xia, Y., Pan, S., Huang, X., Lü, Y., Liu, X., Keller, E. T., Sun, D., Deng, J., & Zhang, J. (2017). Litchi seed extracts diminish prostate cancer progression via induction of apoptosis and attenuation of EMT through Akt/GSK-3β signaling. *Scientific Reports*, *7*(1). https://doi.org/10.1038/srep41656

Guo, K., Yan, Y., Zeng, C., Shen, L., He, Y., & Tan, Z. (2022). Study on Baohe pills regulating intestinal microecology and treating diarrhea of high-fat and high-protein diet mice. *BioMed Research International*, *2022*, 1–8. https://doi.org/10.1155/2022/6891179

Han, P., & Wang, Y. (2019). Effect of modified Sijunzi decoction on pulmonary function and inflammation indexes in children with ventilator-associated severe pneumonia. *Journal of Clinical Medicine in Practice*, (3), 70–72. https://jcmp.yzu.edu.cn/en/article/doi/10.7619/jcmp.201903019

Hayasaka, S., Kodama, T., & Ohira, A. (2012). Traditional Japanese herbal (Kampo) medicines and treatment of ocular diseases: A review. *American Journal of Chinese Medicine*, *40*(05), 887–904. https://doi.org/10.1142/s0192415x12500668

He, A., Wang, W., Yang, X., & Niu, X. (2021). A network pharmacology approach to explore the mechanisms of Artemisiae scopariae Herba for the treatment of chronic hepatitis B. *Evidence-based Complementary and Alternative Medicine*, *2021*, 1–10. https://doi.org/10.1155/2021/6614039

Ho, Y., Wang, C., Hsu, W., Tseng, T., Hsu, C., Kao, M., & Tsai, Y. (2007). Psychoimmunological effects of dioscorea in ovariectomized rats: Role of anxiety level. *Annals of General Psychiatry*, *6*(1). https://doi.org/10.1186/1744-859x-6-21

Hsieh, Y., Yen, M. H., Chiang, Y. W., Yeh, C. F., Chiang, L. C., Shieh, D. E., Yeh, I., & Chang, J. S. (2016). Gan-Lu-Siao-Du-yin, a prescription of traditional Chinese medicine, inhibited enterovirus 71 replication, translation, and virus-induced cell apoptosis. *Journal of Ethnopharmacology*, *185*, 132–139. https://doi.org/10.1016/j.jep.2016.03.034

Hu, Q., Zhu, J., Ji, J., Wei, L., Miao, M., & Ji, H. (2013). Fructus Gardenia extract ameliorates oxonate-induced hyperuricemia with renal dysfunction in mice by regulating organic ion transporters and mOIT3. *Molecules*, *18*(8), 8976–8993. https://doi.org/10.3390/molecules18088976

Huang, X., Chen, C. X., Zhang, X. M., Liu, Y., Xian, W., & Li, Y. M. (2012). Effects of ethanolic extract from Radix Scrophulariae on ventricular remodeling in rats. *Phytomedicine*, *19*(3–4), 193–205. https://doi.org/10.1016/j.phymed.2011.09.079

Huang, K., Su, Y., Sun, M., & Huang, S. (2018). Chinese herbal medicine improves the long-term survival rate of patients with chronic kidney disease in Taiwan: A nationwide retrospective population-based cohort study. *Frontiers in Pharmacology*, *9*. https://doi.org/10.3389/fphar.2018.01117

Ilkhanizadeh, B., Shirpoor, A., Ansari, M. H. K., Nemati, S., & Rasmi, Y. (2016). Protective effects of ginger (*Zingiber officinale*) extract against diabetes-induced heart abnormality in rats. *Diabetes & Metabolism Journal*, *40*(1), 46. https://doi.org/10.4093/dmj.2016.40.1.46

Inagaki, Y., Kido, J., Nishikawa, Y., Kido, R., Sakamoto, E., Bando, M., Naruishi, K., Nagata, T., & Yumoto, H. (2021). Gan-Lu-Yin (Kanroin), traditional Chinese herbal extracts, reduces osteoclast differentiation in vitro and prevents alveolar bone resorption in rat experimental periodontitis. *Journal of Clinical Medicine*, *10*(3), 386. https://doi.org/10.3390/jcm10030386

Ji, H., Kang, N., Chen, T., Lv, L., Ma, X., Wang, F., & Tang, X. (2019). Shen-ling-bai-zhu-san, a spleen-tonifying Chinese herbal formula, alleviates lactose-induced chronic diarrhea in rats. *Journal of Ethnopharmacology*, *231*, 355–362. https://doi.org/10.1016/j.jep.2018.07.031

Jia, J., Li, X., Ren, X., Liu, X., Wang, Y., Dong, Y., Wang, X., Sun, S., Xu, X., Li, X., Song, R., Ma, J., Yu, A., Fan, Q., Wei, J., Yan, X., Wang, X., & She, G. (2021). Sparganii Rhizoma: A review of traditional clinical application, processing, phytochemistry, pharmacology, and toxicity. *Journal of Ethnopharmacology*, *268*, 113571. https://doi.org/10.1016/j.jep.2020.113571

Jo, H., Seo, J., Choi, S. K., & Lee, D. (2022). East Asian Herbal medicine to reduce primary pain and adverse events in cancer patients: A systematic review and meta-analysis with association rule mining to identify core herb combination. *Frontiers in Pharmacology*, *12*. https://doi.org/10.3389/fphar.2021.800571

Kim, H. R., Lee, Y., Kim, T., Lim, R., Hwang, D. Y., Moffat, J. J., Kim, S., Seo, J., & Ka, M. (2020). Asparagus cochinchinensis extract ameliorates menopausal depression in ovariectomized rats under chronic unpredictable mild stress. *BMC Complementary Medicine and Therapies*, *20*(1). https://doi.org/10.1186/s12906-020-03121-0

Kim, J. (2012). Cardiovascular diseases and *Panax ginseng*: A review on molecular mechanisms and medical applications. *Journal of Ginseng Research*, *36*(1), 16–26. https://doi.org/10.5142/jgr.2012.36.1.16

Kim, S., Yook, T. H., & Kim, J. (2017). *Rehmanniae Radix*, an effective treatment for patients with various inflammatory and metabolic diseases: Results from a review of Korean publications. *Journal of Pharmacopuncture*, *20*(2), 81–88. https://doi.org/10.3831/kpi.2017.20.010

Kim, Y. J., Jeon, W., Hwang, Y., & Lee, M. (2021). Inhibitory effects of Gyeji-Tang on MMP-9 activity and the expression of adhesion molecules in IL-4- and TNF-A-stimulated BEAS-2B cells. *Plants, 10*(5), 951. https://doi.org/10.3390/plants10050951

Kimura, Y., Miwa, H., Furukawa, M., & Mizukami, Y. (1996). Relapsing polychondritis presented as inner ear involvement. *Journal of Laryngology & Otology, 110*(2), 154–157. https://doi.org/10.1017/s002221510013302x

Kuboyama, T., Hirotsu, K., Arai, T., Yamasaki, H., & Tohda, C. (2017). Polygalae radix extract prevents axonal degeneration and memory deficits in a transgenic mouse model of Alzheimer's disease. *Frontiers in Pharmacology, 8*. https://doi.org/10.3389/fphar.2017.00805

Kwak, K. I., Kang, J. H., & Lee, H. (2013). The effect of phaseoli semen herbal-acupuncture at KI10 in lipopolysaccharide induced acute nephritis in rats. *Journal of Acupuncture Research, 30*(3), 61–73. https://www.e-jar.org/journal/view.html?pn=vol&uid=2051

Kwon, Y., Son, D., Chung, T., & Lee, Y. (2020). A review of the pharmacological efficacy and safety of licorice root from corroborative clinical trial findings. *Journal of Medicinal Food, 23*(1), 12–20. https://doi.org/10.1089/jmf.2019.4459

Lalert, L., Kruevaisayawan, H., Amatyakul, P., Ingkaninan, K., & Khongsombat, O. (2018). Neuroprotective effect of Asparagus racemosus root extract via the enhancement of brain-derived neurotrophic factor and estrogen receptor in ovariectomized rats. *Journal of Ethnopharmacology, 225*, 336–341. https://doi.org/10.1016/j.jep.2018.07.014

Lam, K. Y. C., Wu, Q., Hu, W., Yao, P., Wang, H., Dong, T. T. X., & Tsim, K. W. (2019). Asarones from Acori Tatarinowii Rhizoma stimulate expression and secretion of neurotrophic factors in cultured astrocytes. *Neuroscience Letters, 707*, 134308. https://doi.org/10.1016/j.neulet.2019.134308

Lee, B. B., Shim, I. S., Lee, H. J., & Hahm, D. H. (2011). *Rehmannia glutinosa* ameliorates scopolamine-induced learning and memory impairment in rats. *Journal of Microbiology and Biotechnology, 21*(8), 874–883. https://doi.org/10.4014/jmb.1104.04012

Lee, G., Chang, C., Wāng, Y., Ma, R., Chen, C., Hsue, Y., Liao, N., & Chang, H. (2021). Chinese herbal medicine SS-1 inhibits T cell activation and abrogates TH responses in Sjögren's syndrome. *Journal of the Formosan Medical Association, 120*(1), 651–659. https://doi.org/10.1016/j.jfma.2020.07.024

Lee, H., Kim, H., Lee, D., Choi, B., & Yang, S. H. (2021). *Scrophulariae radix*: An overview of its biological activities and nutraceutical and pharmaceutical applications. *Molecules, 26*(17), 5250. https://doi.org/10.3390/molecules26175250

Lee, H. J., Spandidos, D. A., Tsatsakis, A., Marginǎ, D., Izotov, B. N., & Yang, S. H. (2019). Neuroprotective effects of *Scrophularia buergeriana* extract against glutamate-induced toxicity in SH-SY5Y cells. *International Journal of Molecular Medicine*. https://doi.org/10.3892/ijmm.2019.4139

Lee, J., & Hyun, M. K. (2018). Herbal medicine (Gegen-decoction) for treating cervical spondylosis: A systematic review and meta-analysis of randomized controlled trials. *European Journal of Integrative Medicine, 18*, 52–58. https://doi.org/10.1016/j.eujim.2017.12.005

Lee, K., Shin, M. S., Ham, I., & Choi, H. (2015). Investigation of the mechanisms of Angelica dahurica root extract-induced vasorelaxation in isolated rat aortic rings. *BMC Complementary and Alternative Medicine, 15*(1). https://doi.org/10.1186/s12906-015-0889-8

Lee, Y., Wang, T., Chen, S., Lin, H., & Tsai, M. (2017). Management of viral oral ulcers in children using Chinese herbal medicine: A report of two cases. *Complementary Therapies in Medicine, 32*, 61–65. https://doi.org/10.1016/j.ctim.2017.04.001

Li, C., Gao, X., Gao, X., Lv, J., Bian, X., Lv, J., Sun, J., Luo, G., & Zhang, H. (2021). Effects of medicine food Fructus *Gardeniae* on liver and kidney functions after oral administration to rats for 12 weeks. *Journal of Food Biochemistry, 45*(7). https://doi.org/10.1111/jfbc.13752

Li, J., Zhang, Y., Liu, S., Li, W., Sun, Y., Cao, H., Wang, S., & Meng, J. (2023). A network pharmacology integrated pharmacokinetics strategy to investigate the pharmacological mechanism of absorbed components from crude and processed Zingiberis Rhizoma on deficiency-cold and hemorrhagic syndrome. *Journal of Ethnopharmacology, 301*, 115754. https://doi.org/10.1016/j.jep.2022.115754

Li, N., Wang, J., Ma, J., Gu, Z. Z., Jiang, C., Yu, L., & Fu, X. (2015). Neuroprotective effects of Cistanches Herba therapy on patients with moderate Alzheimer's disease. *Evidence-based Complementary and Alternative Medicine, 2015*, 1–12. https://doi.org/10.1155/2015/103985

Li, R., Sakwiwatkul, K., Li, Y., & Hu, S. (2009). Enhancement of the immune responses to vaccination against foot-and-mouth disease in mice by oral administration of an extract made from Rhizoma Atractylodis Macrocephalae (RAM). *Vaccine, 27*(15), 2094–2098. https://doi.org/10.1016/j.vaccine.2009.02.002

Li, T., Cheng, S., Lin, X., Peng, L., & Shao, M. (2023). Yue-bi-tang attenuates adriamycin-induced nephropathy edema through decreasing renal microvascular permeability via inhibition of the Cav-1/eNOS pathway. *Frontiers in Pharmacology, 14*. https://doi.org/10.3389/fphar.2023.1138900

Li, X., Cui, J., Yu, Y., Li, W., Hou, Y., Wang, X., Qin, D., Zhao, C., Yao, X., Zhao, J., & Pei, G. (2016). Traditional Chinese nootropic medicine *Radix Polygalae* and its active constituent onjisaponin B reduce B-amyloid production and improve cognitive impairments. *PloS One, 11*(3), e0151147. https://doi.org/10.1371/journal.pone.0151147

Li, Y., Wang, D., Guo, R. S., Ma, B., Miao, L., Sun, M., He, L., Liu, L., Pan, Y., Ren, J., & Liu, J. (2023). Neuroprotective effect of Astragali Radix on cerebral infarction based on proteomics. *Frontiers in Pharmacology, 14*. https://doi.org/10.3389/fphar.2023.1162134

Li, Y., Xiang, M., Rong, R., Hou, L., Zhang, C., & Zhu, Q. (2017). [Inhibitory effect of Glehniae Radix petroleum ether part on TGF-β1-induced epithelial mesenchymal transition in A549 cells]. *Zhongguo Zhong Yao Za Zhi, 42*(9), 1736–1741. [Article in Chinese] https://doi.org/10.19540/j.cnki.cjcmm.20170222.008

Li, Z., Ren, L., Gu, R., Zhou, C., Tong, X., & Hu, J. (2022). The efficacy and safety of Wulingsan modified formulas for chronic heart failure patients: A systematic review and meta-analysis. *Journal of Thoracic Disease, 14*(4), 1232–1242. https://doi.org/10.21037/jtd-22-261

Liao, H., Yen, H., Muo, C., Lee, Y., Wu, M., Chou, L., Sun, M., & Chang, T. (2017). Complementary traditional Chinese medicine use in children with cerebral palsy: A nationwide retrospective cohort study in Taiwan. *BMC Complementary and Alternative Medicine, 17*(1). https://doi.org/10.1186/s12906-017-1668-5

Liew, W. K., Loh, W., Chiang, W. C., Goh, A., Chay, O. M., & Kidon, M. (2015). Pilot study of the use of Yin Qiao San in children with conventional antipyretic hypersensitivity. *Asia Pacific Allergy, 5*(4), 222–229. https://doi.org/10.5415/apallergy.2015.5.4.222

Lim, C., Lim, S., Moon, S. Y., & Cho, S. (2024). Neuroprotective effects of methanolic extract from Chuanxiong Rhizoma in mice with middle cerebral artery occlusion-induced ischemic stroke: Suppression of astrocyte- and microglia-related inflammatory response. *BMC Complementary Medicine and Therapies, 24*(1). https://doi.org/10.1186/s12906-024-04454-w

Lin, C., Chiu, H. E., Wu, S., Tseng, S., Wu, T., Hung, Y., Hsu, C. Y., Chen, H., Hsu, S., Kuo, C., & Hu, W. (2021). Chinese Herbal products for non-motor symptoms of Parkinson's disease in Taiwan: A population-based study. *Frontiers in Pharmacology, 11*. https://doi.org/10.3389/fphar.2020.615657

Liu, C. H., Lin, Y. W., Tang, N. Y., Liu, H. J., Huang, C. Y., & Hsieh, C. L. (2012). Effect of oral administration of *Pheretima aspergillum* (earthworm) in rats with cerebral infarction induced by middle-cerebral artery occlusion. *African Journal of Traditional Complementary and Alternative Medicines, 10*(1). https://doi.org/10.4314/ajtcam.v10i1.11

Liu, F. C., Pan, C., Lai, M. T., Chang, S., Chung, J. G., & Wu, C. H. (2013). Gan-Lu-Yin inhibits proliferation and migration of murine WEHI-3 leukemia cells and tumor growth in BALB/C allograft tumor model. *Evidence-based Complementary and Alternative Medicine, 2013*, 1–13. https://doi.org/10.1155/2013/684071

Liu, J., Peter, K., Shi, D., Zhang, L., Dong, G., Zhang, D., Breiteneder, H., Jakowitsch, J., & Ma, Y. (2014). Traditional formula, modern application: Chinese Medicine formula Sini Tang improves early ventricular remodeling and cardiac function after myocardial infarction in rats. *Evidence-based Complementary and Alternative Medicine, 2014*, 1–10. https://doi.org/10.1155/2014/141938

Liu, X., Xu, H., Zang, Y., Liu, W., & Sun, X. (2022). Radix Rehmannia Glutinosa inhibits the development of renal fibrosis by regulating miR-122-5p/PKM axis. *Am J Transl Res, 14*(1), 103–119. https://pubmed.ncbi.nlm.nih.gov/35173832

Liu, Y. C., Liu, G. Y., & Liu, R. L. (1995). [Effects of *Poria cocos* on ototoxicity induced by kanamycin in guinea-pigs]. *Zhongguo Zhong Xi Yi Jie He Za Zhi, 15*(7), 422–423. [Article in Chinese] https://pubmed.ncbi.nlm.nih.gov/7580066

López-Franco, Ó., Morin, J., Cortés-Sol, A., Molina-Jiménez, T., Del Moral, D. I., Flores-Muñoz, M., Roldán-Roldán, G., Juárez-Portilla, C., & Zepeda, R. C. (2021). Cognitive impairment after resolution of hepatic encephalopathy: A systematic review and meta-analysis. *Frontiers in Neuroscience, 15*. https://doi.org/10.3389/fnins.2021.579263

Luo, H., Li, Q., Flower, A., Lewith, G., & Liu, J. (2012). Comparison of effectiveness and safety between granules and decoction of Chinese herbal medicine: A systematic review of randomized clinical trials. *Journal of Ethnopharmacology, 140*(3), 555–567. https://doi.org/10.1016/j.jep.2012.01.031

Makinodan, M., Yamauchi, T., Tatsumi, K., Okuda, H., Noriyama, Y., Sadamatsu, M., Kishimoto, T., & Wanaka, A. (2009). Yi-Gan San restores behavioral alterations and a decrease of brain glutathione level in a mouse model of schizophrenia. *Journal of Brain Disease, 1*, 1–6. https://doi.org/10.4137/jcnsd.s2255

Meng, X., Liu, X., Ning, C., Ma, J., Zhang, X., Su, X., Ren, K., & Zhang, S. (2021). [Rehmanniae Radix and *Rehmanniae Radix Praeparata* improve diabetes induced by high-fat diet coupled with streptozotocin in mice through AMPK-mediated NF-κB/NLRP3 signaling pathway]. *China Journal of Chinese Materia Medica*, (24), 5627–5640. https://pesquisa.bvsalud.org/portal/resource/pt/wpr-921747

Meng, X., Xie, W., Qiao, X., Liang, T., Xu, X., Sun, G., & Sun, X. (2018). Neuroprotective effects of radix scrophulariae on cerebral ischemia and reperfusion injury via MAPK pathways. *Molecules*, *23*(9), 2401. https://doi.org/10.3390/molecules23092401

Miyaoka, T., Furuya, M., Liaury, K., Wake, R., Kimura, K., Nagahama, M., Kawano, K., Ieda, M., Tsuchie, K., & Horiguchi, J. (2011). Yi-Gan San for treatment of Charles Bonnet syndrome (Visual hallucination due to vision loss). *Clinical Neuropharmacology*, *34*(1), 24–27. https://doi.org/10.1097/wnf.0b013e318 206785a

Miyaoka, T., Furuya, M., Yasuda, H., Hayashia, M., Inagaki, T., & Horiguchi, J. (2008). Yi-gan san for the treatment of borderline personality disorder: An open-label study. *Progress in Neuro-psychopharmacology & Biological Psychiatry*, *32*(1), 150–154. https://doi.org/10.1016/j.pnpbp.2007.07.026

Moon, B. C., & Kim, J. S. (2018). The potential of earthworm and its components as a therapeutic agent for neuronal damage. *Journal of Biomedical and Translational Research*, *19*(3), 58–64. https://doi.org/10.12729/jbtr.2018.19.3.058

Moon, M., Huh, E., Lee, W., Song, E. J., Hwang, D., Lee, T. H., & Oh, M. S. (2017). Coptidis rhizoma prevents heat stress-induced brain damage and cognitive impairment in mice. *Nutrients*, *9*(10), 1057. https://doi.org/10.3390/nu9101057

Murayama, C., Wang, C. C., Michihara, S., & Norimoto, H. (2014). Pharmacological effects of "Jutsu" (Atractylodis rhizome and Atractylodis lanceae rhizome) on 1-(2,5-dimethoxy-4-iodophenyl)-2-aminopropane (DOI)-induced head twitch response in mice (I). *Molecules*, *19*(9), 14979–14986. https://doi.org/10.3390/molecules190914979

Nabil, W. N. N., Zhou, W., Shergis, J. L., Mansu, S., Xue, C. C., & Zhang, A. L. (2015). Management of respiratory disorders in a Chinese medicine teaching clinic in Australia: Review of clinical records. *Chinese Medicine*, *10*(1). https://doi.org/10.1186/s13020-015-0063-8

Ojha, S., Sharma, C., Golechha, M., Bhatia, J., Kumari, S., & Arya, D. S. (2015). Licorice treatment prevents oxidative stress, restores cardiac function, and salvages myocardium in rat model of myocardial injury. *Toxicology and Industrial Health*, *31*(2), 140–152. https://doi.org/10.1177/0748233713491800

Okada, K., Ishimoto, S., Fujimaki, Y., & Yamasoba, T. (2012). Trial of Chinese medicine Wu-Ling-San for acute low-tone hearing loss. *ORL*, *74*(3), 158–163. https://doi.org/10.1159/000337819

Ou, Z., Zhao, M., Xu, Y., Wu, Y., Qin, L., Li, F., Xu, H., & Chen, J. (2023). Huangqi Guizhi Wuwu decoction promotes M2 microglia polarization and synaptic plasticity via Sirt1/NF-κB/NLRP3 pathway in MCAO rats. *Aging*, *15*(19), 10031–10056. https://doi.org/10.18632/aging.204989

Park, W., Yoo, D. M., & So, J. N. (2014). Effects of Ukgansan (Yokukansan in Japanese, Yigansan in Chinese) on the locomotor velocity and glutamate-induce paroxysm in planarian. *KSBB Journal*, *29*(1), 67–71. https://doi.org/10.7841/ksbbj.2014.29.1.67

Qiu, J., Zheng, B., Zhou, H., Ye, C., Shi, M., Shi, S., & Wu, S. (2022). Network pharmacology, molecular docking, and molecular dynamic-based investigation on the mechanism of compound chrysanthemum in the treatment of asthenopia. *Computational and Mathematical Methods in Medicine*, *2022*, 1–18. https://doi.org/10.1155/2022/3444277

Sahni, D., Verma, P., Bhagat, S., & Sharma, V. (2022). Hearing assessment in patients of allergic rhinitis: A study on 200 subjects. *Indian Journal of Otolaryngology and Head and Neck Surgery*, *74*(S1), 125–131. https://doi.org/10.1007/s12070-020-01890-1

Sakata, M., & Egami, H. (2021). Successful treatment of orthostatic dysregulation with Japanese (Kampo) herbal medicine ryokeijutsukanto. *Explore*, *17*(6), 521–524. https://doi.org/10.1016/j.explore.2020.04.003

Sato, Y., Yoshioka, E., Saijo, Y., Miyamoto, T., Azuma, H., Tanahashi, Y., Ito, Y., Kobayashi, S., Minatoya, M., Bamai, Y. A., Yamazaki, K., Ito, S., Miyashita, C., Araki, A., & Kishi, R. (2022). Lower respiratory tract infections and orofacial clefts: A prospective cohort study from the Japan environment and Children's study. *Journal of Epidemiology*, *32*(6), 270–276. https://doi.org/10.2188/jea.je20200438

Shah, S. L., Wahid, F., Khan, N. A., Farooq, U., Shah, A. J., Tareen, S., Ahmad, F., & Khan, T. (2018). Inhibitory effects of *Glycyrrhiza glabra* and its major constituent glycyrrhizin on inflammation-associated corneal neovascularization. *Evidence-based Complementary and Alternative Medicine*, *2018*, 1–8. https://doi.org/10.1155/2018/8438101

Shao, J., Zhou, L., Shao, T., Ding, M., & Jin, Z. (2020). Effectiveness and safety of the Xuefu Zhuyu Tang for post-stroke depression: A systematic review and meta-analysis. *European Journal of Integrative Medicine*, *37*, 101150. https://doi.org/10.1016/j.eujim.2020.101150

Shi, L., An, Y., Cheng, L., Li, Y., Li, H., Wang, C., Lv, Y., Duan, Y., Dai, H., He, C., Zhang, H., Huang, Y., Fu, W., Wang, S., Zhao, B., Wang, Y., & Zhao, Y. (2022). Qingwei San treats oral ulcer subjected to stomach heat syndrome in db/db mice by targeting TLR4/MyD88/NF-κB pathway. *Chinese Medicine*, *17*(1). https://doi.org/10.1186/s13020-021-00565-5

Shih, H., Kaung-Hsiung, C., Chen, F., Chen, C., Chen, S., Lin, Y., & Shibuya, T. (2000). Anti-aging effects of the traditional Chinese medicine Bu-Zhong-Yi-Qi-Tang in mice. *American Journal of Chinese Medicine*, *28*(01), 77–86. https://doi.org/10.1142/s0192415x00000106

Shimizu, I. (2000). Sho-saiko-to: Japanese Herbal medicine for protection against hepatic fibrosis and carcinoma. *Journal of Gastroenterology and Hepatology*, *15*(s1), 84–90. https://doi.org/10.1046/j.1440-1746.2000.02138.x

Su, F., Bai, C., Luo, Y., Zhang, W., Cui, N., Wang, Y., Sun, Y., Zhu, W., Zhao, M., Yang, B., Kuang, H., & Wang, Q. (2022). Cattle bile arisaema aqueous extracts protect against febrile seizures in rats through regulating neurotransmitters and suppressing neuroinflammation. *Frontiers in Pharmacology*, *13*. https://doi.org/10.3389/fphar.2022.889055

Su, S., Ho, T., & Yang, C. (2021). Retrospective evaluation of the curative effect of traditional Chinese medicine on dry eye disease. *Tzu-chi Medical Journal*, *33*(4), 365. https://doi.org/10.4103/tcmj.tcmj_281_20

Takahashi, N., Sato, K., Kiyota, N., Tsuda, S., Murayama, N., & Nakazawa, T. (2023). A ginger extract improves ocular blood flow in rats with endothelin-induced retinal blood flow dysfunction. *Scientific Reports*, *13*(1). https://doi.org/10.1038/s41598-023-49598-w

Tian, C., Chang, Y. C., Liu, X., Zhang, Z., Guo, Y., Lan, Z., Zhang, P., & Liu, M. (2020). Anti-inflammatory activity in vitro, extractive process and HPLC-MS characterization of total saponins extract from *Tribulus terrestris* L. fruits. *Industrial Crops and Products*, *150*, 112343. https://doi.org/10.1016/j.indcrop.2020.112343

Tian, D., Yang, Y., Meng, Y., Han, Z., Wei, M., Zhang, H., Jia, H., & Zou, Z. (2020). Anti-inflammatory chemical constituents of Flos Chrysanthemi Indici determined by UPLC-MS/MS integrated with network pharmacology. *Food & Function*, *11*(7), 6340–6351. https://doi.org/10.1039/d0fo01000f

Tsai, F. J., Ho, T. J., Cheng, C. F., Shiao, Y. T., Chien, W. K., Chen, J. H., Liu, X., Tsang, H., Lin, T. H., Liao, C., Huang, S., Li, J. P., Lin, C. W., Lin, J. G., Lan, Y. C., Liu, Y. H., Hung, C. H., Lin, J., Lin, C., Lai, C. H., Liang, W. M., & Lin, Y. (2017). Characteristics of Chinese herbal medicine usage in ischemic heart disease patients among type 2 diabetes and their protection against hydrogen peroxide-mediated apoptosis in H9C2 cardiomyoblasts. *Oncotarget*, *8*(9), 15470–15489. https://doi.org/10.18632/oncotarget.14657

Tsai, F. J., Li, T. M., Ko, C. H., Cheng, C. F., Ho, T. J., Liu, X., Tsang, H., Lin, T. H., Liao, C., Li, J. P., Huang, S., Lin, J., Lin, C., Liang, W. M., & Lin, Y. (2017). Effects of Chinese herbal medicines on the occurrence of diabetic retinopathy in type 2 diabetes patients and protection of ARPE-19 retina cells by inhibiting oxidative stress. *Oncotarget*, *8*(38), 63528–63550. https://doi.org/10.18632/oncotarget.18846

Tsai, M., Hu, W., Chiang, J., Huang, Y., Chen, S., Hung, Y., & Chen, Y. (2017). Improved medical expenditure and survival with integration of traditional Chinese medicine treatment in patients with heart failure: A nationwide population-based cohort study. *Oncotarget*, *8*(52), 90465–90476. https://doi.org/10.18632/oncotarget.20063

Vahedi-Mazdabadi, Y., Karimpour-Razkenari, E., Akbarzadeh, T., Lotfian, H., Toushih, M., Roshanravan, N., Saeedi, M., & Ostadrahimi, A. (2020). Anti-cholinesterase and neuroprotective activities of sweet and bitter apricot kernels (Prunus armeniaca L.). *Iran J Pharm Res*, *19*(4), 216–224. https://doi.org/10.22037/ijpr.2019.15514.13139

Van Gelderen, C., Bijlsma, J. A., Van Dokkum, W., & Savelkoul, T. J. F. (2000). Glycyrrhizic acid: The assessment of a no effect level. *Human & Experimental Toxicology*, *19*(8), 434–439. https://doi.org/10.1191/096032700682694251

Wang, H., Huang, G., Zhou, S., Lixian, L., Ding, T., Gui, Z., & Chu, W. (2018). Liuwei Dihuang exhibits anti-diabetic effects through inhibiting α-amylase and α-glucosidase. *Med Sci (Paris)*, *34*, 4–7. https://doi.org/10.1051/medsci/201834f101

Wang, R., Chen, Y., Wang, Z., Cao, B., Du, J., Deng, T., Yang, M., & Han, J. (2023). Antidepressant effect of licorice total flavonoids and liquiritin: A review. *Heliyon*, *9*(11), e22251. https://doi.org/10.1016/j.heliyon.2023.e22251

Wang, S.-C. (2019). Therapeutic classes of CHEG formulas. In S.-C. Wang, *Clinical herbal prescriptions: Principles and practices of herbal formulations from deep learning health insurance herbal prescription big data* (pp. 16–89). World Scientific Publishing. https://doi.org/10.1142/11211

Wang, S.-C. (2020). Modern therapeutic uses of CHEG herbs and herb pairs. In S.-C. Wang, *Veterinary herbal pharmacopoeia* (pp. 35–233). Nova Science Publishers. https://doi.org/10.52305/GHTR1903

Wang, S. D., Li, L., Chen, C. L., Lee, S. C., Lin, C. C., Wang, J. Y., & Kao, S. T. (2012). Xiao-Qing-Long-Tang attenuates allergic airway inflammation and remodeling in repetitive dermatogoides pteronyssinus challenged chronic asthmatic mice model. *Journal of Ethnopharmacology*, *142*(2), 531–538. https://doi.org/10.1016/j.jep.2012.05.033

Wang, X., Cheng, Y., Xue, H., Yue, Y., Zhang, W., & Li, X. (2015). Fargesin as a potential β1 adrenergic receptor antagonist protects the hearts against ischemia/reperfusion injury in rats via attenuating oxidative stress and apoptosis. *Fitoterapia, 105*, 16–25. https://doi.org/10.1016/j.fitote.2015.05.016

Wang, X., Su, P., Hao, Q., Zhang, X., Xia, L., & Zhang, Y. (2022). A Chinese classical prescription Guizhi-Fuling Wan in treatment of ovarian cancer: An overview. *Biomedicine & Pharmacotherapy, 153*, 113401. https://doi.org/10.1016/j.biopha.2022.113401

Wang, Y., Lin, Z., Huang, J., Chu, M., Ding, X., Li, W., Mao, Q., & Zhang, B. (2022). An integrated study of Shenling Baizhu San against hyperuricemia: Efficacy evaluation, core target identification and active component discovery. *Journal of Ethnopharmacology, 295*, 115450. https://doi.org/10.1016/j.jep.2022.115450

Wang, Y., Zhou, X., Chen, X., Wang, F., Zhu, W., Yan, D., & Shang, H. (2020). Efficacy and safety of Shengmai injection for chronic heart failure: A Systematic review of randomized controlled trials. *Evidence-based Complementary and Alternative Medicine, 2020*, 1–10. https://doi.org/10.1155/2020/9571627

Wang, Z., Li, L., Lin, L. W., & Qin, H. (2017). Radix Glehniae extract inhibits migration and invasion of lung cancer cells. *Infection International/Infection International (Electronic Edition), 6*(2), 48–53. https://doi.org/10.1515/ii-2017-0159

Wang, S., & Qiu, X. (2019). The efficacy of Xue Fu Zhu Yu prescription for hyperlipidemia: A meta-analysis of randomized controlled trials. *Complementary Therapies in Medicine, 43*, 218–226. https://doi.org/10.1016/j.ctim.2019.02.008

Wei, Y., Li, Y., Wang, S., Xiang, Z., Li, X., Wang, Q., Dong, W., Gao, P., & Dai, L. (2023). Phytochemistry and pharmacology of *Armeniacae semen* Amarum: A review. *Journal of Ethnopharmacology, 308*, 116265. https://doi.org/10.1016/j.jep.2023.116265

Wu, H., Xi, L., Gao, Z., Dai, Z., Lin, M., Fang, T., Zhao, X., Sun, Y., & Pu, X. (2019). Anti-myocardial infarction effects of Radix aconiti lateralis preparata extracts and their influence on small molecules in the heart using matrix-assisted laser Desorption/Ionization–Mass spectrometry imaging. *International Journal of Molecular Sciences, 20*(19), 4837. https://doi.org/10.3390/ijms20194837

Wu, J., Huang, G., Li, Y., & Li, X. (2020). Flavonoids from Aurantii Fructus Immaturus and Aurantii Fructus: Promising phytomedicines for the treatment of liver diseases. *Chinese Medicine, 15*(1). https://doi.org/10.1186/s13020-020-00371-5

Wu, Z., Chen, D., Lin, F., Lin, L., Shuai, O., Wang, J., Qi, L., & Zhang, P. (2015). Effect of bajijiasu isolated from *Morinda officinalis* F. C. how on sexual function in male mice and its antioxidant protection of human sperm. *Journal of Ethnopharmacology, 164*, 283–292. https://doi.org/10.1016/j.jep.2015.02.016

Xiang, X., Cao, N., Chen, F., Qian, L., Wang, Y., Huang, Y., Tian, Y., Xu, D., & Li, W. (2020). Polysaccharide of Atractylodes macrocephala Koidz (PAMK) alleviates cyclophosphamide-induced immunosuppression in mice by upregulating CD28/IP3R/PLCγ-1/AP-1/NFAT signal pathway. *Frontiers in Pharmacology, 11*. https://doi.org/10.3389/fphar.2020.529657

Xiao, Y., Liu, Y., Yu, K., Ouyang, M., Luo, R., & Zhao, X. (2012). Chinese Herbal medicine Liu Jun Zi Tang and Xiang Sha Liu Jun Zi Tang for functional dyspepsia: Meta-analysis of randomized controlled trials. *Evidence-based Complementary and Alternative Medicine, 2012*, 1–7. https://doi.org/10.1155/2012/936459

Xiao, J. R., Wai, C., & To, C. (2014). Potential therapeutic effects of baicalein, baicalin, and wogonin in ocular disorders. *Journal of Ocular Pharmacology and Therapeutics, 30*(8), 605–614. https://doi.org/10.1089/jop.2014.0074

Xie, X., Guo, H., Liu, J., Wang, J., Li, H., & Deng, Z. (2023). Edible and medicinal progress of *Cryptotympana atrata* (Fabricius) in China. *Nutrients, 15*(19), 4266. https://doi.org/10.3390/nu15194266

Xie, Z., Wang, S., Liang, Z., & Zeng, L. (2010). Effect of Zhenwu Tang granule on pressure-overloaded left ventricular myocardial hypertrophy in rats. *World J Emerg Med, 1*(2), 149–153. https://pubmed.ncbi.nlm.nih.gov/25214959

Xiong, Y., Shang, B., Xu, S., Zhao, R., Gou, H., & Wang, C. (2016). Protective effect of Bu-zhong-yi-qi decoction, the water extract of Chinese traditional herbal medicine, on 5-fluorouracil-induced renal injury in mice. *Renal Failure, 38*(8), 1240–1248. https://doi.org/10.1080/0886022x.2016.1209380

Xu, J., Huang, Y., Wei, L., Li, Y., Wang, M., Chen, X., Sui, Y., & Zhao, H. (2015). Wen Dan decoction for hemorrhagic stroke and ischemic stroke. *Complementary Therapies in Medicine, 23*(2), 298–308. https://doi.org/10.1016/j.ctim.2015.01.001

Xu, S., Qiao, X., Peng, P., Zhu, Z., Li, Y., Yu, M., Chen, L., Cai, Y., Xu, J., Shi, X., Proud, C. G., Xie, J., & Shen, K. (2022). Da-Chai-Hu-Tang protects from acute intrahepatic cholestasis by inhibiting hepatic inflammation and bile accumulation via activation of PPARα. *Frontiers in Pharmacology, 13*. https://doi.org/10.3389/fphar.2022.847483

Xu, T., Qin, G., Jiang, W., Zhao, Y., Xu, Y., & Lv, X. (2019). Corrigendum to "6-Gingerol protects heart by suppressing myocardial Ischemia/Reperfusion induced inflammation via the PI3K/Akt-dependent mechanism in rats. *Evidence-based Complementary and Alternative Medicine, 2019*, 1–2. https://doi.org/10.1155/2019/7659701

Xu, W., Xu, L., Deng, B., Leng, J., Tang, N., Zhao, L., Zhou, H. H., Zhao, Z., Yang, Z., Xiao, T. T., Tian, X. Y., Ho, A., Chan, N. W. K., Chow, Y. L., Chow, C. Y., & Xu, M. (2017). The potential impact of *Radix Paeoniae alba* in embryonic development of mice. *Phytotherapy Research, 31*(9), 1376–1383. https://doi.org/10.1002/ptr.5864

Xu, X., Li, H., Huang, B., Wei, Y., Zheng, S., & Li, W. (2013). Efficacy of ethanol extract of *Fructus lycii* and its constituents Lutein/Zeaxanthin in protecting retinal pigment epithelium cells against oxidative stress: In vivo and in vitro models of age-related macular degeneration. *Journal of Ophthalmology, 2013*, 1–10. https://doi.org/10.1155/2013/862806

Yan, P., Mao, W., Jin, L., Fang, M., Liu, X., Lang, J., Lü, J., Cao, B., Shou, Q., & Fu, H. (2020). Crude Radix *Aconiti Lateralis Preparata* (Fuzi) with *Glycyrrhiza* reduces inflammation and ventricular remodeling in mice through the TLR4/NF-κB pathway. *Mediators of Inflammation, 2020*, 1–13. https://doi.org/10.1155/2020/5270508

Yan, X., Lee, S., Li, W., Jang, H., & Kim, Y. H. (2015). Terpenes and sterols from the fruits of Prunus mume and their inhibitory effects on osteoclast differentiation by suppressing tartrate-resistant acid phosphatase activity. *Archives of Pharmacal Research, 38*(2), 186–192. https://doi.org/10.1007/s12272-014-0389-2

Yang, M., Li, X., Zhang, L., Wang, C., Ji, M., Xu, J., Zhang, K., Liu, J., Zhang, C., & Li, M. (2019). Ethnopharmacology, phytochemistry, and pharmacology of the genus *Glehnia*: A systematic review. *Evidence-based Complementary and Alternative Medicine, 2019*, 1–33. https://doi.org/10.1155/2019/1253493

Yang, P., Tian, Y., Deng, W., Cai, X., Liu, W., Li, L., & Huang, H. (2019). Sijunzi decoction may decrease apoptosis via stabilization of the extracellular matrix following cerebral ischaemia-reperfusion in rats. *Experimental and Therapeutic Medicine, 18*(4), 2805–2812. https://doi.org/10.3892/etm.2019.7878

Yang, S., Fu, Q., Deng, H., Liu, Z., Zhong, J., Zhu, X., Wang, Q., Sun, C., & Wu, J. (2021). Mechanisms and molecular targets of the Yu-Ping-Feng powder for allergic rhinitis, based on network pharmacology. *Medicine, 100*(35), e26929. https://doi.org/10.1097/md.0000000000026929

Yang, Y., Yan, X., Wu, R., Li, N., Chu, M., Dong, Y., Fu, S., Shi, J., & Liu, Q. (2022). Network pharmacology and experimental evidence reveal the protective mechanism of Yi-Qi Cong-Ming decoction on age-related hearing loss. *Pharmaceutical Biology, 60*(1), 1478–1490. https://doi.org/10.1080/13880209.2022.2101671

Yi, G., Qiu, Y., Xiao, Y., & Lu, Y. (2014). The usefulness of Xuefu Zhuyu Tang for patients with Angina Pectoris: A meta-analysis and systematic review. *Evidence-based Complementary and Alternative Medicine, 2014*, 1–11. https://doi.org/10.1155/2014/521602

Yip, K. L., Koon, C. M., Chen, Z. Y., Chook, P., Leung, P. C., Schachter, S., Leung, W., Mok, C. T. V., & Leung, H. (2020). The antiepileptic effect of Gastrodiae Rhizoma through modulating overexpression of mTOR and attenuating astrogliosis in pilocarpine mice model. *Epilepsia Open, 5*(1), 50–60. https://doi.org/10.1002/epi4.12372

Yu, X., Cui, Z., Zhou, Z., Shan, T., Li, D., & Cui, N. (2014). Si-Jun-Zi decoction treatment promotes the restoration of intestinal function after obstruction by regulating intestinal homeostasis. *Evidence-based Complementary and Alternative Medicine, 2014*, 1–8. https://doi.org/10.1155/2014/928579

Yuan, H., Zhu, M., Wen, G., Jin, L., Chen, W., Brunk, U. T., & Zhao, M. (2011). Mustard seeds (Sinapis Alba Linn) attenuate azoxymethane-induced colon carcinogenesis. *Redox Report, 16*(1), 38–44. https://doi.org/10.1179/174329211x12968219310918

Yuan, W., & Wang, Q. (2019). Perioperative acupuncture medicine. *Chinese Medical Journal, 132*(6), 707–715. https://doi.org/10.1097/cm9.0000000000000123

Yuan, Z., Du, W., He, X., Zhang, D., & He, W. (2020). *Tribulus terrestris* ameliorates oxidative stress-induced ARPE-19 cell injury through the PI3K/Akt-Nrf2 signaling pathway. *Oxidative Medicine and Cellular Longevity, 2020*, 1–14. https://doi.org/10.1155/2020/7962393

Yue, Y., Gao, M., Deng, Y., Shao, J., & Sun, Y. (2021). Efficacy and safety of modified Yunu-Jian in patients with periodontitis: A meta-analysis. *Evidence-based Complementary and Alternative Medicine, 2021*, 1–9. https://doi.org/10.1155/2021/5147439

Zhang, Q., Li, R., Liu, J., Peng, W., Fan, W., Gao, Y., Wei, J., & Wu, C. (2020). Efficacy and tolerability of Guizhi-Shaoyao-Zhimu decoction in gout patients: A systematic review and meta-analysis. *Pharmaceutical Biology, 58*(1), 1032–1043. https://doi.org/10.1080/13880209.2020.1823426

Zhang, R., Liu, Z., Li, C., Hu, S., Liu, L., Wang, J., & Mei, Q. (2009). Du-Zhong (*Eucommia ulmoides* Oliv.) cortex extract prevent OVX-induced osteoporosis in rats. *Bone, 45*(3), 553–559. https://doi.org/10.1016/j.bone.2008.08.127

Zhang, W., Zhao, Z., Chang, L., Cao, Y., Wang, S., Kang, C., Wang, H., Zhou, L., Huang, L., & Guo, L. (2021). Atractylodis *Rhizoma*: A review of its traditional uses, phytochemistry, pharmacology, toxicology and quality control. *Journal of Ethnopharmacology, 266*, 113415. https://doi.org/10.1016/j.jep.2020.113415

Zhang, X., Jiang, R., Zhang, X., Dong, X., Xue, S., & Li, F. (2022). Effect of *Rehmanniae Radix* combined with *Scrophulariae Radix* on renal microinflammation in diabetic nephropathy rats based on NF-κB pathway. *International Journal of Traditional Chinese Medicine*, (6): 49–55. https://pesquisa.bvsalud.org/gim/resource/en,au:%22Martins%20Neto,%20Viviana%22/wpr-930098

Zhang, Y., Liu, T., Zhang, L., Pu, Z., Zheng, Y., & Hua, H. (2022). Wendan decoction in the treatment of nonalcoholic fatty liver disease: A systematic review and meta-analysis. *Frontiers in Pharmacology, 13*. https://doi.org/10.3389/fphar.2022.1039611

Zhang, Y., Qian, X., Sun, X., Lin, C., Jing, Y., Yao, Y., Ma, Z., Kuai, M., Lü, Y., Kong, X., Chen, Q., Wu, X., Zhao, X., Li, Y., & Bian, H. (2018). Liuwei Dihuang, a traditional Chinese medicinal formula, inhibits proliferation and migration of vascular smooth muscle cells via modulation of estrogen receptors. *International Journal of Molecular Medicine, 42*(1), 31–40. https://doi.org/10.3892/ijmm.2018.3622

Zhang, Y., Wang, M., Yang, J., & Li, X. (2018). The effects of the honey-roasting process on the pharmacokinetics of the six active compounds of licorice. *Evidence-based Complementary and Alternative Medicine, 2018*, 1–9. https://doi.org/10.1155/2018/5731276

Zhang, Z., & Liu, Z. (2022). The research progress of Chinese medicinal food therapy on infertility. *Food Therapy & Health Care, 4*(1), 4. https://doi.org/10.53388/fthc20220124004

Zhao, H., Feng, Y., Wang, M., Wang, J., Liu, T., & Yu, J. (2022). The Angelica dahurica: A review of traditional uses, phytochemistry and pharmacology. *Frontiers in Pharmacology, 13*. https://doi.org/10.3389/fphar.2022.896637

Zhao, H., Ji, Z., Liu, C., & Yu, X. (2015). Neuroprotection and mechanisms of atractylenolide III in preventing learning and memory impairment induced by chronic high-dose homocysteine administration in rats. *Neuroscience, 290*, 485–491. https://doi.org/10.1016/j.neuroscience.2015.01.060

Zhao, Y., Lei, P., Chen, D., Feng, Y., & Xu, B. (2013). Renal metabolic profiling of early renal injury and renoprotective effects of *Poria cocos* epidermis using UPLC Q-TOF/HSMS/MS^E. *Journal of Pharmaceutical and Biomedical Analysis, 81–82*, 202–209. https://doi.org/10.1016/j.jpba.2013.03.028

Zhao, Y., Zhang, Y., Kong, H., Cheng, G., Qu, H., & Zhao, Y. (2022). Protective effects of carbon dots derived from Armeniacae Semen Amarum Carbonisata against acute lung injury induced by lipopolysaccharides in rats. *International Journal of Nanomedicine, 17*, 1–14. https://doi.org/10.2147/ijn.s338886

Zheng, M., Liu, C., Fan, Y., Shi, D., & Jian, W. (2019). Total glucosides of paeony (TGP) extracted from *Radix Paeoniae Alba* exerts neuroprotective effects in MPTP-induced experimental parkinsonism by regulating the cAMP/PKA/CREB signaling pathway. *Journal of Ethnopharmacology, 245*, 112182. https://doi.org/10.1016/j.jep.2019.112182

Zheng, N., Dai, J., Cao, H., Sun, S., Fang, J., Li, Q., Su, S., Zhang, Y., Qiu, M., & Huang, S. (2013). Current understanding on antihepatocarcinoma effects of Xiao Chai Hu Tang and its constituents. *Evidence-based Complementary and Alternative Medicine, 2013*, 1–14. https://doi.org/10.1155/2013/529458

Zhou, F., Su, Z., Li, Q., Wang, R., Liao, Y., Zhang, M., & Li, J. (2022). Characterization of bacterial differences induced by cleft-palate-related spatial heterogeneity. *Pathogens, 11*(7), 771. https://doi.org/10.3390/pathogens11070771

Zhou, Y., Wang, C., Kou, J., Wang, M., Rong, X., Pu, X., Xie, X., Han, G., & Pang, X. (2021). *Chrysanthemi Flos* extract alleviated acetaminophen-induced rat liver injury via inhibiting oxidative stress and apoptosis based on network pharmacology analysis. *Pharmaceutical Biology, 59*(1), 1376–1385. https://doi.org/10.1080/13880209.2021.1986077

Zhu, J., Tong, H., Ye, X., Zhang, J., Yi, H., Yang, M., Zhong, L., & Gong, Q. (2020). The effects of low-dose and high-dose decoctions of *Fructus aurantii* in a rat model of functional dyspepsia. *Medical Science Monitor, 26*. https://doi.org/10.12659/msm.919815

Zhu, X., Zhao, Z., Hu, X., Luo, X., Long, X., Jiang, S., & Wang, H. (2022). Application of Buzhong Yiqi decoction combined with biological mesh during rehabilitation after inguinal hernia repairment. *Science & Technology Review, 40*(23), 72–77. http://www.kjdb.org/EN/10.3981/j.issn.1000-7857.2022.23.009

Zhu, Y., Zhao, J., Han, Q., Wang, Z., Wang, Z., Dong, X., Li, J., Liu, L., & Shen, X. (2018). The effect and mechanism of Chinese herbal formula Sini Tang in heart failure after myocardial infarction in rats. *Evidence-based Complementary and Alternative Medicine, 2018*, 1–7. https://doi.org/10.1155/2018/5629342

2 GMP Herbal Medicine for Rare Neurologic Diseases

Neurologic disorders can affect the brain and nerves throughout the body including the spinal cord and other nerves. Examples of neurologic disorders are epilepsy, sleep disorders, ataxia, pain, muscle weakness, and neurodegeneration such as Alzheimer's disease and Parkinson's disease. Neurons of the central nervous system rarely regenerate; neurologic conditions can thus persist. The causes of two-thirds of the rare neurologic diseases of this chapter involve genetic mutations, many of which are inherited. Furthermore, the onset ages of the diseases vary from infancy to late adulthood.

The GMP single herbs and multi-herb formulas that are frequently discussed for the neurologic diseases of this chapter are Rhubarb Root and Rhizome (Dàhuáng), Licorice Root (Gāncǎo), Aconite Accessory Root (Fùzǐ), Chinese Wild Ginger (Xìxīn), Siler Root (Fángfēng), Astragalus Root (Huángqí), White Peony Root (Báisháo), Golden Thread Root (Huánglián), Poria (Fúlíng), Scutellaria Root (Huángqín), Chinese Angelica Root (female Ginseng; Dāngguī), Dried Ginger Rhizome (Gānjiāng), Red Peony Root (Chìsháo), Relax the Channels and Invigorate the Blood Decoction (Shūjīnghuóxuètāng), Enrich the Kidneys and Improve Vision Decoction (Zīshènmíngmùtāng), Licorice, Wheat and Jujube Decoction (Gāncǎoxiǎomàidàzǎotāng), Bupleurum plus Dragon Bone and Oyster Shell Decoction (Cháihújiālónggǔmǔlìtāng), Lycium, Chrysanthemum and Rehmannia Pill (Qǐjúdìhuángwán), Tonify the Middle and Augment the Qi Decoction (Bǔzhōngyìqìtāng), Peony and Licorice Decoction (Sháoyàogāncǎotāng), Angelica Pubescens and Taxillus Decoction (Dúhuójìshēngtāng), Tangkuei Decoction for Frigid Extremities (Dāngguīsìnìtāng), Generalized Pain Dispel Stasis Decoction (Shēntòngzhúyūtāng), and Tonify Yang and Restore Five Decoction (Bǔyánghuánwǔtāng). Many of the herbs are known to affect the nerves. For example, the neuropharmacological effects of processed Fùzǐ on depression, epilepsy, and dementia were reviewed and summarized (Zhao et al., 2020). Many of the formulas are known to relieve neuralgia. Moreover, we note that acupuncture is frequently prescribed, along with the herbal regimens, for the conditions of this chapter.

2.1 NEURALGIC AMYOTROPHY

Neuralgic amyotrophy is caused by a mutated gene on chromosome 17 or an abnormal autoimmune reaction. Either way, it affects the network of nerves called the brachial plexus that serves the upper extremities of the body, triggering an episode of neuralgic pain and muscle weakness in one or two shoulders and arms that can last for a month.

Huángqí (cf. Section 1.9) supplements Qi and is used for symptoms of the mother, chest, nerves, skin, and intestines (Wang, 2020). Wēilíngxiān, or Radix et Rhizoma Clematidis, "removes rheumatism, opens meridians" and was reviewed to relieve rheumatism pain, cervical spondylopathy, and scapulohumeral periarthritis (Lin et al., 2021). Huángqín (cf. Section 1.6) "quenches fire and detoxifies," consisting of flavones that are antitumor, hepatoprotective, antibacterial, antiviral, antioxidant, anticonvulsant, and neuroprotective (Zhao et al., 2016). Huángqíwǔwùtāng (cf. Section 1.5) contains Huángqí. Shēntòngzhúyūtāng translates word-for-word to "decoction for body pain and blood stasis." Gānlùyǐn (cf. Section 1.38) bears Huángqín. Xièhuángsǎn "quenches Spleen-Stomach latent fire" and is used for diseases of the oral soft tissues, excluding lesions specific for gingiva and the tongue (Wang, 2019).

DOI: 10.1201/9781032726625-2

TABLE 2.1

GMP Herbal Medicines for a 25-Year-Old Adult with Neuralgic Amyotrophy

Neuralgic amyotrophy (OrphaCode: 2901)

A disease with a prevalence of ~3 in 10,000

Major susceptibility factor: septin 9 (*SEPTIN9* / Entrez: 10801) at 17q25.3

Autosomal dominant, Not applicable

Polyneuropathy, Muscle weakness, Arthralgia, EMG abnormality

Sprengel anomaly, Paresthesia, Scapular winging

Narrow mouth, Cleft palate, Round face, Acrocyanosis, Respiratory insufficiency, Neurological speech impairment, Sleep disturbance, Short stature, Peripheral neuropathy

Adult

Polyneuropathy (357.82), Muscle weakness (D018908), Arthralgia (D018771):

Huángqíwǔwùtāng 5g + dāngguīsìnìtāng 5g + jīxuèténg 2-0g + dānshēn 1-0g + zhúrú 1-0g + sāngzhī 1-0g + jiānghuáng 1-0g + acupuncture.

Dāngguīsìnìtāng 5g + huángqí 2-1g + jīxuèténg 1-0g + fùzǐ 1-0g + shēngjiāng 0g + wúzhūyú 0g.

Huángqí 5g + dāngguī 3-2g + zhìgāncǎo 2g + wǔwèizǐ 2-1g.

Huángqí 5g + jīxuèténg 5g + chìsháo 4g + sāngzhī 4g + qínjiāo 4g + dāngguī 4g + chuānxiōng 2g + jiānghuáng 2g.

Huángqí 5g + jīxuèténg 5g + gǒuqǐzǐ 4g + dāngguī 4g + wǔlíngzhī 4-3g + bājǐtiān 3-2g + tùsīzǐ 3-0g + fùpénzǐ 3-0g.

Fángfēng 5g + qiānghuó 5g + hòupò 5g + zhǐshí 5g + huángqín 1g + huánglián 1g + dàhuáng 0g.

Paresthesia (D010292):

Shēntòngzhúyūtāng 5g + dāngguīniántòngtāng 2-0g + huángbò 1-0g + cāngzhú 1-0g + yītiáogēn 0g + chuānqí 0g + mùguā 0g + xùduàn 0g + acupuncture.

Shēntòngzhúyūtāng 5g + sháoyàogāncǎotāng 2-0g + niúxī 1-0g + yánhúsuǒ 1-0g + acupuncture.

Shēntòngzhúyūtāng 5g + shūjīnghuóxuètāng 5-0g + yánhúsuǒ 1-0g + acupuncture.

Wēilíngxiān 5g + chuānshānlóng 5g + sānqī 4g + mùguā 4g + niúxī 4g + hónghuā 4g + huángbò 4g + wǔjiāpí 4g + gǒujǐ 4-0g + dàhuáng 2-0g.

Wēilíngxiān 5g + báizhú 3g + qiānghuó 3g + xiāngfù 3g + huángqín 3g + cāngzhú 3g + tiānnánxīng 2g + bànxià 2g + gāncǎo 2g + shēngjiāng 2g + fúlíng 2g + chénpí 2g.

Wēilíngxiān 5g + chuānshānlóng 5g + mùtōng 3g + xìngrén 3g + chìfúlíng 3g + fángfēng 3g + qiānghuó 3g + guìzhī 3g + qínjiāo 3g + huángqín 3g + dāngguī 3g + gégēn 3g + gāncǎo 2g.

Cleft palate (749.0), Neurological speech impairment (D013064):

Gānlùyǐn 5g + qīngwèisǎn 5g + xuánshēn 1g + tiānhuā 1-0g + shígāo 1-0g + shíhú 1-0g + dìhuáng 1-0g + màiméndōng 1-0g.

Gānlùyǐn 5g + qīngwèisǎn 5g + yínqiàosǎn 5g + tiānhuā 1g + xuánshēn 1g.

Dǎochìsǎn 5g + xuánshēn 1g + gāncǎo 0g.

Xièhuángsǎn 5g.

Yùnǔjiān 5g + gānlùyǐn 5g + xuánshēn 1g + sāngbáipí 1g + liánqiáo 1g.

Huángqín 5g + báizhǐ 4g + zhìgāncǎo 2g + shārén 2g + tiānhuā 2g + dàhuáng 1g.

Huángqín 5g + báizhǐ 4g + tiānhuā 3-2g + gāncǎo 3-2g + shārén 3-2g + dàhuáng 1-0g.

Xuánshēn 5g + dìhuáng 5g + màiméndōng 5g + yùzhú 5-4g + hòupò 5-4g + zhǐshí 5-4g + shāshēn 5-0g + dàhuáng 2-0g.

Báizhǐ 5g + zhìgāncǎo 3g + shārén 3g + huángqín 3g + tiānhuā 2g + xìxīn 2g + dàhuáng 0g.

Huángbò 5g + shārén 4g + shānzhīzǐ 2g + dìhuáng 2g + bǎihé 2g + dàndòuchǐ 2g + gāncǎo 2g + chìsháo 2g + ējiāo 2g + huángqín 2g + jiānghuáng 2g + jiāngcán 2g + chántuì 2g + dàhuáng 0g + huánglián 0g.

2.2 YOUNG-ONSET PARKINSON DISEASE

The average onset age of Parkinson's disease in the West is early 60s. However, patients with young-onset Parkinson disease (YOPD), start to have symptoms in their 20s. The cause of YOPD is more likely to be genetic than that of late onset Parkinson disease. Patients with YOPD usually still have roles to play in society; therefore, management of YOPD is more challenging. Table 2.2 shows the prescriptions for symptoms including dyskinesia which is very common in YOPD patients.

Bǔzhōngyìqìtāng, translated to "decoction to nourish interior and benefit Qi," carries Huángqí. Mǔlì, i.e., Concha Ostreae, contains caffeine as one of its key compounds (Yang et al., 2012). Caffeine consumption at a low to moderate dose can benefit schizophrenia patients experiencing negative and cognitive symptoms (Huang & Sperlágh, 2021). Fùzǐ (cf. Section 1.16) is listed as one of the common medicinals in TCM for the prevention and treatment of Parkinson's disease (Zheng, 2009). Máhuángfùzǐxìxīntāng is a formula containing Fùzǐ as one of its major constituent herbs. Báizhú (cf. Section 1.21) was summarized to have effects on the central

---

TABLE 2.2

GMP Herbal Medicines for a 45-Year-Old Adult with Young-Onset Parkinson Disease

Young-onset Parkinson disease (OrphaCode: 2828)

A disease with a prevalence of ~3 in 10,000

Disease-causing germline mutation(s): synaptojanin 1 (*SYNJ1* / Entrez: 8867) at 21q22.11

Candidate gene tested: synuclein alpha (*SNCA* / Entrez: 6622) at 4q22.1

Disease-causing germline mutation(s): PTEN induced kinase 1 (*PINK1* / Entrez: 65018) at 1p36.12

Candidate gene tested: ubiquitin C-terminal hydrolase L1 (*UCHL1* / Entrez: 7345) at 4p13

Candidate gene tested: HtrA serine peptidase 2 (*HTRA2* / Entrez: 27429) at 2p13.1

Disease-causing germline mutation(s) (loss of function): podocalyxin like (*PODXL* / Entrez: 5420) at 7q32.3

Candidate gene tested: leucine rich repeat kinase 2 (*LRRK2* / Entrez: 120892) at 12q12

Disease-causing germline mutation(s): parkin RBR E3 ubiquitin protein ligase (*PRKN* / Entrez: 5071) at 6q26

Disease-causing germline mutation(s): Parkinsonism associated deglycase (*PARK7* / Entrez: 11315) at 1p36.23

Disease-causing germline mutation(s) (loss of function): vacuolar protein sorting 13 homolog C (*VPS13C* / Entrez: 54832) at 15q22.2

Disease-causing germline mutation(s) (loss of function): DnaJ heat shock protein family (Hsp40) member C6 (*DNAJC6* / Entrez: 9829) at 1p31.3

Autosomal recessive

Rigidity

Depression, Hallucinations, Apathy, Tremor, Postural instability, Dyskinesia

Color vision defect, Dementia, Impaired social interactions, Short attention span, Anxiety, Spasticity, Dystonia, Hyperreflexia, Diarrhea, Nausea, Constipation, Bradykinesia, Gait imbalance, Gastroparesis, Muscle spasm, Hyposmia, Abnormal autonomic nervous system physiology, Restless legs, Panic attack, Female sexual dysfunction, Male sexual dysfunction, Cognitive impairment, Insomnia

Adult

Rigidity (D009127):

Bǔzhōngyìqìtāng 5g + liùwèidìhuángwán 4-0g + dùzhòng 1-0g + bǔgǔzhī 1-0g + xùduàn 1-0g.

Bǔzhōngyìqìtāng 5g + jìshēngshènqìwán 5-0g + dānshēn 1-0g + dùzhòng 1-0g.

Bǔzhōngyìqìtāng 5g + sìnìtāng 2-0g + ròuguì 1-0g + zhìgāncǎotāng 1-0g.

Bǔzhōngyìqìtāng 5g + guīpítāng 5-0g.

Guìzhītāng 5g + xìngrén 1g + hòupò 1g.

Máhuángfùzǐxìxīntāng 5g + báizhú 2g + fùzǐ 2g + báisháo 2g + fúlíng 2g + dǎngshēn 1g + shēngjiāng 1g + dàhuáng 0g.

Huángqí 5g + chìsháo 1g + fángfēng 1g + xìxīn 1-0g + huánglián 1-0g + dàhuáng 0g.

Hallucinations (D006212), Tremor (D014202), Dyskinesia (333.82):

Gāncǎoxiǎomàidàzǎotāng 5g + cháihújiālónggǔmǔlìtāng 5g + wēndǎntāng 5-0g + yuǎnzhì 1g + shíchāngpú 1-0g + héhuānpí 1-0g + bǎihé 1-0g + fúshén 1-0g.

Gāncǎoxiǎomàidàzǎotāng 5g + yìgānsǎn 5g + héhuānpí 1g + yùjīn 1g.

Gāncǎoxiǎomàidàzǎotāng 5g + sháoyàogāncǎotāng 5g + cháihújiālónggǔmǔlìtāng 5-0g.

Yìgānsǎn 5g + sháoyàogāncǎotāng 5g + shūjīnghuóxuètāng 5g + acupuncture.

Mǔlì 5g + zhìgāncǎo 5g + gānjiāng 5g + cāngzhú 5g + fùzǐ 3g + dàhuáng 0g.

Mǔlì 5g + gāncǎo 4-3g + báisháo 4-3g + shúdìhuáng 4-3g + biējiǎ 4-3g + màiméndōng 3g + ējiāo 2g + huǒmárén 2g + fúshén 2-0g.

Bǎihé 5g + xuánshēn 4-3g + bèimǔ 4-3g + tiānhuā 4-0g + dìhuáng 4-0g + wūyào 3-0g + niúbàngzǐ 2-0g + shègān 2-0g + mǔlì 2-0g.

(Continued)

TABLE 2.2 *(Continued)*

GMP Herbal Medicines for a 45-Year-Old Adult with Young-Onset Parkinson Disease

Color vision defect (368.53, 368.5, 368.52, 368.51, 368.54, 368.55), Spasticity (D009128), Dystonia (D004421), Hyperreflexia (D012021), Diarrhea (D003967), Nausea (D009325), Constipation (564.0), Bradykinesia (D018476), Gastroparesis (536.3), Muscle spasm (D009120), Restless legs (333.94):

Zīshènmíngmùtāng 5g + juémíngzǐ 1g + gǒuqǐzǐ 1-0g + júhuā 1-0g + gǔjīngcǎo 1-0g + chēqiánzǐ 1-0g.	Fùzǐ 5g + fúlíng 5g + gānjiāng 5g + gāncǎo 3g + dǎngshēn 3g.
Zīshènmíngmùtāng 5g + bǔzhōngyìqìtāng 5g + gǒuqǐzǐ 2g + júhuā 2g + dàhuáng 0g.	Fúlíng 5g + fùzǐ 5-4g + dǎngshēn 5-3g + báisháo 5-3g + báizhú 5-2g.
Zīshènmíngmùtāng 5g + xǐgānmíngmùtāng 4g + dàhuáng 1-0g.	Gǒuqǐzǐ 5g + júhuā 5g + dìhuáng 2g + fángfēng 2g + dāngguī 2g + xìxīn 1g + huánglián 1g.
Wǔlíngsǎn 5g + fùzǐ 1g + huángqín 1g + tiáowèichéngqìtāng 1g.	Huángqí 5g + gǒuqǐzǐ 1g + júhuā 1g + chìsháo 1g + fángfēng 1g + xìxīn 1g + huánglián 1g.
Guìzhītāng 5g + báizhú 1g + fùzǐ 1g + dàhuáng 0g.	Júhuā 5g + zhǐqiào 2g.
Guìzhītāng 5g + báisháo 1g + shēngjiāng 1g + dàhuáng 0g.	

and autonomic nervous systems (Zhang et al., 2021). Zīshènmíngmùtāng was introduced in Section 1.29 for the eye.

2.3 IDIOPATHIC HYPERSOMNIA

Idiopathic hypersomnia is a chronic neurologic condition, with which patients feel sleepy during the daytime even though their nighttime sleep is normal and undisturbed. They take long naps in the day and have a hard time waking up from the naps, which are unrefreshing. The cause of idiopathic hypersomnia is unknown.

Huángjīng, or Rhizoma Polygonati, "replenishes Qi, nourishes yin, drenches the Lung, fortifies the Spleen, tonifies the Kidney" and was reviewed to have antifatigue and antiaging effects (Wang et al., 2023). Bànxià, i.e., Rhizoma Pinelliae Praeparatum, was shown to be sedative, hypnotic, and anticonvulsant in mice probably through its effect on the GABAergic system (Wu et al., 2011). Traditional Chinese medicine believes that an individual retaining excessive body fluids can feel sleepy. Wǔlíngsǎn helps body fluid metabolism and warms up yang. Note that Wǔlíngsǎn was found to improve insomnia, even though the improvement did not differ significantly compared with patients receiving a placebo (Lin et al., 2013).

TABLE 2.3

GMP Herbal Medicines for a 22-Year-Old Adult with Idiopathic Hypersomnia

Idiopathic hypersomnia (OrphaCode: 33208)

A disease with a prevalence of ~3 in 10,000

Unknown

Excessive daytime somnolence, Sleep disturbance, Hypersomnia

All ages

Hypersomnia (327.13):

Wǔlíngsǎn 5g + báisháo 1g + fùzǐ 1-0g + guìzhī 1-0g + táorén 1-0g + tiáowèichéngqìtāng 1-0g + dǐdāngtāng 1-0g.	Huángjīng 5g.
	Gāncǎo 5g + yánhúsuǒ 5g + fùzǐ 5g + gǒuqǐzǐ 5g + gānjiāng 5g + júhuā 5g.
	Gāncǎo 5g + báizhú 5g + báisháo 5g + báibiǎndòu 5g + fúlíng 5g + huángqí 5g + dàzǎo 2g + shēngjiāng 2g.
	Gāncǎo 5g + báisháo 5g + shíhú 5g + chēqiánzǐ 5g + fúlíng 5g + màiméndōng 5-0g + huángqí 5-0g + dǎngshēn 5-0g.
	Bànxià 5g + fúlíng 5g + fùzǐ 4g + xìxīn 2g + dàhuáng 2g.

2.4　CHARCOT-MARIE-TOOTH DISEASE TYPE 1A

Charcot-Marie-Tooth disease type 1A, or microduplication 17p12, is the most common type of Charcot-Marie-Tooth disease. It is a hereditary peripheral neuropathy caused by a duplication in the *PMP22* gene at 17p12, whose over-expression leads to abnormal structure and function of the myelin sheath that wraps around nerve axons.

Sāngzhī (Ramulus Mori) has been extensively used as an antirheumatic agent in TCM. It was shown to be highly analgesic and anti-inflammatory in mice with inflammatory pain (Zhang & Shi, 2010) and is used today for pain in joints and disorders of muscles, ligaments, and fascia (Wang, 2020). Cumulative use of GMP herbal extract granules of Jīxuèténg (Caulis Spatholobi), Xùduàn (Radix Dipsaci), Dùzhòng (cf. Section 1.4), Dānshēn (cf. Section 1.61), Shūjīnghuóxuètāng, Sháoyàogāncǎotāng, or Shēntòngzhúyūtāng was found to be correlated with a reduced risk of osteoporotic fracture in sarcopenia patients in a duration-dependent manner (Chen et al., 2023). We note that acupuncture is frequently prescribed along with TCM herbal medicine for the relief of musculoskeletal pain.

TABLE 2.4
GMP Herbal Medicines for a Seven-Year-Old Child with Charcot-Marie-Tooth Disease Type 1A

Charcot-Marie-Tooth disease type 1A (OrphaCode: 101081)

A disease with a prevalence of ~3 in 10,000

Disease-causing germline mutation(s): peripheral myelin protein 22 (*PMP22* / Entrez: 5376) at 17p12

Autosomal dominant

Hyporeflexia, Gait disturbance, Pes cavus, Distal muscle weakness, Distal sensory impairment, Skeletal muscle atrophy, Decreased motor nerve conduction velocity, Decreased sensory nerve conduction velocity, Demyelinating peripheral neuropathy, Sensory ataxia

Gait imbalance, Kyphoscoliosis, Paresthesia, Acute demyelinating polyneuropathy, Calf muscle hypertrophy, Diaphragmatic weakness, Spontaneous pain sensation, Shoulder pain

Childhood

Skeletal muscle atrophy (D009133), Sensory ataxia (D001259):

Juānbìtāng 5g + sháoyàogāncǎotāng 3-0g + yánhúsuǒ 1-0g + rǔxiāng 1-0g + sāngzhī 1-0g + jīxuèténg 1-0g + dǎodìwúgōng 1-0g + acupuncture.

Huángqíwǔwùtāng 5g + dānshēn 1g + zhúrú 1g + sāngzhī 1g + dāngguī 1g + jiānghuáng 1g + acupuncture.

Sāngzhī 5g + chìsháo 1g + hónghuā 1g + táorén 1g + zélán 1g + acupuncture.

Sāngzhī 5g + jīxuèténg 5g + chìsháo 4g + qínjiāo 4g + dāngguī 4g + chuānxiōng 2g + jiānghuáng 2g.

Sāngzhī 5g + gégēn 5g + jiānghuáng 5g + jīxuèténg 5g + acupuncture.

Sāngzhī 5g + sāngjìshēng 5g + gǔsuìbǔ 5g + xùduàn 5g + dùzhòng 3g + yánhúsuǒ 2g.

Fùzǐ 5g + xìxīn 5g + dàhuáng 4g + bànxià 4g + fúlíng 4g.

Fùzǐ 5g + báizhú 3g + báisháo 3g + fúlíng 3g + dǎngshēn 3g.

Paresthesia (D010292), Shoulder pain (D020069):

Shēntòngzhúyūtāng 5g + sháoyàogāncǎotāng 2-0g + rǔxiāng 1-0g + yánhúsuǒ 1-0g + acupuncture.

Shēntòngzhúyūtāng 5g + shūjīnghuóxuètāng 5-0g + niúxī 2-0g + yánhúsuǒ 2-0g + acupuncture.

Xiǎohuóluòdān 5g + shūjīnghuóxuètāng 5g + niúxī 2-0g + yánhúsuǒ 2-0g + acupuncture.

Wēilíngxiān 5g + chuānshānlóng 5g + sānqī 4g + mùguā 4g + niúxī 4g + hónghuā 4g + huángbò 4g + gǒujǐ 4-0g + dàhuáng 1-0g.

Wēilíngxiān 5g + báizhú 3g + qiānghuó 3g + xiāngfù 3g + huángqín 3g + cāngzhú 3g + tiānnánxīng 2g + bànxià 2g + gāncǎo 2g + shēngjiāng 2g + fúlíng 2g + chénpí 2g.

Wēilíngxiān 5g + chuānshānlóng 5g + mùtōng 3g + xìngrén 3g + chìfúlíng 3g + fángfēng 3g + qiānghuó 3g + guìzhī 3g + qínjiāo 3g + huángqín 3g + dāngguī 3g + gégēn 3g + gāncǎo 2g.

2.5 NARCOLEPSY TYPE 1

Narcolepsy is a chronic neurological condition associated with dysregulation of sleep-wake cycles, resulting in excessive daytime sleepiness and abnormal rapid eye movement (REM) sleep. Patients with narcolepsy can fall asleep suddenly while they are eating, talking, walking, or driving. The cause of narcolepsy is unknown but is believed to involve many factors, including autoimmunity,

TABLE 2.5
GMP Herbal Medicines for a 15-Year-Old Adolescent with Narcolepsy Type 1

Narcolepsy type 1 (OrphaCode: 2073)

A disease with a prevalence of ~2 in 10,000

Major susceptibility factor: hypocretin neuropeptide precursor (*HCRT* / Entrez: 3060) at 17q21.2

Major susceptibility factor: major histocompatibility complex, class II, DR beta 1 (*HLA-DRB1* / Entrez: 3123) at 6p21.32

Major susceptibility factor: major histocompatibility complex, class II, DQ beta 1 (*HLA-DQB1* / Entrez: 3119) at 6p21.32

Major susceptibility factor: myelin oligodendrocyte glycoprotein (*MOG* / Entrez: 4340) at 6p22.1

Major susceptibility factor: TNF superfamily member 4 (*TNFSF4* / Entrez: 7292) at 1q25.1

Major susceptibility factor: purinergic receptor P2Y11 (*P2RY11* / Entrez: 5032) at 19p13.2

Major susceptibility factor: zinc finger protein 365 (*ZNF365* / Entrez: 22891) at 10q21.2

Major susceptibility factor: cathepsin H (*CTSH* / Entrez: 1512) at 15q25.1

Unknown

Hallucinations, Excessive daytime sleepiness, Sleep disturbance, Cataplexy, Transient global amnesia

Abnormality of the eye, Abnormality of vision, Abnormal rapid eye movement sleep

Syncope, Slurred speech, Obesity

Childhood, Adolescent, Adult

Hallucinations (D006212), Transient global amnesia (437.7):

Gāncǎoxiǎomàidàzǎotāng 5g + wēndǎntāng 5g + héhuānpí 1g + yèjiāoténg 1g + yuǎnzhì 1g + suānzǎorén 1g.

Cháihújiālóngǔmǔlìtāng 5g + gāncǎoxiǎomàidàzǎotāng 5-4g + wēndǎntāng 5-0g + shíchāngpú 2-0g + yuǎnzhì 2-0g + dānshēn 1-0g + yùjīn 1-0g + héhuānpí 1-0g + bǎihé 1-0g + suānzǎorén 1-0g.

Yìgānsǎn 5g + wēndǎntāng 5g + héhuānpí 1g + bǎihé 1g + yèjiāoténg 1g.

Yìgānsǎn 5g + gāncǎoxiǎomàidàzǎotāng 2g + bǎihé 1g + yèjiāoténg 1g + fúshén 1g.

Abnormality of the eye (379.90):

Qǐjúdìhuángwán 5g + xǐgānmíngmùtāng 5g + zīshènmíngmùtāng 5-0g + gǔjīngcǎo 1-0g + mùzéicǎo 1-0g + juémíngzǐ 1-0g + mìménghuā 1-0g + júhuā 1-0g.

Zīshènmíngmùtāng 5g + qǐjúdìhuángwán 5-4g + gǒuqǐzǐ 1-0g + júhuā 1-0g + gǔjīngcǎo 1-0g.

Qǐjúdìhuángwán 5g + bǔzhōngyìqìtāng 5g.

Syncope (D013575), Obesity (278.00):

Shēngmàiyǐn 5g + bǔzhōngyìqìtāng 5-0g + jìshēngshènqìwán 5-0g.

Shēngmàiyǐn 5g + xuèfǔzhúyūtāng 5-0g.

Shēngmàiyǐn 5g + zhēnwǔtāng 5-0g.

Shēngmàiyǐn 5g + zhìgāncǎotāng 5-0g.

Yùzhú 5g + sìnìtāng 5g + mázǐrénwán 5g.

Shíjuémíng 5g + mǔlì 2g + bèimǔ 1g + fángfēng 1g + jīngjiè 1g + fúlíng 1g + gégēn 1g + huòxiāng 1g + xùduàn 1-0g + wǔlíngzhī 0g + bājǐtiān 0g + yìzhìrén 0g + yuǎnzhì 0g + zàojiāocì 0g + cāngěrzǐ 0g.

Mǔlì 5g + cháihú 4g + gāncǎo 3g + guìzhī 3g + tiānhuā 2g + gānjiāng 2g + huángqín 2g.

Mǔlì 5g + gāncǎo 4-3g + báisháo 4-3g + shúdìhuáng 4-3g + biējiǎ 4-3g + màiméndōng 3g + ējiāo 2g + huǒmárén 2g + fúshén 2-0g.

Zhúrú 5g + júhóng 5g + báidòukòu 2g + rénshēn 1g + shēngjiāng 1g + gānjiāng 1g + huángqín 1g + huánglián 0g.

Gǒuqǐzǐ 5g + júhuā 5g + dìhuáng 4-3g + dānggu ī 4-3g + fángfēng 3-2g + niúbàngzǐ 3-0g + shègān 3-0g + xìxīn 2-1g + huánglián 2-1g.

Xuánshēn 5g + yùzhú 5g + dìhuáng 5g + shāshēn 5g + hòupò 5g + zhǐshí 5g + màiméndōng 5g + dàhuáng 1-0g.

Bǎihé 5g + zhīmǔ 5-3g + tiānhuā 3-1g + xuánshēn 3-1g + bèimǔ 3-1g + wūyào 3-0g + mǔlì 2-0g + niúbàngzǐ 2-0g + shègān 2-0g + zhīmǔ 1-0g.

Shānzhā 5g + dānshēn 5g + héshǒuwū 5g + juémíngzǐ 5g + hóngqū 5g + zéxiè 5g.

Héyè 5g + cǎojuémíng 3g + máhuáng 3g + zéxiè 3g + shígāo 2g + chēqiánzǐ 2g + hǔzhàng 2g.

infection, and gene mutations. Narcolepsy type 1, also known as Gélineau disease or narcolepsy-cataplexy, is a common subtype of narcolepsy where narcolepsy can cooccur with muscle weakness triggered by emotions.

Shíjuémíng (Concha Haliotidis) lowers blood pressure through effects on calcium channel regulation in rats (Chen et al., 2013) and is used for headaches, sleep disturbances, and essential hypertension (Wang, 2020). Both Shíjuémíng and Mǔlì are among the "Liver-pacifying" medicinals that were reviewed to pass through the blood-brain barrier, act directly on neurons, and provide protective effects against brain diseases (Lee et al., 2018). Bǎihé (Bulbus Lilii) "nourishes yin, moistens the Lung, stops coughing, clears the Heart, anchors the mind" and is used today for sleep disturbances and coughs (Wang, 2020). We will see the use of Shēngmàiyǐn for syncope in Chapter 14 on rare cardiac diseases.

2.6   NARCOLEPSY TYPE 2

Cataplexy is sudden and brief bouts of muscle weakness triggered by strong emotions such as anger, fear, anxiety and laughter when one is awake. Narcolepsy type 2 is narcolepsy without cataplexy and with normal levels of orexin in the brain, which is a neuropeptide that regulates food intake and wakefulness.

Mǔlì, annotated in the text of Section 2.2, "normalizes the Liver and subdues an overacting yang," with its modern uses including sleep disturbances (Wang, 2020). Gāncǎoxiǎomàidàzǎotāng has been a formula for the treatment of "visceral agitation" (i.e., organic mania) in TCM and is used today for insomnia, depression, irritable bowel syndrome, anxiety, and menopause. It was summarized to improve the outcomes of such neuropsychiatric disorders as acute psychological stress, post-traumatic stress disorders, unpredictable mild stress depression, and prenatal depression in animal models (Kim et al., 2017).

TABLE 2.6
GMP Herbal Medicines for a 36-Year-Old Adult with Narcolepsy Type 2

Narcolepsy type 2 (OrphaCode: 83465)

A disease with a prevalence of ~2 in 10,000

Candidate gene tested: hypocretin neuropeptide precursor (*HCRT* / Entrez: 3060) at 17q21.2

Major susceptibility factor: major histocompatibility complex, class II, DR beta 1 (*HLA-DRB1* / Entrez: 3123) at 6p21.32

Major susceptibility factor: major histocompatibility complex, class II, DQ beta 1 (*HLA-DQB1* / Entrez: 3119) at 6p21.32

Major susceptibility factor: zinc finger protein 365 (*ZNF365* / Entrez: 22891) at 10q21.2

Unknown

Hallucinations, Excessive daytime somnolence, Sleep disturbance, Insomnia

Behavioral abnormality

Childhood, Adolescent, Adult

Hallucinations (D006212):

Gāncǎoxiǎomàidàzǎotāng 5g + cháihújiālónggǔmǔlìtāng 5g + wēndǎntāng 5-0g + zhúrú 1-0g + yèjiāoténg 1-0g + héhuānpí 1-0g + fúshén 1-0g + yuǎnzhì 1-0g + bózǐrén 1-0g + bǎihé 1-0g + xiāngfù 1-0g + yùjīn 1-0g.

Gāncǎoxiǎomàidàzǎotāng 5g + xiāoyáosǎn 5g + bǎihé 1g + dānshēn 1-0g + xiāngfù 1-0g + yùjīn 1-0g + héhuānpí 1-0g + yuǎnzhì 1-0g.

Bǎihé 5g + tiānhuā 3g + xuánshēn 3g + bèimǔ 3g + wūyào 3-0g + zhīmǔ 3-0g + niúbàngzǐ 2g + shègān 2g + mǔlì 2-1g.

Mǔlì 5g + gāncǎo 4g + báisháo 4g + shúdìhuáng 4g + biējiǎ 4g + màiméndōng 3g + ējiāo 2g + fúshén 2g + huǒmárén 2g.

Mǔlì 5g + biējiǎ 5g + shānzhūyú 3g + wūméi 2g + qīnghāo 1g + qínjiāo 1g.

Zhúrú 5g + ējiāo 5g + jiégěng 5g + sāngbáipí 5g + huángqín 5g.

2.7 PUDENDAL NEURALGIA

Pudendal neuralgia, also known as Alcock syndrome, is a chronic pelvic pain or numbness due to entrapment of a main nerve in the pelvic floor called the pudendal nerve. The pudendal nerve can be damaged or compressed by surgery, injury, childbirth, or tumor.

TABLE 2.7

GMP Herbal Medicines for a 59-Year-Old Adult with Pudendal Neuralgia

Pudendal neuralgia (OrphaCode: 60039)

A disease with a prevalence of ~2 in 10,000

Not applicable

Impotence, Constipation, Episodic abdominal pain, Paresthesia, Back pain, Abdominal colic, Dyspareunia, Scrotal pain, Vulvodynia, Pollakisuria, Dysuria

Adult

Constipation (564.0), Paresthesia (D010292), Back pain (D001416), Abdominal colic (D003085), Dysuria (D053159):

Dàcháihútāng 5g + mázǐrénwán 5g.

Mùxiāngbīnglángwán 5g + mázǐrénwán 5g + tiáowèichéngqìtāng 5-0g + dàhuáng 2-0g + hòupò 2-0g + zhǐshí 2-0g.

Zhēnwǔtāng 5g + mázǐrénwán 5g + dàhuáng 1g.

Mázǐrénwán 5g + tiáowèichéngqìtāng 5g + xuánshēn 1g + dìhuáng 1g + màiméndōng 1g + táorén 1g.

Gāncǎo 5g + hòupò 5-0g + zhǐshí 5-0g + dàhuáng 2-1g.

Fùzǐ 5g + guìzhī 5g + huánglián 5g + huángqín 4g + dàhuáng 1g.

Hòupò 5g + zhǐshí 5g + dàhuáng 1g + acupuncture.

Gāncǎo (cf. Section 1.1) helps digestion, including constipation (Wang, 2020). Dàcháihútāng (cf. Section 1.22) "resolves external pathogens and purges internal stagnation." Its modern uses include chronic liver disease and cirrhosis (Wang, 2019). Mùxiāngbīnglángwán "moves Qi, conducts stagnation, purges heat, passes stools" and is used for functional digestive disorders (Wang, 2019). We note that pain can be alleviated by acupuncture (Kelly & Willis, 2019).

2.8 LENNOX-GASTAUT SYNDROME

Lennox-Gastaut syndrome is a complex, severe childhood-onset epilepsy characterized by a pattern of slow-spike wave brain electrical activities in or between seizures. Lennox-Gastaut syndrome can be caused by gene mutations or by perinatal brain damage such as central nervous system infection, brain malformation, and brain tumor.

TABLE 2.8

GMP Herbal Medicines for a Four-Year-Old Child with Lennox-Gastaut Syndrome

Lennox-Gastaut syndrome (OrphaCode: 2382)

A disease with a prevalence of ~1 in 10,000

Disease-causing germline mutation(s): cut like homeobox 2 (*CUX2* / Entrez: 23316) at 12q24.11-q24.12

Disease-causing germline mutation(s): sodium voltage-gated channel alpha subunit 1 (*SCN1A* / Entrez: 6323) at 2q24.3

Candidate gene tested: mitogen-activated protein kinase 10 (*MAPK10* / Entrez: 5602) at 4q21.3

Disease-causing germline mutation(s): chromodomain helicase DNA binding protein 2 (*CHD2* / Entrez: 1106) at 15q26.1

Disease-causing germline mutation(s): dynamin 1 (*DNM1* / Entrez: 1759) at 9q34.11

Disease-causing germline mutation(s): gamma-aminobutyric acid type A receptor subunit beta3 (*GABRB3* / Entrez: 2562) at 15q12

Disease-causing germline mutation(s) (gain of function): calcium voltage-gated channel subunit alpha1 A (*CACNA1A* / Entrez: 773) at 19p13.13

Disease-causing germline mutation(s) (loss of function): calcium voltage-gated channel subunit alpha1 A (*CACNA1A* / Entrez: 773) at 19p13.13

(Continued)

TABLE 2.8 *(Continued)*
GMP Herbal Medicines for a Four-Year-Old Child with Lennox-Gastaut Syndrome

Autosomal dominant, Multigenic/multifactorial, Not applicable

Intellectual disability, Encephalopathy, EEG with focal sharp slow waves

Behavioral abnormality, Aggressive behavior, Autistic behavior, Hyperactivity, Mental deterioration, Myoclonus, Bilateral
  tonic-clonic seizure, EEG abnormality, Abnormal brainstem morphology, Falls, Atypical absence seizure, Generalized
  tonic seizures, Atonic seizure, Personality disorder

Generalized myoclonic seizures, Focal-onset seizure

Infancy, Childhood

Intellectual disability (D008607), Encephalopathy (348.30, 348.9):

Sāngjúyǐn 5g + zhǐqiào 1-0g + jílí 1-0g + chántuì 1-0g + júhuā 1-0g. Yínqiàosǎn 5g + zhǐqiào 1g.	Zhǐqiào 5-3g + chántuì 5-2g + jílí 5-0g. Gāncǎo 5g + báizhǐ 5g + shārén 5g + dàhuáng 0g.

Hyperactivity (D006948), Myoclonus (D009207), Bilateral tonic-clonic seizure (D012640), Personality disorder
  (301.82, 301.81):

Bǔzhōngyìqìtāng 5g + shānzhā 1-0g +
  shénqū 1-0g + màiyá 1-0g + gāncǎo 1-0g.
	Dàzǎo 5g + gāncǎo 5g + báisháo 5g + bǎihé 5g + ējiāo 5g + fúxiǎomài 5g +
	  fúshén 5g + màiméndōng 5g + suānzǎorén 5g + dǎngshēn 5g.
	Dàzǎo 5g + gāncǎo 5g + xìngrén 5g + jiégěng 5g + kuǎndōnghuā 5g + zǐwǎn
	  5g + tínglìzǐ 5g + máhuáng 3g + wǔwèizǐ 2g + xìxīn 1g + gānjiāng 1-0g.
	Huángqí 5g + zhìgāncǎo 3g + wǔwèizǐ 1g + dāngguī 0g.
	Huángqí 5g + chìsháo 1g + fángfēng 1g + xìxīn 0g + huánglián 0g.

Zhǐqiào (cf. Sections 1.31 and 1.54) was shown to exhibit rapid antidepressant-like effects, like
ketamine, in mice (Wu et al., 2021). Sāngyè (Folium Mori), the major herb in Sāngjúyǐn, and Fructus
Mori mixture was shown to recover the cognitive deficits in high-fat diet induced obese mice by
regulating neural and synaptic activities (Kim et al., 2015). Dàzǎo (Fructus Jujubae) "replenishes
interior, benefits Qi, nourishes Blood, and calms the spirit." Dàzǎo has been used alone or with
other herbs in a formula as a tranquilizer. It was reviewed to protect neuronal cells against neu-
rotoxin stress, stimulate neuronal differentiation, increase expression of neurotrophic factors, and
promote memory and learning (Chen et al., 2017a).

2.9 IDIOPATHIC INTRACRANIAL HYPERTENSION

Idiopathic intracranial hypertension (IIH), also known as pseudotumor cerebri, is increased pressure
around the brain. Increased pressure can compress the tissue and nerve, causing pain in the head, neck,
and shoulders and it also causes problems with vision. Although the pathophysiology of IIH is unknown,
increased blood flow to the brain and/or decreased venous drainage of cerebral blood are theorized.

TABLE 2.9
**GMP Herbal Medicines for a 30-Year-Old Woman with Idiopathic Intracranial
Hypertension**

Idiopathic intracranial hypertension (OrphaCode: 238624)

A disease with a prevalence of ~1 in 10,000

Not applicable

Headache, Increased intracranial pressure

Papilledema, Obesity, Allergy

Visual loss, Photophobia, Blurred vision, Diplopia, Vomiting, Nausea, Sleep disturbance, Scintillating scotoma,
  Abnormal emotion/affect behavior

Adult, Elderly

(Continued)

TABLE 2.9 *(Continued)*

GMP Herbal Medicines for a 30-Year-Old Woman with Idiopathic Intracranial Hypertension

Headache (D006261):

Wǔlíngsǎn 5g + báisháo 1-0g + fùzǐ 1-0g + huángqín 1-0g + tiáowèichéngqìtāng 0g + dǐdāngtāng 0g.
Guìzhītāng 5g + gégēn 1g + dàhuáng 0g.

Gāncǎo 5g + báizhú 5g + báisháo 5g + zhīmǔ 5g + liánqiáo 5g + huáshí 5g + dāngguī 5g + dǎngshēn 5g.

Gāncǎo 5g + báizhǐ 5g + huángqín 5g + shārén 5-3g + tiānhuā 2-0g + xìxīn 2-0g + dàhuáng 1-0g.

Papilledema (362.83, 377.0, 377.01), Obesity (278.00):

Jiāwèixiāoyáosǎn 5g + qǐjúdìhuángwán 5g + dānshēn 1g + chēqiánzǐ 1g + chōngwèizǐ 1-0g + nǚzhēnzǐ 1-0g + tùsīzǐ 1-0g + niúxī 1-0g.
Sāngjúyǐn 5g + jiāwèixiāoyáosǎn 5-0g + zhǐqiào 2-1g + jílí 2-1g + chántuì 2-0g + júhuā 1-0g.

Gāncǎo 5g + zhīmǔ 5-4g + huángqín 5-0g + dàhuáng 0g + huánglián 0g.
Shānzhīzǐ 5g + zhīmǔ 4-3g + dìhuáng 3-0g + gāncǎo 2-0g + dàzǎo 1-0g + huánglián 1-0g + dàhuáng 0g.

Photophobia (D020795), Diplopia (D004172), Vomiting (D014839), Nausea (D009325), Scintillating scotoma (D012607):

Wúzhūyútāng 5g + máhuángfùzǐxìxīntāng 3-2g + fùzǐ 1g + gānjiāng 1g.
Yínqiàosǎn 5g + júhuā 2-1g + zhǐqiào 1-0g + jílí 1-0g.
Guìzhītāng 5g + wúzhūyútāng 3g + fùzǐ 1g + gānjiāng 1g.

Chántuì 5g + zhǐqiào 5-4g + jílí 5-3g.
Júhuā 5g + chántuì 5-0g + zhǐqiào 4-3g + jílí 4-1g.

Wǔlíngsǎn contains herbs that "promote urination, improve digestion and resolve pathogen-induced fever and headache," achieving "diuresis and yang-warming." Shānzhīzǐ (cf. Section 1.39), being bitter in TCM taste and cold in TCM nature, "quenches fires lingering in the body." Modern research finds it to decrease fat percentage and BMI in middle-aged obese women (Shin & Huh, 2014). Wúzhūyútāng "warms interior, replenishes deficiency, lowers ascent, stops vomiting" and is used today for migraines (Wang, 2019), which makes one sensitive to light.

2.10 STEINERT MYOTONIC DYSTROPHY

Steinert myotonic dystrophy, also known as myotonic dystrophy type 1, is a progressive muscular dystrophy, affecting multi-systems including the skeleton, distal muscle, eye and heart. Steinert myotonic dystrophy is caused by an increased number of trinucleotide repeats at the end of the *DMPK* gene, whose products play a role in muscle contraction and relaxation.

TABLE 2.10

GMP Herbal Medicines for a 30-Year-Old Adult with Steinert Myotonic Dystrophy

Steinert myotonic dystrophy (OrphaCode: 273)

A disease with a prevalence of ~1 in 10,000

Disease-causing germline mutation(s): DM1 protein kinase (*DMPK* / Entrez: 1760) at 19q13.32

Autosomal dominant

Muscle weakness

Excessive daytime somnolence, Distal muscle weakness, Myotonia with warm-up phenomenon, Posterior subcapsular cataract, Cardiac conduction abnormality, EMG: myotonic discharges

Behavioral abnormality, Gait disturbance, Abnormal rapid eye movement sleep, Obstructive sleep apnea, Myalgia, Atrial fibrillation, Prolonged QRS complex, Poor fine motor coordination, Foot dorsiflexor weakness, Prolonged PR interval, Fatigue, Fatigable weakness of bulbar muscles, Weakness of facial musculature, Impairment in personality functioning, Cognitive impairment, Hypersomnia, Abnormality of masticatory muscle

(Continued)

TABLE 2.10 *(Continued)*

GMP Herbal Medicines for a 30-Year-Old Adult with Steinert Myotonic Dystrophy

Male hypogonadism, Testicular atrophy, Decreased fertility, Neck muscle weakness, Astigmatism, Hypermetropia, Ophthalmoplegia, Depression, Autistic behavior, Short attention span, Anxiety, Impotence, Hypergonadotropic hypogonadism, Diabetes mellitus, Hyperinsulinemia, Insulin resistance, Secondary hyperparathyroidism, Cholelithiasis, Intellectual disability, mild, Dysarthria, Global developmental delay, Mental deterioration, Neonatal hypotonia, Specific learning disability, Facial diplegia, Bilateral ptosis, Decreased fetal movement, Polyhydramnios, Mood changes, Alopecia, Talipes equinovarus, Diarrhea, Constipation, Respiratory insufficiency, Cerebral cortical atrophy, Early balding, Abnormal cerebral white matter morphology, Falls, Respiratory insufficiency due to muscle weakness, Respiratory failure, Elevated hepatic transaminase, Abnormality of thyroid physiology, Hypercholesterolemia, Skeletal muscle atrophy, Distal amyotrophy, Proximal muscle weakness, Neck flexor weakness, Intestinal pseudo-obstruction, Supraventricular tachycardia, Respiratory failure requiring assisted ventilation, Intellectual disability, borderline, Reduced visual acuity, Limited extraocular movements, Feeding difficulties in infancy, Diaphragmatic weakness, Peripheral neuropathy, Impaired visuospatial constructive cognition, Tented upper lip vermilion, Mild fetal ventriculomegaly, Nasogastric tube feeding in infancy, Paranoia, Handgrip myotonia, Myotonia of the jaw, Myotonia of the upper limb, Left ventricular systolic dysfunction, Decreased serum testosterone level, Abnormality of the tongue muscle, Oral-pharyngeal dysphagia

Antenatal, Neonatal, Infancy, Childhood, Adolescent, Adult

Muscle weakness (D018908):

Dúhuójìshēngtāng 5g + niúxī 1g + mòyào 1g + rǔxiāng 1g + yánhúsuǒ 1g + fùzǐ 1g + guìzhī 1g + jīxuèténg 1g + acupuncture.

Dúhuójìshēngtāng 5g + shūjīnghuóxuètāng 4g + sháoyàogāncǎotāng 4-0g + acupuncture.

Dúhuójìshēngtāng 5g + shūjīnghuóxuètāng 4g + yánhúsuǒ 1g + mòyào 1-0g + rǔxiāng 1-0g + niúxī 1-0g + dùzhòng 1-0g + acupuncture.

Báizhú 5g + fùzǐ 5-3g + báisháo 5-3g + fúlíng 5-3g + dǎngshēn 5-2g + cháihú 5-0g + tiānhuā 2-0g + shēngjiāng 2-0g + guìzhī 2-0g + huángqín 2-0g + gāncǎo 1-0g + mǔlì 1-0g + gānjiāng 1-0g + dàhuáng 0g.

Báizhú 5g + fúlíng 5g + zhìgāncǎo 3g + gānjiāng 3g + niúxī 2g + fùzǐ 2g + guìzhī 2g.

Obstructive sleep apnea (327.23), Myalgia (D063806), Atrial fibrillation (427.31), Fatigue (D005221), Hypersomnia (327.13):

Cháihújiālónggǔmǔlìtāng 5g + tiānhuā 1g + guìzhī 1g.

Cháihújiālónggǔmǔlìtāng 5g + guālóurén 1g + xièbái 1-0g + dǐdāngtāng 1-0g + dàhuáng 0g.

Gāncǎo 5g + zhǐqiào 5-3g + guìzhī 5-3g + táorén 5-3g + dàhuáng 1-0g + hónghuā 1-0g.

Gāncǎo 5g + shēngjiāng 5g + guìzhī 5g + báizhú 5-0g + fùzǐ 5-0g + fúlíng 5-0g + ròuguì 5-0g.

Huángqí 5g + gāncǎo 2g + zhīmǔ 2g + jiégěng 2g + shēngmá 1g + cháihú 1g.

Astigmatism (367.2), Hypermetropia (367.0), Ophthalmoplegia (378.56), Diabetes mellitus (250), Dysarthria (D004401), Polyhydramnios (657.0), Alopecia (704.0), Talipes equinovarus (754.51), Diarrhea (D003967), Constipation (564.0), Elevated hepatic transaminase (573.9), Skeletal muscle atrophy (D009133), Intestinal pseudo-obstruction (560.1):

Jiāwèixiāoyáosǎn 5g + zhǐqiào 3-2g + jílí 3-2g + sāngbáipí 2-0g.

Zhúyèshígāotāng 5g + júhuā 2g + zhǐqiào 1g + jílí 1g.

Gǒuqǐzǐ 5g + júhuā 5g + dāngguī 5g + dìhuáng 4g + fángfēng 4g + xìxīn 2g + huánglián 2g + dàhuáng 0g.

Zhǐqiào 5g + jílí 5-4g + chántuì 5-4g + júhuā 5-0g + júhóng 5-0g + sīguāluò 4-0g.

Dúhuójìshēngtāng was concluded to be safe and effective for the treatment of lumbar disc herniation in a systematic review and meta-analysis of randomized controlled trials (Xiong et al., 2020). Cháihújiālónggǔmǔlìtāng "mediates Shaoyang, subdues panic, calms the mind" and is used today for general symptoms, neurotic disorders, and essential hypertension (Wang, 2019). The TCM Shaoyang syndrome is caused by "external heat evils (i.e., pathogens) intruding into the interior," manifesting an alternating chillness and fever, full and discomfort chest, bitter mouth, dry throat, dizziness, upsetting, vomiting, and lack of appetite. Cháihújiālónggǔmǔlìtāng was shown to significantly improve circadian rhythm and sleep disturbance in mice with chronic kidney disease by regulating orexin-A (Cao et al., 2023).

2.11 FAMILIAL OR SPORADIC HEMIPLEGIC MIGRAINE

Hemiplegic migraine is tense and pulsing pain starting in a region of the head, such as the eye or temple, accompanied by weakness in one side of the body, which is considered one of the migraine aura symptoms. Hemiplegic migraine is caused by mutations in genes whose products are part of

---

TABLE 2.11
GMP Herbal Medicines for a 12-Year-Old Child with Familial or Sporadic Hemiplegic Migraine

Familial or sporadic hemiplegic migraine (OrphaCode: 569)

A disease with a prevalence of ~1 in 10,000

Disease-causing germline mutation(s): sodium voltage-gated channel alpha subunit 1 (*SCN1A* / Entrez: 6323) at 2q24.3

Disease-causing germline mutation(s): calcium voltage-gated channel subunit alpha1 A (*CACNA1A* / Entrez: 773) at 19p13.13

Disease-causing germline mutation(s): ATPase Na+/K+ transporting subunit alpha 2 (*ATP1A2* / Entrez: 477) at 1q23.2

Disease-causing germline mutation(s): proline rich transmembrane protein 2 (*PRRT2* / Entrez: 112476) at 16p11.2

Autosomal dominant

Muscle weakness, Migraine with aura, Neurological speech impairment, EEG abnormality, Focal motor seizure, Focal sensory seizure

Hearing impairment, Scotoma, Diplopia, Dysarthria, Hemiparesis, Confusion, Tongue fasciculations, Postural instability, Cerebral edema, Vertigo, Increased CSF protein, Paresthesia, Involuntary movements, Progressive gait ataxia, Dissociated sensory loss, Complex febrile seizure, Facial tics, CSF pleocytosis, Metamorphopsia, Photopsia, CSF lymphocytic pleiocytosis

Tinnitus, Coma, Cerebellar atrophy, Hemiplegia, Dysphasia, Impaired thermal sensitivity, Facial paralysis, Gaze-evoked horizontal nystagmus, Distal upper limb muscle weakness, Vertical nystagmus, Spontaneous pain sensation, EEG with generalized sharp slow waves, Seesaw nystagmus, Nuchal rigidity, Decreased vigilance, Alien limb phenomenon

Childhood

Muscle weakness (D018908), Migraine with aura (346.0), Neurological speech impairment (D013064), Focal sensory seizure (345.9):

Xiǎocháihútāng 5g + xìngrén 4-2g + hǎigé 4-2g + xīnyí 1g + jiégěng 1-0g + máhuáng 1-0g.

Yìgānsǎn 5g + chuānxiōng 2g + báizhǐ 2g.

Gōuténgsǎn 5g + chuānxiōng 1g + báizhǐ 1g.

Tiānmá 5g + gāncǎo 5g + báisháo 5g + dìhuáng 5g + hángjú 5g + xiàkūcǎo 5g + gōuténg 5g + niúxī 3g + báizhǐ 3g + màiméndōng 3g + dāngguī 3g + mànjīngzǐ 3g + gǎoběn 3g.

Tiānmá 5g + gāncǎo 5g + báisháo 5g + dìhuáng 5g + bǎihé 5g + ējiāo 5g + bózǐrén 5g + fúshén 5g + màiméndōng 5g + suānzǎorén 5g + gōuténg 5-0g.

Gāncǎo 5g + báizhǐ 5g + shārén 5g + dàhuáng 1-0g.

Fángfēng 5g + qiānghuó 5g + hòupò 3g + zhǐshí 3g + dàhuáng 0g.

Hearing impairment (D003638), Scotoma (D012607), Diplopia (D004172), Dysarthria (D004401), Hemiparesis (D010291), Confusion (D003221), Tongue fasciculations (D005207), Vertigo (386.2), Paresthesia (D010292), Metamorphopsia (D014786):

Línguìshùgāntāng 5g + zhēnwǔtāng 5-0g + bànxià 1-0g + shēngjiāng 1-0g + dàhuáng 0g.

Línguìshùgāntāng 5g + zhēnwǔtāng 3-0g + fùzǐ 1-0g + wǔwèizǐ 1-0g + gānjiāng 1-0g + xìxīn 1-0g + dàhuáng 0g.

Rénshēn 5g + cōngbái 4g + fùzǐ 3g + gānjiāng 3g + ròuguì 2g + wúzhūyú 2g + xìxīn 2g.

Rénshēn 5g + báizhú 5-4g + huángqín 5-0g + gānjiāng 5-0g + dàhuáng 0g.

Tinnitus (D014012), Coma (D003128), Hemiplegia (343.4), Facial paralysis (D005158), Vertical nystagmus (379.53, 379.55, 379.50):

Wǔlíngsǎn 5g + línguìshùgāntāng 5g + bànxià 1g + shēngjiāng 1g + fùzǐ 1-0g + acupuncture.

Sìnìtāng 5g + gǒuqǐzǐ 1g + júhuā 1g + dàhuáng 0g.

Guìzhītāng 5g + xìngrén 1-0g + hòupò 1-0g + bànxià 1-0g + dàhuáng 0g.

Dàhuáng 5g + gāncǎo 5g + báizhǐ 5g + shārén 5g + huángqín 5-0g.

Gāncǎo 5g + hòupò 5-0g + zhǐshí 5-0g + dàhuáng 1-0g.

sodium or calcium ion channels on the cell membrane or involved in neurotransmitter release for neuronal excitability. Germline mutations of these genes cause familial hemiplegic migraine, while *de novo* mutations of these genes cause sporadic hemiplegic migraine.

Tiānmá (cf. Section 1.22) "calms Wind, stops convulsions, inhibits Liver yang, dispels Wind, opens collaterals" and was summarized to be anticonvulsive, antioxidant, antidepressant, mono-amines modulating, GABAergic regulating, BDNF modulating, neuroprotective, and anti-inflammatory (Chen & Sheen, 2011). It is used today for an array of cerebroneural conditions, including headaches, sleep disturbances, vertiginous syndromes and labyrinthine disorders, con-cussions, paralysis agitans, migraines, dizziness and giddiness, quadriplegia, and Ménière's disease (Wang, 2020).

2.12 AICARDI-GOUTIÈRES SYNDROME

Aicardi-Goutières syndrome (AGS), also known as encephalopathy with intracranial calcifica-tion and chronic lymphocytosis of cerebrospinal fluid, is characterized by loss of white matter and deposits of calcium in the brain, affecting the brain and immune system. Most cases of AGS are caused by mutations in the genes whose products degrade one-stranded DNA and RNA when they are no longer needed in the cell.

Chuānwū (Radix Aconiti praeparata) "dispels Wind, removes dampness, disperses coldness and stops pain." It was reviewed to be anti-inflammatory, analgesic, and antitumor (Li et al., 2019a) and is used today for lumbago, hypertension, myalgia/myositis, chest pain, and monoplegia (Wang,

---

TABLE 2.12

GMP Herbal Medicines for a One-Year-Old Infant with Aicardi-Goutières Syndrome

Aicardi-Goutières syndrome (OrphaCode: 51)

A disease with a prevalence of ~1 in 10,000

Disease-causing germline mutation(s): LSM11, U7 small nuclear RNA associated (*LSM11* / Entrez: 134353) at 5q33.3

Disease-causing germline mutation(s): RNA, U7 small nuclear 1 (*RNU7-1* / Entrez: 100147744) at 12p13.31

Disease-causing germline mutation(s): SAM and HD domain containing deoxynucleoside triphosphate triphosphohydrolase 1 (*SAMHD1* / Entrez: 25939) at 20q11.23

Disease-causing germline mutation(s): ribonuclease H2 subunit A (*RNASEH2A* / Entrez: 10535) at 19p13.13

Disease-causing germline mutation(s): ribonuclease H2 subunit B (*RNASEH2B* / Entrez: 79621) at 13q14.3

Disease-causing germline mutation(s): ribonuclease H2 subunit C (*RNASEH2C* / Entrez: 84153) at 11q13.1

Disease-causing germline mutation(s): adenosine deaminase RNA specific (*ADAR* / Entrez: 103) at 1q21.3

Disease-causing germline mutation(s): three prime repair exonuclease 1 (*TREX1* / Entrez: 11277) at 3p21.31

Disease-causing germline mutation(s) (gain of function): interferon induced with helicase C domain 1 (*IFIH1* / Entrez: 64135) at 2q24.2

Autosomal dominant, Autosomal recessive

Spasticity, Global developmental delay, Hypertonia, Porencephaly, Arrhinencephaly, Intellectual disability, profound, Multifocal cerebral white matter abnormalities

Increased CSF interferon alpha, Chilblain lesions, Brain atrophy, Increased serum interferon-gamma level, Microcephaly, Eyelid coloboma, Irritability, Dry skin, Seizure, Dystonia, Hepatosplenomegaly, Unexplained fevers, Abnormality of extrapyramidal motor function, Hypoplasia of the corpus callosum, Ventriculomegaly, Difficulty walking, Loss of speech, Developmental regression, Leukodystrophy, Cerebral calcification, Elevated hepatic transaminase, Autoimmunity, Large beaked nose, Short stature, Hemiplegia/hemiparesis, Extrapyramidal muscular rigidity, Muscular hypotonia of the trunk, Chronic CSF lymphocytosis

Micropenis, Low-set ears, Abnormality of eye movement, Glaucoma, Ptosis, Nystagmus, Diabetes mellitus, Hypothyroidism, Cutis marmorata, Acrocyanosis, Developmental glaucoma, Tremor, Plagiocephaly, Arthritis, Hoarse voice, Cardiomegaly, Spastic paraparesis, Headache, Spastic tetraplegia, Scoliosis, Multiple joint contractures, Muscle stiffness, Neonatal alloimmune thrombocytopenia, Prolonged neonatal jaundice, Demyelinating peripheral neuropathy, Abnormal pyramidal sign, Panniculitis, Raynaud phenomenon

Neonatal, Infancy

(Continued)

TABLE 2.12 *(Continued)*

GMP Herbal Medicines for a One-Year-Old Infant with Aicardi-Goutières Syndrome

Spasticity (D009128), Hypertonia (D009122), Intellectual disability, profound (D008607):

Dāngguīsìnìtāng 5g + shēngjiāng 2-1g + báizhú 2-0g + fùzǐ 2-0g + báisháo 2-0g + fúlíng 2-0g + wúzhūyú 2-0g + dǎngshēn 1-0g + gānjiāng 1-0g + dàhuáng 0g.

Chuānwū 5g + wǔlíngzhī 5-2g + tiānnánxīng 5-2g + mùxiāng 5-2g + gāncǎo 5-2g + dìlóng 5-2g + yánhúsuǒ 5-2g + táorén 5-2g + huíxiāng 5-2g + chénpí 5-2g + dāngguī 5-2g + acupuncture.

Seizure (345.9), Dystonia (D004421), Difficulty walking (D051346), Elevated hepatic transaminase (573.9):

Yìgānsǎn 5g + cháihújiālónggǔmǔlìtāng 5g + tiānmá 2-0g + shíchāngpú 2-0g + yuǎnzhì 2-0g.

Yìgānsǎn 5g + wēndǎntāng 5g + shíchāngpú 1g + yuǎnzhì 1g.

Xiǎocháihútāng 5g + tiānmá 1g + shíchāngpú 1g + yuǎnzhì 1g.

Gāncǎo 5g + báizhǐ 2-0g + shārén 2-0g + dàhuáng 1-0g.

Zhìgāncǎo 5g + shārén 5g + dàhuáng 0g.

Huángqí 5-0g + gāncǎo 5-0g.

Glaucoma (365), Ptosis (374.3), Nystagmus (379.53, 379.55, 379.50), Diabetes mellitus (250), Hypothyroidism (244.9), Tremor (D014202), Hoarse voice (D006685), Spastic paraparesis (D020336), Headache (D006261), Spastic tetraplegia (344.00), Panniculitis (729.30):

Zīshènmíngmùtāng 5g + xǐgānmíngmùtāng 5-0g + xiàkūcǎo 1g + cǎojuémíng 1g + nǚzhēnzǐ 1-0g + hànliáncǎo 1-0g + mìménghuā 1-0g.

Qǐjúdìhuángwán 5g + xǐgānmíngmùtāng 5-0g + zīshènmíngmùtāng 5-0g + jiāwèixiāoyáosǎn 5-0g + nǚzhēnzǐ 1g + juémíngzǐ 1g + xiàkūcǎo 1g + mìménghuā 1-0g + gǔjīngcǎo 1-0g + hànliáncǎo 1-0g + chēqiánzǐ 1-0g + acupuncture.

Dàhuáng 5g + gāncǎo 5g + báizhǐ 5g + shārén 5g + huángqín 5g + huánglián 5-0g + gǒuqǐzǐ 2-0g + júhuā 2-0g.

Gǒuqǐzǐ 5g + júhuā 5g + dìhuáng 4g + dāngguī 4g + fángfēng 4-2g + huángqín 4-0g + xìxīn 2-1g + huánglián 2-1g + dàhuáng 1-0g.

2020). Note that unprocessed Chuānwū and Fùzǐ are toxic (Chan et al., 2021). Dāngguīsìnìtāng "nourishes Blood, disperses coldness, warms channels, opens collaterals" and is used today for diffuse diseases of connective tissue (Wang, 2019). Both Xǐgānmíngmùtāng and Zīshènmíngmùtāng are traditional formulas for ophthalmic disorders, as we will see their frequent uses in Chapter 6.

2.13 CHARCOT-MARIE-TOOTH DISEASE TYPE 4G

Charcot-Marie-Tooth disease is a hereditary motor and sensory neuropathy affecting peripheral nerves. It is characterized by progressive loss of muscles and sensation in the distal lower limbs. Different gene mutations give different Charcot-Marie-Tooth disease subtypes. Charcot-Marie-Tooth disease type 4G is associated with a mutation in the upstream region of the *HK1* gene, whose products catalyze the first step in glucose metabolism.

TABLE 2.13

GMP Herbal Medicines for a Ten-Year-Old Child with Charcot-Marie-Tooth Disease Type 4G

Charcot-Marie-Tooth disease type 4G (OrphaCode: 99953)

A disease with a prevalence of ~1 in 10,000

Disease-causing germline mutation(s): hexokinase 1 (*HK1* / Entrez: 3098) at 10q22.1

Autosomal recessive

Areflexia, Abnormality of the foot, Impaired vibratory sensation, Distal sensory impairment, Decreased motor nerve conduction velocity, Peripheral axonal neuropathy, Distal sensory loss of all modalities, Demyelinating peripheral neuropathy, Decreased distal sensory nerve action potential, Distal lower limb muscle weakness, Peripheral demyelination, Motor conduction block

Abnormality of the hand, Pes cavus, Talipes equinovarus, Difficulty walking, Distal amyotrophy, Proximal muscle weakness, Lower limb amyotrophy, Distal upper limb muscle weakness, Upper limb amyotrophy, Impaired tactile sensation

Gait imbalance, Progressive inability to walk, Scoliosis, Impaired pain sensation, Pes valgus

Childhood, Adolescent

(Continued)

TABLE 2.13 *(Continued)*

GMP Herbal Medicines for a Ten-Year-Old Child with Charcot-Marie-Tooth Disease Type 4G

Areflexia (D012021):

Qīngshǔyìqìtāng 5g + huòxiāngzhèngqìsǎn 5-0g + gégēnhuángqínhuángliántāng 3-0g.

Qīngshǔyìqìtāng 5g + huòxiāngzhèngqìsǎn 5-0g + píngwèisǎn 2-0g.

Qīngshǔyìqìtāng 5g + xiāngrúyǐn 4-0g + gégēn 1-0g.

Qīngshǔyìqìtāng 5g + shēngmàiyǐn 4-0g.

Shēngmá 5g + xuánshēn 5g + dìhuáng 5g + hòupò 5g + zhǐshí 5g + màiméndōng 5g + dàhuáng 0g.

Shēngmá 5g + gāncǎo 5g + dìhuáng 5g + dāngguī 5g + shúdìhuáng 5g + hónghuā 2g + táorén 2g.

Shēngmá 5g + chìsháo 5g + qiánhú 5g + sāngbáipí 5g + cháihú 5g + jīngjiè 5g + huángqín 5g + gégēn 5g.

Shēngmá 5g + gāncǎo 5g + báizhú 5g + cháihú 5g + chénpí 5g + huángqí 5g + dāngguī 5g + dǎngshēn 5g + fúlíng 5-0g.

Talipes equinovarus (754.51), Difficulty walking (D051346):

Zhènggǔzǐjīndān 5g + shūjīnghuóxuètāng 5-0g + acupuncture.

Zhènggǔzǐjīndān 5g + sháoyàogāncǎotāng 5-0g + acupuncture.

Guīlùèrxiānjiāo 5g + acupuncture.

Shūjīnghuóxuètāng 5g + acupuncture.

Gǔsuìbǔ 5g + xùduàn 5-2g + bǔgǔzhī 5-0g + jīxuèténg 2-0g + acupuncture.

Niúxī 5g + báisháo 5g + guìzhī 5g + gǔsuìbǔ 5g + dāngguī 5g + mùguā 4g + xùduàn 4g + mòyào 2g + rǔxiāng 2g.

Shēngmá (Rhizoma Cimicifugae) was found to protect against neurotoxicity in mice with Parkinson's disease by modulating oxidative stress and neuroinflammation in the brain (Cordaro et al., 2023). Qīngshǔyìqìtāng contains Shēngmá and Huángqí. Gǔsuìbǔ (Rhizoma Drynariae), which is translated to "bone fracture repairing," improves bone healing, as we will see in Chapter 10. Xùduàn (cf. Section 2.4) was demonstrated to prevent microgravity-induced bone loss in rats (Niu et al., 2015) and is used today for lumbago (Wang, 2020). Bǔgǔzhī (Fructus Psoraleae) "replenishes yang of the Kidney," which governs bone development and growth in TCM.

2.14 ACUTE TRANSVERSE MYELITIS

Acute transverse myelitis is inflammation on both sides of a spinal cord section with rapid onset of symptoms. The damaged segment of the spinal cord affects the body function at that level and below. Acute transverse myelitis can be caused by viral/bacterial/fungal infection or a disease such as multiple sclerosis.

TABLE 2.14

GMP Herbal Medicines for a 40-Year-Old Adult with Acute Transverse Myelitis

Acute transverse myelitis (OrphaCode: 139417)

A disease with a prevalence of ~8 in 100,000

Not applicable

Muscle weakness, Abnormality of extrapyramidal motor function, Increased CSF protein, Sensory impairment, CSF pleocytosis, Abnormal autonomic nervous system physiology

Urinary retention, Urinary incontinence, Hypertension, Spasticity, Orthostatic hypotension, Meningitis, Gait disturbance, Hyperreflexia, Fever, Constipation, Subarachnoid hemorrhage, Paraparesis, Upper motor neuron dysfunction, Impaired vibratory sensation, Gastroparesis, Paralytic ileus, Immunodeficiency, Systemic lupus erythematosus, Urinary bladder sphincter dysfunction, Autoimmunity, Paresthesia, Back pain, Upper limb muscle weakness, Babinski sign, Abnormality of temperature regulation, Autonomic bladder dysfunction, CNS demyelination, Distal lower limb muscle weakness, Muscle flaccidity, Paraplegia, Impaired proprioception, Dissociated sensory loss, Decreased circulating copper concentration, Hypoglycorrhachia, Fatigue, Dysesthesia, Abscess, Nuchal rigidity, Severe viral infection, Invasive parasitic infection, Abnormal libido, Extrapulmonary tuberculosis, Disseminated nontuberculous mycobacterial infection, Vitamin B12 deficiency

Infancy, Childhood, Adolescent, Adult, Elderly

(Continued)

TABLE 2.14 *(Continued)*
GMP Herbal Medicines for a 40-Year-Old Adult with Acute Transverse Myelitis

Muscle weakness (D018908), Sensory impairment (D006987):

Dúhuójìshēngtāng 5g + sháoyàogāncǎotāng 4-0g + mùguā 1-0g + niúxī 1-0g + acupuncture.

Dúhuójìshēngtāng 5g + shūjīnghuóxuètāng 4-0g + acupuncture.

Máhuángfùzǐxìxīntāng 5g + báizhú 2g + fùzǐ 2g + báisháo 2g + fúlíng 2g + gānjiāng 1g + dǎngshēn 1g + gāncǎo 1g.

Báizhú 5g + fùzǐ 5g + báisháo 5-4g + fúlíng 5-4g + dǎngshēn 5-2g + cháihú 5-0g + tiānhuā 2-0g + guìzhī 2-0g + huángqín 2-0g + shēngjiāng 2-0g + dàhuáng 2-0g + gāncǎo 1-0g + mǔlì 1-0g + gānjiāng 1-0g.

Báizhú 5g + fúlíng 5g + zhìgāncǎo 3g + gānjiāng 3g + niúxī 2g + fùzǐ 2g + guìzhī 2g.

Urinary incontinence (D014549), Hypertension (401-405.99), Spasticity (D009128), Meningitis (322.9), Hyperreflexia (D012021), Fever (D005334), Constipation (564.0), Paraparesis (D020335), Gastroparesis (536.3), Paralytic ileus (560.1), Immunodeficiency (279.3), Systemic lupus erythematosus (710.0), Paresthesia (D010292), Back pain (D001416), Muscle flaccidity (D009123), Paraplegia (344.1), Fatigue (D005221), Dysesthesia (D010292):

Bǔzhōngyìqìtāng 5g + dàhuáng 2-0g.

Dǐdāngtāng 5-3g + táohéchéngqìtāng 5-0g +dàhuáng 2-0g + gāncǎo 1-0g.

Qiānghuó 5g + hòupò 5-3g + zhǐshí 5-3g + dàhuáng 1-0g + huángqín 1-0g + huánglián 1-0g.

Qiānghuó (Rhizoma et Radix Notopterygii) "reduces coldness, scatters wind, removes dampness, stops pain" and is used today for fever, rhinitis, hypertensive heart and renal disease, and headache (Wang, 2020). Dǐdāngtāng "removes blood stasis of the lower body" and is used today for essential hypertension and disorder of joint (Wang, 2019). Táohéchéngqìtāng has been used for the relief of "blood stored in the lower body" and is used today for hemorrhoids (Wang, 2019).

2.15 MYASTHENIA GRAVIS

Myasthenia gravis, also known as acquired myasthenia, is an autoimmune disease of the synapse that transmits signals from a motor neuron to a muscle fiber for muscle contraction. Myasthenia gravis is caused by attacks of antibodies on the neurotransmitter receptors on the surface of the muscle cells.

TABLE 2.15
GMP Herbal Medicines for a 50-Year-Old Adult with Myasthenia Gravis

Myasthenia gravis (OrphaCode: 589)

A disease with a prevalence of ~8 in 100,000

Multigenic/multifactorial, Not applicable

Muscle weakness

Ptosis, Ophthalmoparesis, Diplopia, Abnormality of the thymus, Dysarthria, Bulbar palsy, Dysphagia, Dyspnea, Single fiber EMG abnormality, Acetylcholine receptor antibody positivity, Muscle specific kinase antibody positivity, Myositis

Hearing impairment, Hyperthyroidism, Hashimoto thyroiditis, Rheumatoid arthritis, Systemic lupus erythematosus, Glycosuria, Paresthesia, Primary adrenal insufficiency, Hyperacusis, Raynaud phenomenon

All ages

Muscle weakness (D018908):

Dúhuójìshēngtāng 5g + shūjīnghuóxuètāng 4g + sháoyàogāncǎotāng 4-0g + acupuncture.

Dúhuójìshēngtāng 5g + sháoyàogāncǎotāng 3-0g + dùzhòng 1-0g + gǔjǐ 1-0g + gǔsuìbǔ 1-0g + jīxuèténg 1-0g + xùduàn 1-0g + niúxī 0g.

Báizhú 5g + fùzǐ 5g + báisháo 5-4g + fúlíng 5-4g + dǎngshēn 5-2g + cháihú 5-0g + tiānhuā 2-0g + guìzhī 2-0g + huángqín 2-0g + wǔwèizǐ 2-0g + xìxīn 2-0g + gāncǎo 1-0g + mǔlì 1-0g + gānjiāng 1-0g + dàhuáng 1-0g.

Báizhú 5g + fúlíng 5-3g + zhìgāncǎo 3g + gānjiāng 3g + niúxī 3-2g + fùzǐ 3-2g + guìzhī 3-2g + dàhuáng 0g.

(Continued)

TABLE 2.15 *(Continued)*

GMP Herbal Medicines for a 50-Year-Old Adult with Myasthenia Gravis

Ptosis (374.3), Ophthalmoparesis (378.56), Diplopia (D004172), Dysarthria (D004401), Bulbar palsy (335.22), Dyspnea (D004417):

Zīshènmíngmùtāng 5g + qǐjúdìhuángwán 5-4g + nǚzhēnzǐ 1-0g + hànliáncǎo 1-0g + cǎojuémíng 1-0g + mìmēnghuā 1-0g + juémíngzǐ 1-0g + gǒuqǐzǐ 1-0g + xiàkūcǎo 1-0g + chēqiánzǐ 1-0g + jílí 1-0g.

Báizhǐ 5g + huángqín 5g + zhìgāncǎo 3g + shārén 3g + guālóugēn 2g + xìxīn 1g + dàhuáng 0g.
Báizhǐ 5g + huángqín 5-3g + gāncǎo 5-2g + shārén 5-2g + tiānhuā 2-0g + xìxīn 2-0g + guālóugēn 2-0g + dàhuáng 1g.

Hearing impairment (D003638), Rheumatoid arthritis (714.0), Systemic lupus erythematosus (710.0), Paresthesia (D010292), Hyperacusis (D012001):

Guìzhīsháoyàozhīmǔtāng 5g + dāngguīniántòngtāng 5g + niúxī 1g + huángbò 1g + cāngzhú 1g + yìyǐrén 1-0g + acupuncture.
Dāngguīniántòngtāng 5g + jìshēngshènqìwán 4-2g + shūjīnghuóxuètāng 2-0g + fóshǒugān 1g.

Chuānwū 5g + yánhúsuǒ 5-2g + wǔlíngzhī 2g + tiānnánxīng 2g + mùxiāng 2g + dìlóng 2g + táorén 2g + huíxiāng 2g + chénpí 2g + dāngguī 2g + gāncǎo 2-0g.
Fùzǐ 5g + báizhú 5-3g + cháihú 5-3g + báisháo 4-2g + fúlíng 4-2g + tiānhuā 2g + dǎngshēn 2g + huángqín 2-1g + shēngjiāng 2-0g + guìzhī 1g + gāncǎo 1g + mǔlì 1g + gānjiāng 1g.

Báisháo (cf. Section 1.65) extract was shown to markedly improve motor coordination of experimental parkinsonism in mice (Zheng et al., 2019). Yánhúsuǒ (Rhizoma Corydalis) was reviewed and summarized to have analgesic, antiarrhythmic, antipeptic ulcer, and hypnotic effects (Zhang et al., 2020a) and is used for peptic ulcers, dysmenorrhea, chest pain, and Klippel-Feil syndrome (Wang, 2020). Guìzhīsháoyàozhīmǔtāng treats rheumatoid arthritis, as we will see in Chapter 3 on rheumatologic diseases.

2.16 SPORADIC ADULT-ONSET ATAXIA OF UNKNOWN ETIOLOGY

Sporadic adult-onset ataxia of unknown etiology (SAOA), also known as idiopathic late-onset cerebellar ataxia, is a non-genetic neurodegeneration of the cerebellum manifesting slow progressive impairment and loss of muscle coordination. SAOA can arise from new and recent mutations in a gene or as a result of an underlying condition such as chronic alcoholism, vitamin deficiency, or hypothyroidism.

Dàzhēnjiāotāng "dispels Wind, clears heat, recuperates Qi/Blood, nourishes Blood/muscles" and is used today for arthropathies, late effects of cerebrovascular disease, and paralytic syndromes

TABLE 2.16

GMP Herbal Medicines for a 56-Year-Old Adult with Sporadic Adult-Onset Ataxia of Unknown Etiology

Sporadic adult-onset ataxia of unknown etiology (OrphaCode: 247234)

A disease with a prevalence of ~8 in 100,000

Not applicable

Abnormality of eye movement, Ataxia, Gait ataxia

Visual loss, Macular degeneration, Gaze-evoked nystagmus, Memory impairment, Dysautonomia, Abnormal vestibulo-ocular reflex, Impaired smooth pursuit, Cerebellar cortical atrophy

Hypomimic face, Sensory neuropathy, Spasticity, Dysarthria, Abnormal cranial nerve morphology, Parkinsonism, Hyperreflexia, Dysphagia, Rigidity, Dysdiadochokinesis, Akinesia, Resting tremor, Shuffling gait, Babinski sign

Adult, Elderly

Ataxia (D002524), Gait ataxia (D020234):

Dàzhēnjiāotāng 5g + dāngguīniántòngtāng 5g + sháoyàogāncǎotāng 4g + yánhúsuǒ 1-0g + hòupò 1-0g.

Huángqí 5g + chìsháo 1-0g + fángfēng 1-0g + xìxīn 1-0g + huánglián 1-0g + dàhuáng 0g.

(Continued)

TABLE 2.16 *(Continued)*
GMP Herbal Medicines for a 56-Year-Old Adult with Sporadic Adult-Onset Ataxia of Unknown Etiology

Memory impairment (D008569):

Sìnìtāng 5g + gānlùyǐn 5g.

Sìnìtāng 5g + píngwèisǎn 5g + xiāngshāliùjūnzǐtāng 5g.

Sìnìtāng 5g + shēngmàiyǐn 5g + zhìgāncǎotāng 5g.

Sìnìtāng 5g + bànxià 1g + fúlíng 1-0g + wúzhūyú 1-0g + dàhuáng 0g.

Gānjiāng 5g + rénshēn 4-2g + bànxià 4-2g.

Spasticity (D009128), Dysarthria (D004401), Hyperreflexia (D012021), Rigidity (D009127), Resting tremor (D014202), Shuffling gait (D020233):

Dāngguīsìnìtāng 5g + fùzǐ 1g + gānjiāng 1-0g.

Dāngguīsìnìtāng 5g + sìnìtāng 4-0g + shēngjiāng 1g + wúzhūyú 1-0g.

Chuānwū 5g + shúdìhuáng 5g + gāncǎo 3g + báisháo 3g + máhuáng 3g + huángqí 3g + báijièzǐ 2g + dàhuáng 1g + shēngjiāng 1g + huánglián 0g.

Chuānwū 5g + wǔlíngzhǐ 2g + tiānnánxīng 2g + mùxiāng 2g + gāncǎo 2g + dìlóng 2g + yánhúsuǒ 2g + táorén 2g + huíxiāng 2g + chénpí 2g + dāngguī 2g + acupuncture.

(Wang, 2019). Gānjiāng (cf. Sections 1.15 and 1.46) was shown to ameliorate morphine-induced memory impairment in rats (Gomar et al., 2014) and neuroinflammation-associated memory dysfunction in mice (Im et al., 2022). Sìnìtāng is made of Zhìgāncǎo, Gānjiāng, and Fùzǐ.

2.17   ANGELMAN SYNDROME

Angelman syndrome is a complex genetic disorder of the nervous system characterized by delayed development, intellectual disability, language impairment, ataxia, and seizures. Most cases of Angelman syndrome are caused by deletion or mutation in a region of the maternally derived chromosome 15 containing the *UBE3A* gene whose products play roles in synaptic plasticity through regulation of protein synthesis and degradation at the junctions between nerve cells. The genetic changes occur randomly during egg formation or early embryogenesis and are thus not inherited.

TABLE 2.17
GMP Herbal Medicines for a Three-Year-Old Child with Angelman Syndrome

Angelman syndrome (OrphaCode: 72)

A malformation syndrome with a prevalence of ~7 in 100,000

Disease-causing germline mutation(s) (loss of function): ubiquitin protein ligase E3A (*UBE3A* / Entrez: 7337) at 15q11.2

Role: the phenotype of small nuclear ribonucleoprotein polypeptide N (*SNRPN* / Entrez: 6638) at 15q11.2

Role: the phenotype of ubiquitin protein ligase E3A (*UBE3A* / Entrez: 7337) at 15q11.2

Role: the phenotype of ATPase phospholipid transporting 10A (putative) (*ATP10A* / Entrez: 57194) at 15q12

Role: the phenotype of OCA2 melanosomal transmembrane protein (*OCA2* / Entrez: 4948) at 15q12-q13.1

Not applicable, Unknown

Microcephaly, Behavioral abnormality, Autistic behavior, Inappropriate laughter, Delayed speech and language development, Hyperactivity, Seizure, Ataxia, Motor delay, Tremor, Cerebral cortical atrophy, Broad-based gait, Neurological speech impairment, EEG abnormality, Sleep disturbance, Poor speech, Intellectual disability, severe, Severe global developmental delay, Self-injurious behavior

Wide mouth, Astigmatism, Strabismus, Hypopigmentation of the skin, Obesity, Abnormal facial shape, Constipation, Gastroesophageal reflux, Fair hair, Drooling, Polyphagia, Scoliosis, Sleep-wake cycle disturbance, Iris hypopigmentation, Infantile muscular hypotonia, Protruding tongue, Abnormality of the gastrointestinal tract, Feeding difficulties, Recurrent hand flapping

(Continued)

TABLE 2.17 *(Continued)*

GMP Herbal Medicines for a Three-Year-Old Child with Angelman Syndrome

Mandibular prognathia, Ptosis, Hypermetropia, Optic disc pallor, Myopia, Keratoconus, Nystagmus, Amblyopia, Optic atrophy, Widely spaced teeth, Aggressive behavior, Anxiety, Poor eye contact, Myoclonus, Absent speech, Vomiting, Dysphagia, Poor suck, Generalized myoclonic seizures, Status epilepticus, Inability to walk, Flat occiput, Cerebral dysmyelination, Atypical absence seizure, Pes valgus, Precocious puberty in females, Atonic seizure, Gastrostomy tube feeding in infancy, Delayed menarche, Happy demeanor, Nasogastric tube feeding, Tongue thrusting

Infancy

Delayed speech and language development (D007805), Hyperactivity (D006948), Seizure (345.9), Ataxia (D002524), Tremor (D014202):

Yìgānsǎn 5g + guìzhījiālónggǔmǔlìtāng 5g + yuǎnzhì 1g.

Yìgānsǎn 5g + cháihújiālónggǔmǔlìtāng 5g + tiānmá 2-0g + gōuténg 2-0g.

Xiǎojiànzhōngtāng 5g + shānzhā 1g + shénqū 1g + màiyá 1g + jīnèijīn 1g.

Gāncǎoxiǎomàidàzǎotāng 5g + tiānmá 1g + shíchāngpú 1g + yuǎnzhì 1g + acupuncture.

Dàhuáng 5g + gāncǎo 5g + báizhǐ 5-0g + shārén 5-0g.

Gāncǎo 5g + báizhǐ 5-0g + shārén 5-0g + dàhuáng 1-0g.

Huángqí 5g + chìsháo 1g + fángfēng 1g + xìxīn 1-0g + huánglián 1-0g + dàhuáng 0g.

Astigmatism (367.2), Strabismus (378.7, 378.6, 378.31), Obesity (278.00), Constipation (564.0), Gastroesophageal reflux (530.81), Polyphagia (D006963), Abnormality of the gastrointestinal tract (520-579.99):

Sāngjúyǐn 5g + cāngěrsǎn 5g + chántuì 1g + zhǐqiào 0g.

Sāngjúyǐn 5g + zhǐqiào 2-0g + jílí 2-0g.

Hángjú 5g + gǒuqǐzǐ 5g + shíchāngpú 3-2g + yuǎnzhì 3-2g + nǚzhēnzǐ 2-0g + gāncǎo 2-0g + dàhuáng 1-0g.

Chántuì 5-4g + jílí 5-4g + júhuā 4-0g + júhóng 4-0g.

Ptosis (374.3), Hypermetropia (367.0), Myopia (367.1), Keratoconus (371.6), Nystagmus (379.53, 379.55, 379.50), Amblyopia (368.01, 368.00), Optic atrophy (377.1), Myoclonus (D009207), Vomiting (D014839):

Qǐjúdìhuángwán 5g + zīshènmíngmùtāng 5g + nǚzhēnzǐ 2g + hànliáncǎo 2g + cǎojuémíng 2g.

Yìqìcōngmíngtāng 5g + qǐjúdìhuángwán 5-4g + nǚzhēnzǐ 2-0g + juémíngzǐ 2-0g + gǒuqǐzǐ 2-0g + tùsīzǐ 2-0g + hànliáncǎo 2-0g + cǎojuémíng 2-0g + chōngwèizǐ 1-0g + shíchāngpú 1-0g + yuǎnzhì 1-0g + acupuncture.

Gǒuqǐzǐ 5g + shíchāngpú 4-3g + hángjú 4-2g + yuǎnzhì 4-2g + nǚzhēnzǐ 2-0g + liánqiáo 2-0g + gāncǎo 2-0g.

Compounds in Dàhuáng (cf. Section 1.30) were summarized to be neuroprotective, in vivo and in vitro, in a range of central nervous system diseases including cerebral ischemic stroke, intracerebral hemorrhage, traumatic brain injury, brain tumor, Alzheimer's disease, depression, epilepsy, neuropathic pain, diabetic encephalopathy, lead poisoning, and encephalitis (Li et al., 2019b).

2.18 SUNCT SYNDROME

SUNCT syndrome, i.e., short-lasting unilateral neuralgiform headache attacks with conjunctival injection and tearing, is characterized by brief and frequent bursts of moderate to severe pain near the eye or temple on one side of the head accompanied by eye redness and watering. The cause of SUNCT syndrome is not well understood but may involve abnormal hypothalamic activations.

Chuānxiōngchádiàosǎn "dispels Wind, clears heat, stops pain" and is used today for migraine (Wang, 2019). Shānzhūyú (Fructus Corni) has traditionally been used to "replenish the Liver and Kidney." It was reviewed to be hypoglycemic, antioxidant, anti-inflammatory, anticancer, neuroprotective, hepatoprotective, and nephroprotective (Dong et al., 2018) and is used today for a wide range of conditions including vision, circulation, reproduction, sleep, respiration, digestion, and metabolism (Wang, 2020). Zhēnrénhuómìngyǐnqùchuānshānjiǎ "clears heat, neutralizes pathogens, reduces swelling, destroys hardening, activates circulation, stops pain" and is used for diseases of sebaceous glands and hemorrhoids (Wang, 2019). Note that

TABLE 2.18

GMP Herbal Medicines for a 55-Year-Old Man with SUNCT Syndrome

SUNCT syndrome (OrphaCode: 57145)

A disease with a prevalence of ~7 in 100,000

Not applicable

Epiphora, Conjunctival hyperemia, Episodic pain

Ptosis, Restlessness, Agitation, Hyperhidrosis, Episodic hyperhidrosis, Migraine, Flushing, Rhinorrhea, Increased tear production, Trigeminal neuralgia

Facial edema, Photophobia, Miosis, Facial erythema, Nasal obstruction, Nausea, Ear pain, Jaw pain, Palpebral edema Adult

Epiphora (375.2, 375):

Qǐjúdìhuángwán 5g + zīshènmíngmùtāng 5-0g + mùzéicǎo 1-0g + cǎojuémíng 1-0g + mìmēnghuā 1-0g + gǔjīngcǎo 1-0g + chēqiánzǐ 1-0g + juémíngzǐ 1-0g.

Júhuā 5g + gǒuqǐzǐ 5-3g + dìhuáng 3-2g + fángfēng 3-2g + dāngguī 3-2g + huánglián 2-1g + xìxīn 2-0g.

Ptosis (374.3), Migraine (346), Trigeminal neuralgia (350.1):

Tiānmágōuténgyǐn 5g + qǐjúdìhuángwán 5g + dānshēn 1g + báijiāngcán 1g + dìlóng 1-0g + xiàkūcǎo 1-0g + báizhǐ 1-0g + xiōngqióng 1-0g.

Báizhǐ 5g + huángqín 5-0g + gāncǎo 4-3g + shārén 4-3g + guālóugēn 2-0g + tiānhuā 1-0g + xìxīn 1-0g + dàhuáng 1-0g.

Chuānxiōngchádiàosǎn 5g + xuèfǔzhúyūtāng 5-0g + jiāwèixiāoyáosǎn 4-0g + báijiāngcán 1g + hángjú 1g + mànjīngzǐ 1-0g + gǒuqǐzǐ 1-0g + acupuncture.

Huángqín 5g + báizhǐ 4g + zhìgāncǎo 2g + shārén 2g + guālóugēn 2g + xìxīn 1g + dàhuáng 0g.

Xǐgānmíngmùtāng 5g + qǐjúdìhuángwán 4g + xiōngqióng 1g + gǎoběn 1g.

Photophobia (D020795), Miosis (D015877), Facial erythema (695.3), Nausea (D009325), Ear pain (D004433):

Xiāofēngsǎn 5g + zhēnrénhuómìngyǐnqùchuānshānjiǎ 5g + báixiānpí 2g.

Shānzhūyú 5g + shānyào 5g + dìhuáng 5g + mǔdānpí 5g + fúlíng 5g + zéxiè 5g.

Xiāofēngsǎn 5g + lóngdǎnxiègāntāng 5g + zhēnrénhuómìngyǐnqùchuānshānjiǎ 4-0g + báixiānpí 1g + yúxīngcǎo 1-0g + yìyǐrén 1-0g + dìfūzǐ 1-0g + mǔdānpí 1-0g + chìsháo 1-0g + tǔfúlíng 1-0g + kǔshēngēn 1-0g.

Dānshēn 5g + gāncǎo 5g + báisháo 5g + shíhú 5g + bǎihé 5g + chēqiánzǐ 5g + fúlíng 5g + chénpí 5g + huángqí 5g + dǎngshēn 5g.

Zhēnrénhuómìngyǐnqùchuānshānjiǎ 5g + lóngdǎnxiègāntāng 5g + tǔfúlíng 1g + púgōngyīng 1g.

Báizhú 5g + fùzǐ 5g + cháihú 5g + báisháo 4g + fúlíng 4g + tiānhuā 2g + dǎngshēn 2g + guìzhī 2g + huángqín 2g + zhǐshí 2-0g + gāncǎo 1g + mǔlì 1g + gānjiāng 1g.

Zhēnrénhuómìngyǐn means "immortal life-sustaining drink" and qùchuānshānjiǎ means "excluding Manidae." Species within the Manidae family are endangered. When modern formulation of Zhēnrénhuómìngyǐn does not include Manidae, it is called Zhēnrénhuómìngyǐnqùchuānshānjiǎ. The indications of Zhēnrénhuómìngyǐn and Zhēnrénhuómìngyǐnqùchuānshānjiǎ are the same (Wang, 2019).

2.19 KENNEDY DISEASE

Kennedy disease, also known as X-linked bulbospinal muscular atrophy, is a neuromuscular disease characterized by progressive weakness and wasting of the muscles close to the trunk, including the face and throat. Kennedy disease is caused by an increased number of repeats in the *AR* gene, which encodes androgen receptors to activate androgen-responsive genes in various types of cells in the body, including the skeletal muscle and central nervous system.

Bājǐtiān (cf. Section 1.58) "replenishes Kidney yang, strengthens muscles and bones, dispels rheumatism," and has long been used in TCM for bone protection as well as andrological and gynecological healthcare. It is used today for male infertility and impotence of organic origin (Wang, 2020). Bāwèidìhuángwán "warms/nourishes the lower body, supplements Kidney yang" and is

TABLE 2.19

GMP Herbal Medicines for a 35-Year-Old Man with Kennedy Disease

Kennedy disease (OrphaCode: 481)

A disease with a prevalence of ~6 in 100,000

Disease-causing germline mutation(s): androgen receptor (*AR* / Entrez: 367) at Xq12

X-linked recessive

Decreased fertility, Gynecomastia, Hypotonia, Dysarthria, Hyporeflexia, Gait disturbance, Dysphonia, Skeletal muscle atrophy, Abnormality of movement, Erectile dysfunction

Testicular atrophy, Abnormal circulating lipid concentration, Type II diabetes mellitus

Adult

Gynecomastia (778.7), Hypotonia (D009123), Dysarthria (D004401), Dysphonia (D055154), Skeletal muscle atrophy (D009133):

Bāwèidìhuángwán 5g + bǔzhōngyìqìtāng 5g + bājǐtiān 1g + ròucōngróng 1g + yínyánghuò 1-0g + tùsīzǐ 1-0g + bǔgǔzhī 1-0g.

Liùwèidìhuángwán 5g + bǔzhōngyìqìtāng 5g + bājǐtiān 1g + ròucōngróng 1g + yínyánghuò 1g + tùsīzǐ 1g.

Yòuguīwán 5g + jìshēngshènqìwán 5g + bājǐtiān 1g + ròucōngróng 1g + yínyánghuò 1g + acupuncture.

Guìzhījiālónggǔmǔlìtāng 5g + bāwèidìhuángwán 3g + bājǐtiān 1g + ròucōngróng 1g + yínyánghuò 1g + bǔgǔzhī 1g.

Bājǐtiān 5g + dìhuáng 5g + dùzhòng 5g + guìzhī 5g + dǎngshēn 5g + xùduàn 5g + huángqín 5-0g + chuānxiōng 4-0g.

Fùzǐ 5g + gānjiāng 5g + cōngbái 5g + rénshēn 2-0g + ròuguì 2-0g + wúzhūyú 2-0g + xìxīn 2-0g.

Gāncǎo 5g + shārén 5g + huángbò 5g + wúzhūyú 2g + yánhúsuǒ 2g + fùzǐ 2g.

used today for diabetes mellitus, disorders of back, and chronic glomerulonephritis (Wang, 2019). Yòuguīwán was shown to enhance sperm fertilizing ability in normal male mice (Jiang et al., 2014).

2.20 INFANTILE SPASMS SYNDROME

Infantile spasms syndrome, also called West syndrome, is characterized by sudden and brief spasms of the baby that occur in clusters. Any brain damage due to brain trauma, brain malformation, brain infection, brain tumor, chromosomal abnormalities, genetic mutations, and metabolic disease can cause infantile spasms syndrome.

TABLE 2.20

GMP Herbal Medicines for a One-Year-Old Infant with Infantile Spasms Syndrome

Infantile spasms syndrome (OrphaCode: 3451)

A clinical syndrome with a prevalence of ~6 in 100,000

Disease-causing germline mutation(s): neurotrophic receptor tyrosine kinase 2 (*NTRK2* / Entrez: 4915) at 9q21.33

Disease-causing germline mutation(s): WD repeat domain 45 (*WDR45* / Entrez: 11152) at Xp11.23

Disease-causing germline mutation(s): sodium voltage-gated channel alpha subunit 2 (*SCN2A* / Entrez: 6326) at 2q24.3

Disease-causing germline mutation(s): cyclin dependent kinase like 5 (*CDKL5* / Entrez: 6792) at Xp22.13

Disease-causing germline mutation(s): aristaless related homeobox (*ARX* / Entrez: 170302) at Xp21.3

Disease-causing germline mutation(s): phosphatidylinositol glycan anchor biosynthesis class A (*PIGA* / Entrez: 5277) at Xp22.2

Disease-causing germline mutation(s): spectrin alpha, non-erythrocytic 1 (*SPTAN1* / Entrez: 6709) at 9q34.11

Disease-causing germline mutation(s) (loss of function): phospholipase C beta 1 (*PLCB1* / Entrez: 23236) at 20p12.3

Disease-causing germline mutation(s) (gain of function): glutamate ionotropic receptor NMDA type subunit 2B (*GRIN2B* / Entrez: 2904) at 12p13.1

Disease-causing germline mutation(s): ST3 beta-galactoside alpha-2,3-sialyltransferase 3 (*ST3GAL3* / Entrez: 6487) at 1p34.1

Disease-causing germline mutation(s): salt inducible kinase 1 (*SIK1* / Entrez: 150094) at 21q22.3

Disease-causing germline mutation(s): phosphatase and actin regulator 1 (*PHACTR1* / Entrez: 221692) at 6p24.1

(Continued)

TABLE 2.20 *(Continued)*

GMP Herbal Medicines for a One-Year-Old Infant with Infantile Spasms Syndrome

Disease-causing germline mutation(s): GTP binding elongation factor GUF1 (*GUF1* / Entrez: 60558) at 4p12
Disease-causing germline mutation(s): canopy FGF signaling regulator 3 (*CNPY3* / Entrez: 10695) at 6p21.1
Autosomal dominant, Autosomal recessive, X-linked recessive
Myoclonus, Developmental regression, Hypsarrhythmia, Infantile spasms
Abnormality of the nervous system, Abnormality of skin morphology
Neonatal, Infancy, Childhood

Myoclonus (D009207):

Sānbìtāng 5g + bǔzhōngyìqìtāng 2-0g.	Wēilíngxiān 5g + chuānshānlóng 5g + mùguā 4g + niúxī 4g + hónghuā 4g +
Sānbìtāng 5g + shūjīnghuóxuètāng 5-0g.	huángbò 4g + sānqī 4-0g + wǔjiāpí 4-0g + dàhuáng 4-0g.
Sānbìtāng 5g + dúhuójìshēngtāng 5-0g.	Chántuì 5g + jílí 5-4g + zhǐqiào 4-0g.

Chántuì (cf. Section 1.54), an animal traditional Chinese medicine, is the cast-off shell of a cicada. It has the effect of "dispelling wind-heat, promoting skin eruption, stopping itching, removing nebula, improving vision, and relieving convulsions." It was shown to be anticonvulsive, sedative, and hypothermic in rats (Hsieh et al., 1991). Sānbìtāng treats paralysis resulting from "wind, coldness and dampness" and is used today for osteoarthrosis and allied disorders (Wang, 2019).

2.21 TIBIAL MUSCULAR DYSTROPHY

Tibial muscular dystrophy, also known as Udd myopathy or distal titinopathy, is wasting of the muscles at the front of the lower leg. Tibial muscular dystrophy is caused by mutations in the *TTN* gene, whose products constitute part of the basic contractile unit called the sarcomere in a muscle fiber.

Shūjīnghuóxuètāng "relaxes muscles, invigorates Blood" and is used today for disorders of soft tissues and joints (Wang, 2019). Acupuncture as an adjuvant to medication was shown to enhance the efficacy of medication in patients with myasthenia gravis (Zhang et al., 2019a), which causes weakness of the voluntary muscles.

TABLE 2.21

GMP Herbal Medicines for a 35-Year-Old Adult with Tibial Muscular Dystrophy

Tibial muscular dystrophy (OrphaCode: 609)
A disease with a prevalence of ~6 in 100,000
Disease-causing germline mutation(s): titin (*TTN* / Entrez: 7273) at 2q31.2
Autosomal dominant, Autosomal recessive
Difficulty walking, Myopathy, Steppage gait, EMG: myopathic abnormalities, Increased variability in muscle fiber diameter, Centrally nucleated skeletal muscle fibers, Rimmed vacuoles, Mildly elevated creatine kinase, Foot dorsiflexor weakness, Peroneal muscle atrophy, Increased muscle lipid content, Ankle weakness
Clumsiness, Quadriceps muscle weakness, Proximal muscle weakness in lower limbs
Adult

Difficulty walking (D051346), Myopathy (359.9), Steppage gait (D020233):

Shūjīnghuóxuètāng 5g + dúhuójìshēngtāng 5-0g + dāngguīsìnìtāng 5-0g + acupuncture.	Báizhú 5g + fúlíng 4g + niúxī 3g + zhìgāncǎo 3g + zhǐshí 3g + guìzhī 3g + fùzǐ 2g + dàhuáng 0g.
Zhēnwǔtāng 5g + fùzǐ 1g + gānjiāng 1g + tiáowèichéngqìtāng 0g.	Báizhú 5g + báisháo 5-4g + fúlíng 5-4g + dǎngshēn 5-3g + fùzǐ 5-3g + cháihú 5-0g + tiānhuā 2-0g + guìzhī 2-0g + huángqín 2-0g + shēngjiāng 2-0g + suānzǎorén 2-0g + gāncǎo 1-0g + mǔlì 1-0g + gānjiāng 1-0g.
Dāngguīsìnìtāng 5g + fùzǐ 1g + shēngjiāng 1g + wúzhūyú 1g.	

2.22 PROGRESSIVE SUPRANUCLEAR PALSY

Progressive supranuclear palsy is deterioration and death of neuron cells in specific volumes of the brain, including the brainstem, where tau proteins accumulate. The cause of progressive supranuclear palsy is unknown; however, damage of the nerve cells by free radicals, a by-product of cellular metabolism, is hypothesized.

Wūyàoshùnqìsǎn "leads Qi, dispels Wind, dissipates congelation, moves stasis" and is used today for paralytic syndromes including facial nerve disorders and trigeminal nerve disorders (Wang, 2019). Mùguā (Fructus Chaenomelis) "relaxes muscles, activates collaterals, removes dampness, harmonizes the Stomach" and is used today for disorders of muscles, ligaments, and fascia (Wang, 2020).

TABLE 2.22

GMP Herbal Medicines for a 65-Year-Old Adult with Progressive Supranuclear Palsy

Progressive supranuclear palsy (OrphaCode: 683)

A disease with a prevalence of ~5 in 100,000

Not applicable

Supranuclear gaze palsy, Supranuclear ophthalmoplegia, Dysphagia, Postural instability, Unsteady gait, Falls, Neuronal loss in central nervous system, Abnormal synaptic transmission, Impulsivity

Vertical supranuclear gaze palsy, Slow saccadic eye movements, Blepharospasm, Depression, Delayed speech and language development, Dystonia, Bradykinesia, Cerebral cortical atrophy, Gliosis, Pseudobulbar signs, Memory impairment, Aphasia, Cognitive impairment

Abnormality of eye movement, Dementia, Tremor, Rigidity

Adult, Elderly

Unsteady gait (D020233):	
Shēntòngzhúyūtāng 5g + shūjīnghuóxuètāng 5g + yánhúsuǒ 1g + niúxī 1-0g + guìzhī 1-0g + acupuncture.	Chuānwū 5g + wǔlíngzhī 2g + tiānnánxīng 2g + mùxiāng 2g + gāncǎo 2g + dìlóng 2g + yánhúsuǒ 2g + táorén 2g + huíxiāng 2g + chénpí 2g + dāngguī 2g + acupuncture.
Dàzhēnjiāotāng 5g + dāngguīniāntòngtāng 5g + sháoyàogāncǎotāng 4g.	Wēilíngxiān 5g + báizhú 3g + qiānghuó 3g + xiāngfù 3g + huángqín 3g + cāngzhú 3g + tiānnánxīng 2g + bànxià 2g + gāncǎo 2g + shēngjiāng 2g + fúlíng 2g + chénpí 2g.
	Wēilíngxiān 5g + chuānshānlóng 5g + sānqī 4g + mùguā 4g + niúxī 4g + hónghuā 4g + huángbò 4g + dàhuáng 1-0g.

Blepharospasm (333.81), Delayed speech and language development (D007805), Dystonia (D004421), Bradykinesia (D018476), Memory impairment (D008569), Aphasia (D001037):	
Wūyàoshùnqìsǎn 5g + huángqíwǔwùtāng 5g + dānshēn 1g + jīxuèténg 1g + acupuncture.	Huángqí 5g + chìsháo 1-0g + fángfēng 1-0g + xìxīn 1-0g + huánglián 1-0g + dàhuáng 0g + acupuncture.
Wūyàoshùnqìsǎn 5g + bǔyánghuánwǔtāng 5g + sānqī 1-0g + dānshēn 1-0g + tiānmá 1-0g + acupuncture.	

Tremor (D014202), Rigidity (D009127):	
Sānbìtāng 5g + dúhuójìshēngtāng 5g + shūjīnghuóxuètāng 5-0g + acupuncture.	Mùguā 5g + niúxī 5g + wēilíngxiān 5g + chuānshānlóng 5g + hónghuā 5g + huángbò 5g.
Sānbìtāng 5g + shūjīnghuóxuètāng 5-2g + mùguā 1-0g + niúxī 1-0g + acupuncture.	Chuānwū 5g + shúdìhuáng 5g + gāncǎo 3g + báisháo 3g + máhuáng 3g + huángqí 3g + báijièzǐ 2g + dàhuáng 1g + shēngjiāng 1g.

2.23 RETT SYNDROME

Rett syndrome is a neurodevelopmental condition affecting female cognition with a characteristic disease course consisting of the following four stages: normal growth, regression, plateau, and deterioration in movement. Rett syndrome is caused by mutations in the *MECP2* gene, whose products,

TABLE 2.23

GMP Herbal Medicines for a One-Year-Old Girl with Rett Syndrome

Rett syndrome (OrphaCode: 778)

A disease with a prevalence of ~5 in 100,000

Disease-causing germline mutation(s): methyl-CpG binding protein 2 (*MECP2* / Entrez: 4204) at Xq28
X-linked dominant

Progressive microcephaly, Stereotypy, Global developmental delay, Gait disturbance, Absent speech, Developmental regression, Abnormal pattern of respiration, Stereotypical hand wringing, High-pitched cry

Seizure, Dystonia, Failure to thrive, Bradykinesia, EEG abnormality, Difficulty walking, Skeletal muscle atrophy, Limb apraxia

Agitation, Cholecystitis, Hyperammonemia, Increased serum lactate, Sleep disturbance, Increased CSF lactate, Inability to walk, Scoliosis, Increased serum pyruvate, Infantile muscular hypotonia, Abnormal autonomic nervous system physiology, Increased serum leptin

Infancy

Stereotypy (307.3):

Shēnlíngbáizhúsǎn 5g + gāncǎoxiǎomàidàzǎotāng 5-0g + shānzhā 1-0g + shénqū 1-0g + màiyá 1-0g + jīnèijīn 1-0g + wūméi 1-0g.

Wēndǎntāng 5g + shānzhā 1g + shénqū 1g + màiyá 1g.

Gāncǎo 5g + hòupò 5g + zhǐshí 5g + dàhuáng 1g.

Gāncǎo 5g + shārén 5-0g + báizhǐ 5-0g + dàhuáng 1-0g.

Xuánshēn 5g + dìhuáng 5g + màiméndōng 5g + dàhuáng 0g + hòupò 0g + zhǐshí 0g.

Seizure (345.9), Dystonia (D004421), Bradykinesia (D018476), Difficulty walking (D051346), Skeletal muscle atrophy (D009133):

Yìgānsǎn 5g + cháihújiālónggǔmǔlìtāng 5-0g + gāncǎoxiǎomàidàzǎotāng 3-0g + shíchāngpú 1-0g + fúshén 1-0g + yuǎnzhì 1-0g.

Cháihújiālónggǔmǔlìtāng 5g + gāncǎoxiǎomàidàzǎotāng 5-0g + shēnlíngbáizhúsǎn 5-0g + shíchāngpú 2-1g + yuǎnzhì 2-1g + héhuānpí 1-0g.

Gāncǎoxiǎomàidàzǎotāng 5g + cháihújiālónggǔmǔlìtāng 5g + wēndǎntāng 5-0g.

Gāncǎo 5g + báizhǐ 5-0g + shārén 5-0g + huángqín 5-0g + dàhuáng 1-0g.

Gāncǎo 5g + hòupò 4g + zhǐshí 4g + dàhuáng 1g.

Cholecystitis (575.10), Hyperammonemia (D022124) [Disorders of urea cycle metabolism (270.6)]:

Bāzhèngsǎn 5g + wǔlínsǎn 5g + dǐdāngtāng 5-2g.

Sháoyàogāncǎotāng 5g + tiānhuā 2g + xuánshēn 2g + mǔlì 2g + màiméndōng 2g + fùzǐ 1g.

Niúbàngzǐ 5g + zàojiǎocì 5g + rǔxiāng 5g + gǒujǐ 5g + fùzǐ 5g + dàhuáng 3-2g.

Bànxià 5g + fúlíng 5g + fùzǐ 5-3g + xìxīn 5-3g + dàhuáng 2-1g.

which are abundant in brain cells, regulate the activities of many other genes through an epigenetic mechanism called DNA methylation.

Shēnlíngbáizhúsǎn was shown to ameliorate colitis in mice by restoring the disturbed gut microbiota (Gao et al., 2024). Its use for stereotypy in Table 2.23 is supposed to be based on the gut-brain axis, through which animal behaviors and gut bacteria compositions are connected (Morais et al., 2020). An alkaloid in Yìgānsǎn (cf. Sections 1.1, 1.43, and 1.57) was found to reduce seizures in mice (Xie et al., 2020). Niúbàngzǐ (Fructus Arctii) was shown to attenuate diabetic kidney disease in mice (Zhong et al., 2019). Bāzhèngsǎn "relieves stranguria by diuresis" and is used today for chronic glomerulonephritis and cystitis (Wang, 2019).

2.24 JUVENILE ABSENCE EPILEPSY

Juvenile absence epilepsy (JAE) refers to a sudden, brief loss of, or reduction in, responsiveness to the environment associated with abnormal electric conductivity in the brain that first begins in one's adolescence. The exact cause of JAE is not known, although mutations in the *EFHC1* gene, whose

TABLE 2.24

GMP Herbal Medicines for an 11-Year-Old Child with Juvenile Absence Epilepsy

Juvenile absence epilepsy (OrphaCode: 1941)

A disease with a prevalence of ~5 in 100,000

Major susceptibility factor: EF-hand domain containing 1 (*EFHC1* / Entrez: 114327) at 6p12.2

Multigenic/multifactorial, Unknown

Bilateral tonic-clonic seizure, Generalized-onset seizure, EEG with polyspike wave complexes

Abnormality of the mouth, Abnormality of eye movement

Generalized non-motor (absence) seizure, Febrile seizures

Adolescent

Bilateral tonic-clonic seizure (D012640):

Tiānwángbǔxīndān 5g + cháihújiālónggǔmǔlìtāng 5g + shíchāngpú 1g + fúshén 1g + yuǎnzhì 1g.

Tiānwángbǔxīndān 5g + jiāwèixiāoyáosǎn 5g + gāncǎoxiǎomàidàzǎotāng 5-0g + xīnyíqīngfèitāng 5-0g + shíchāngpú 1-0g + yuǎnzhì 1-0g + héhuānpí 1-0g + yèjiāoténg 1-0g.

Fúshén 5g + diàoténggōu 5g + gégēn 2g + gǎoběn 2g + chìsháo 1g + cháihú 1g + jīngjiè 1g + xùduàn 1g.

Fúshén 5g + gōuténg 5g + shāshēn 4-0g + xuánshēn 4-0g + gégēn 2g + gǎoběn 2g + chìsháo 1g + jīngjiè 1g + xùduàn 1g + yùzhú 1-0g + mànjīngzǐ 1-0g + cháihú 1-0g.

Suānzǎorén 5g + yèjiāoténg 2g + fúshén 2g + shíchāngpú 1g + yuǎnzhì 1g + wǔwèizǐ 0g.

Yèjiāoténg 5g + diàoténggōu 5g + màiméndōng 5g + gāncǎo 2g + báisháo 2g + dìhuáng 2g + juémíngzǐ 2g + fúlíng 2g + suānzǎorén 2g.

Febrile seizures (D003294) [Febrile convulsions (simple), unspecified (780.31)]:

Sháoyàogāncǎotāng 5g + èrchéntāng 3g + gégēn 2g + fúshén 1g.

Sháoyàogāncǎotāng 5g + shūjīnghuóxuètāng 5g + mùguā 1-0g + niúxī 1-0g.

Sháoyàogāncǎotāng 5g + bǔzhōngyìqìtāng 5g.

Sháoyàogāncǎotāng 5g + gégēntāng 5g.

Fúxiǎomài 5g + dàzǎo 2g + gāncǎo 2g + báisháo 2-1g + gānjiāng 2-0g.

products interact with other proteins for calcium ion movement important for signaling between the nerve cells in the brain, are suspected.

Fúshén (Poria cum Radix Pini) "strengthens the Spleen, soaks dampness, calms the Heart, tranquilizes the mind" and was shown to improve the neuropsychological assessment results in patients with amnestic mild cognitive impairment (Choi et al., 2020). Tiānwángbǔxīndān "cultivates the Heart, calms the mind, nourishes yin, and clears heat." It was suggested to be effective for insomnia in a systematic review and meta-analysis (Yang et al., 2019) and is used today for neurotic disorders (Wang, 2019). Fúxiǎomài (Fructus Tritici Levis) "arrests sweating, benefits Qi, clears heat" and has been used for night sweats. Sháoyàogāncǎotāng "modulates Qi/Blood, alleviates cramps, and stops pain."

2.25 NARP SYNDROME

NARP syndrome, also known as neuropathy-ataxia-retinitis pigmentosa syndrome, is a mitochondrial disorder affecting the nervous system and the retina. NARP syndrome is caused by mutations in the *MT-ATP6* gene in mitochondrial DNA, which encodes a subunit of an enzyme that converts energy from food to ATP, through a process called oxidative phosphorylation, in mitochondria.

Wǔlíngsǎn and Língguìshùgāntāng were annotated in Section 1.35 to treat acute low-tone sensorineural hearing loss and orthostatic dysregulation induced dizziness, respectively. Furthermore, Wǔlíngsǎn was reported to treat Ménière's disease (Hirata, 1994; Ye, 1999).

TABLE 2.25
GMP Herbal Medicines for a 12-Year-Old Child with NARP Syndrome

NARP syndrome (OrphaCode: 644)

A disease with a prevalence of ~5 in 100,000

Disease-causing germline mutation(s): mitochondrially encoded ATP synthase membrane subunit 6 (*MT-ATP6* / Entrez: 4508) at mitochondria

Mitochondrial inheritance

Hearing impairment, Rod-cone dystrophy, Optic disc pallor, Blindness, Nystagmus, Dementia, Irritability, Sensory neuropathy, Constriction of peripheral visual field, Retinal arteriolar tortuosity, Seizure, Ataxia, Global developmental delay, Ventriculomegaly, Cerebral cortical atrophy, Headache, Muscle spasm, Babinski sign, Proximal muscle weakness, Myoclonic spasms, Short stature, Corticospinal tract atrophy, Progressive gait ataxia, Retinal pigment epithelial mottling, Intellectual disability, severe, Abnormal basal ganglia MRI signal intensity, Abnormal visual field test

Childhood

Hearing impairment (D003638), Nystagmus (379.53, 379.55, 379.50), Seizure (345.9), Ataxia (D002524), Headache (D006261), Muscle spasm (D009120):

Wǔlíngsǎn 5g + língguìshùgāntāng 5g + chēqiánzǐ 1g + niúxī 1-0g + chōngwèizǐ 1-0g.	Gāncǎo 5g + huángqín 5g + huángbò 5g + huánglián 1g + dàhuáng 0g.
Língguìshùgāntāng 5g + zīshènmíngmùtāng 5g + shíchāngpú 1g + juémíngzǐ 1g + yuǎnzhì 1g.	Gāncǎo 5g + gānjiāng 5g + dàhuáng 5-0g + báizhú 5-0g + fúlíng 5-0g + fùzǐ 5-0g + gǒuqǐzǐ 5-0g + júhuā 5-0g.
Língguìshùgāntāng 5g + qǐjúdìhuángwán 3g + niúxī 1g + chēqiánzǐ 1g + qīngxiāngzǐ 1g + chōngwèizǐ 1g + mìménghuā 1g + gǔjīngcǎo 1g.	Huángqí 5g + chìsháo 0g + fángfēng 0g + xìxīn 0g + huánglián 0g.

2.26 TYPICAL NEMALINE MYOPATHY

Typical nemaline myopathy is a congenital neuromuscular disorder characterized by facial and skeletal muscle weakness and the presence of thread-like or rod-like structures in muscle fibers when viewed under the microscope. Most cases of typical nemaline myopathy are attributed to mutations in the *NEB* gene, whose products interact with other proteins in muscle cells to generate mechanical forces for skeletal muscle contraction.

TABLE 2.26
GMP Herbal Medicines for a One-Year-Old Infant with Typical Nemaline Myopathy

Typical nemaline myopathy (OrphaCode: 171436)

A disease with a prevalence of ~5 in 100,000

Disease-causing germline mutation(s): actin alpha 1, skeletal muscle (*ACTA1* / Entrez: 58) at 1q42.13

Disease-causing germline mutation(s): cofilin 2 (*CFL2* / Entrez: 1073) at 14q13.1

Disease-causing germline mutation(s): tropomyosin 2 (*TPM2* / Entrez: 7169) at 9p13.3

Disease-causing germline mutation(s): nebulin (*NEB* / Entrez: 4703) at 2q23.3

Disease-causing germline mutation(s) (loss of function): kelch like family member 41 (*KLHL41* / Entrez: 10324) at 2q31.1

Disease-causing germline mutation(s) (loss of function): leiomodin 3 (*LMOD3* / Entrez: 56203) at 3p14.1

Autosomal dominant, Autosomal recessive

High palate, Hyporeflexia, Gait disturbance, Neonatal hypotonia, Respiratory insufficiency, Limb-girdle muscle weakness, Axial muscle weakness, Increased variability in muscle fiber diameter, Neck flexor weakness, Type 1 muscle fiber predominance, Foot dorsiflexor weakness, Facial palsy, Fatigable weakness of distal limb muscles

Narrow face, Micrognathia, Short neck, Ptosis, Pectus excavatum, Narrow chest, Facial diplegia, Flexion contracture, Polyhydramnios, Hypokinesia, Waddling gait, Scoliosis, Arthrogryposis multiplex congenita, Hip dislocation, Genu valgum, Nocturnal hypoventilation, Genu varum, Myopathy, Elevated circulating creatine kinase concentration, Spinal rigidity, Hyperlordosis, Nemaline bodies, Feeding difficulties, Fatigable weakness of respiratory muscles, Fatiguable weakness of proximal limb muscles

Neonatal

(Continued)

TABLE 2.26 *(Continued)*

GMP Herbal Medicines for a One-Year-Old Infant with Typical Nemaline Myopathy

Neonatal hypotonia (D009123), Facial palsy (351.0):

Xiǎoxùmìngtāng 5g + acupuncture.

Wūyàoshùnqìsǎn 5g + xiǎoxùmìngtāng 5-0g + acupuncture.

Bǔyánghuánwǔtāng 5g + acupuncture.

Guìzhītāng 5g + xìngrén 1g + hòupò 1g + dàhuáng 0g.

Báizhǐ 5g + zhìgāncǎo 5g + shārén 5g + dàhuáng 0g + acupuncture.

Báizhǐ 5g + gāncǎo 5-3g + shārén 5-3g + dàhuáng 0g + acupuncture. Zhǐqiào 5g.

Ptosis (374.3), Hypokinesia (D018476), Waddling gait (D020233), Myopathy (359.9):

Shēnlíngbáizhúsǎn 5g + xiāngshāliùjūnzǐtāng 5-0g.

Shēnlíngbáizhúsǎn 5g + yùpíngfēngsǎn 2-0g + shénqū 1g + màiyá 1-0g + shānzhā 1-0g + gāncǎo 1-0g.

Shēnlíngbáizhúsǎn 5g + bǎohéwán 2-0g + shānzhā 1g + shénqū 1g + màiyá 1g + gāncǎo 1-0g.

Báizhǐ 5g + shārén 5g + huángqín 5-0g + gāncǎo 3-2g + dàhuáng 1-0g.

Báizhǐ (cf. Section 1.7) was shown to reinforce the anti-migraine activity of Chuānxiōng (cf. Section 1.26) in rats (Feng et al., 2018). Xiǎoxùmìngtāng (cf. Section 1.17) was shown to dramatically alleviate learning and memory deficits and motor and coordination dysfunction in rats with bilateral common carotid artery occlusion (Wang et al., 2019). Shēnlíngbáizhúsǎn was demonstrated in rats to improve dyspeptic symptoms and also amend the dysregulated composition and function of the microbial community in the digestive tract (Zhang et al., 2019b). Gut-modulating TCM products such as Shēnlíngbáizhúsǎn may influence mood, cognition, and mental health of the patient through the gut-brain axis.

2.27 EARLY-ONSET AUTOSOMAL DOMINANT ALZHEIMER DISEASE

Early-onset autosomal dominant Alzheimer disease, also known as familial Alzheimer disease, is Alzheimer disease that affects more than one family members in more than one generation with the age of onset consistently before 65. Many cases of early-onset autosomal dominant Alzheimer disease are associated with mutations in the *PSEN1* gene, whose products cleave proteins, such as amyloid-beta precursor proteins, into pieces. Accumulation of a longer form of amyloid-beta is found in Alzheimer disease brains.

TABLE 2.27

GMP Herbal Medicines for a 45-Year-Old Adult with Early-Onset Autosomal Dominant Alzheimer Disease

Early-onset autosomal dominant Alzheimer disease (OrphaCode: 1020)

A disease with a prevalence of ~5 in 100,000

Candidate gene tested: ATP binding cassette subfamily A member 7 (*ABCA7* / Entrez: 10347) at 19p13.3

Candidate gene tested: triggering receptor expressed on myeloid cells 2 (*TREM2* / Entrez: 54209) at 6p21.1

Disease-causing germline mutation(s): presenilin 1 (*PSEN1* / Entrez: 5663) at 14q24.2

Disease-causing germline mutation(s): presenilin 2 (*PSEN2* / Entrez: 5664) at 1q42.13

Disease-causing germline mutation(s): amyloid beta precursor protein (*APP* / Entrez: 351) at 21q21.3

Disease-causing germline mutation(s): sortilin related receptor 1 (*SORL1* / Entrez: 6653) at 11q24.1

Biomarker tested: translocase of outer mitochondrial membrane 40 (*TOMM40* / Entrez: 10452) at 19q13.32

Autosomal dominant

Agitation, Dementia, Hallucinations, Seizure, Hypertonia, Confusion, Parkinsonism, Myoclonus, Cerebral cortical atrophy, Neurofibrillary tangles, Memory impairment, Language impairment, Deposits immunoreactive to beta-amyloid protein, Abnormal social behavior, Neurodevelopmental abnormality

(Continued)

TABLE 2.27 *(Continued)*

GMP Herbal Medicines for a 45-Year-Old Adult with Early-Onset Autosomal Dominant Alzheimer Disease

Disinhibition

Abnormality of vision, Oculomotor apraxia, Intellectual disability, Ataxia, Apraxia, Aphasia, Finger agnosia, Dysgraphia, Abnormality of higher mental function, Semantic dementia

Adult

Hallucinations (D006212), Seizure (345.9), Hypertonia (D009122), Confusion (D003221), Myoclonus (D009207), Memory impairment (D008569), Language impairment (D007806):

Gāncǎoxiǎomàidàzǎotāng 5g + cháihújiālónggǔmǔlìtāng 5g + wēndǎntāng 5-0 + bǎihé 1-0g + bózǐrén 1-0g + fúshén 1-0g. Gāncǎoxiǎomàidàzǎotāng 5g + yìgānsǎn 5g + cháihújiālónggǔmǔlìtāng 5-0g + fúshén 1-0g + yuǎnzhì 1-0g.	Mǔlì 5g + gāncǎo 4-3g + báisháo 4-3g + shúdìhuáng 4-3g + biējiǎ 4-3g + màiméndōng 3g + ējiāo 2g + huǒmárén 2g + fúshén 2-0g. Huángqí 5g + chìsháo 1g + fángfēng 1g + xìxīn 1g + huánglián 1g + dàhuáng 0g.

Intellectual disability (D008607), Ataxia (D002524), Apraxia (D001072), Aphasia (D001037), Finger agnosia (D000377), Dysgraphia (D000381):

Huángqíwǔwùtāng 5g + dāngguīsìnìtāng 5-0g + sāngzhī 2-1g + dānshēn 2-0g + zhúrú 2-0g + jiānghuáng 2-0g + jīxuèténg 1-0g + acupuncture. Huángqíwǔwùtāng 5g + bǔyánghuánwǔtāng 5g + jīxuèténg 1g.	Huángqí 5g + chìsháo 1g + fángfēng 1-0g + xìxīn 1-0g + huánglián 1-0g + dàhuáng 0g.

A systematic review and meta-analysis of randomized controlled trials suggested that adding Gāncǎoxiǎomàidàzǎotāng (cf. Sections 1.3, 1.42, and 2.6) to antidepressants reduces side effects and enhances efficacy of antidepressants (Yeung et al., 2014). Huángqí (cf. Sections 1.9, 1.68, and 2.1) plus conventional treatment was found to improve the symptoms of myasthenia gravis, a neuromuscular disorder, in a systematic review and meta-analysis of randomized clinical trials (Zhu et al., 2022).

2.28 PROXIMAL SPINAL MUSCULAR ATROPHY

Proximal spinal muscular atrophy, or SMA, is weakness and wasting of the muscles close to the center of the body due to loss of motor neurons. SMA is caused by mutations in the *SMN1* gene, whose products help maintain motor neurons in the brainstem and spinal cord for the transmission of signals between the brain and the skeletal muscles. Mutations in the *SMN2* gene modify the affected muscles and onset age of SMA.

TABLE 2.28

GMP Herbal Medicines for a 35-Year-Old Adult with Proximal Spinal Muscular Atrophy

Proximal spinal muscular atrophy (OrphaCode: 70)

A disease with a prevalence of ~5 in 100,000

Modifying germline mutation: survival of motor neuron 2, centromeric (*SMN2* / Entrez: 6607) at 5q13.2

Modifying germline mutation: NLR family apoptosis inhibitory protein (*NAIP* / Entrez: 4671) at 5q13.2

Disease-causing germline mutation(s): survival of motor neuron 1, telomeric (*SMN1* / Entrez: 6606) at 5q13.2

Autosomal recessive

Skeletal muscle atrophy, Proximal muscle weakness

Bulbar palsy, Areflexia, Tongue fasciculations, Reduced tendon reflexes, Dysphagia, Poor suck, Recurrent aspiration pneumonia, Difficulty walking, Distal muscle weakness, Inability to walk, Neonatal respiratory distress, Respiratory insufficiency due to muscle weakness, Axial muscle weakness, Difficulty climbing stairs, Quadriceps muscle weakness, Intercostal muscle weakness, Recurrent infections due to aspiration, Difficulty running, Fatigue, Weakness of facial musculature, Triceps weakness

(Continued)

TABLE 2.28 *(Continued)*

GMP Herbal Medicines for a 35-Year-Old Adult with Proximal Spinal Muscular Atrophy

Hypotonia, Global developmental delay, Motor delay, Neonatal hypotonia, Facial diplegia, Flexion contracture, Decreased fetal movement, Atrial septal defect, Constipation, Gastroesophageal reflux, Restrictive ventilatory defect, Poor head control, Gastroparesis, Scoliosis, Hypoventilation, Hip dislocation, Multiple joint contractures, Respiratory failure, Thoracic kyphosis, Difficulty standing, Knee flexion contracture, Absent patellar reflexes, Distal upper limb muscle weakness, Distal lower limb muscle weakness

All ages

Skeletal muscle atrophy (D009133):

Juānbìtāng 5g + sháoyàogāncǎotāng 3-0g + niúxī 1-0g + rǔxiāng 1-0g + yánhúsuǒ 1-0g + dǎodìwúgōng 1-0g + acupuncture.	Bànxià 5g + fúlíng 5g + fùzǐ 5-4g + xìxīn 5-2g + dàhuáng 2-1g + acupuncture.
Juānbìtāng 5g + shūjīnghuóxuètāng 4-0g + sāngzhī 1-0g + jīxuèténg 1-0g + acupuncture.	Fóshǒugān 5g + fúlíng 5g + guìzhī 5-4g + gānjiāng 2g + gāncǎo 2-1g + shārén 1-0g.

Bulbar palsy (335.22), Areflexia (D012021), Tongue fasciculations (D005207), Difficulty walking (D051346), Fatigue (D005221):

Bǔyánghuánwǔtāng 5g + huángqíwǔwùtāng 5-0g + dānshēn 2-1g + niúxī 2-1g + jīxuèténg 1-0g + acupuncture.	Huángqí 5g + chìsháo 1g + fángfēng 1g + xìxīn 1-0g + huánglián 1-0g.
Dúhuójìshēngtāng 5g + bǔyánghuánwǔtāng 5-0g + acupuncture.	Shúdìhuáng 5g + báizhú 4g + fùzǐ 4g + báisháo 3g + fúlíng 3g + báijièzǐ 2g + dǎngshēn 2g + gāncǎo 1g + shēngjiāng 1g + máhuáng 1g + huánglián 0g.
	Dìlóng 5g + táorén 5g + huángbò 5g + dāngguī 5g + gāncǎo 2g + ròuguì 2g + máhuáng 2g + sūmù 2g + chuānwū 1g + acupuncture.

Hypotonia (D009123), Constipation (564.0), Gastroesophageal reflux (530.81), Gastroparesis (536.3), Hypoventilation (D007040):

Lǐzhōngtāng 5g + mázǐrénwán 2g + tiáowèichéngqìtāng 2-0g + fùzǐ 1-0g + mǔlì 1-0 + dàhuáng 0g.	Běishāshēn 5g + yùzhú 5g + xuánshēn 5-0g + dìhuáng 5-0g + hòupò 5-0g + zhǐshí 5-0g + màiméndōng 5-0g + dàhuáng 1-0g.
Xuánfùdàizhěshítāng 5g + mázǐrénwán 2g + báijí 1g + hǎipiāoxiāo 1g + táohéchéngqìtāng 1g.	
Huángqíwǔwùtāng 5g + shēnlíngbáizhúsǎn 4g + fùzǐ 1g + dàhuáng 0g.	

Fóshǒugān (Fructus Citri Sarcodactylis) "soothes the Liver, resolves depression, regulates Qi, harmonizes interior, dries dampness, dissolves phlegm" and is used today to improve digestion (Wang, 2020). Its fermented derivative was shown to improve the growth performance of broiler chickens by improving intestinal digestive enzyme activity and gut microbial diversity (Zhou et al., 2023). Juānbìtāng "benefits Qi, activates circulation, dispels wind, removes dampness" and is used today for peripheral enthesopathies and allied syndromes (Wang, 2019). Lǐzhōngtāng is used today for functional digestive disorder (Wang, 2019).

2.29 OCULOPHARYNGEAL MUSCULAR DYSTROPHY

Oculopharyngeal muscular dystrophy, or OPMD, refers to weakness of the eyelid muscles and throat muscles, manifesting droopy eyelids and difficulty swallowing. Mutations in the *PABPN1* gene produce nonfunctional *PABPN1* proteins in muscle cells. Nonfunctional *PABPN1* proteins clump and kill muscle cells, causing OPMD.

A Huángqín decoction, made of Huángqín, Báisháo, Gāncǎo, and Dàzǎo, was shown to improve motor coordination, muscle strength, and mitochondrial dysfunction in rats with Parkinson's disease (Gao et al., 2022). Báizhǐ was annotated in Section 1.7 for the relief of facial paralysis.

TABLE 2.29

GMP Herbal Medicines for a 40-Year-Old Adult with Oculopharyngeal Muscular Dystrophy

Oculopharyngeal muscular dystrophy (OrphaCode: 270)

A disease with a prevalence of ~5 in 100,000

Disease-causing germline mutation(s): poly(A) binding protein nuclear 1 (*PABPN1* / Entrez: 8106) at 14q11.2
Autosomal dominant, Autosomal recessive

Ptosis, Abnormality of the pharynx, Ophthalmoplegia, Myopathy, Ragged-red muscle fibers, Elevated circulating creatine
 kinase concentration, Spondylolisthesis, Rimmed vacuoles, Abnormal muscle fiber morphology

Mask-like facies

Adult, Elderly

Ptosis (374.3), Ophthalmoplegia (378.56), Myopathy (359.9):

Jiāwèixiāoyáosǎn 5g + qǐjúdìhuángwán 5g + cǎojuémíng 1g +
 mìmēnghuā 1-0g + xuánshēn 1-0g + xiàkūcǎo 1-0g + nǚzhēnzǐ
 1-0g + hànliáncǎo 1-0g + tùsīzǐ 1-0g.
Qǐjúdìhuángwán 5g + zīshènmíngmùtāng 5g +
 jiāwèixiāoyáosǎn 5-0g + mùzéicǎo 1-0g + juémíngzǐ 1-0g.

Báizhǐ 5g + huángqín 5g + gāncǎo 3-2g + shārén 3-2g +
 guālóugēn 2-0g + dàhuáng 1-0g.
Huángqín 5g + báizhǐ 4g + shārén 3g + tiānhuā 2g +
 dàhuáng 0g.
Huángqín 5g + báizhǐ 3g + zhìgāncǎo 2g + shārén 2g +
 guālóugēn 2g + xìxīn 1g + dàhuáng 0g.

2.30 EARLY-ONSET CEREBELLAR ATAXIA WITH RETAINED TENDON REFLEXES

Early-onset cerebellar ataxia with retained tendon reflexes (EOCARR), also known as Harding ataxia, is characterized by association of progressive cerebellar ataxia with above-average response in the upper and lower limbs during a reflex test. The gene that causes EOCARR has not been identified, although its genomic locus was mapped. The inheritance pattern of EOCARR was found to be autosomal recessive.

The whole extract of Gāncǎo was shown to improve the neurologic symptoms of patients with acute ischemic stroke in a randomized, double-blind, placebo-controlled study (Ravanfar et al., 2016). Guìzhītāng's major component, Guìzhī (Ramulus Cinnamomi), is "perspiration inducing, muscle relaxing, warm to open meridians, and helping yang to disperse." Guìzhī was shown to protect the prefrontal cortex of rats against oxidative damage (Zheng et al., 2015).

TABLE 2.30

GMP Herbal Medicines for a Nine-Year-Old Child with Early-Onset Cerebellar Ataxia with Retained Tendon Reflexes

Early-onset cerebellar ataxia with retained tendon reflexes (OrphaCode: 1177)

A disease with a prevalence of ~5 in 100,000

Autosomal recessive

Progressive cerebellar ataxia

Nystagmus, Dysarthria, Dysphagia, Sensory impairment, Lower limb hypertonia, Hyperactive patellar reflex, Progressive
 gait ataxia, Abnormal pyramidal sign, Hyperreflexia in upper limbs, Jerky ocular pursuit movements

Pes cavus, Lower limb spasticity, Scoliosis, Abnormal EKG, Generalized amyotrophy, Lower limb muscle weakness,
 Impaired visuospatial constructive cognition, Cognitive impairment, Decreased/absent ankle reflexes

Childhood, Adolescent, Adult

Dysarthria (D004401), Sensory impairment (D006987):

Guìzhītāng 5g + báisháo 1g + dàhuáng 0g.
Guìzhītāng 5g + xìngrén 1g + hòupò 1g + dàhuáng 0g.
Zhēnwǔtāng 5g + fùzǐ 1g + gānjiāng 1g + dǐdāngtāng 0g.

Gāncǎo 5g + báizhǐ 5-0g + shārén 5-0g + dàhuáng 1-0g.
Gāncǎo 5g + hòupò 5-3g + zhǐshí 5-3g + dàhuáng 0g.
Gāncǎo 5g + báisháo 5g + shúdìhuáng 5g + biējiǎ 5g +
 màiméndōng 4g + ējiāo 3g + huǒmárén 2g.

2.31 ADNP SYNDROME

ADNP syndrome, also known as Helsmoortel-van der Aa syndrome, is characterized by intellectual disability and autism spectrum disorder. ADNP syndrome is caused by mutations in the *ADNP* gene, whose products control the activity of other genes important for brain development by dynamically unpacking chromatin structures to allow DNA transcriptional machinery proteins accessible to the DNA in the nucleus.

Fùpénzǐ (Fructus Rubi) "benefits the Liver/Kidney, retains semen, absorbs urine, improves eyesight" and is used for urinary frequency, urinary incontinence, and so on (Wang, 2020). The

---

TABLE 2.31

GMP Herbal Medicines for a Three-Year-Old Child with ADNP Syndrome

ADNP syndrome (OrphaCode: 404448)

A malformation syndrome with a prevalence of ~5 in 100,000

Disease-causing germline mutation(s): activity dependent neuroprotector homeobox (*ADNP* / Entrez: 23394) at 20q13.13

Unknown

Urinary incontinence, Autistic behavior, Impaired social interactions, Delayed speech and language development, Global developmental delay, Neurological speech impairment

Obsessive-compulsive behavior, Anxiety, Abnormality of finger, Joint laxity, Gastroesophageal reflux, Polyphagia, Attention deficit hyperactivity disorder, Infantile muscular hypotonia, Moderate global developmental delay, Severe global developmental delay, Abnormality of brain morphology, Chronic constipation, Abnormal temper tantrums, Oral-pharyngeal dysphagia

Recurrent urinary tract infections, Thick lower lip vermilion, Thin upper lip vermilion, Trigonocephaly, Smooth philtrum, Low-set ears, Protruding ear, Astigmatism, Strabismus, Hypermetropia, Aggressive behavior, Single transverse palmar crease, Plagiocephaly, Bilateral ptosis, Abnormality of the nail, Abnormality of toe, Sandal gap, Truncal obesity, Vomiting, Cerebral atrophy, Hypoplasia of the corpus callosum, Ventriculomegaly, Sleep disturbance, Developmental regression, Recurrent upper respiratory tract infections, Aspiration, Short stature, Impaired mastication, Advanced eruption of teeth, Wide intermamillary distance, Focal white matter lesions, Microtia, High anterior hairline, Polydactyly, Mild global developmental delay, Gastrostomy tube feeding in infancy, Abnormality of cardiovascular system morphology, Cerebral visual impairment, Slanting of the palpebral fissure

Infancy, Childhood

Urinary incontinence (D014549), Delayed speech and language development (D007805), Neurological speech impairment (D013064):

Sāngpiāoxiāosǎn 5g + bǔzhōngyìqìtāng 5-0g + yìzhìrén 1-0g + fùpénzǐ 1-0g.	Shānzhīzǐ 5g + báimáogēn 5g + zhīzǐ 5g + jīnyínhuā 2g + huángqín 2g + huángbò 2g + huánglián 2g + hǎipiāoxiāo 2-0g.
	Fùpénzǐ 5g + xiǎohuíxiāng 2g + wúzhūyú 2g + zéxiè 2g + sāngpiāoxiāo 1g + huángqí 1g + xùduàn 1g + tiānméndōng 1g.
	Xiǎohuíxiāng 5g + mùxiāng 5g + shārén 5g + ròudòukòu 3g + hòupò 3g + chénpí 3g + láifúzǐ 3g + gǔyá 3g.

Obsessive-compulsive behavior (300.3), Gastroesophageal reflux (530.81), Polyphagia (D006963):

Yìgānsǎn 5g + gāncǎoxiǎomàidàzǎotāng 2g + cháihújiālónggǔmǔlìtāng 2-0g + shíchāngpú 1-0g + yuǎnzhì 1-0g + suānzǎorén 1-0g + mǔlì 0g + lónggǔ 0g.	Bànxià 5g + gāncǎo 5g + fúlíng 5g + gānjiāng 5g.
	Huángqín 5g + gāncǎo 2g + báizhǐ 2g + shārén 2g + liánqiáo 2g + zhīzǐ 1g + dàhuáng 1g.
Liùwèidìhuángwán 5g + shēnlíngbáizhúsǎn 5g + shānzhā 0g + shénqū 0g + màiyá 0g.	Gāncǎo 5g + báizhǐ 5g + shārén 5-3g + dàhuáng 1-0g.
Wēndǎntāng 5g + gāncǎoxiǎomàidàzǎotāng 3g + shíchāngpú 1g + yuǎnzhì 1g.	

Astigmatism (367.2), Strabismus (378.7, 378.6, 378.31), Truncal obesity (D056128), Vomiting (D014839), Polydactyly (755.0), Cerebral visual impairment (377.75):

Qǐjúdìhuángwán 5g + yìqìcōngmíngtāng 5-0g.	Jílí 5g + zhǐqiào 5-2g + chántuì 5-0g.
Qǐjúdìhuángwán 5g + zīshènmíngmùtāng 5-0g.	
Sāngjúyǐn 5g + zhǐqiào 2-1g + chántuì 2-0g + jílí 1-0g.	

bioactive compounds in Wēndǎntāng were reviewed to show potential in treating patients with neurological and psychiatric disorders (Pradhan et al., 2022). Sāngjúyǐn, combined with two other formulas, was found to relieve the dry eye symptom of patients with Sjögren's syndrome in a randomized, double-blind, crossover, placebo-controlled trial (Chang et al., 2021).

2.32 FRAGILE X-ASSOCIATED TREMOR/ATAXIA SYNDROME

Fragile X-associated tremor/ataxia syndrome (FXTAS syndrome) is characterized by involuntary, rhythmic muscle contractions during a voluntary movement, followed by the development of impaired muscle coordination and balance. FXTAS syndrome is caused by mutations in the *FMR1* gene, whose products play roles in the development of synapses between the neurons in the brain and regulate synaptic plasticity, which is essential for learning and memory.

Dāngguīniāntòngtāng "dispels Wind, eliminates dampness, clears heat, stops pain" and is used today for gout and disorder of the joints (Wang, 2019). Guìzhījiālónggǔmǔlìtāng (cf. Section 1.4) is derived from the combination of Guìzhītāng, Lónggǔ, and Mǔlì, in which Lónggǔ (Os Draconis) was shown in mice to be anxiolytic (Chen et al., 2022a). Guìzhījiālónggǔmǔlìtāng is used for neurotic

---

TABLE 2.32

GMP Herbal Medicines for a 50-Year-Old Man with Fragile X–Associated Tremor/Ataxia Syndrome

Fragile X-associated tremor/ataxia syndrome (OrphaCode: 93256)

A malformation syndrome with a prevalence of ~5 in 100,000

Disease-causing germline mutation(s) (gain of function): fragile X messenger ribonucleoprotein 1 (*FMR1* / Entrez: 2332) at Xq27.3

X-linked dominant

Dementia, Ataxia, Dysarthria, Gait disturbance, Dysmetria, Gait ataxia, Intention tremor, Cerebral cortical atrophy, Memory impairment, Inertia

Depression, Obsessive-compulsive behavior, Anxiety, Impotence, Hyporeflexia, Muscle weakness, Rigidity, Dysautonomia, Urinary bladder sphincter dysfunction, Peripheral neuropathy, Dysesthesia, Diffuse cerebellar atrophy, Pollakisuria

Hypothyroidism, Hypertension, Parkinsonism, Dysphagia, Bradykinesia, Abnormal brain stem morphology, Bowel incontinence, Hypotension, Myalgia

Adult

Ataxia (D002524), Dysarthria (D004401), Gait ataxia (D020234), Intention tremor (D014202), Memory impairment (D008569):

Dàzhēnjiāotāng 5g + sānbìtāng 5g + dāngguīniāntòngtāng 5-0g.

Dàzhēnjiāotāng 5g + dāngguīniāntòngtāng 5g + sháoyàogāncǎotāng 4-0g + yánhúsuǒ 1-0g + dàhuáng 1-0g.

Huángqí 5g + chìsháo 2-0g + fángfēng 2-0g + xìxīn 1-0g + huánglián 1-0g.

Obsessive-compulsive behavior (300.3), Muscle weakness (D018908), Rigidity (D009127), Dysesthesia (D010292):

Guìzhījiālónggǔmǔlìtāng 5g + wǔwèizǐ 1g + bózǐrén 1g + yuǎnzhì 1-0g + suānzǎorén 1-0g.

Dāngguīsìnìtāng 5g + shēngjiāng 1g + wúzhūyú 1g.

Dāngguīsìnìtāng 5g + wúzhūyú 1g + gānjiāng 1g + fùzǐ 1g + wūméi 1g.

Dúhuójìshēngtāng 5g + dùzhòng 1g + gǒujǐ 1g + gǔsuìbǔ 1g + jīxuèténg 1g + xùduàn 1g.

Báizhú 5g + fùzǐ 5g + cháihú 5g + báisháo 4g + fúlíng 4g + tiānhuā 2g + dǎngshēn 2g + guìzhī 2g + huángqín 2g + wǔwèizǐ 2-0g + xìxīn 2-0g + shēngjiāng 2-0g + gāncǎo 1g + mǔlì 1g + gānjiāng 1g.

Gāncǎo 5g + báisháo 5g + shíhú 5g + bǎihé 5g + chēqiánzǐ 5g + fúlíng 5g + màiméndōng 5g.

Hypothyroidism (244.9), Hypertension (401-405.99), Bradykinesia (D018476), Myalgia (D063806):

Tiānmágōuténgyǐn 5g + xuèfǔzhúyūtāng 5g + tiānwángbǔxīndān 5-0g + dānshēn 1g + xiàkūcǎo 1-0g.

Tiānmágōuténgyǐn 5g + zhībódìhuángwán 5-4g + jiāwèixiāoyáosǎn 5-0g + dānshēn 1g + xiàkūcǎo 1g.

Bànxià 5g + ējiāo 5g + zǐcǎo 5g + dǎngshēn 5g + fùzǐ 3g + gānjiāng 3g.

Qiānghuó 5g + hòupò 5g + zhǐshí 5g + huánglián 3-1g + huángqín 2-1g + dàhuáng 1g.

disorders and general symptoms (Wang, 2019). Bànxià (cf. Section 2.3) was shown to inhibit human papillary thyroid carcinoma cells (Du et al., 2019).

2.33 CHARCOT-MARIE-TOOTH DISEASE TYPE 1B

Charcot-Marie-Tooth disease type 1B, or CMT1B, is a peripheral nervous system disorder characterized by weakness and wasting of the muscles and reduced sensation in the forearms, hands, lower legs, and feet. CMT1B is caused by mutations in the *MPZ* gene, whose products produce myelin in Schwann cells, which form a sheath around nerve axons for efficient transmission of electric impulses along nerve fibers.

Báizhú (cf. Section 1.21, 1.63, and 2.2) was shown to stimulate mitochondrial function and energy metabolism in myotubes derived from mice (Song et al., 2015). Rénshēn (cf. Sections 1.15 and 1.61) "supplements Qi, replenishes the Spleen, benefits the Lung, engenders fluid" and is used today for rhinitis, vertiginous syndromes and labyrinthine disorders, heart disease, palpitations, and coughs (Wang, 2020). Wēilíngxiān has traditionally been used for numbness and pain and was prescribed in Section 2.1 for paresthesia.

TABLE 2.33
GMP Herbal Medicines for a 40-Year-Old Adult with Charcot-Marie-Tooth Disease Type 1B

Charcot-Marie-Tooth disease type 1B (OrphaCode: 101082)

A disease with a prevalence of ~5 in 100,000

Disease-causing germline mutation(s): myelin protein zero (*MPZ* / Entrez: 4359) at 1q23.3

Autosomal dominant

Muscle weakness

Hearing impairment, Abnormal pupil morphology, Decreased nerve conduction velocity, Areflexia, Scoliosis, Increased CSF protein, Skeletal muscle atrophy, Elevated circulating creatine kinase concentration, Peripheral dysmyelination, Peripheral axonal neuropathy, Skeletal muscle hypertrophy

Motor delay, Sensory impairment

Infancy, Childhood, Adolescent, Adult

Muscle weakness (D018908):	
Dúhuójìshēngtāng 5g + shūjīnghuóxuètāng 4g + acupuncture.	Báizhú 5g + fùzǐ 5g + báisháo 5-4g + fúlíng 5-4g + dǎngshēn 5-2g + cháihú 5-0g + tiānhuā 2-0g + guìzhī 2-0g + huángqín 2-0g + wǔwèizǐ 2-0g + xìxīn 2-0g + shēngjiāng 2-0g + gāncǎo 1-0g + mǔlì 1-0g + gānjiāng 1-0g.
Dúhuójìshēngtāng 5g + dùzhòng 1g + gǒujǐ 1g + gǔsuìbǔ 1g.	
Dúhuójìshēngtāng 5g + jìshēngshènqìwán 5-0g + niúxī 1g + jīxuèténg 1g + mùguā 1-0g + dùzhòng 1-0g + mòyào 1-0g + rǔxiāng 1-0g + yánhúsuǒ 1-0g + fùzǐ 1-0g + guìzhī 1-0g.	Báizhú 5g + fúlíng 5g + zhìgāncǎo 3g + gānjiāng 3g + niúxī 2g + fùzǐ 2g + guìzhī 2g.

Hearing impairment (D034381), Areflexia (D012021), Skeletal muscle atrophy (D009133):	
Língguìshùgāntāng 5g + bànxià 1-0g + fùzǐ 1-0g + shārén 1-0g + gānjiāng 1-0g + xìxīn 1-0g + dàhuáng 0g.	Rénshēn 5g + bànxià 5-4g + gānjiāng 5-4g + huángqín 2-0g + huánglián 2-0g + dàhuáng 1-0g.
	Rénshēn 5g + báizhú 5g + huángqín 5-0g + báisháo 5-0g + fùzǐ 5-0g + fúlíng 5-0g.

Sensory impairment (D006987):	
Shēntòngzhúyūtāng 5g + dāngguīniāntòngtāng 5-0g + huángbò 1-0g + cāngzhú 1-0g + acupuncture.	Wēilíngxiān 5g + chuānshānlóng 5g + sānqī 4g + mùguā 4g + niúxī 4g + hónghuā 4g + huángbò 4g + dàhuáng 1-0g.
Shēntòngzhúyūtāng 5g + shūjīnghuóxuètāng 5-0g + niúxī 1-0g + yánhúsuǒ 1-0g + lùlùtōng 1-0g + acupuncture.	Wēilíngxiān 5g + báizhú 3g + qiānghuó 3g + xiāngfù 3g + huángqín 3g + cāngzhú 3g + tiānnánxīng 2g + bànxià 2g + gāncǎo 2g + shēngjiāng 2g + fúlíng 2g + chénpí 2g.

2.34 FACIOSCAPULOHUMERAL DYSTROPHY

Facioscapulohumeral dystrophy, also known as Landouzy-Dejerine myopathy, refers to progressive weakness and wasting of the muscles of the face, shoulder girdle, and upper arms. Facioscapulohumeral dystrophy is caused by contraction of the repeats in the *DUX4* gene, whose products activate other genes important for myogenesis during early embryonic development.

TABLE 2.34

GMP Herbal Medicines for a 22-Year-Old Adult with Facioscapulohumeral Dystrophy

Facioscapulohumeral dystrophy (OrphaCode: 269)

A disease with a prevalence of ~4 in 100,000

Modifying germline mutation: DNA methyltransferase 3 beta (*DNMT3B* / Entrez: 1789) at 20q11.21

Candidate gene tested: double homeobox 4 (*DUX4* / Entrez: 100288687) at 4q35.2

Candidate gene tested: double homeobox 4 like 1 (pseudogene) (*DUX4L1* / Entrez: 22947) at 4q35.2

Candidate gene tested: FSHD region gene 1 (*FRG1* / Entrez: 2483) at 4q35.2

Disease-causing germline mutation(s): structural maintenance of chromosomes flexible hinge domain containing 1 (*SMCHD1* / Entrez: 23347) at 18p11.32

Modifying germline mutation: structural maintenance of chromosomes flexible hinge domain containing 1 (*SMCHD1* / Entrez: 23347) at 18p11.32

Autosomal dominant

Mask-like facies, Skeletal muscle atrophy, Elevated circulating creatine kinase concentration, Hyperlordosis, EMG abnormality

Sensorineural hearing impairment, Abnormal eyelash morphology, Abnormal retinal vascular morphology, Palpebral edema

Malformation of the heart and great vessels

All ages

Skeletal muscle atrophy (D009133):

Juānbìtāng 5g + sháoyàogāncǎotāng 4-0g + sháoyàogāncǎotāng 4-0g + sāngzhī 1-0g + jīxuèténg 1-0g + yánhúsuǒ 1-0g + acupuncture.	Fóshǒugān 5g + guìzhī 5-4g + fúlíng 5-4g + máhuáng 4-0g + gānjiāng 3-0g + gāncǎo 1-0g.

Sensorineural hearing impairment (389.1):

Zīshèntōngěrtāng 5g + yìqìcōngmíngtāng 4-0g + shíchāngpú 1-0g + yuǎnzhì 1-0g + acupuncture. Yìqìcōngmíngtāng 5g + liùwèidìhuángwán 2g + shíchāngpú 1g + yuǎnzhì 1g. Tōngqiàohuóxuètāng 5g + shíchāngpú 1g + yuǎnzhì 1g.	Cōngbái 5g + fùzǐ 2g + gānjiāng 2g + rénshēn 2-1g + xìxīn 2-1g + ròuguì 1g + wúzhūyú 1g + bànxià 1-0g + dàhuáng 0g. Huángbò 5g + shārén 4g + shānzhīzǐ 2g + dìhuáng 2g + bǎihé 2g + dàndòuchǐ 2g + gāncǎo 2g + chìsháo 2g + ējiāo 2g + huángqín 2g + jiānghuáng 2g + jiāngcán 2g + chántuì 2g + dàhuáng 0g + huánglián 0g.

The organo-sulfur compounds in Cōngbái (Bulbus Allii Fistulosi) or garlic were shown to reduce the long-term effects of noise in rats (Şahin et al., 2018). Huángbò (cf. Section 1.61) was shown to reduce ear edema in mice through anti-inflammatory effects (Xian et al., 2011). Zīshèntōngěrtāng "nourishes the Kidney, opens the ear" and is used today for disorders of the ear (Wang, 2019). Tōngqiàohuóxuètāng "activates circulation, opens orifices" and is used for disorders of lipoid metabolism and essential hypertension (Wang, 2019).

2.35 BEHAVIORAL VARIANT OF FRONTOTEMPORAL DEMENTIA

Behavioral variant of frontotemporal dementia (bv-FTD) is characterized by changes in personality and decline in socially acceptable behaviors due to the loss of neuronal cells in the frontal and temporal lobes of the brain. Mutations in the *MAPT* gene are the first identified association with

TABLE 2.35

GMP Herbal Medicines for a 55-Year-Old Adult with Behavioral Variant of Frontotemporal Dementia

Behavioral variant of frontotemporal dementia (OrphaCode: 275864)

A disease with a prevalence of ~4 in 100,000

Major susceptibility factor: transmembrane protein 106B (*TMEM106B* / Entrez: 54664) at 7p21.3

Disease-causing germline mutation(s): presenilin 1 (*PSEN1* / Entrez: 5663) at 14q24.2

Major susceptibility factor: charged multivesicular body protein 2B (*CHMP2B* / Entrez: 25978) at 3p11.2

Major susceptibility factor: triggering receptor expressed on myeloid cells 2 (*TREM2* / Entrez: 54209) at 6p21.1

Major susceptibility factor: valosin containing protein (*VCP* / Entrez: 7415) at 9p13.3

Major susceptibility factor: microtubule associated protein tau (*MAPT* / Entrez: 4137) at 17q21.31

Major susceptibility factor: granulin precursor (*GRN* / Entrez: 2896) at 17q21.31

Disease-causing germline mutation(s): sequestosome 1 (*SQSTM1* / Entrez: 8878) at 5q35.3

Major susceptibility factor: C9orf72-SMCR8 complex subunit (*C9orf72* / Entrez: 203228) at 9p21.2

Autosomal dominant

Thickened nuchal skin fold, Behavioral abnormality, Hyperorality, Restlessness, Aggressive behavior, Inappropriate behavior, Restrictive behavior, Stereotypy, Disinhibition, Irritability, Personality changes, Lack of insight, Mental deterioration, Frontotemporal dementia, Memory impairment, Dysphasia, Loss of speech, Dyscalculia, Poor speech, Frontotemporal cerebral atrophy, Dyslexia, Dysgraphia, Echolalia, Emotional blunting, Perseveration

Abnormal cerebral white matter morphology, EEG with continuous slow activity, Collectionism, Abnormal brain FDG positron emission tomography

Psychosis, Apathy, Gait disturbance, Hyperreflexia, Bilateral tonic-clonic seizure, Abnormality of extrapyramidal motor function, Mutism, Fasciculations, Astrocytosis, Upper motor neuron dysfunction, Abulia

Adult

Stereotypy (307.3), Memory impairment (D008569), Dyslexia (315.01), Dysgraphia (D000381), Echolalia (D004454):

Cháihújiālónggǔmǔlìtāng 5g + suānzǎoréntāng 5g + tiānwángbǔxīndān 5-0g + yèjiāoténg 2g + fúshén 2g + yuǎnzhì 2-0g.

Lǐzhōngtāng 5g + suānzǎoréntāng 4-0g + mǔlì 2-0g + fùzǐ 2-0g.

Dìhuáng 5g + bǎihé 5g + yèjiāoténg 5g + bózǐrén 5g + fúxiǎomài 5g + fúshén 5g + màiméndōng 5g + suānzǎorén 5g + huángqín 5-0g + shíchāngpú 3-0g + yuǎnzhì 3-0g + gāncǎo 3-0g.

Huángqín 5g + báizhǐ 4-3g + gāncǎo 3-2g + shārén 3-2g + tiānhuā 1-0g + dàhuáng 1-0g + guālóugēn 1-0g.

Psychosis (295.4, 295.7), Hyperreflexia (D012021), Bilateral tonic-clonic seizure (D012640), Mutism (D009155), Fasciculations (D005207):

Gāncǎoxiǎomàidàzǎotāng 5g + wēndǎntāng 5g + guìzhījiālónggǔmǔlìtāng 5-0g + cháihújiālónggǔmǔlìtāng 5-0g + shíchāngpú 2-0g + yuǎnzhì 2-0g + yùjīn 1-0g.

Gāncǎoxiǎomàidàzǎotāng 5g + guìzhījiālónggǔmǔlìtāng 5g + shíchāngpú 1g + yuǎnzhì 1g + yùjīn 1g.

Gāncǎoxiǎomàidàzǎotāng 5g + wēndǎntāng 4g + fúshén 1g + yuǎnzhì 1g.

Bǎihé 5g + zhīmǔ 5-3g + xuánshēn 3-0g + bèimǔ 3-0g + mǔlì 3-0g + huánglián 3-0g + huángqín 2-0g + dàhuáng 1-0g.

Mǔlì 5g + gāncǎo 4g + báisháo 4g + shúdìhuáng 4g + biējiǎ 4g + màiméndōng 3g + ējiāo 2g + huǒmárén 2g + fúshén 2-0g.

bv-FTD. The *MAPT* gene encodes a protein called tau, which assembles and stabilizes the cytoskeleton of the nerve cells in the brain.

Yèjiāoténg (Caulis Polygoni Multiflori) "nourishes and calms the mind" and is used today for sleep disturbances and headaches (Wang, 2020). Bózǐrén (Semen Platycladi) was shown to have anxiolytic effects in chronic unpredictable mild-stress-induced mice through regulation of lipid metabolism and neuroactive ligand-receptor interaction (Xie et al., 2023). Zhīmǔ (Rhizoma Anemarrhenae) is cool in TCM nature; it was shown to protect cells derived from rat adrenal medullary pheochromocytoma (Piwowar et al., 2020) and to prevent and alleviate Alzheimer's disease in rats (Wang et al., 2022).

2.36 AMYOTROPHIC LATERAL SCLEROSIS

Amyotrophic lateral sclerosis (ALS), also known as Charcot disease or Lou Gehrig disease, is characterized by a progressive loss of the motor neurons in the brain and spinal cord for the control of voluntary muscles. Most ALS cases are sporadic. Among the heritable ALS, many are caused by mutations in the *C9orf72* gene, whose products help process RNA in the pre-synaptic terminals at the tip of nerve cells for neuron communications.

TABLE 2.36

GMP Herbal Medicines for a 65-Year-Old Adult with Amyotrophic Lateral Sclerosis

Amyotrophic lateral sclerosis (OrphaCode: 803)

A disease with a prevalence of ~4 in 100,000

Disease-causing germline mutation(s): cyclin F (*CCNF* / Entrez: 899) at 16p13.3

Candidate gene tested: TATA-box binding protein associated factor 15 (*TAF15* / Entrez: 8148) at 17q12

Candidate gene tested: EPH receptor A4 (*EPHA4* / Entrez: 2043) at 2q36.1

Disease-causing germline mutation(s): annexin A11 (*ANXA11* / Entrez: 311) at 10q22.3

Disease-causing germline mutation(s): cilia and flagella associated protein 410 (*CFAP410* / Entrez: 755) at 21q22.3

Disease-causing germline mutation(s): GLE1 RNA export mediator (*GLE1* / Entrez: 2733) at 9q34.11

Major susceptibility factor: NIMA related kinase 1 (*NEK1* / Entrez: 4750) at 4q33

Major susceptibility factor: glycosyltransferase 8 domain containing 1 (*GLT8D1* / Entrez: 55830) at 3p21.1

Disease-causing germline mutation(s): coiled-coil-helix-coiled-coil-helix domain containing 10 (*CHCHD10* / Entrez: 400916) at 22q11.23

Disease-causing germline mutation(s): D-amino acid oxidase (*DAO* / Entrez: 1610) at 12q24.11

Major susceptibility factor: ataxin 2 (*ATXN2* / Entrez: 6311) at 12q24.12

Disease-causing germline mutation(s): charged multivesicular body protein 2B (*CHMP2B* / Entrez: 25978) at 3p11.2

Disease-causing germline mutation(s): superoxide dismutase 1 (*SOD1* / Entrez: 6647) at 21q22.11

Major susceptibility factor: triggering receptor expressed on myeloid cells 2 (*TREM2* / Entrez: 54209) at 6p21.1

Disease-causing germline mutation(s): VAMP associated protein B and C (*VAPB* / Entrez: 9217) at 20q13.32

Disease-causing germline mutation(s): valosin containing protein (*VCP* / Entrez: 7415) at 9p13.3

Major susceptibility factor: neurofilament heavy chain (*NEFH* / Entrez: 4744) at 22q12.2

Disease-causing germline mutation(s): optineurin (*OPTN* / Entrez: 10133) at 10p13

Candidate gene tested: dynactin subunit 1 (*DCTN1* / Entrez: 1639) at 2p13.1

Disease-causing germline mutation(s): TAR DNA binding protein (*TARDBP* / Entrez: 23435) at 1p36.22

Disease-causing germline mutation(s): FIG4 phosphoinositide 5-phosphatase (*FIG4* / Entrez: 9896) at 6q21

Disease-causing germline mutation(s): FUS RNA binding protein (*FUS* / Entrez: 2521) at 16p11.2

Disease-causing germline mutation(s): angiogenin (*ANG* / Entrez: 283) at 14q11.2

Disease-causing germline mutation(s): matrin 3 (*MATR3* / Entrez: 9782) at 5q31.2

Major susceptibility factor: peripherin (*PRPH* / Entrez: 5630) at 12q13.12

Disease-causing germline mutation(s): paraoxonase 1 (*PON1* / Entrez: 5444) at 7q21.3

Disease-causing germline mutation(s): paraoxonase 2 (*PON2* / Entrez: 5445) at 7q21.3

Disease-causing germline mutation(s): paraoxonase 3 (*PON3* / Entrez: 5446) at 7q21.3

Disease-causing germline mutation(s): sequestosome 1 (*SQSTM1* / Entrez: 8878) at 5q35.3

Disease-causing germline mutation(s): ubiquilin 2 (*UBQLN2* / Entrez: 29978) at Xp11.21

Disease-causing germline mutation(s): C9orf72-SMCR8 complex subunit (*C9orf72* / Entrez: 203228) at 9p21.2

Disease-causing germline mutation(s): profilin 1 (*PFN1* / Entrez: 5216) at 17p13.2

Major susceptibility factor: TANK binding kinase 1 (*TBK1* / Entrez: 29110) at 12q14.2

Disease-causing germline mutation(s): heterogeneous nuclear ribonucleoprotein A1 (*HNRNPA1* / Entrez: 3178) at 12q13.13

Modifying germline mutation: PPARG coactivator 1 alpha (*PPARGC1A* / Entrez: 10891) at 4p15.2

Disease-causing germline mutation(s): erb-b2 receptor tyrosine kinase 4 (*ERBB4* / Entrez: 2066) at 2q34

Major susceptibility factor: unc-13 homolog A (*UNC13A* / Entrez: 23025) at 19p13.11

Autosomal dominant, Autosomal recessive, Not applicable

Amyotrophic lateral sclerosis

(Continued)

TABLE 2.36 *(Continued)*

GMP Herbal Medicines for a 65-Year-Old Adult with Amyotrophic Lateral Sclerosis

Neurodegeneration, Generalized muscle weakness, Motor neuron atrophy

Xerostomia, Emotional lability, Depression, Anxiety, Spasticity, Dyspnea, Functional respiratory abnormality, Respiratory failure, Skeletal muscle atrophy, Muscle spasm, Paralysis, Fatigue, Pain, Fatigable weakness of bulbar muscles, Fatigable weakness of swallowing muscles, Fatigable weakness of respiratory muscles

Agitation, Nausea and vomiting, Laryngospasm

Adult

Amyotrophic lateral sclerosis (335.20):

Bǔyánghuánwǔtāng 5g + dúhuójìshēngtāng 5-0g + dānshēn 1-0g + niúxī 1-0g + wēilíngxiān 1-0g + jīxuèténg 1-0g + acupuncture.	Shúdìhuáng 5g + báizhú 4g + fùzǐ 4g + báisháo 3g + fúlíng 3g + báijièzǐ 2g + dǎngshēn 2g + shēngjiāng 1g + máhuáng 1g + dàhuáng 1-0g + gāncǎo 1-0g + huánglián 0g.
Huángqíwǔwùtāng 5g + shūjīnghuóxuètāng 4g + sāngzhī 1g + jīxuèténg 1g.	Shúdìhuáng 5g + báizhú 3-2g + qiànshí 3-2g + yìyǐrén 3-2g + shānzhūyú 2-1g + báijièzǐ 2-1g + dùzhòng 2-1g + wǔwèizǐ 2-0g + dǎngshēn 2-0g + guìzhī 2-0g + fúlíng 2-0g + júhóng 1g + yìzhìrén 1-0g + rénshēn 1-0g + ròuguì 1-0g + shārén 1-0g.

Neurodegeneration (D009410) [Other cerebral degenerations (331)]:

Bǔyánghuánwǔtāng 5g + liùwèidìhuángwán 3-0g + dānshēn 1g + shíchāngpú 1g + yuǎnzhì 1g + tiānmá 1-0g + gōuténg 1-0g + acupuncture.	Huángqí 5g + chìsháo 2-0g + fángfēng 2-0g + xìxīn 1-0g + huánglián 1-0g + dàhuáng 0g.

Spasticity (D009128), Dyspnea (D004417), Skeletal muscle atrophy (D009133), Muscle spasm (D009120), Paralysis (D010243), Fatigue (D005221), Pain (D010146):

Dāngguīsìnìtāng 5g + dúhuójìshēngtāng 5-0g + shēngjiāng 2-0g + wúzhūyú 2-0g + niúxī 1-0g + fùzǐ 1-0g + acupuncture.	Chuānwū 5g + shúdìhuáng 5g + gāncǎo 3g + báisháo 3g + máhuáng 3g + huángqí 3g + báijièzǐ 2g + dàhuáng 1g + shēngjiāng 1g + huánglián 0g.
	Chuānwū 5g + wǔlíngzhī 2g + tiānnánxīng 2g + mùxiāng 2g + gāncǎo 2g + dìlóng 2g + yánhúsuǒ 2g + táorén 2g + huíxiāng 2g + chénpí 2g + dāngguī 2g + acupuncture.

Shúdìhuáng (cf. Section 1.71) "supplements Blood, nourishes yin, benefits essence, fills marrow," and was shown to ameliorate cognitive dysfunction and brain histopathological changes in Alzheimer's disease mice (Su et al., 2023). Bǔyánghuánwǔtāng "replenishes Qi, invigorates Blood, opens collaterals" and was shown to reduce the infarct area and ameliorate neurofunctional defects in rats with transient focal cerebral ischemia (Chen et al., 2020). Notice that Bǔyánghuánwǔtāng contains Huángqí and Chìsháo (Radix Paeoniae Rubra).

2.37 CHRONIC INFLAMMATORY DEMYELINATING POLYNEUROPATHY

Chronic inflammatory demyelinating polyneuropathy refers to inflammation of multiple peripheral nerves and spinal nerve roots, causing damage to the myelin sheaths of nerve fibers and impairment of the motor and sensory functions of the arms and legs. Chronic inflammatory demyelinating polyneuropathy is an autoantibody-mediated autoimmune disorder.

Chuānshānlóng (Rhizoma Dioscoreae Nipponicae) "soothes muscles, enlivens Blood, dispels Wind, and stops pain." It was shown to relieve synovial inflammation in rats with gouty arthritis (Lu et al., 2014); it is used today for myalgia, myositis, and pain in joints (Wang, 2020). Compounds isolated from Fúlíng (cf. Sections 1.21 and 1.66) were shown to be anti-inflammatory in a mouse macrophage cell line (Lee et al., 2017). Adjunctive use of GMP-concentrated Shūjīnghuóxuètāng extract granules was found to be associated with a lower risk of overall mortality, readmission, and reoperation in patients with a hip fracture (Cheng et al., 2019).

TABLE 2.37
GMP Herbal Medicines for a 50-Year-Old Man with Chronic Inflammatory Demyelinating Polyneuropathy

Chronic inflammatory demyelinating polyneuropathy (OrphaCode: 2932)

A disease with a prevalence of ~4 in 100,000

Not applicable

Decreased nerve conduction velocity, Areflexia, Unsteady gait, Paresthesia, Sensory impairment, Segmental peripheral demyelination/remyelination, Peripheral neuropathy, Sensory ataxia, Peripheral demyelination, Motor conduction block, Fatiguable weakness of proximal limb muscles, Abnormal nerve conduction velocity

Difficulty walking, Falls, Difficulty climbing stairs, Hand muscle weakness

Spontaneous pain sensation

Childhood, Adolescent, Adult, Elderly

Areflexia (D012021), Unsteady gait (D020233), Paresthesia (D010292), Sensory impairment (D006987), Sensory ataxia (D001259):

Bǔzhōngyìqìtāng 5g + bǔyánghuánwǔtāng 5-0g + chuānxiōng 1-0g + dānshēn 1-0g + jīxuèténg 1-0g + fùzǐ 0g + acupuncture.	Wēilíngxiān 5g + chuānshānlóng 5g + sānqī 4g + mùguā 4g + niúxī 4g + hónghuā 4g + huángbò 4g + gǒujǐ 4-0g + dàhuáng 1-0g.
Bǔzhōngyìqìtāng 5g + dúhuójìshēngtāng 5-0g.	Wēilíngxiān 5g + báizhú 3g + qiānghuó 3g + xiāngfù 3g + huángqín 3g + cāngzhú 3-0g + tiānnánxīng 2g + bànxià 2g + gāncǎo 2g + shēngjiāng 2g + fúlíng 2g + chénpí 2g.

Difficulty walking (D051346):

Shūjīnghuóxuètāng 5g + juānbìtāng 5g + sháoyàogāncǎotāng 4-0g + yánhúsuǒ 1-0g + wēilíngxiān 1-0g + acupuncture.	Fúlíng 5g + báisháo 4g + fùzǐ 4g + dǎngshēn 4g + báizhú 1g.
Shūjīnghuóxuètāng 5g + dúhuójìshēngtāng 5g + acupuncture.	Fúlíng 5g + bànxià 3g + fùzǐ 3g + xìxīn 2g + dàhuáng 1-0g.
Huángqíwǔwùtāng 5g + bǔyánghuánwǔtāng 5g + sāngzhī 1g + jīxuèténg 1g.	Chuānwū 5g + wǔlíngzhī 2g + tiānnánxīng 2g + mùxiāng 2g + gāncǎo 2g + dìlóng 2g + yánhúsuǒ 2g + táorén 2g + huíxiāng 2g + chénpí 2g + dāngguī 2g.

2.38 WORSTER-DROUGHT SYNDROME

Worster-Drought syndrome, also known as congenital suprabulbar paresis, is a permanent movement condition affecting the muscles in the head and neck for speaking, swallowing, and chewing. Worster-Drought syndrome is believed to be due to inadequate development of the motor neurons in the brain of the fetus, although no obvious causes during gestation or at birth were identified and families with a history of the condition were found.

TABLE 2.38
GMP Herbal Medicines for a Six-Year-Old Boy with Worster-Drought Syndrome

Worster-Drought syndrome (OrphaCode: 3465)

A malformation syndrome with a prevalence of ~4 in 100,000

Autosomal dominant, Not applicable

Abnormal cranial nerve morphology, Neurological speech impairment

Hyperreflexia, Cognitive impairment

Microcephaly, Sensorineural hearing impairment, Seizure, Tetraplegia

Childhood

Neurological speech impairment (D013064):

Gānlùxiāodúdān 5g + xīnyíqīngfèitāng 5g + cāngěrsǎn 5-0g + yínqiàosǎn 3-0g + gāncǎo 0g.	Běishāshēn 5g + xuánshēn 5g + yùzhú 5g + dìhuáng 5g + hòupò 5g + zhǐshí 5g + màiméndōng 5g + dàhuáng 1-0g.
Gānlùxiāodúdān 5g + bǎohéwán 5g.	Xuánshēn 5g + dìhuáng 5g + hòupò 5g + zhǐshí 5g + màiméndōng 5g + dàhuáng 0g.
Gānlùxiāodúdān 5g + jīngfángbàidúsǎn 5g + gāncǎo 1-0g + jiégěng 1-0g.	

(Continued)

TABLE 2.38 *(Continued)*
GMP Herbal Medicines for a Six-Year-Old Boy with Worster-Drought Syndrome

Hyperreflexia (D012021):

Yùpíngfēngsǎn 5g + xiāngshāliùjūnzǐtāng 5-0g + shēnlíngbáizhúsǎn 5-0g + bǔzhōngyìqìtāng 5-0g + wǔwèizǐ 1-0g.

Sāngpiāoxiāosǎn 5g + bǔzhōngyìqìtāng 5g + fùpénzǐ 2g.

Dàzǎo 5g + gāncǎo 5g + báisháo 5g + bǎihé 5g + ējiāo 5g + fúxiǎomài 5g + fúshén 5g + màiméndōng 5g + suānzǎorén 5g + gégēn 5-0g + shúdìhuáng 5-0g + dǎngshēn 5-0g.

Shēngmá 5g + xuánshēn 5g + dìhuáng 5g + hòupò 5g + zhǐshí 5g + màiméndōng 5g + gāncǎo 2-0g + dàhuáng 1-0g.

Xiǎohuíxiāng 5g + mùxiāng 5g + qiānghuó 5g + fùzǐ 5g + gānjiāng 5g + dúhuó 5g.

Sensorineural hearing impairment (389.1), Seizure (345.9), Tetraplegia (344.00):

Cháihújiālónggǔmǔlìtāng 5g + wēndǎntāng 5-0g + yìqìcōngmíngtāng 5-0g + gāncǎoxiǎomàidàzǎotāng 4-0g + shíchāngpú 2-1g + yuǎnzhì 2-1g + tiānmá 1-0g + acupuncture.

Liùwèidìhuángwán 5g + bǔzhōngyìqìtāng 5g + tiānmá 1g + shíchāngpú 1g + yuǎnzhì 1g + acupuncture.

Liùwèidìhuángwán 5g + guìzhījiālónggǔmǔlìtāng 5g + shíchāngpú 1g + yuǎnzhì 1g.

Huángqín 5g + báizhǐ 4-3g + gāncǎo 2g + shārén 2g + tiānhuā 1g + dàhuáng 0g + acupuncture.

Xuánshēn 5g + dìhuáng 5g + màiméndōng 5g + hòupò 2-1g + zhǐshí 2-1g + dàhuáng 1g.

Běishāshēn was introduced in Section 1.6 to be yin-nourishing. Indeed, it was shown to promote cell proliferation, neuroblast differentiation, and neuronal maturation in the hippocampus of adult mice (Park et al., 2018). Gānlùxiāodúdān was demonstrated to inhibit the replication of coxsackie-viruses in cultured cells (He et al., 1998). Jīngfángbàidúsǎn was shown to alleviate motor paralysis in mice with autoimmune encephalomyelitis (Choi et al., 2015). Yùpíngfēngsǎn contains Fángfēng (Radix Saposhnikoviae), which was shown to serve as a guiding herb to the cerebral tissue in rats (Wang et al., 2021). Sāngpiāoxiāosǎn contains Yuǎnzhì, Fúshén, and Shíchāngpú, which were identified to be the common herbs for memory disorders since ancient times (May et al., 2013).

2.39 ATTRV30M AMYLOIDOSIS

ATTRV30M amyloidosis, also known as familial amyloid polyneuropathy type I or transthyretin amyloid neuropathy, is a progressive peripheral (sensory and motor) and autonomic neuropathy and can manifest large deposits of amyloid fibrils in the medullary zone of the kidney and tubules. It is

TABLE 2.39
GMP Herbal Medicines for a 39-Year-Old Adult with ATTRV30M Amyloidosis

ATTRV30M amyloidosis (OrphaCode: 85447)

A disease with a prevalence of ~4 in 100,000

Disease-causing germline mutation(s): transthyretin (*TTR* / Entrez: 7276) at 18q12.1

Autosomal dominant

Nephropathy, Polyneuropathy, Abnormal test result

Impotence, Cardiomyopathy, Cardiomegaly, Atrioventricular block, Weight loss, Diarrhea, Constipation, Dysautonomia, Arrhythmia, Constrictive median neuropathy, Abnormal renal physiology, Vitreous floaters

Adult

Polyneuropathy (357.82):

Sháoyàogāncǎotāng 5g + shūjīnghuóxuètāng 5g + dāngguīniàntòngtāng 5-0g + dúhuójìshēngtāng 5-0g + gégēntāng 5-0g + acupuncture.

Huángqí 5g + jīxuèténg 5g + wǔlíngzhī 4g + gǒuqǐzǐ 4g + dāngguī 4g + tùsīzǐ 3g + fùpénzǐ 3g + bājǐtiān 2g.

Huángqí 5g + chìsháo 1-0g + fángfēng 1-0g + xìxīn 0g + huánglián 0g + dàhuáng 0g.

(Continued)

TABLE 2.39 *(Continued)*

GMP Herbal Medicines for a 39-Year-Old Adult with ATTRV30M Amyloidosis

Cardiomyopathy (425, 425.9), Atrioventricular block (426.10), Weight loss (D015431), Diarrhea (D003967), Constipation (564.0):

Zhìgāncǎotāng 5g + shēngmàiyǐn 5-4g + dānshēn 2-1g + yùjīn 2-1g + sānqī 1-0g + xiāngfù 1-0g + yuǎnzhì 1-0g.

Shēngmàiyǐn 5g + sìnìtāng 4g + dānshēn 1g + yùjīn 1g.

Sìnìtāng 5g + gānlùyǐn 5g + yùzhú 2g + mázǐrénwán 1g.

Mǔlì 5g + fúlíng 5g + dàfùpí 4g + gāncǎo 4g + sāngbáipí 4g + hǎipiāoxiāo 4g + jílí 4g + sānléng 3g + wǔlíngzhī 3g + éshù 3g + zǐsūyè 3g + yuǎnzhì 3-0g + xīnyí 2-0g + cāngěrzǐ 2-0g.

Dǎngshēn 5g + fùzǐ 4g + gānjiāng 4g + gāncǎo 3g.

Dàhuáng 5g + fùzǐ 5g + xìxīn 5g + máhuáng 5g.

Gāncǎo 5g + dàhuáng 3g + hòupò 3g + zhǐshí 3g.

caused by a methionine for valine substitution at residue 30 of the transthyretin protein, encoded by the *TTR* gene, resulting in amyloid aggregates of misfolded transthyretin monomers in multiple tissues and organs.

As one of the most frequently used formulas for the treatment of pain-related diseases in TCM, Sháoyàogāncǎotāng was shown to be anti-inflammatory and antinociceptive in rats with arthritic pain (Sui et al., 2016). Sháoyàogāncǎotāng was also demonstrated to exert an analgesic effect on thermal hyperalgesia in rats with paclitaxel-induced peripheral neuropathy (Chen et al., 2022b). Shēngmàiyǐn was shown to protect against ferroptosis and cardiotoxicity in mice (Meng et al., 2023).

2.40 HEREDITARY NEUROPATHY WITH LIABILITY TO PRESSURE PALSIES

Hereditary neuropathy with liability to pressure palsies (HNPP) is also known as tomaculous neuropathy, heterozygous microdeletion 17p11.2p12, potato-grubbing palsy, or tulip-bulb digger's palsy. HNPP is characterized by recurrent episodes of tingling, numbness, or pain in the wrists, elbows, knees, fingers, or feet due to compression of peripheral nerves. Examples of the activities that compress the nerves include kneeling during potato grubbing and tulip-bulb digging. HNPP is caused by deletion or mutations in the *PMP22* gene whose products not only make up myelin but help the nerve recover from compression.

TABLE 2.40

GMP Herbal Medicines for a 20-Year-Old Adult with Hereditary Neuropathy with Liability to Pressure Palsies

Hereditary neuropathy with liability to pressure palsies (OrphaCode: 640)

A malformation syndrome with a prevalence of ~3 in 100,000

Disease-causing germline mutation(s): peripheral myelin protein 22 (*PMP22* / Entrez: 5376) at 17p12

Role: the phenotype of peripheral myelin protein 22 (*PMP22* / Entrez: 5376) at 17p12

Autosomal dominant

Decreased motor nerve conduction velocity, Peripheral neuropathy

Scoliosis, Paresthesia

Hyporeflexia, Vocal cord paralysis, Abnormality of the voice, Pes cavus, Respiratory insufficiency, Cranial nerve paralysis

Infancy, Childhood, Adolescent, Adult, Elderly

Paresthesia (D010292):

Shēntòngzhúyūtāng 5g + shūjīnghuóxuètāng 4-0g + yánhúsuǒ 1-0g + lùlùtōng 1-0g + jīxuèténg 1-0g + acupuncture.

Shēntòngzhúyūtāng 5g + sháoyàogāncǎotāng 2-0g + yánhúsuǒ 1-0g + wēilíngxiān 1-0g + acupuncture.

Wēilíngxiān 5g + chuānshānlóng 5g + sānqī 4g + mùguā 4g + niúxī 4g + hónghuā 4g + huángbò 4g + gǒujǐ 4-0g + dàhuáng 1-0g.

Wēilíngxiān 5g + báizhú 3g + qiānghuó 3g + xiāngfù 3g + huángqín 3g + cāngzhú 3g + tiānnánxīng 2g + bànxià 2g + gāncǎo 2g + shēngjiāng 2g + fúlíng 2g + chénpí 2g.

(Continued)

TABLE 2.40 *(Continued)*

GMP Herbal Medicines for a 20-Year-Old Adult with Hereditary Neuropathy with Liability to Pressure Palsies

Vocal cord paralysis (D014826), Cranial nerve paralysis (352.9):

Guìzhītāng 5g + gégēn 2-0g + bànxià 1g + xìngrén 1-0g + hòupò 1-0g + shēngjiāng 1-0g + guìzhī 1-0g + báisháo 1-0g + dàhuáng 0g.	Báizhǐ 5g + gāncǎo 4g + shārén 4g + huángqín 4g + guālóugēn 2g + dàhuáng 1g + xìxīn 1-0g.
Guìzhītāng 5g + báizhú 2g + fùzǐ 2g + báisháo 2g + fúlíng 2g + dǎngshēn 1g + shēngjiāng 1g + dàhuáng 0g.	Gāncǎo 5g + dìlóng 5g + fángfēng 5g + jiégěng 5g + jīngjiè 5g + yúxīngcǎo 5g + bòhé 5g + jiāngcán 5g.
	Gāncǎo 5g + jiégěng 5g + xuánshēn 3g + bèimǔ 3g + mǔlì 3-2g + liánqiáo 3-2g + zhīzǐ 2g.

Báizhǐ (cf. Section 1.7) extract was shown to improve functional recovery of rats after spinal cord injury through inhibition of inflammation and oxidative stress (Moon et al., 2012). The herb pair Báizhǐ and Chuānxiōng was introduced in Section 2.26 to be anti-migraine and the molecular mechanisms were elucidated (Thanh et al., 2022). Báizhǐ alone was also shown to ameliorate migraines in rats, likely by modulating the levels of vasoactive substances (Sun et al., 2017). Modern clinical applications of Guìzhītāng include throat disease and nervous system disease (Feng et al., 2018).

2.41 MULTIPLE SYSTEM ATROPHY

Multiple system atrophy (MSA) is characterized by progressive impairment in movement and balance and dysfunction of the autonomic nervous system, which regulates involuntary bodily functions such as blood pressure and bladder control. MSA can be explained in pathophysiology by progressive loss of function of the glial cells that support the nerve cells in the movement and autonomic-control centers of the brain. MSA is found in some populations to be associated with

TABLE 2.41

GMP Herbal Medicines for a 55-Year-Old Adult with Multiple System Atrophy

Multiple system atrophy (OrphaCode: 102)

A disease with a prevalence of ~3 in 100,000

Major susceptibility factor: coenzyme Q2, polyprenyltransferase (*COQ2* / Entrez: 27235) at 4q21.23

Multigenic/multifactorial, Not applicable

Gaze-evoked nystagmus, Dysarthria, Parkinsonism, Constipation, Rigidity, Gait ataxia, Bradykinesia, Progressive cerebellar ataxia, Postural instability, Postural tremor, Orofacial dyskinesia, Resting tremor, Frequent falls, Dysautonomia, Abnormal rapid eye movement sleep, Axial dystonia, Orthostatic hypotension due to autonomic dysfunction, Autonomic bladder dysfunction, Abnormal pyramidal sign, Autonomic erectile dysfunction, Stridor, Central sleep apnea, Abnormal brain FDG positron emission tomography, Orthostatic syncope, Female anorgasmia, Raynaud phenomenon, Camptocormia

Adult

Dysarthria (D004401), Constipation (564.0), Rigidity (D009127), Gait ataxia (D020234), Bradykinesia (D018476), Postural tremor (D014202), Orofacial dyskinesia (333.82), Resting tremor (D014202), Stridor (D012135):

Máhuángfùzǐxìxīntāng 5g + fùzǐ 3g + guìzhī 3g + gānjiāng 3-2g + dàzǎo 2g + zhìgāncǎo 2g + báizhú 2-0g + wēilíngxiān 2-0g + zhìgāncǎotāng 2-0g.	Dàhuáng 5g + gāncǎo 5g + báizhǐ 5g + shārén 5g + huángqín 5-0g.
	Dàhuáng 5g + fùzǐ 5g + xìxīn 5g.
Máhuángfùzǐxìxīntāng 5g + fùzǐ 3g + guìzhī 3g + gānjiāng 3-2g + báizhú 2g + wúzhūyú 2g + zhìgāncǎotāng 2-0g.	Dàhuáng 5g + huǒmárén 5g + dìhuáng 5g + shārén 5g + zhǐqiào 5g + huáihuā 5g + huòxiāng 5g + zéxiè 2g.
	Qiānghuó 5g + hòupò 5g + zhǐshí 5g + dàhuáng 1g + huángqín 1g + huánglián 1g.

mutations in the *COQ2* gene, whose products are involved in the production of coenzyme Q10, which is an antioxidant protecting cells from damage of the free radicals resulting from cellular energy generation.

The neuroprotective effects of Dàhuáng on the central nervous system were introduced and summarized in Section 2.17. Huǒmárén (Fructus Cannabis) was shown to exhibit beneficial effects on the learning and memory of aging rats (Chen et al., 2017b); it was also shown to alleviate constipation and accelerate the recovery of colitis injury in rats (Li, 2018). Qiānghuó (cf. Section 2.14) was shown to protect human neuroblastoma cells from oxidative damage (Ma et al., 2022). Máhuángfùzǐxìxīntāng was demonstrated to relieve a depressive-like state in mice through inhibition of inflammasome and enhancement of neurogenesis (Jing et al., 2019).

2.42 ACUTE INFLAMMATORY DEMYELINATING POLYRADICULONEUROPATHY

Acute inflammatory demyelinating polyradiculoneuropathy (AIDP), also known as Guillain-Barré syndrome, is an acute inflammatory demyelinating polyradiculoneuropathic form. AIDP is characterized by progressive weakness and numbness of the muscles in the lower extremities in the initial phase of the condition lasting for a few weeks, followed by plateauing and then recovery of the symptoms. AIDP is thought to be due to attacks of macrophages toward the myelin of the peripheral nerves, triggered by a viral/bacterial infection or vaccination.

Processed Chuānwū (cf. Section 2.12) was shown to reduce both peripherally and centrally induced pain in mice through elevation of hepatic antioxidative enzymes to eradicate free radicals (Lai et al., 2012). Shēntòngzhúyūtāng (cf. Sections 2.1 and 2.4) was shown in rats to inhibit the viability, inflammatory response, migration, invasion, cell cycle transition, and to promote apoptosis of fibroblast-like synoviocytes (Han et al., 2021), which initiate and drive synovial inflammation and joint damage in rheumatoid arthritis.

TABLE 2.42

GMP Herbal Medicines for a 43-Year-Old Man with Acute Inflammatory Demyelinating Polyradiculoneuropathy

Acute inflammatory demyelinating polyradiculoneuropathy (OrphaCode: 98916)

A disease with a prevalence of ~3 in 100,000

Major susceptibility factor: peripheral myelin protein 22 (*PMP22* / Entrez: 5376) at 17p12

Multigenic/multifactorial, Not applicable

Acute demyelinating polyneuropathy

Hyporeflexia, Generalized hypotonia, Recurrent fever, Drooling, Unsteady gait, EMG: neuropathic changes, Sleepy facial expression, Distal lower limb muscle weakness, Dysesthesia, Impaired oropharyngeal swallow response

Onion bulb formation

All ages

Unsteady gait (D020233), Dysesthesia (D010292):

Shēntòngzhúyūtāng 5g + shūjīnghuóxuètāng 5g + acupuncture.	Chuānwū 5g + wǔlíngzhī 2g + tiānnánxīng 2g + mùxiāng 2g + gāncǎo 2g + dìlóng 2g + yánhúsuǒ 2g + táorén 2g + huíxiāng 2g + chénpí 2g + dāngguī 2g + acupuncture.
Shēntòngzhúyūtāng 5g + dúhuójìshēngtāng 5g + acupuncture.	Chuānwū 5g + shúdìhuáng 5g + gāncǎo 3g + báisháo 3g + máhuáng 3g + huángqí 3g + báijièzǐ 2g + dàhuáng 1g + shēngjiāng 1g + huánglián 0g.
Shēntòngzhúyūtāng 5g + dāngguīniántòngtāng 5g + huángbò 1g + cāngzhú 1g + acupuncture.	
Shēntòngzhúyūtāng 5g + sháoyàogāncǎotāng 4g + yánhúsuǒ 1g + wēilíngxiān 1g + acupuncture.	Wēilíngxiān 5g + báizhú 3g + qiānghuó 3g + xiāngfù 3g + huángqín 3g + cāngzhú 3g + tiānnánxīng 2g + bànxià 2g + gāncǎo 2g + shēngjiāng 2g + fúlíng 2g + chénpí 2g.

2.43 CEREBRAL AUTOSOMAL DOMINANT ARTERIOPATHY-SUBCORTICAL INFARCTS-LEUKOENCEPHALOPATHY

Cerebral autosomal dominant arteriopathy-subcortical infarcts-leukoencephalopathy (CADASIL), also called hereditary multi-infarct dementia, is characterized by recurrent ischemic stroke, migraine with aura, and seizures due to abnormality and death of the smooth muscle cells of the small blood vessels. CADASIL is caused by mutations in the *NOTCH3* gene, whose products are receptors on the cell surface to turn on genes in the nucleus within cells in response to extracellular signals important for normal function and survival of vascular smooth muscle cells.

Oral use of Chinese herbal medicine, including Chuānxiōng, Báizhǐ, Báisháo, Tiānmá, Dāngguī (Radix Angelicae Sinensis), Xìxīn (Radix et Rhizoma Asari), and Gōuténg (Ramulus Uncariae Cum Uncis), was found to decrease the frequency of episodic migraine attacks in adults in a systematic review and meta-analysis of randomized controlled trials (Lyu et al., 2020). Chuānxiōngchádiàosǎn is made up of Chuānxiōng, Qiānghuó, Báizhǐ, Xìxīn, Bòhé (Herba Menthae), Jīngjiè (Spica Schizonepetae), Fángfēng, and Gāncǎo. Máxìnggānshítāng (cf. Section 1.47) "soothes the Lung, quenches heat, stops coughing, quells asthma" and is used for symptoms involving respiratory system and other chest symptoms such as asthma (Wang, 2019).

TABLE 2.43

GMP Herbal Medicines for a 47-Year-Old Adult with Cerebral Autosomal Dominant Arteriopathy-Subcortical Infarcts-Leukoencephalopathy

Cerebral autosomal dominant arteriopathy-subcortical infarcts-leukoencephalopathy (OrphaCode: 136)

A disease with a prevalence of ~3 in 100,000

Disease-causing germline mutation(s): notch receptor 3 (*NOTCH3* / Entrez: 4854) at 19p13.12

Autosomal dominant

Leukoencephalopathy, Abnormal cerebral white matter morphology, Lacunar stroke, Multifocal hyperintensity of cerebral white matter on MRI

Apathy, Stroke, Mood changes, Migraine, Migraine with aura, Transient ischemic attack, Cerebral ischemia, Cognitive impairment

Depression, Dementia, Anxiety, Diabetes mellitus, Hypertension, Seizure, Spasticity, Dysarthria, Gait disturbance, Confusion, Encephalopathy, Parkinsonism, Cerebral hemorrhage, Dysphagia, Ischemic stroke, Intracranial hemorrhage, Hemiplegia, Motor deterioration, Memory impairment, Language impairment, Loss of consciousness, Recurrent subcortical infarcts, Impaired visuospatial constructive cognition, Stress urinary incontinence, Brain atrophy, Bradyphrenia, Arterial stenosis

Adult

Migraine with aura (346.0):

Chuānxiōngchádiàosǎn 5g + qiānghuó 1-0g + júhuā 1-0g + mànjīngzǐ 1-0g + báizhǐ 1-0g + fángfēng 1-0g + jīngjiè 1-0g.
Gégēntāng 5g + chuānxiōng 1g + báizhǐ 1g + jīngjiè 1-0g.

Tiānmá 5g + báisháo 5g + dìhuáng 5g + mànjīngzǐ 5g + gōuténg 5g + niúxī 3g + bànxià 3g + báizhǐ 3g + hángjú 3g + màiméndōng 3g + dāngguī 3g + gǎoběn 3g + tiānhuā 3-0g + zhǐqiào 3-0g + chénpí 3-0g + xìxīn 2g.

Diabetes mellitus (250), Hypertension (401-405.99), Seizure (345.9), Spasticity (D009128), Dysarthria (D004401), Confusion (D003221), Encephalopathy (348.30, 348.9), Intracranial hemorrhage (D020300), Hemiplegia (343.4), Memory impairment (D008569), Language impairment (D007806), Loss of consciousness (D014474), Stress urinary incontinence (D014550):

Máxìnggānshítāng 5g + fùzǐ 2g + hòupò 2g + zhǐshí 2g + dàhuáng 1-0g + xìxīn 1-0g.
Fùzǐ 5g + báizhú 4g + báisháo 4g + fúlíng 4g + gānjiāng 4g + dǎngshēn 4g + tiáowèichéngqìtāng 1g.
Bǔyánghuánwǔtāng 5g + báihǔjiārénshēntāng 5-0g + fùzǐ 2-1g + báizhú 2-0g + báisháo 2-0g + fúlíng 2-0g + dǎngshēn 1-0g + shēngjiāng 1-0g + gānjiāng 1-0g + dàhuáng 0g.

Qiānghuó 5g + hòupò 5g + zhǐshí 5g + dàhuáng 1-0g + huángqín 1-0g + huánglián 1-0g.

2.44 BENIGN ADULT FAMILIAL MYOCLONIC EPILEPSY

Benign adult familial myoclonic epilepsy (BAFME), also called familial cortical myoclonic tremor and epilepsy, is characterized by tremors and jerks of the hand provoked by posture or action, and seizures. BAFME in some populations is mapped to the *SAMD12* gene, whose products are predicted to be involved in the receptor tyrosine kinase signaling pathway, important for cell proliferation and differentiation.

Jīxuèténg (cf. Section 2.4) was shown to promote neuronal survival and level of brain-derived neurotrophic factor by reducing glial activation, oxidative stress, and apoptosis in the ipsilateral cortex of rats subject to focal ischemic stroke/reperfusion injury (Park et al., 2017). Suānzǎorén

TABLE 2.44
GMP Herbal Medicines for a 25-Year-Old Adult with Benign Adult Familial Myoclonic Epilepsy

Benign adult familial myoclonic epilepsy (OrphaCode: 86814)

A disease with a prevalence of ~3 in 100,000

Disease-causing germline mutation(s): sterile alpha motif domain containing 12 (*SAMD12* / Entrez: 401474) at 8q24.11-q24.12

Disease-causing germline mutation(s): YEATS domain containing 2 (*YEATS2* / Entrez: 55689) at 3q27.1

Disease-causing germline mutation(s): catenin delta 2 (*CTNND2* / Entrez: 1501) at 5p15.2

Disease-causing germline mutation(s): contactin 2 (*CNTN2* / Entrez: 6900) at 1q32.1

Disease-causing germline mutation(s) (gain of function): adrenoceptor alpha 2B (*ADRA2B* / Entrez: 151) at 2q11.2

Disease-causing germline mutation(s): membrane associated ring-CH-type finger 6 (*MARCHF6* / Entrez: 10299) at 5p15.2

Autosomal dominant

Myoclonus, EEG abnormality, Hand tremor

Generalized-onset seizure, Focal-onset seizure

Intellectual disability, Headache, Amaurosis fugax

All ages

Myoclonus (D009207):

Sānbìtāng 5g + shūjīnghuóxuètāng 5g + liùwèidìhuángwán 5-0g + dúhuójìshēngtāng 5-0g + niúxī 1-0g + yánhúsuǒ 1-0g + acupuncture.

Sānbìtāng 5g + shàngzhōngxiàtōngyòngtòngfēngwán 5g + huǒmárén 1g + niúxī 1g.

Jīxuèténg 5g + chìsháo 1g + hónghuā 1g + táorén 1g + zélán 1g + acupuncture.

Jīxuèténg 5g + héshǒuwū 4g + chìsháo 4g + nǚzhēnzǐ 2g + hànliáncǎo 2g + xiāngfù 2g + yùjīn 2g + cháihú 1g.

Jīxuèténg 5g + huángqí 4g + dāngguī 3g + gǒuqǐzǐ 3-2g + wǔlíngzhī 2g + tùsīzǐ 2g + fùpénzǐ 2g + bājǐtiān 2g.

Generalized-onset seizure (D012640):

Tiānwángbǔxīndān 5g + cháihújiālónggǔmǔlìtāng 5g + suānzǎoréntāng 5g + héhuānpí 1g + yèjiāoténg 1g.

Tiānwángbǔxīndān 5g + jiāwèixiāoyáosǎn 5g + gāncǎoxiǎomàidàzǎotāng 5-0g + suānzǎoréntāng 5-0g + yèjiāoténg 1-0g + fúshén 1-0g + yuǎnzhì 1-0g + suānzǎorén 1-0g.

Suānzǎoréntāng 5g + yèjiāoténg 1g + bózǐrén 1g + fúshén 1g + yuǎnzhì 1g.

Fúshén 5g + gōuténg 5g + xuánshēn 4-0g + shāshēn 4-0g + gégēn 2g + gǎoběn 2g + chìsháo 1g + jīngjiè 1g + xùduàn 1g + chuānxiōng 1-0g + yánhúsuǒ 1-0g + mànjīngzǐ 1-0g.

Suānzǎorén 5g + yèjiāoténg 2g + fúshén 2g + shíchāngpú 1g + yuǎnzhì 1g + wǔwèizǐ 0g.

Yèjiāoténg 5g + diàoténggōu 5g + màiméndōng 5g + gāncǎo 2g + báisháo 2g + dìhuáng 2g + juémíngzǐ 2g + fúlíng 2g + suānzǎorén 2g.

Intellectual disability (D008607), Headache (D006261), Amaurosis fugax (D020757):

Huángqíwǔwùtāng 5g + juānbìtāng 5-0g + dānshēn 1-0g + zhúrú 1-0g + sāngzhī 1-0g + qínjiāo 1-0g + gōuténg 1-0g + fùzǐ 0g + acupuncture.

Huángqíwǔwùtāng 5g + dāngguīsìnìtāng 5-0g + dānshēn 2-0g + zhúrú 2-0g + sāngzhī 2-0g + jiānghuáng 2-0g + fùzǐ 0g + acupuncture.

Huángqí 5g + chìsháo 1-0g + fángfēng 1-0g + xìxīn 1-0g + huánglián 1-0g + dàhuáng 0g.

(Semen Ziziphi Spinosae) was shown to be antiepileptogenic in rats by alleviating traumatic epilepsy-induced oxidative stress and inflammatory responses (Lu et al., 2022). Use of Diàoténggōu (Ramulus Uncariae Cum Uncis) for migraines was reviewed (Chong et al., 2021). Héhuānpí (Cortex Albiziae) was shown to be anxiolytic in rats (Kim et al., 2004). Huángqíwǔwùtāng (cf. Sections 1.5 and 1.68) was proposed for the management of post-stroke-related numbness and weakness in a computational molecular docking analysis (Lee et al., 2022).

2.45 DUCHENNE MUSCULAR DYSTROPHY

Duchenne muscular dystrophy (DMD), also known as severe dystrophinopathy, Duchenne type, is characterized by weakness and wasting of skeletal and heart muscles that get worse quickly. DMD is caused by mutations in the *DMD* gene, whose products are a component of a large complex that bridges the muscle cell cytoskeleton and extracellular matrix for proper development and organization of muscle fibers.

Dàfùpí (Pericarpium Arecae) was shown to be hypotensive in rats (Inokuchi et al., 1986). Sāngbáipí (Cortex Mori) was demonstrated to alleviate myocardial damages such as cardiac hypertrophy and fibrosis in diabetic rats by regulating endoplasmic reticulum stress (Lian et al., 2017). Hǎigé, i.e., clam, was shown to ameliorate triglyceride and cholesterol metabolism in rats (Laurent et al., 2013). Xuèfǔzhúyūtāng (cf. Section 1.70) "invigorates Blood, disperses stasis, moves Qi, stops pain" and is used today for disorders of lipoid metabolism and essential hypertension (Wang, 2019).

TABLE 2.45

GMP Herbal Medicines for a Four-Year-Old Boy with Duchenne Muscular Dystrophy

Duchenne muscular dystrophy (OrphaCode: 98896)

A disease with a prevalence of ~3 in 100,000

Disease-causing germline mutation(s): dystrophin (*DMD* / Entrez: 1756) at Xp21.2-p21.1

Modifying germline mutation: latent transforming growth factor beta binding protein 4 (*LTBP4* / Entrez: 8425) at 19q13.2

X-linked recessive

Delayed speech and language development, Global developmental delay, Motor delay, Specific learning disability, Flexion contracture, Cardiomyopathy, Respiratory insufficiency, Waddling gait, Scoliosis, Skeletal muscle atrophy, Elevated circulating creatine kinase concentration, Progressive muscle weakness, Proximal muscle weakness, Calf muscle hypertrophy, Cognitive impairment

Childhood

Delayed speech and language development (D007805), Cardiomyopathy (425, 425.9), Waddling gait (D020233), Skeletal muscle atrophy (D009133):

Shēngmàiyǐn 5g + xuèfǔzhúyūtāng 5g + dānshēn 2g + chuānqí 1g + báijí 1g + guìzhī 1g + guālóurén 1-0g + xièbái 1-0g + mázǐrénwán 1-0g.

Shēngmàiyǐn 5g + shēnlíngbáizhúsǎn 5g + shānzhā 2g + shénqū 2g + màiyá 2g.

Bǔzhōngyìqìtāng 5g + shēngmàiyǐn 5-0g + shíchāngpú 1-0g + yuǎnzhì 1-0g.

Dàfùpí 5g + mǔlì 5g + sāngbáipí 5g + hǎigé 5g + hǎipiāoxiāo 5g + shénqū 5g + fúlíng 5g + chénpí 5g + màiyá 5g + gégēn 5g + cāngěrzǐ 5-0g + jílí 5-0g.

Hǎigé 5g + mǔlì 4-3g + sāngbáipí 4-3g + dàfùpí 4-2g + fúlíng 4-0g + zǐsūyè 4-0g + jílí 4-0g + wǔlíngzhī 2g + gāncǎo 2-0g + hànliáncǎo 2-0g + xīnyí 2-0g + zhīmǔ 2-0g + huángbò 2-0g + cāngěrzǐ 2-0g + bīngláng 2-0g + bǎibù 1-0g.

Mǔlì 5g + sāngbáipí 5g + shénqū 5g + fúlíng 5g + chénpí 5g + gégēn 5g + dàxiǎojì 3g + wǔlíngzhī 3g + dìyú 3g + hǎigé 3g + bǎibù 1g.

2.46 HUNTINGTON DISEASE

Huntington disease, also called Huntington chorea, is characterized by changes in movement, emotions, and mentality, manifesting involuntary jerking and twitching, irritability, depression, and decline in thinking and reasoning. Huntington disease is caused by neuron death in the brain due

TABLE 2.46

GMP Herbal Medicines for a 39-Year-Old Adult with Huntington Disease

Huntington disease (OrphaCode: 399)

A disease with a prevalence of ~3 in 100,000

Disease-causing germline mutation(s) (gain of function): huntingtin (*HTT* / Entrez: 3064) at 4p16.3

Modifying germline mutation: solute carrier family 2 member 3 (*SLC2A3* / Entrez: 6515) at 12p13.31

Autosomal dominant

Mental deterioration, Hyperreflexia, Chorea

Abnormality of eye movement, Agitation, Depression, Aggressive behavior, Obsessive-compulsive behavior, Disinhibition, Irritability, Hallucinations, Anxiety, Apathy, Delusions, Seizure, Gait disturbance, Dystonia, Myoclonus, Weight loss, Bradykinesia, Gait imbalance, Clumsiness, Memory impairment, Difficulty walking, Hypokinesia, Generalized muscle weakness, Involuntary movements, Abnormality of the sense of smell, Poor fine motor coordination, Speech articulation difficulties, Staring gaze, Hostility, Bradyphrenia, Abnormal libido

Excessive daytime somnolence, Cerebral atrophy, Rigidity, Clonus, Mutism, Caudate atrophy, Abnormal cerebral white matter morphology, Inability to walk, Polyphagia, Abnormality of cholesterol metabolism, Babinski sign, Impaired visuospatial constructive cognition, Choking episodes, Alcoholism, Suicidal ideation, Degeneration of the striatum, Decreased body mass index, Insomnia, Oral-pharyngeal dysphagia

Childhood, Adolescent, Adult, Elderly

Hyperreflexia (D012021), Chorea (D002819):

Qīngshǔyìqìtāng 5g + huòxiāngzhèngqìsǎn 5-2g + shēngmàiyǐn 2-0g + huáshí 1-0g.

Qīngshǔyìqìtāng 5g + shēngmàiyǐn 4-3g + tiānhuā 1-0g.

Qīngshǔyìqìtāng 5g + gānlùxiāodúdān 1g.

Shēngmá 5g + xuánshēn 5g + yùzhú 5g + dìhuáng 5g + hòupò 5g + zhǐshí 5g + màiméndōng 5g + dàhuáng 0g.

Shēngmá 5g + chìsháo 5g + qiánhú 5g + sāngbáipí 5g + cháihú 5g + jīngjiè 5g + huángqín 5g + gégēn 5g.

Shēngmá 5g + gāncǎo 5g + báizhú 5g + cháihú 5g + chénpí 5g + huángqí 5g + dāngguī 5g + dǎngshēn 5g + shúdìhuáng 5-0g.

Dàzǎo 5g + bànxià 5g + shēngjiāng 5g + báisháo 5g + zhǐshí 5g + cháihú 5g + huángqín 5g + dàhuáng 0g.

Obsessive-compulsive behavior (300.3), Hallucinations (D006212), Seizure (345.9), Dystonia (D004421), Myoclonus (D009207), Weight loss (D015431), Bradykinesia (D018476), Memory impairment (D008569), Difficulty walking (D051346), Hypokinesia (D018476):

Gāncǎoxiǎomàidàzǎotāng 5g + wēndǎntāng 5g + cháihújiālónggǔmǔlìtāng 5-0g + shíchāngpú 1-0g + héhuānpí 1-0g + yuǎnzhì 1-0g + yùjīn 1-0g.

Gāncǎoxiǎomàidàzǎotāng 5g + cháihújiālónggǔmǔlìtāng 5g + bǎihé 1-0g + bózǐrén 1-0g + fúshén 1-0g + yuǎnzhì 1-0g.

Gāncǎoxiǎomàidàzǎotāng 5g + yìgānsǎn 5g + héhuānpí 1-0g + bǎihé 1-0g + fúshén 1-0g.

Mǔlì 5g + gāncǎo 4g + báisháo 4g + shúdìhuáng 4g + biējiǎ 4g + màiméndōng 3g + ējiāo 2g + huǒmárén 2g + fúshén 2-0g.

Bǎihé 5g + zhīmǔ 3g + huángqín 2g + huánglián 2g + dàhuáng 0g.

Bǎihé 5g + zhīmǔ 3g + tiānhuā 2g + xuánshēn 2g + mǔlì 2g + bèimǔ 2g + niúbàngzǐ 1g + shègān 1g.

Rigidity (D009127), Mutism (D009155), Abnormal cerebral white matter morphology (D049292) [Leukodystrophy 330.0)], Polyphagia (D006963):

Bǔzhōngyìqìtāng 5g + guīpítāng 5-0g + xiānhècǎo 1-0g + dùzhòng 1-0g + xùduàn 1-0g.

Bǔzhōngyìqìtāng 5g + liùwèidìhuángwán 4-0g + dùzhòng 1-0g + sāngjìshēng 1-0g + tùsīzǐ 1-0g + xùduàn 1-0g + acupuncture.

Bǔzhōngyìqìtāng 5g + jìshēngshènqìwán 5-0g + dānshēn 1-0g + dùzhòng 1-0g + bǔgǔzhī 1-0g.

Huángqí 5g + dǎngshēn 5-0g + chuānxiōng 2-1g + shēngmá 2-1g + báizhǐ 2-1g + zhìgāncǎo 2-1g + cháihú 2-1g + dāngguī 2-1g + chénpí 2-0g + shēngmá 1-0g + báizhú 1-0g.

Huángqí 5g + dǎngshēn 5-0g + báisháo 4-2g + chuānxiōng 4-0g + dìhuáng 4-0g + huángqín 4-0g + dāngguī 4-0g + guìzhī 2-0g + fùzǐ 2-0g + shēngjiāng 1-0g + dàhuáng 0g.

to aggregates of toxic fragments of faulty proteins made from the *HTT* gene, which contains extra repeats inherited from a parent. As the repeat passes down from generation to generation, the number of repeats in the *HTT* gene can increase. The onset age becomes earlier with the increased *HTT* repeats in the offspring.

Shēngmá and Qīngshǔyìqìtāng are introduced in Section 2.13 for areflexia. Use of Huòxiāngzhèngqìsǎn was found to be associated with a lower risk of early neurologic deterioration in patients with acute ischemic stroke (Huang et al., 2020). Bǎihé (cf. Section 2.5) was shown to promote hippocampal neurogenesis and enhance memory retention in mice (Park et al., 2023). Cháihújiālónggǔmǔlìtāng (cf. Sections 1.30 and 2.10) was concluded to be effective in the treatment of depression in a meta-analysis of randomized controlled trials, improving symptoms such as anxiety and insomnia with fewer side effects (Zhao et al., 2023). Bǔzhōngyìqìtāng (cf. Sections 1.34, 1.68, 1.71, and 2.2) was shown to modulate the immune reaction in muscles and neurons to delay disease progression in mice with amyotrophic lateral sclerosis (Cai & Yang, 2019), which is characterized by motor neuron cell death and muscle paralysis.

2.47 PROGRESSIVE NON-FLUENT APHASIA

Progressive non-fluent aphasia (PNFA), also called agramatic variant of primary progressive aphasia, is a language-based dementia characterized by reduced speech output with poor grammar and laborious and clumsy talking. Individuals with PNFA have difficulties finding and saying the right words, although they know what they want to say and may understand what others are saying. Patients end up uttering very short sentences with less than four words or becoming mute. PNFA is a form of frontotemporal lobar degeneration that occurs sporadically or can be caused by mutations in the *C9orf72* or *GRN* gene.

TABLE 2.47

GMP Herbal Medicines for a 60-Year-Old Adult with Progressive Non-Fluent Aphasia

Progressive non-fluent aphasia (OrphaCode: 100070)

A disease with a prevalence of ~2 in 100,000

Major susceptibility factor: transmembrane protein 106B (*TMEM106B* / Entrez: 54664) at 7p21.3

Disease-causing germline mutation(s): presenilin 1 (*PSEN1* / Entrez: 5663) at 14q24.2

Major susceptibility factor: charged multivesicular body protein 2B (*CHMP2B* / Entrez: 25978) at 3p11.2

Major susceptibility factor: triggering receptor expressed on myeloid cells 2 (*TREM2* / Entrez: 54209) at 6p21.1

Major susceptibility factor: valosin containing protein (*VCP* / Entrez: 7415) at 9p13.3

Major susceptibility factor: microtubule associated protein tau (*MAPT* / Entrez: 4137) at 17q21.31

Major susceptibility factor: granulin precursor (*GRN* / Entrez: 2896) at 17q21.31

Major susceptibility factor: C9orf72-SMCR8 complex subunit (*C9orf72* / Entrez: 203228) at 9p21.2

Multigenic/multifactorial, Not applicable

Thickened nuchal skin fold, Mental deterioration, Frontotemporal dementia, Memory impairment, Dysphasia, Aphasia, Frontotemporal cerebral atrophy, Grammar-specific speech disorder, Temporal cortical atrophy, Spoken Word Recognition Deficit

Depression, Anxiety, Apraxia, Abnormal cerebral white matter morphology, Alexia, EEG with continuous slow activity, Abnormal brain FDG positron emission tomography

Behavioral abnormality, Restlessness, Personality changes, Parkinsonism, Abnormality of extrapyramidal motor function, Mutism, Abnormal lower motor neuron morphology, Motor aphasia, Astrocytosis, Dysgraphia, Perseveration, Senile plaques

Adult

Memory impairment (D008569), Aphasia (D001037):

Sìnìtāng 5g + rénshēn 1-0g + bànxià 1-0g + jiégěng Gānjiāng 5g + bànxià 3-2g + rénshēn 3-0g + dàhuáng 0g.
1-0g + dàhuáng 0g.

Sìnìtāng 5g + lǐzhōngtāng 4g + ròuguì 1g +
zhìgāncǎotāng 1g.

(Continued)

TABLE 2.47 *(Continued)*
GMP Herbal Medicines for a 60-Year-Old Adult with Progressive Non-Fluent Aphasia

Apraxia (D001072), Abnormal cerebral white matter morphology (D049292) [Leukodystrophy 330.0)], Alexia (315.01):

Bǔzhōngyìqìtāng 5g + bǔyánghuánwǔtāng 5g + shíchāngpú 1g + yuǎnzhì 1g + tiānmá 1-0g + sānqī 1-0g + dānshēn 1-0g.

Bǔzhōngyìqìtāng 5g + jìshēngshènqìwán 5g + dānshēn 1g + shíchāngpú 1g + yuǎnzhì 1g + yùjīn 1g + acupuncture.

Huángqín 5g + báizhǐ 4-3g + gāncǎo 2g + shārén 2g + tiānhuā 1-0g + zhīzǐ 1-0g + liánqiáo 1-0g + dàhuáng 1-0g + acupuncture.

Huángqí 5g + chìsháo 1g + fángfēng 1g + dàhuáng 0g + xìxīn 0g + huánglián 0g.

Mutism (D009155), Motor aphasia (D001039), Dysgraphia (D000381):

Bǔzhōngyìqìtāng 5g + jìshēngshènqìwán 5-0g + dùzhòng 1-0g + xùduàn 1-0g.

Bǔzhōngyìqìtāng 5g + wǔlíngsǎn 1-0g + fùzǐ 0g.

Bǔzhōngyìqìtāng 5g + sìnìtāng 2-0g.

Dàzǎo 5g + gāncǎo 5g + shēngjiāng 5g + báisháo 5g + báizhú 5-0g + báibiǎndòu 5-0g + fúlíng 5-0g + huángqí 5-0g + bànxià 5-0g + zhǐshí 5-0g + cháihú 5-0g + huángqín 5-0g.

Dàzǎo 5g + tínglìzǐ 5g + zhǐshí 3g + chénpí 3g.

Dàzǎo 5g + shēngjiāng 5g + zhìgāncǎo 5g + hòupò 5g + zhǐshí 5g + guìzhī 5g + dàhuáng 0g.

Wūméi 5g + ròuguì 1g + fùzǐ 1g + gānjiāng 1g + xìxīn 1g + huángbò 1g + huánglián 1g + dāngguī 1g + dǎngshēn 1g.

Sìnìtāng was shown to prevent depression-like behavior in rats exposed to chronic unpredictable stress, likely through modulating corticotropin-releasing hormone mRNA expression in the hypothalamus (Guo et al., 2009). Prophylactic administration of Bǔzhōngyìqìtāng was shown to reduce brain infarct volume and improve neurological function and behavior in a cerebral ischemia mouse model through regulating intestinal microbiota (Li et al., 2022). Bǔzhōngyìqìtāng contains Huángqí, Rénshēn, Báizhú, Zhìgāncǎo, Dāngguī, Chénpí (Pericarpium Citri Reticulatae), Shēngmá, Cháihú, Shēngjiāng, and Dàzǎo.

2.48 NEUROMYELITIS OPTICA SPECTRUM DISORDER

Neuromyelitis optica spectrum disorder (NMOSD), also known as Devic disease, is characterized by recurrent episodes of spinal cord inflammation and unilateral or bilateral optic nerve inflammation. NMOSD is caused by autoantibody-mediated immune attacks on an abundant water channel protein or a myelination protein in the central nervous system.

Huángqí (cf. Sections 1.68, 1.9, 2.1, and 2.27) was shown to prevent deterioration of autoimmune encephalomyelitis in mice through orchestrated multiple pathways, including immunoregulation, antioxidation, anti-neuroinflammation, and anti-neuroapoptosis (He et al., 2014). Gāncǎo

---

TABLE 2.48
GMP Herbal Medicines for a 35-Year-Old Woman with Neuromyelitis Optica Spectrum Disorder

Neuromyelitis optica spectrum disorder (OrphaCode: 71211)

A disease with a prevalence of ~2 in 100,000

Multigenic/multifactorial

Functional abnormality of the bladder, Visual loss, Neuronal loss in central nervous system, Sensory impairment, Paraplegia, Peripheral demyelination, Myelitis, Autoimmune antibody positivity, Optic neuritis, Ocular pain

Abnormality of brain morphology

Nausea, Respiratory failure, CSF pleocytosis, Recurrent singultus

Childhood, Adolescent, Adult, Elderly

(Continued)

TABLE 2.48 *(Continued)*
GMP Herbal Medicines for a 35-Year-Old Woman with Neuromyelitis Optica Spectrum Disorder

Sensory impairment (D006987), Paraplegia (344.1), Optic neuritis (377.3), Ocular pain (D058447):

Qǐjúdìhuángwán 5g + shūjīnghuóxuètāng 5g + dúhuójìshēngtāng 5g + acupuncture.	Huángqí 5g + chìsháo 1-0g +
Qǐjúdìhuángwán 5g + zīshènmíngmùtāng 5g + acupuncture.	fángfēng 1-0g + xìxīn 0g +
Xuèfǔzhúyūtāng 5g + qǐjúdìhuángwán 5g + dānshēn 1g + acupuncture.	huánglián 0g + acupuncture.
Qǐjúdìhuángwán 5g + bǔyánghuánwǔtāng 5g + nǚzhēnzǐ 1g + hànliáncǎo 1g + acupuncture.	

Nausea (D009325), Recurrent singultus (D006606):

Wǔlíngsǎn 5g + píngwèisǎn 5g.	Zhìgāncǎo 5g + hòupò 5-0g + zhǐshí
Lǐzhōngtāng 5g + wǔlíngsǎn 5-0g + fùzǐ 2-0g + bànxià 1-0g + shārén 1-0g + fúlíng 1-0g.	5-0g + běishāshēn 4-0g + xuánshēn
Wǔlíngsǎn 5g + jiāwèixiāoyáosǎn 5g + xiāngshāliùjūnzǐtāng 5g + yánhúsuǒ 1g + xiāngfù 1g.	4-0g + yùzhú 4-0g + dìhuáng 4-0g + màiméndōng 4-0g + dàhuáng 1-0g.
Língguìshùgāntāng 5g + báisháo 1g + fùzǐ 1g + gānjiāng 1g.	

(cf. Section 1.1) was found to be among the most commonly used Chinese herbal medicine for chemotherapy-induced nausea and vomiting (Lv et al., 2018). Lǐzhōngtāng (cf. Section 2.28) was shown to alleviate serious gastric mucosal ulcerations in rats (Song et al., 2020).

2.49 FRIEDREICH ATAXIA

Friedreich ataxia is a hereditary ataxia characterized by loss of leg reflexes and difficulty balancing, walking, and speaking. Friedreich ataxia is caused by repeat expansion in the noncoding region of the *FXN* gene, whose products are required for proper mitochondrial functioning. The repeat expansion silences the *FXN* gene, causing degeneration of the cells that particularly depend on cellular energy production such as nerve cells and heart cells.

Sānbìtāng (cf. Section 2.20) granules were shown to protect against joint synovial tissue injury in rats with arthritis (Zhang et al., 2020b). The mechanisms and safety of Gāncǎo for neurodegenerative disorders and neurologic deficits subsequent to cerebrovascular accidents were recently reviewed (Zulfugarova et al., 2023). Rénshēn (cf. Section 2.33) was demonstrated to ameliorate

TABLE 2.49
GMP Herbal Medicines for a 12-Year-Old Child with Friedreich Ataxia

Friedreich ataxia (OrphaCode: 95)

A disease with a prevalence of ~2 in 100,000

Disease-causing germline mutation(s) (loss of function): frataxin (*FXN* / Entrez: 2395) at 9q21.11

Autosomal recessive

Gait ataxia

Dysarthria, Limb ataxia, Gait imbalance, Babinski sign, Hand muscle atrophy, Impaired proprioception

Abnormal saccadic eye movements, Nystagmus, Optic atrophy, Dysmetria, Muscle weakness, Cardiomyopathy, Abnormality of the foot, Pes cavus, Intention tremor, Areflexia of lower limbs, Falls, Scoliosis, Urinary bladder sphincter dysfunction, Sensory axonal neuropathy, Poor fine motor coordination, Cervical spinal cord atrophy, Impaired visually enhanced vestibulo-ocular reflex

Hearing impairment, Diabetes mellitus, Spasticity, Dystonia, Dysphagia, Chorea, Inability to walk, Incomprehensible speech, Decreased motor nerve conduction velocity, Reduced visual acuity

Childhood, Adolescent

(Continued)

TABLE 2.49 *(Continued)*

GMP Herbal Medicines for a 12-Year-Old Child with Friedreich Ataxia

Gait ataxia (D020234):

Sānbìtāng 5g + shūjīnghuóxuètāng 5g + yánhúsuǒ 1-0g + jīxuèténg 1-0g + acupuncture.

Sānbìtāng 5g + shàngzhōngxiàtōngyòngtòngfēngwán 4g + huǒmárén 1g + niúxī 1g.

Sānbìtāng 5g + dúhuójìshēngtāng 5g.

Jīxuèténg 5g + huángqí 4g + gǒuqǐzǐ 3g + dāngguī 3g + wǔlíngzhī 2g + tùsīzǐ 2g + fùpénzǐ 2g + bājǐtiān 2g.

Jīxuèténg 5g + nǚzhēnzǐ 3g + báisháo 3g + héshǒuwū 3g + hànliáncǎo 3g + yínyánghuò 3g + tùsīzǐ 3g + xiāngfù 2g + yùjīn 2g + cháihú 1g.

Huángqí 5g + chìsháo 1g + fángfēng 1g + xìxīn 0g + huánglián 0g.

Jīxuèténg 5g + chìsháo 1g + hónghuā 1g + táorén 1g + zélán 1g.

Dysarthria (D004401), Limb ataxia (D001259):

Guìzhītāng 5g + báisháo 1-0g + xìngrén 1-0g + hòupò 1-0g + dàhuáng 0g.

Gānjiāng 5g + rénshēn 3-2g + bànxià 3-2g + dàhuáng 0g.

Gāncǎo 5g + báizhǐ 5g + shārén 5g + dàhuáng 0g.

Gāncǎo 5g + báizhú 5g + báisháo 5g + báibiǎndòu 5g + fúlíng 5g + huángqí 5g + dàzǎo 2g + shēngjiāng 2g.

Nystagmus (379.53, 379.55, 379.50), Optic atrophy (377.1), Dysmetria (D002524), Muscle weakness (D018908), Cardiomyopathy (425, 425.9), Intention tremor (D014202):

Zīshènmíngmùtāng 5g + yìqìcōngmíngtāng 4g + xuèfǔzhúyūtāng 2g.

Qǐjúdìhuángwán 5g + zīshènmíngmùtāng 5-4g + yìqìcōngmíngtāng 2-0g + dānshēn 1g + chēqiánzǐ 1-0g + cǎojuémíng 1-0g + chōngwèizǐ 1-0g + tùsīzǐ 1-0g + acupuncture.

Gǒuqǐzǐ 5g + júhuā 5g + dāngguī 5g + shúdìhuáng 5g + fángfēng 4g + xìxīn 2g + huánglián 2g.

Gǒuqǐzǐ 5g + júhuā 5g + dìhuáng 4-3g + fángfēng 4-3g + dāngguī 4-3g + xìxīn 2-0g + huánglián 2-0g + dàhuáng 0g.

Hearing impairment (D034381), Diabetes mellitus (250), Spasticity (D009128), Dystonia (D004421), Chorea (D002819):

Wǔlíngsǎn 5g + língguìshùgāntāng 5-4g + jìshēngshènqìwán 5-0g + niúxī 1-0g + chēqiánzǐ 1-0g.

Zhēnwǔtāng 5g + fùzǐ 1g + gānjiāng 1g + tiáowèichéngqìtāng 1g + dàhuáng 0g.

Wǔlíngsǎn 5g + báizhǐ 1g + fùfāngdānshēnpiàn 1g + gāncǎo 0g.

Rénshēn 5g + báizhú 5g + shārén 5g + gānjiāng 5g + bànxià 4g + zhìgāncǎo 4g + fúlíng 4g + dàhuáng 2g.

Rénshēn 5g + gānjiāng 5g + huángqín 5-0g + bànxià 5-0g + huánglián 5-0g + dàhuáng 1-0g.

Fùzǐ 5g + xìxīn 4g + dàhuáng 3g + bànxià 3g + fúlíng 3g.

auditory cortex injury associated with military aviation noise-induced hearing loss in guinea pigs (Chen et al., 2020). Zhēnwǔtāng was shown to alleviate proteinuria and renal damage in rats with diabetic nephropathy (Cai et al., 2010).

2.50 PROGRESSIVE MYOCLONIC EPILEPSY TYPE 1

Progressive myoclonic epilepsy type 1, also known as Unverricht-Lundborg disease, is characterized by convulsions, violent jerks triggered by outside stimuli, and muscle stiffening, followed by loss of consciousness and then rhythmic jerks of the limbs. Progressive myoclonic epilepsy type 1 is caused by repeat expansions in the promoter of the *CSTB* gene, whose products inhibit lysosomal proteases and thus help protect proteins from cutting by the proteases that leak out of the lysosomes.

Dàzhēnjiāotāng (cf. Section 2.16) contains Qínjiāo (Radix Gentianae Macrophyllae) as the major herb. Qínjiāo was shown to exert anti-inflammatory effects on gouty arthritis in hyperuricemic rats (Yang et al., 2023). Furthermore, Dàzhēnjiāotāng was formulated for hyperkinesia with regard to the wind in meridians and collaterals by Liu Wansu (AD 1110–1200), a TCM physician in the Jin dynasty of China (Liu & Wang, 2017). Xiǎocháihútāng was reviewed to be effective and promising for the treatment of depression due to Shaoyang stagnation (Sun et al., 2023). Xiǎocháihútāngqùrénshēn is for Shaoyang syndrome without Qi deficiency. Bǎihégùjīntāng contains Bǎihé (and Dìhuáng) as the

TABLE 2.50
GMP Herbal Medicines for a Nine-Year-Old Child with Progressive Myoclonic Epilepsy Type 1

Progressive myoclonic epilepsy type 1 (OrphaCode: 308)

A malformation syndrome with a prevalence of ~2 in 100,000

Disease-causing germline mutation(s): cystatin B (*CSTB* / Entrez: 1476) at 21q22.3

Disease-causing germline mutation(s): scavenger receptor class B member 2 (*SCARB2* / Entrez: 950) at 4q21.1

Disease-causing germline mutation(s): prickle planar cell polarity protein 1 (*PRICKLE1* / Entrez: 144165) at 12q12

Autosomal recessive

Myoclonus, Limb ataxia, EEG with polyspike wave complexes, Morning myoclonic jerks

Ataxia, Dysarthria, Intention tremor

Dementia, Cutaneous photosensitivity, Intellectual disability

Childhood, Adolescent

Myoclonus (D009207), Limb ataxia (D001259):

Sānbìtāng 5g + shūjīnghuóxuètāng 5-0g + acupuncture.
Sānbìtāng 5g + sháoyàogāncǎotāng 5-0g + shēntòngzhúyūtāng 5-0g + dúhuójìshēngtāng 5-0g + dàfēngténg 2-0g + shíhúsuī 2-0g + jīxuèténg 2-0g.

Jīxuèténg 5g + chìsháo 1g + hónghuā 1g + táorén 1g + zélán 1g + acupuncture.
Jīxuèténg 5g + huángqí 4g + dāngguī 4-3g + gǒuqǐzǐ 3g + wǔlíngzhī 3-2g + tùsīzǐ 3-2g + fùpénzǐ 3-2g + bājǐtiān 2g.
Wēilíngxiān 5g + chuānshānlóng 5g + wǔjiāpí 4g + mùguā 4g + niúxī 4g + gǒujǐ 4g + hónghuā 4g + huángbò 4g.

Ataxia (D002524), Dysarthria (D004401), Intention tremor (D014202):

Dàzhēnjiāotāng 5g + dāngguīniàntòngtāng 5g + sháoyàogāncǎotāng 4-2g + yánhúsuǒ 1-0g.
Dàzhēnjiāotāng 5g + jiāwèipíngwèisǎn 2g.

Huángqí 5g + chìsháo 1-0g + fángfēng 1-0g + xìxīn 0g + huánglián 0g + dàhuáng 0g.

Intellectual disability (D008607):

Xiǎocháihútāngqùrénshēn 5g + bǎihégùjīntāng 2-1g + qínjiāobiējiǎsǎn 2-0g + qínjiāo 1-0g + biējiǎ 1-0g + wūméi 0g.

Xuánshēn 5g + dìhuáng 5g + màiméndōng 5g + hòupò 5-2g + zhǐshí 5-2g + gāncǎo 1-0g + dàhuáng 0g.
Běishāshēn 5g + xuánshēn 5g + yùzhú 5g + dìhuáng 5g + màiméndōng 5g + hòupò 5-4g + zhǐshí 5-4g + dàhuáng 1-0g.

monarch (and minister) herb. The Bǎihé and Dìhuáng pair was shown to significantly attenuate the depressive phenotype in mice under chronic, unpredicted mild stress (Zhang et al., 2020c).

2.51 CHILDHOOD DISINTEGRATIVE DISORDER

Childhood disintegrative disorder, also known as dementia infantilis or Heller syndrome, is characterized by at least 2 years of normal development followed by a profound loss of language, social and motor skills, including bowel and bladder control, that have already been learned. The cause

TABLE 2.51
GMP Herbal Medicines for a Three-Year-Old Child with Childhood Disintegrative Disorder

Childhood disintegrative disorder (OrphaCode: 168782)

A disease with a prevalence of ~2 in 100,000

Not applicable

Autistic behavior, Mental deterioration, Progressive language deterioration, Abnormal emotion/affect behavior

Urinary incontinence, Stereotypy, Impaired social interactions, Anxiety, Absent speech, Bowel incontinence, Social and occupational deterioration

Motor deterioration, Developmental regression, Intellectual disability, severe, Dementia

Childhood

(Continued)

TABLE 2.51 *(Continued)*
GMP Herbal Medicines for a Three-Year-Old Child with Childhood Disintegrative Disorder

Urinary incontinence (D014549), Stereotypy (307.3):

Gāncǎoxiǎomàidàzǎotāng 5g + cháihújiālónggǔmǔlìtāng 5g + wēndǎntāng 5-0g + shíchāngpú 2-0g + yuǎnzhì 2-0g.

Gāncǎoxiǎomàidàzǎotāng 5g + bǎohéwán 5g + gāncǎo 0g.

Shēnlíngbáizhúsǎn 5g + gāncǎoxiǎomàidàzǎotāng 5-0g + shānzhā 2-1g + shénqū 2-1g + màiyá 2-1g.

Yùzhú 5g + shāshēn 5g + hòupò 5-2g + zhǐshí 5-2g + màiméndōng 5-0g + dàhuáng 1-0g.

Xuánshēn 5g + dìhuáng 5g + màiméndōng 5g + hòupò 5-2g + zhǐshí 5-2g + dàhuáng 1g.

---

of childhood disintegrative disorder is unknown, although the underlying mechanism is believed to be organic.

In a retrospective review of hemorrhagic and ischemic stroke patient recovery, acupuncture plus GMP herbal extract granules including Shíchāngpú (cf. Sections 1.36 and 1.53), Dàhuáng (cf. Sections 1.30 and 2.17), Yùzhú (cf. Section 1.5), and Yuǎnzhì (cf. Sections 1.41 and 1.60), integrated with conventional rehabilitation, was found to better improve stroke patients' functional recovery at the early subacute phase (Tseng et al., 2022).

2.52 BECKER MUSCULAR DYSTROPHY

Becker muscular dystrophy (BMD), also known as Becker dystrophinopathy, is characterized by progressive weakness and wasting of the skeletal muscles, including the legs and pelvis, and heart muscles. BMD is caused by mutations in the *DMD* gene, whose products are found in the skeletal and heart muscles to stabilize and protect muscle fibers after repeated contraction and relaxation with use. The onset age, symptoms, and progression of BMD are later, milder, and slower than those of Duchenne muscular dystrophy (cf. Section 2.45) due to different mutations in the *DMD* gene that retain some function of the dystrophin protein in the muscle.

Fúlíng (cf. Sections 1.21, 1.66, and 2.37) was shown in aging rats to promote the production of hyaluronic acid (Chao et al., 2023), whose levels correlate dynamically with skeletal muscle growth and repair (Calve et al., 2012). Gāncǎo flavonoid oil supplement was shown to increase the muscle mass in the body trunk of the elderly in a randomized, double-blind, placebo-controlled

---

TABLE 2.52
GMP Herbal Medicines for a 10-Year-Old Boy with Becker Muscular Dystrophy

Becker muscular dystrophy (OrphaCode: 98895)

A disease with a prevalence of ~2 in 100,000

Disease-causing germline mutation(s): dystrophin (*DMD* / Entrez: 1756) at Xp21.2-p21.1

X-linked recessive

Difficulty walking, Myoglobinuria, Elevated circulating creatine kinase concentration, Myalgia, Exercise intolerance, Difficulty climbing stairs, Abnormal urinary color

Muscle weakness, Falls, Abnormality of the lower limb, Elevated hepatic transaminase, Muscle spasm, Fatigue

Pes planus, Skeletal muscle atrophy, Toe walking

Childhood

Difficulty walking (D051346), Myalgia (D063806):

Shūjīnghuóxuètāng 5g + dúhuójìshēngtāng 5-0g + acupuncture.

Zhēnwǔtāng 5g + gānjiāng 1g + fùzǐ 1-0g + tiáowèichéngqìtāng 1-0g + wǔwèizǐ 1-0g + xìxīn 1-0g + dàhuáng 0g.

Fúlíng 5-4g + fùzǐ 5-3g + xìxīn 5-1g + bànxià 4-3g + dàhuáng 4-0g.

Chuānwū 5g + xiǎohuíxiāng 1g + wǔlíngzhī 1g + tiānnánxīng 1g + mùxiāng 1g + yánhúsuǒ 1g + táorén 1g + chénpí 1g + dāngguī 1g.

(Continued)

TABLE 2.52 *(Continued)*

GMP Herbal Medicines for a 10-Year-Old Boy with Becker Muscular Dystrophy

Muscle weakness (D018908), Elevated hepatic transaminase (573.9), Muscle spasm (D009120), Fatigue (D005221):

Jiāwèixiāoyáosǎn 5g + zhìgāncǎotāng 5g + dānshēn 1g + yùjīn 1g + xiāngfù 1-0g + shíchāngpú 1-0g + yuǎnzhì 1-0g.

Xiǎocháihútāng 5g + liùwèidìhuángwán 5g + xiāngshāliùjūnzǐtāng 5g.

Jiāwèixiāoyáosǎn 5g + xiāngshāliùjūnzǐtāng 5-0g + bǔzhōngyìqìtāng 4-0g + shānzhā 1g + shénqū 1g + màiyá 1g.

Báizhú 5g + báisháo 5g + shíhú 5g + chēqiánzǐ 5g + fúlíng 5g + huángqí 5g + dǎngshēn 5g + gāncǎo 3g + yīnchén 3g.

Gāncǎo 5g + báizhú 5g + báisháo 5g + báibiǎndòu 5g + fúlíng 5g + huángqí 5g + dāngguī 5-0g + dǎngshēn 5-0g + dàzǎo 3-0g + shēngjiāng 3-0g.

Gāncǎo 5g + báizhǐ 5g + shārén 5g + dàhuáng 0g.

Skeletal muscle atrophy (D009133):

Èrshùtāng 5g + shūjīnghuóxuètāng 5g + sháoyàogāncǎotāng 5-0g + acupuncture.

Huángqíwǔwùtāng 5g + sháoyàogāncǎotāng 4-2g + sāngzhī 1g + jīxuèténg 1-0g + jiānghuáng 1-0g.

Guìzhītāng 5g + xìngrén 1g + hòupò 1g + acupuncture.

Fóshǒugān 5g + guìzhī 5-4g + fúlíng 5-4g + gānjiāng 3-2g + gāncǎo 2-1g.

Huángqí 5g + chìsháo 1g + fángfēng 1g + xìxīn 0g + huánglián 0g.

Shēngjiāng 5g + báisháo 5g + guìzhī 5g + dàzǎo 4g + zhìgāncǎo 3g + dàhuáng 1g.

---

trial (Kinoshita et al., 2017). Èrshùtāng "dries dampness, dissolves phlegm, relaxes meridians, stops pain" and is used today for peripheral enthesopathies and allied syndromes (Wang, 2019).

2.53   MULTIFOCAL MOTOR NEUROPATHY

Multifocal motor neuropathy (MMN), also known as multifocal motor neuropathy with conduction block, is characterized by progressive weakness, cramps, and wasting of the muscles of the arms and legs in association with deficient transmission of nerve impulses to the affected muscles without sensory loss. MMN is caused by autoantibodies targeting a fatty material on the cellular surface of peripheral nerve cells.

Huángqí (cf. Section 1.9) plus Dānshēn (cf. Section 1.61) was shown to be effective for the treatment of skeletal muscle injury in aerobics athletes (Zhang & Dong, 2018). Wūyàoshùnqìsǎn (cf. Section 2.22) was shown to be effective for the treatment of facial nerve paralysis in dogs (Eom et al., 2008). Note that both Huángqíwǔwùtāng and Bǔyánghuánwǔtāng contain Huángqí. Zhúrú

TABLE 2.53

GMP Herbal Medicines for a 45-Year-Old Man with Multifocal Motor Neuropathy

Multifocal motor neuropathy (OrphaCode: 641)

A disease with a prevalence of ~2 in 100,000

Unknown

Progressive distal muscle weakness

Reduced tendon reflexes, Fasciculations, Increased CSF protein, Progressive muscle weakness, Muscle spasm, Limb muscle weakness, Functional motor deficit, Abnormality of ganglioside metabolism, Limited wrist extension, Weakness of long finger extensor muscles, Motor conduction block

Adult

Fasciculations (D005207), Muscle spasm (D009120):

Huángqíwǔwùtāng 5g + bǔyánghuánwǔtāng 5g + dānshēn 1g + zhúrú 1g + sāngzhī 1g + jiānghuáng 1-0g + jīxuèténg 1-0g + acupuncture.

Wūyàoshùnqìsǎn 5g + bǔyánghuánwǔtāng 5g + huángqíwǔwùtāng 5-0g + dānshēn 1-0g + niúxī 1-0g + acupuncture.

Wūyàoshùnqìsǎn 5g + shūjīnghuóxuètāng 4g + dānshēn 1g + yánhúsuǒ 1g + acupuncture.

Huángqí 5g + chìsháo 1g + fángfēng 1g + xìxīn 1-0g + huánglián 1-0g.

(Caulis Bambusae in Taenia) was demonstrated to be neuroprotective and anti-neuroinflammatory in mouse hippocampal cells and mouse microglial cells (Eom et al., 2012).

2.54 PRIMARY LATERAL SCLEROSIS

Primary lateral sclerosis (PLS), also called adult-onset primary lateral sclerosis, is a malfunction of the nerve cells in the cerebral cortex and brain stem that carry instructions from the brain to the muscles, characterized by progressive weakness and stiffness of the muscles in the legs, arms, and at the base of the brain. The cause of PLS is unclear and may involve both genetic and environmental factors.

TABLE 2.54

GMP Herbal Medicines for a 50-Year-Old Man with Primary Lateral Sclerosis

Primary lateral sclerosis (OrphaCode: 35689)

A disease with a prevalence of ~2 in 100,000

Disease-causing germline mutation(s): SPG7 matrix AAA peptidase subunit, paraplegin (*SPG7* / Entrez: 6687) at 16q24.3

Autosomal dominant, Autosomal recessive, Not applicable

Spasticity, Abnormal upper motor neuron morphology, Upper motor neuron dysfunction, Babinski sign, Generalized hyperreflexia

Dysphagia, Spastic gait, Pseudobulbar signs, Loss of speech, Spastic dysarthria, EMG: chronic denervation signs, Progressive spastic paraparesis, Weakness due to upper motor neuron dysfunction

Atrophy of the spinal cord, Motor axonal neuropathy, Cervical spinal cord atrophy

Adult, Elderly

Spasticity (D009128):

Dāngguīsìnìtāng 5g + dúhuójìshēngtāng 5g + niúxī 1g + dùzhòng 1-0g.

Dāngguīsìnìtāng 5g + sìnìtāng 3-0g + shēngjiāng 1g + wúzhūyú 1g + jīxuèténg 1-0g + fùzǐ 1-0g + gānjiāng 1-0g.

Chuānwū 5g + wǔlíngzhī 2g + tiānnánxīng 2g + mùxiāng 2g + gāncǎo 2g + dìlóng 2g + yánhúsuǒ 2g + táorén 2g + huíxiāng 2g + chénpí 2g + dāngguī 2g + acupuncture.

Chuānwū 5g + shúdìhuáng 5g + gāncǎo 3g + báisháo 3g + máhuáng 3g + huángqí 3g + báijièzǐ 2g + dàhuáng 1g + shēngjiāng 1g + huánglián 0g.

Spastic gait (D020233), Spastic dysarthria (D004401):

Shēntòngzhúyūtāng 5g + shūjīnghuóxuètāng 5g + dúhuójìshēngtāng 5-0g + yánhúsuǒ 1-0g + jīxuèténg 1-0g + acupuncture.

Shēntòngzhúyūtāng 5g + sháoyàogāncǎotāng 3g + niúxī 1g + mòyào 1g + rǔxiāng 1g + acupuncture.

Sānbìtāng 5g + shūjīnghuóxuètāng 5g + acupuncture.

Wēilíngxiān 5g + báizhú 3g + qiānghuó 3g + xiāngfù 3g + huángqín 3g + cāngzhú 3g + tiānnánxīng 2g + bànxià 2g + gāncǎo 2g + shēngjiāng 2g + fúlíng 2g + chénpí 2g.

Chuānwū 5g + yánhúsuǒ 5g + xiǎohuíxiāng 2g + wǔlíngzhī 2g + tiānnánxīng 2g + mùxiāng 2g + dìlóng 2g + táorén 2g + chénpí 2g + dāngguī 2g.

A compound isolated from Wǔlíngzhī (Faeces Trogopterori), i.e., epifriedelanol, was shown to attenuate the secondary injury in traumatic brain injury rats through reducing serum cytokines and oxidative stress (Li et al., 2018). Dāngguīsìnìtāng (cf. Section 2.12) was demonstrated to prevent sciatic neuropathy in diabetic rats (Liu et al., 2016) and its therapeutic mechanisms for peripheral nerve injury were elucidated (Zhang et al., 2023). An injection of Wēilíngxiān (cf. Sections 2.1 and 2.33) distillates to the acupoint Zusanli (ST36) was shown to treat inflammatory pain in rats (Hwang et al., 2008).

2.55 SPINOCEREBELLAR ATAXIA TYPE 1

Spinocerebellar ataxia type 1 (SCA1) is a progressive movement condition characterized by poor coordination and balance and difficulties speaking and swallowing. SCA1 is caused by trinucleotide repeat expansion of the *ATXN1* gene, whose products are involved in gene transcription in the

TABLE 2.55

GMP Herbal Medicines for a 35-Year-Old Adult with Spinocerebellar Ataxia Type 1

Spinocerebellar ataxia type 1 (OrphaCode: 98755)

A disease with a prevalence of ~2 in 100,000

Disease-causing germline mutation(s): ataxin 1 (*ATXN1* / Entrez: 6310) at 6p22.3

Autosomal dominant

Progressive cerebellar ataxia, Peripheral neuropathy

Abnormality of eye movement, Slow saccadic eye movements, Dysarthria, Cerebellar atrophy, Gait disturbance, Dystonia, Slurred speech, Dysphagia, Bradykinesia, Chorea, Memory impairment, Bulbar signs, Loss of Purkinje cells in the cerebellar vermis, Atrophy/Degeneration affecting the brainstem, Abnormality of somatosensory evoked potentials, Abnormal flash visual evoked potentials, Upgaze palsy, Staring gaze, Inertia, Abnormal nerve conduction velocity, Cognitive impairment

Ophthalmoparesis, Nystagmus, Optic atrophy, Hyporeflexia, Generalized hypotonia, Dysmetria, Dysdiadochokinesis, Gait imbalance, Postural tremor, Abnormal brainstem morphology, Fasciculations, Respiratory failure, Skeletal muscle atrophy, Hyperactive deep tendon reflexes, Hypermetric saccades, Impaired proprioception, Abnormality of masticatory muscle

All ages

Dysarthria (D004401), Dystonia (D004421), Bradykinesia (D018476), Chorea (D002819), Memory impairment (D008569):

Bǔzhōngyìqìtāng 5g + shēngmàiyǐn 2-0g + fùzǐ 0g.
Guìzhītāng 5g + bànxià 1g.

Huángqí 5g + chìsháo 1g + fángfēng 1g + xìxīn 1-0g + huánglián 1-0g.
Huángqí 5g + zhìgāncǎo 4g + wǔwèizǐ 1g + dāngguī 1g.
Huángqí 5g + gāncǎo 4g + wǔwèizǐ 2g + dāngguī 1g.

Ophthalmoparesis (378.56), Nystagmus (379.53, 379.55, 379.50), Optic atrophy (377.1), Dysmetria (D002524), Postural tremor (D014202), Fasciculations (D005207), Skeletal muscle atrophy (D009133):

Zīshènmíngmùtāng 5g + qǐjúdìhuángwán 4g + dānshēn 1g + mùzéicǎo 1-0g + juémíngzǐ 1-0g + niúxī 1-0g + chēqiánzǐ 1-0g + qīngxiāngzǐ 1-0g + chōngwèizǐ 1-0g + mìménghuā 1-0g.
Bǔyánghuánwǔtāng 5g + zīshènmíngmùtāng 5-0g + gǒuqǐzǐ 1-0g + júhuā 1-0g + dānshēn 1-0g.

Gǒuqǐzǐ 5g + júhuā 5g + dāngguī 5g + shúdìhuáng 5g + fángfēng 4g + xìxīn 2g + huánglián 2g + dàhuáng 1g.
Gǒuqǐzǐ 5g + júhuā 5g + dìhuáng 4-3g + dāngguī 4-3g + fángfēng 4-2g + xìxīn 2-1g + huánglián 2-1g.

---

nucleus. The protein products of the repeat expanded *ATXN1* gene have an abnormal three-dimensional structure that aggregates and damages the cells in the cerebellum, causing SCA1. The longer the repeat expansion, the earlier the disease onset.

Zhìgāncǎo (cf. Sections 1.11 and 1.25), i.e., honey-roasted Gāncǎo, has effects on the brain. For example, it was shown to inhibit proliferation, cell locomotion, cell cycle progression, and induce apoptosis in human glioblastoma cells in vitro (Lin et al., 2022). Guìzhītāng "restores yin-yang balance, modulates nutrition-defense homeostasis" and is applied to not only infectious diseases but other miscellaneous conditions. Note that Guìzhītāng contains Zhìgāncǎo. Shēngmàiyǐn (cf. Section 2.39) was shown to protect brain impairment in endotoxin-induced shock rats (Zhang et al., 2010).

2.56   SPINOCEREBELLAR ATAXIA TYPE 2

Spinocerebellar ataxia type 2 (SCA2) is a progressive movement disorder marked by impaired coordination and balance, speaking and swallowing difficulties, repetitive and uncontrolled eye movement, and slowed and jerky movements of both eyes between directions. SCA2 is associated with long repeat expansion in the *ATXN2* gene whose products are involved in cell eating and drinking called endocytosis.

TABLE 2.56

GMP Herbal Medicines for a 30-Year-Old Adult with Spinocerebellar Ataxia Type 2

Spinocerebellar ataxia type 2 (OrphaCode: 98756)

A disease with a prevalence of ~2 in 100,000

Disease-causing germline mutation(s): ataxin 2 (*ATXN2* / Entrez: 6311) at 12q24.12

Autosomal dominant

Progressive cerebellar ataxia, Abnormality of the substantia nigra

Slow saccadic eye movements, Supranuclear ophthalmoplegia, Nystagmus, Dementia, Dysarthria, Hyporeflexia, Generalized hypotonia, Dystonia, Gait ataxia, Chorea, Postural tremor, Fasciculations, Abnormality of the spinocerebellar tracts, Muscle spasm, Olivopontocerebellar hypoplasia, Spinal cord posterior columns myelin loss, Cerebellar Purkinje layer atrophy, Abnormal cell morphology, Kinetic tremor

Ophthalmoparesis, Parkinsonism, Cerebral cortical atrophy, Abnormal cortical gyration, Hyperactive deep tendon reflexes, Cerebral white matter atrophy

All ages

Nystagmus (379.53, 379.55, 379.50), Dysarthria (D004401), Dystonia (D004421), Gait ataxia (D020234), Chorea (D002819), Postural tremor (D014202), Fasciculations (D005207), Muscle spasm (D009120), Kinetic tremor (D014202):

Zīshènmíngmùtāng 5g + xǐgānmíngmùtāng 4-0g + gǒuqǐzǐ 2-0g + júhuā 2-0g.

Zīshènmíngmùtāng 5g + qǐjúdìhuángwán 4-0g + gǒuqǐzǐ 2-0g + júhuā 2-0g + chēqiánzǐ 1-0g + gǔjīngcǎo 1-0g.

Gǒuqǐzǐ 5g + júhuā 5g + dìhuáng 4-3g + fángfēng 4-3g + dāngguī 4-3g + xìxīn 2-1g + huánglián 2-1g + dàhuáng 0g.

Huángqí 5g + chìsháo 1g + fángfēng 1g + xìxīn 0g + huánglián 0g.

Ophthalmoparesis (378.56):

Jīngfángbàidúsǎn 5g + gégēntāng 5g + yínqiàosǎn 5-0g.

Rénshēnbàidúsǎn 5g + gégēntāng 5g + huǒmárén 2g + dúhuó 1g + fúshén 1g.

Guìzhītāng 5g + rénshēn 1g + bànxià 1g + gānjiāng 1g.

Báizhǐ 5g + gāncǎo 5-3g + júhuā 5-0g + shārén 3-2g + dàhuáng 3-0g + huánglián 2-0g.

Shēngmá 5g + chìsháo 5g + qiánhú 5g + sāngbáipí 5g + cháihú 5g + jīngjiè 5g + huángqín 5g + gégēn 5g.

Rénshēnbàidúsǎn "induces sweating, releases exterior, scatters Wind, and dispels dampness." It was shown in vitro to be an immune activator (Huh et al., 2023) and is used for migraines and chronic bronchitis (Wang, 2019). GMP-concentrated Gégēntāng extract granules (cf. Section 1.38) were found to significantly lower headache severity in patients with a common cold (Chou et al., 2022). Gégēntāng granules were also shown to reduce aqueous flare elevation in patients after complicated cataract surgery (Ikeda et al., 2002).

2.57 SPINOCEREBELLAR ATAXIA TYPE 3

Spinocerebellar ataxia type 3 (SCA3) is also known as Azorean disease of the nervous system, Machado-Joseph disease, or Nigro-spino-dentatal degeneration with nuclear ophthalmoplegia. SCA3 is an inherited ataxia characterized by spasticity, tremor, and stiffening of muscles; difficulty speaking and swallowing; paralysis of extraocular muscles; and eye bulging. SCA3 is caused by repeat expansion in the *ATXN3* gene, whose products participate in cellular protein quality control pathways in many tissues including neuronal tissues. The length of repeat expansion correlates positively and negatively with severity and onset age of the disease, respectively.

Oral pre-administration of food containing Xǐgānmíngmùtāng was shown to suppress the elevation of aqueous flare in pigmented rabbits (Nagaki et al., 2001). Jiégěng (Radix Platycodonis) "soothes the Lung, dissolves phlegm, benefits the throat, drains pus" and is used for coughs and chronic nasopharyngitis (Wang, 2020). Jiégěngtāng "dispels phlegm, drains pus, benefits Qi, nourishes Blood" and is used for allergic rhinitis and symptoms involving the head and neck (Wang, 2019). Jiégěngtāng comprises Jiégěng and Gāncǎo as the major herbs.

TABLE 2.57

GMP Herbal Medicines for a 40-Year-Old Adult with Spinocerebellar Ataxia Type 3

Spinocerebellar ataxia type 3 (OrphaCode: 98757)

A disease with a prevalence of ~2 in 100,000

Disease-causing germline mutation(s): ataxin 3 (*ATXN3* / Entrez: 4287) at 14q32.12

Autosomal dominant

Proptosis, Progressive external ophthalmoplegia, Nystagmus, Diplopia, Delayed speech and language development, Dysarthria, Dystonia, Hyperreflexia, Abnormality of extrapyramidal motor function, Progressive cerebellar ataxia, Clumsiness, Skeletal muscle atrophy, Abnormal pyramidal sign

Vocal cord paralysis, Vestibular dysfunction, Abnormality of temperature regulation

Childhood, Adolescent, Adult

Proptosis (376.30), Progressive external ophthalmoplegia (378.72), Nystagmus (379.53, 379.55, 379.50), Diplopia (D004172), Delayed speech and language development (D007805), Dysarthria (D004401), Dystonia (D004421), Hyperreflexia (D012021), Skeletal muscle atrophy (D009133):

Xǐgānmíngmùtāng 5g + zīshènmíngmùtāng 5g + bǔzhōngyìqìtāng 5-0g + xuánshēn 1-0g + mǔlì 1-0g + xiàkūcǎo 1-0g + mìmēnghuā 1-0g.

Xuánshēn 5g + dìhuáng 5g + gǒuqǐzǐ 5g + júhuā 5g + dāngguī 5-4g + fángfēng 4g + xìxīn 2-1g + huánglián 2-1g.

Xǐgānmíngmùtāng 5g + zīshènmíngmùtāng 5g + jiāwèixiāoyáosǎn 5-0g + qǐjúdìhuángwán 5-0g.

Gǒuqǐzǐ 5g + júhuā 5g + dìhuáng 5-3g + fángfēng 5-3g + dāngguī 5-2g + xìxīn 2-1g + huánglián 2-1g.

Zīshènmíngmùtāng 5g + qǐjúdìhuángwán 4g + xiàkūcǎo 1g + cǎojuémíng 1g.

Vocal cord paralysis (D014826):

Jiégěngtāng 5g + xuánshēn 2g + bèimǔ 2g + dàzǎo 2-1g + shēngjiāng 2-1g + liánqiáo 2-1g + mǔlì 2-0g + zhīzǐ 1-0g + shānzhīzǐ 1-0g + dàhuáng 0g.

Gāncǎo 5g + jiégěng 5g + xuánshēn 4-2g + bèimǔ 4-2g + mǔlì 4-2g + liánqiáo 4-2g + zhīzǐ 2g + xìngrén 2-0g.

REFERENCES

Cai, M., & Yang, E. J. (2019). Hochu-Ekki-To improves motor function in an amyotrophic lateral sclerosis animal model. *Nutrients, 11*(11), 2644. https://doi.org/10.3390/nu11112644

Cai, Y., Chen, J., Jiang, J., Cao, W., & He, L. (2010). Zhen-wu-tang, a blended traditional Chinese herbal medicine, ameliorates proteinuria and renal damage of streptozotocin-induced diabetic nephropathy in rats. *Journal of Ethnopharmacology, 131*(1), 88–94. https://doi.org/10.1016/j.jep.2010.06.004

Calve, S., Isaac, J., Gumucio, J. P., & Mendias, C. L. (2012). Hyaluronic acid, HAS1, and HAS2 are significantly upregulated during muscle hypertrophy. *American Journal of Physiology - Cell Physiology, 303*(5), C577–C588. https://doi.org/10.1152/ajpcell.00057.2012

Cao, X., Peng, X., Li, G., Ding, W., Wang, K., Wang, X., Xiong, Y., Xiong, W., Lv, F., & Song, M. (2023). Chaihu-Longgu-Muli decoction improves sleep disorders by restoring orexin-A function in CKD mice. *Frontiers in Endocrinology, 14*. https://doi.org/10.3389/fendo.2023.1206353

Chan, Y. K., Wang, N., & Feng, Y. (2021). The toxicology and detoxification of aconitum: Traditional and modern views. *Chinese Medicine, 16*(1). https://doi.org/10.1186/s13020-021-00472-9

Chang, C., Wu, P., Lin, J., Wu, Y. J., Luo, S., Hsue, Y., Lan, J., Pan, T., Wu, Y., Yu, K., Wei, Y., & Chang, H. (2021). Herbal formula SS-1 increases tear secretion for Sjögren's syndrome. *Frontiers in Pharmacology, 12*. https://doi.org/10.3389/fphar.2021.645437

Chao, C., Kuo, H., Huang, H., Cheng, M., Chao, H., Lu, S. C., Lin, H., Wang, C., Chang, T., & Wu, C. (2023). *Poria cocos* lanostane triterpenoids extract promotes collagen and hyaluronic acid production in D-galactose-induced aging rats. *Life, 13*(11), 2130. https://doi.org/10.3390/life13112130

Chen, C., Zhao, C., Wang, X., Li, W., & Chen, X. (2013). Mechanism and effect of shijueming (Concha Haliotidis) on serum calcium in spontaneously hypertensive rats. *Journal of Traditional Chinese Medicine, 33*(3), 373–377. https://pubmed.ncbi.nlm.nih.gov/24024335

Chen, J., Xiao-Yan, L., Li, Z., Qi, A., Yao, P., Zhou, Z., Dong, T. T. X., & Tsim, K. W. K. (2017a). A review of dietary *Ziziphus jujuba* fruit (Jujube): Developing health food supplements for brain protection. *Evidence-Based Complementary and Alternative Medicine, 2017*, 1–10. https://doi.org/10.1155/2017/3019568

Chen, K., Wu, K., Hueng, D., Huang, K., & Pang, C. (2020). Anti-inflammatory effects of powdered product of Bu Yang Huan Wu decoction: Possible role in protecting against transient focal cerebral ischemia. *International Journal of Medical Sciences*, *17*(12), 1854–1863. https://doi.org/10.7150/ijms.46581

Chen, N., Liu, C., Lin, W., Ding, Y., Bian, Z., Huang, L., Huang, H., Yu, K., Chen, S., Sun, Y., Wei, L., Peng, J., & Pan, S. (2017b). Extract of Fructus Cannabis ameliorates learning and memory impairment induced by D-galactose in an aging rats model. *Evidence-Based Complementary and Alternative Medicine*, *2017*, 1–13. https://doi.org/10.1155/2017/4757520

Chen, P., & Sheen, L. (2011). Gastrodiae Rhizoma (天麻 tiān má): A review of biological activity and anti-depressant mechanisms. *Journal of Traditional and Complementary Medicine*, *1*(1), 31–40. https://doi.org/10.1016/s2225-4110(16)30054-2

Chen, W., Livneh, H., Li, H., Wang, Y., Lu, M., Tsai, T., & Chien, K. (2023). Use of Chinese herbal medicine was related to lower risk of osteoporotic fracture in sarcopenia patients: Evidence from population-based health claims. *International Journal of General Medicine*, *16*, 3345–3354. https://doi.org/10.2147/ijgm.s416705

Chen, X., Ji, S., Liu, Y., Xue, X., Xu, J., Gu, Z., Deng, S., Liu, C., Wang, H., Chang, Y., & Wang, X. (2020). Ginsenoside RD ameliorates auditory cortex injury associated with military aviation noise-induced hearing loss by activating SIRT1/PGC-1A signaling pathway. *Frontiers in Physiology*, *11*. https://doi.org/10.3389/fphys.2020.00788

Chen, Y., Lu, R., Wang, Y., & Gan, P. (2022b). Shaoyao Gancao decoction ameliorates paclitaxel-induced peripheral neuropathy via suppressing TRPV1 and TLR4 signaling expression in rats. *Drug Design, Development and Therapy*, *16*, 2067–2081. https://doi.org/10.2147/dddt.s357638

Chen, Y., Xiong, W., Zhang, Y., Bai, X., Cheng, G., Zhang, Y., Chen, R., Guo, Y., Kong, H., Zhang, Y., Qu, H., & Zhao, Y. (2022a). Carbon dots derived from Os draconis and their anxiolytic effect. *International Journal of Nanomedicine*, *17*, 4975–4988. https://doi.org/10.2147/ijn.s382112

Cheng, C. F., Lin, Y., Tsai, F. J., Li, T. M., Lin, T. H., Liao, C., Huang, S., Liu, X., Li, M. J., Ban, B., Liang, W. M., & Lin, J. (2019). Effects of Chinese herbal medicines on the risk of overall mortality, readmission, and reoperation in hip fracture patients. *Frontiers in Pharmacology*, *10*. https://doi.org/10.3389/fphar.2019.00629

Choi, J., Lee, M. J., Jang, M., Kim, E., Shim, I., Kim, H., Lee, S., Lee, S. W., Kim, Y. O., & Cho, I. (2015). An oriental medicine, Hyungbangpaedok-San attenuates motor paralysis in an experimental model of multiple sclerosis by regulating the T cell response. *PloS One*, *10*(10), e0138592. https://doi.org/10.1371/journal.pone.0138592

Choi, Y., Kim, Y. E., Jerng, U. M., Kim, H., Lee, S. I., Kim, G., Cho, S., Kang, H. W., Jung, I. C., Han, K., & Lee, J. (2020). Korean traditional medicine in treating patients with mild cognitive impairment: A multicenter prospective observational case series. *Evidence-Based Complementary and Alternative Medicine*, *2020*, 1–12. https://doi.org/10.1155/2020/4323989

Chong, C., Zhong, Z., Vong, C. T., Wang, S., Lu, J., Zhong, H., Su, H., & Wang, Y. (2021). The potentials of uncariae ramulus cum uncis for the treatment of migraine: Targeting CGRP in the trigeminovascular system. *Current Neuropharmacology*, *19*(7), 1090–1100. https://doi.org/10.2174/1570159x18666201029150937

Chou, P., Tai, C., Tang, Y., Chen, Y., Lin, K., & Wang, C. (2022). A real-world study on Ge Gen Tang in combination with herbal medicines for relieving common cold-associated symptoms. *Evidence-Based Complementary and Alternative Medicine*, *2022*, 1–10. https://doi.org/10.1155/2022/4790910

Cordaro, M., D'Amico, R., Fusco, R., Genovese, T., Peritore, A. F., Gugliandolo, E., Crupi, R., Di Paola, D., Interdonato, L., Impellizzeri, D., Cuzzocrea, S., Di Paola, R., & Siracusa, R. (2023). Actaea racemosa L. Rhizome protect against MPTP-induced neurotoxicity in mice by modulating oxidative stress and neuroinflammation. *Antioxidants*, *12*(1), 40. https://doi.org/10.3390/antiox12010040

Dong, Y., Feng, Z., Chen, H., Wang, F. S., & Lu, J. (2018). *Corni Fructus*: A review of chemical constituents and pharmacological activities. *Chinese Medicine*, *13*(1). https://doi.org/10.1186/s13020-018-0191-z

Du, Z., Wang, Q., Ma, G., Jiao, J., Jiang, D., Xiao, Z., Qiu, M., & Liu, S. (2019). Inhibition of Nrf2 promotes the antitumor effect of *Pinelliae rhizome* in papillary thyroid cancer. *Journal of Cellular Physiology*, *234*(8), 13867–13877. https://doi.org/10.1002/jcp.28069

Eom, C.-S., Jeon, H.-G., Kim, S.-H., Yoon, H.-I., Kim, M.-C., & Kim, D.-H. (2008). Therapeutic effect of Oyaksungisan in dogs with facial nerve paralysis. *Journal of Veterinary Clinics*, *25*(4), 245–248. https://www.e-jvc.org/journal/view.html?uid=1256

Eom, H. W., Park, S. Y., Kim, Y. H., Seong, S. J., Jin, M. L., Ryu, E. Y., Kim, M. J., & Lee, S. J. (2012). Bambusae Caulis in Taeniam modulates neuroprotective and anti-neuroinflammatory effects in hippocampal and microglial cells via HO-1- and Nrf-2-mediated pathways. *International Journal of Molecular Medicine*, *30*(6), 1512–1520. https://doi.org/10.3892/ijmm.2012.1128

Feng, B., Fang, Y.-T., & Xu, R.-S. (2018). Research progress in modern clinical application and mechanism of Guizhi decoction. *China Journal of Chinese Materia Medica*, (24), 2442–2447. https://pesquisa.bvsalud.org/portal/resource/pt/wpr-687437

Feng, S., He, X., Pei-Ru, Z., Zhao, J., Huang, C., & Hu, Z. (2018). A metabolism-based synergy for total coumarin extract of radix *Angelicae dahuricae* and ligustrazine on migraine treatment in rats. *Molecules*, 23(5), 1004. https://doi.org/10.3390/molecules23051004

Gao, L., Cao, M., Du, G., & Qin, X. (2022). Huangqin decoction exerts beneficial effects on rotenone-induced rat model of Parkinson's disease by improving mitochondrial dysfunction and alleviating metabolic abnormality of mitochondria. *Frontiers in Aging Neuroscience*, 14. https://doi.org/10.3389/fnagi.2022.911924

Gao, Q., Tian, W., Yang, H., Hu, H., Zheng, J., Yao, X., Hu, H., & Hu, H. (2024). Shen-Ling-Bai-Zhu-San alleviates the imbalance of intestinal homeostasis in dextran sodium sulfate-induced colitis mice by regulating gut microbiota and inhibiting the NLRP3 inflammasome activation. *Journal of Ethnopharmacology*, 319, 117136. https://doi.org/10.1016/j.jep.2023.117136

Gomar, A., Hosseini, A., & Mirazi, N. (2014). Memory enhancement by administration of ginger (Zingiber officinale) extract on morphine-induced memory impairment in male rats. *Journal of Acute Disease*, 3(3), 212–217. https://doi.org/10.1016/s2221-6189(14)60047-0

Guo, J., Huo, H., Li, L., Guo, S., & Ting-Liang, J. (2009). Sini Tang prevents depression-like behavior in rats exposed to chronic unpredictable stress. *American Journal of Chinese Medicine*, 37(02), 261–272. https://doi.org/10.1142/s0192415x0900693x

Han, Y., Wang, J., Meng, J., Lin, J., Yan, C., & Wang, Y. (2021). Shentong Zhuyu decoction inhibits inflammatory response, migration, and invasion and promotes apoptosis of rheumatoid arthritis fibroblast-like synoviocytes via the MAPK p38/PPARγ/CTGF pathway. *BioMed Research International*, 2021, 1–13. https://doi.org/10.1155/2021/6187695

He, Y., Du, M., Shi, H., Huang, F., Liu, H., Wu, H., Zhang, B., Dou, W., Wu, X., & Wang, Z. (2014). Astragalosides from *Radix astragali* benefits experimental autoimmune encephalomyelitis in C57BL/6 mice at multiple levels. *BMC Complementary and Alternative Medicine*, 14(1). https://doi.org/10.1186/1472-6882-14-313

He, Y., Wu, C., & Zhao, G. (1998). [Experimental study on inhibitory effect of Ganlu Xiaodu Dan on coxackie virus in vitro]. *Zhongguo Zhong Xi Yi Jie He Za Zhi*, 18(12), 737–40. [Article in Chinese] https://pubmed.ncbi.nlm.nih.gov/11475722

Hirata, K. (1994). Two cases of Ménière's disease to which Wu-Ling-San showed higher efficacy. *Prog Med*, 14, 3238–3239. [Article in Japanese]

Hsieh, M., Peng, W., Yeh, F. T., Tsai, H., & Chang, Y. S. (1991). Studies on the anticonvulsive, sedative and hypothermic effects of Periostracum Cicadae extracts. *Journal of Ethnopharmacology*, 35(1), 83–90. https://doi.org/10.1016/0378-8741(91)90136-2

Huang, L., & Sperlágh, B. (2021). Caffeine consumption and schizophrenia: A highlight on adenosine receptor–independent mechanisms. *Current Opinion in Pharmacology*, 61, 106–113. https://doi.org/10.1016/j.coph.2021.09.003

Huang, Z., Lin, J., Zhang, C., Dai, Y., Lin, S., & Liu, X. (2020). Effect of Huoxiang Zhengqi pill on early neurological deterioration in patients with acute ischemic stroke undergoing recanalization therapy and predictive effect of Essen score. *Evidence-Based Complementary and Alternative Medicine*, 2020, 1–6. https://doi.org/10.1155/2020/6912015

Huh, G., Oh, Y., Jeon, Y., Kang, K. S., Kim, S. N., Jung, S. H., Kim, S. H., & Kim, Y. (2023). Insampaedok-San extract exerts an immune-enhancing effect through NF-κB p65 pathway activation. *BioMed Research International*, 2023, 1–13. https://doi.org/10.1155/2023/5458504

Hwang, H., Kim, S., Lee, H., Kim, Y., Shim, I., Park, H., Choi, W., Kim, J., & Hahm, D. (2008). Analgesic effect of Clematidis Radix (CR) herb-acupuncture in a rat model of pain and inflammation. *Oriental Pharmacy and Experimental Medicine*, 7(5), 501–508. https://doi.org/10.3742/opem.2008.7.5.501

Ikeda, N., Hayasaka, S., Nagaki, Y., Hayasaka, Y., Kadoi, C., & Matsumoto, M. (2002). Effects of Kakkon-to and Sairei-to on aqueous flare elevation after complicated cataract surgery. *American Journal of Chinese Medicine*, 30(02n03), 347–353. https://doi.org/10.1142/s0192415x02000375

Im, H., Ju, I. G., Kim, J. H., Lee, S., & Oh, M. S. (2022). Trichosanthis semen and Zingiberis rhizoma mixture ameliorates lipopolysaccharide-induced memory dysfunction by inhibiting neuroinflammation. *International Journal of Molecular Sciences*, 23(22), 14015. https://doi.org/10.3390/ijms232214015

Inokuchi, J., Okabe, H., Yamauchi, T., Nagamatsu, A., Nonaka, G., & Nishioka, I. (1986). Antihypertensive substance in seeds of *Areca catechu* L. *Life Sciences*, 38(15), 1375–1382. https://doi.org/10.1016/0024-3205(86)90470-4

Jiang, X., Yie, S., Xia, Z., Den, Y., Liang, X., Hu, X., Li, L., Li, Q., Cao, S., & Lu, H. (2014). Effect of You Gui Wan on mouse sperm fertilising ability in vivo and in vitro. *Andrologia, 46*(3), 283–289. https://doi.org/10.1111/and.12075

Jing, W., Song, S., Sun, H., Chen, Y., Zhao, Q., Zhang, Y., Dai, G., & Ju, W. (2019). Mahuang-Fuzi-Xixin decoction reverses depression-like behavior in LPS-induced mice by regulating NLRP3 inflammasome and neurogenesis. *Neural Plasticity, 2019*, 1–13. https://doi.org/10.1155/2019/1571392

Kelly, R. B., & Willis, J. (2019). Acupuncture for pain. *American Family Physician, 100*(2), 89–96. https://pubmed.ncbi.nlm.nih.gov/31305037

Kim, H. G., Jeong, H. U., Park, G., Kim, H., Lim, Y., & Oh, M. S. (2015). *Mori Folium* and *Mori Fructus* mixture attenuates high-fat diet-induced cognitive deficits in mice. *Evidence-Based Complementary and Alternative Medicine, 2015*, 1–8. https://doi.org/10.1155/2015/379418

Kim, S. R., Lee, H. W., Jun, J. H., & Ko, B. (2017). Effects of herbal medicine (Gan mai da Zao decoction) on several types of neuropsychiatric disorders in an animal model: A systematic review. *Journal of Pharmacopuncture, 20*(1), 5–9. https://doi.org/10.3831/kpi.2017.20.005

Kim, W. K., Jung, J. W., Ahn, N. Y., Oh, H. R., Lee, B. K., Oh, J. K., Cheong, J. H., Chun, H. S., & Ryu, J. H. (2004). Anxiolytic-like effects of extracts from Albizzia julibrissin bark in the elevated plus-maze in rats. *Life Sciences, 75*(23), 2787–2795. https://doi.org/10.1016/j.lfs.2004.05.024

Kinoshita, T., Matsumoto, A., Yoshino, K., & Furukawa, S. (2017). The effects of licorice flavonoid oil with respect to increasing muscle mass: A randomized, double-blind, placebo-controlled trial. *Journal of the Science of Food and Agriculture, 97*(8), 2339–2345. https://doi.org/10.1002/jsfa.8044

Lai, M., Liu, I., Liou, S., & Chang, Y. (2012). Radix Aconiti Kusnezoffii exhibits an antinociceptive activity involvement at central and peripheral nervous system. *Journal of Food and Drug Analysis, 20*(2), 501–509. https://doi.org/10.6227/jfda.2012200211

Laurent, T., Okuda, Y., Chijimatsu, T., Umeki, M., Kobayashi, S., Kataoka, Y., Tatsuguchi, I., Mochizuki, S., & Oda, H. (2013). Freshwater clam extract ameliorates triglyceride and cholesterol metabolism through the expression of genes involved in hepatic lipogenesis and cholesterol degradation in rats. *Evidence-Based Complementary and Alternative Medicine, 2013*, 1–10. https://doi.org/10.1155/2013/830684

Lee, K., Joo, H., Sun, M., Kim, M., Kim, B., Lee, B., Cho, J., Jung, J., Park, J., & Bu, Y. (2018). Review on the characteristics of liver-pacifying medicinal in relation to the treatment of stroke: From scientific evidence to traditional medical theory. *Journal of Traditional Chinese Medicine, 38*(1), 139–150. https://doi.org/10.1016/j.jtcm.2018.01.003

Lee, S., Hung, A., Li, H., & Yang, A. W. H. (2022). Mechanisms of action of a herbal formula Huangqi Guizhi Wuwu Tang for the management of post-stroke related numbness and weakness: A computational molecular docking study. *Journal of Evidence-Based Integrative Medicine, 27*, 2515690X2210829. https://doi.org/10.1177/2515690x221082989

Lee, S., Lee, D., Lee, S. O., Ryu, J., Choi, S., Kang, K. S., & Kim, K. (2017). Anti-inflammatory activity of the sclerotia of edible fungus, *Poria cocos* Wolf and their active lanostane triterpenoids. *Journal of Functional Foods, 32*, 27–36. https://doi.org/10.1016/j.jff.2017.02.012

Li, H.-B. (2018). Scientific research of laxative action of Cannabis Fructus based on intestinal environment adjustment. *Chinese Traditional and Herbal Drugs*, (24), 3334–3342. https://pesquisa.bvsalud.org/portal/resource/pt/wpr-851837

Li, Q., Cao, M., Wei, Z., Mei, J., Zhang, Y., Li, M., Li, M., Zhang, Y., & Wang, Z. (2022). The protective effect of Buzhong Yiqi decoction on ischemic stroke mice and the mechanism of gut microbiota. *Frontiers in Neuroscience, 16*. https://doi.org/10.3389/fnins.2022.956620

Li, S., Li, R., Zeng, Y., Meng, X., Wen, C., & Zheng, S. (2019a). [Chemical components and pharmacological action of Aconiti Radix]. *Zhongguo Zhong Yao Za Zhi, 44*(12), 2433–2443. [Article in Chinese] https://doi.org/10.19540/j.cnki.cjcmm.20190221.004

Li, S., Zhang, Q., & Li, P. (2018). Protective effects of epifriedelinol in a rat model of traumatic brain injury assessed with histological and hematological markers. *Translational Neuroscience, 9*(1), 38–42. https://doi.org/10.1515/tnsci-2018-0008

Li, X., Chu, S., Liu, Y., & Chen, N. (2019b). Neuroprotective effects of anthraquinones from rhubarb in central nervous system diseases. *Evidence-Based Complementary and Alternative Medicine, 2019*, 1–12. https://doi.org/10.1155/2019/3790728

Lian, J., Chen, J., Yuan, Y., Chen, J., Sayed, M., Lin, L., Zhu, Y., Li, S., & Bu, S. (2017). Cortex Mori Radicis extract attenuates myocardial damages in diabetic rats by regulating ERS. *Biomedicine & Pharmacotherapy, 90*, 777–785. https://doi.org/10.1016/j.biopha.2017.03.097

Lin, T., Wang, L., Zhang, Y., Zhang, J., Zhou, D., Fang, F., Liu, L., Liu, B., & Jiang, Y. (2021). Uses, chemical compositions, pharmacological activities and toxicology of Clematidis Radix et Rhizome – A review. *Journal of Ethnopharmacology*, *270*, 113831. https://doi.org/10.1016/j.jep.2021.113831

Lin, T., Wu, T., Tzou, R., Hsu, Y., Lee, K., & Tsai, T. (2022). Radix glycyrrhizae Preparata induces cell cycle arrest and induced caspase-dependent apoptosis in Glioblastoma multiforme. *Neurology International*, *14*(4), 804–823. https://doi.org/10.3390/neurolint14040066

Lin, Y., Wang, X., Ren, Y., Hu, W., Sun, S., Jiao, H., Song, X., Yuan, Z., Zheng, Y., Guo, Z., & He, J. (2013). Efficacy and safety of Wuling capsule, a single herbal formula, in Chinese subjects with insomnia: A multicenter, randomized, double-blind, placebo-controlled trial. *Journal of Ethnopharmacology*, *145*(1), 320–327. https://doi.org/10.1016/j.jep.2012.11.009

Liu, P., Bian, Y., Zhang, H., & Ai-Ming, J. (2016). Preventive effects of the Chinese herbal medicine prescription Tangkuei decoction for frigid extremities on sciatic neuropathy in streptozotocin-induced diabetic rats. *Evidence-Based Complementary and Alternative Medicine*, *2016*, 1–11. https://doi.org/10.1155/2016/9138328

Liu, Z., & Wang, L. (2017). Hyperkinesia in ancient China: Perspectives and prescriptions. *CNS Spectrums*, *22*(3), 251–253. https://doi.org/10.1017/s1092852916000560

Lu, F., Liu, L., Yu, D., Li, X., Zhou, Q., & Liu, S. (2014). Therapeutic effect of Rhizoma Dioscoreae Nipponicae on gouty arthritis based on the SDF-1/CXCR 4 and p38 MAPK pathway: An in vivo and in vitro study. *Phytotherapy Research*, *28*(2), 280–288. https://doi.org/10.1002/ptr.4997

Lu, W., Wu, Z., Zhang, C., Gao, T., Ling, X., Xu, M., Wang, W., Jin, X., Li, K., Chen, L., Wang, J., & Sun, Z. (2022). Jujuboside A exhibits an antiepileptogenic effect in the rat model via protection against traumatic epilepsy-induced oxidative stress and inflammatory responses. *Evidence-Based Complementary and Alternative Medicine*, *2022*, 1–9. https://doi.org/10.1155/2022/7792791

Lv, C., Shi, C., Li, L., Wen, X., & Chen, X. (2018). Chinese herbal medicines in the prevention and treatment of chemotherapy-induced nausea and vomiting. *Current Opinion in Supportive and Palliative Care*, *12*(2), 174–180. https://doi.org/10.1097/spc.0000000000000348

Lyu, S., Zhang, C. S., Guo, X., Zhang, A. L., Sun, J., Lu, C., Xue, C. C., & Luo, X. (2020). Oral Chinese Herbal medicine as prophylactic treatment for episodic migraine in adults: A systematic review and meta-analysis of randomized controlled trials. *Evidence-Based Complementary and Alternative Medicine*, *2020*, 1–20. https://doi.org/10.1155/2020/5181587

Ma, L., Chai, T., Wang, C., Zheng, Y., Ma, L., Meng, X., Wang, K., Wang, W., Farimani, M. M., Sang, C., & Yang, J. (2022). Four new compounds with cytotoxic and neuroprotective activity from *Notopterygium incisum*. *Phytochemistry Letters*, *49*, 138–144. https://doi.org/10.1016/j.phytol.2022.03.007

May, B. H., Lu, C., Lu, Y., Zhang, A. L., & Xue, C. C. (2013). Chinese herbs for memory disorders: A review and systematic analysis of classical herbal literature. *Journal of Acupuncture and Meridian Studies*, *6*(1), 2–11. https://doi.org/10.1016/j.jams.2012.11.009

Meng, P., Chen, Z., Sun, T., Wu, L., Wang, Y., Guo, T., Yang, J., & Zhu, J. (2023). Sheng-Mai-Yin inhibits doxorubicin-induced ferroptosis and cardiotoxicity through regulation of Hmox1. *Aging*, *15*(19), 10133–10145. https://doi.org/10.18632/aging.205062

Moon, Y. J., Lee, J. Y., Oh, M. S., Pak, Y. K., Park, K., Oh, T. H., & Yune, T. Y. (2012). Inhibition of inflammation and oxidative stress by *Angelica dahuricae* radix extract decreases apoptotic cell death and improves functional recovery after spinal cord injury. *Journal of Neuroscience Research*, *90*(1), 243–256. https://doi.org/10.1002/jnr.22734

Morais, L. H., Schreiber, H. L., & Mazmanian, S. K. (2020). The gut microbiota–brain axis in behaviour and brain disorders. *Nature Reviews. Microbiology*, *19*(4), 241–255. https://doi.org/10.1038/s41579-020-00460-0

Nagaki, Y., Hayasaka, S., Kadoi, C., Matsumoto, M., Nakamura, N., & Hayasaka, Y. (2001). Effects of Orengedoku-to and Senkanmeimoku-to, traditional herbal medicines, on the experimental herbal medicines, on the experimental elevation of aqueous flare in pigmental rabbits. *American Journal of Chinese Medicine*, *29*(01), 141–147. https://doi.org/10.1142/s0192415x01000150

Niu, Y., Li, C., Pan, Y., Li, Y., Kong, X., Wang, S., Zhai, Y., Wu, X., Wu, F., & Mei, Q. (2015). Treatment of Radix Dipsaci extract prevents long bone loss induced by modeled microgravity in hindlimb unloading rats. *Pharmaceutical Biology*, *53*(1), 110–116. https://doi.org/10.3109/13880209.2014.911920

Park, H. R., Lee, H., Cho, W., & Ma, J. Y. (2023). Pro-neurogenic effects of Lilii Bulbus on hippocampal neurogenesis and memory. *Biomedicine & Pharmacotherapy*, *164*, 114951. https://doi.org/10.1016/j.biopha.2023.114951

Park, H. R., Lee, H., Lee, J., Yim, N., Gu, M., & Ma, J. Y. (2017). Protective effects of *Spatholobi caulis* extract on neuronal damage and focal ischemic stroke/reperfusion injury. *Molecular Neurobiology*, *55*(6), 4650–4666. https://doi.org/10.1007/s12035-017-0652-x

Park, J. H., Shin, B. N., Ahn, J. H., Cho, J. H., Lee, T., Lee, J. C., Jeon, Y. H., Kang, I. J., Yoo, K., Hwang, I. K., Lee, C. H., Noh, Y., Kim, S., Won, M., & Kim, J. D. (2018). *Glehnia littoralis* extract promotes neurogenesis in the hippocampal dentate gyrus of the adult mouse through increasing expressions of brain-derived neurotrophic factor and tropomyosin-related kinase B. *Chinese Medical Journal, 131*(6), 689–695. https://doi.org/10.4103/0366-6999.226894

Piwowar, A., Rembiałkowska, N., Rorbach-Dolata, A., Garbiec, A., Ślusarczyk, S., Dobosz, A., Długosz, A., Marchewka, Z., Matkowski, A., & Saczko, J. (2020). *Anemarrhenae asphodeloides rhizoma* extract enriched in Mangiferin protects PC12 cells against a neurotoxic agent-3-nitropropionic acid. *International Journal of Molecular Sciences, 21*(7), 2510. https://doi.org/10.3390/ijms21072510

Pradhan, S. K., Li, Y., Gantenbein, A. R., Angst, F., Lehmann, S., & Shaban, H. (2022). Wen Dan Tang: A potential Jing Fang decoction for headache disorders? *Medicines, 9*(3), 22. https://doi.org/10.3390/medicines9030022

Ravanfar, P., Namazi, G., Atigh, M., Zafarmand, S., Hamedi, A., Salehi, A., Izadi, S., & Borhani-Haghighi, A. (2016). Efficacy of whole extract of licorice in neurological improvement of patients after acute ischemic stroke. *Journal of Herbal Medicine, 6*(1), 12–17. https://doi.org/10.1016/j.hermed.2015.12.001

Şahin, M. M., Uğur, M. B., Karamert, R., Aytekin, S., Kabiş, B., Düzlü, M., Seymen, C. M., Elmas, Ç., Gökdoğan, Ç., & Ünlü, S. (2018). Evaluation of effect of garlic aged extracts and vitamin B12 on noise-induced hearing loss. *Noise & Health, 20*(97), 232. https://www.ncbi.nlm.nih.gov/pmc/articles/PMC6924192

Shin, J. S., & Huh, Y. S. (2014). Effect of intake of gardenia fruits and combined exercise of middle-aged obese women on hormones regulating energy metabolism. *Journal of Exercise Nutrition & Biochemistry, 18*(1), 41–49. https://doi.org/10.5717/jenb.2014.18.1.41

Song, H., Hou, X., Zeng, M., Chen, X., Chen, X., Yang, T., Xu, F., Peng, J., Peng, Q., Cai, X., & Yu, R. (2020). Traditional Chinese medicine Li-Zhong-Tang accelerates the healing of indomethacin-induced gastric ulcers in rats by affecting TLR-2/MyD88 signaling pathway. *Journal of Ethnopharmacology, 259*, 112979. https://doi.org/10.1016/j.jep.2020.112979

Song, M. J., Kang, S. Y., Oh, T. W., Kumar, R. V., Jung, H. W., & Park, Y. (2015). The roots of *Atractylodes macrocephala* Koidzumi enhanced glucose and lipid metabolism in C2C12 myotubes via mitochondrial regulation. *Evidence-Based Complementary and Alternative Medicine, 2015*, 1–10. https://doi.org/10.1155/2015/643654

Su, Y., Liu, N., Sun, R., Ma, J., Li, Z., Wang, P., Ma, H., Sun, Y., Song, J., & Zhang, Z. (2023). Radix Rehmanniae Praeparata (Shu Dihuang) exerts neuroprotective effects on ICV-STZ-induced Alzheimer's disease mice through modulation of INSR/IRS-1/AKT/GSK-3β signaling pathway and intestinal microbiota. *Frontiers in Pharmacology, 14*. https://doi.org/10.3389/fphar.2023.1115387

Sui, F., Zhou, H., Meng, J., Du, X., Sui, Y., Zhou, Z., Cheng, D., Wang, Z., Wang, W., Li, D., Hai, M., Huo, H., & Ting-Liang, J. (2016). A Chinese herbal decoction, Shaoyao-Gancao Tang, exerts analgesic effect by down-regulating the TRPV1 channel in a rat model of arthritic pain. *American Journal of Chinese Medicine, 44*(07), 1363–1378. https://doi.org/10.1142/s0192415x16500762

Sun, C., Gao, M., & Qiao, M. (2023). Research progress of traditional Chinese medicine compound "Xiaochaihu decoction" in the treatment of depression. *Biomedicine & Pharmacotherapy, 159*, 114249. https://doi.org/10.1016/j.biopha.2023.114249

Sun, J., He, L., Sun, J., Liu, H., Chen, J., & Wang, C. (2017). Chemical composition and antimigraine activity of essential oil of *Angelicae dahuricae* radix. *Journal of Medicinal Food, 20*(8), 797–803. https://doi.org/10.1089/jmf.2016.3898

Thanh, C. D., Van Men, C., Kim, H. M., & Kang, J. S. (2022). Network pharmacology-based investigation on therapeutic mechanisms of the *Angelica dahurica* radix and *Ligusticum chuanxiong* Rhizoma herb pair for anti-migraine effect. *Plants, 11*(17), 2196. https://doi.org/10.3390/plants11172196

Tseng, C., Hsu, P., Lee, C., Huang, H., Lan, C., Hsieh, T., Liu, G., Kuo, C., Wang, M., & Hsieh, P. (2022). Acupuncture and traditional Chinese herbal medicine integrated with conventional rehabilitation for post-stroke functional recovery: A retrospective cohort study. *Frontiers in Neuroscience, 16*. https://doi.org/10.3389/fnins.2022.851333

Wang, H., Dai, J., He, Y., Xia, Z., Chen, X., Hong, Z., & Chai, Y. (2022). Therapeutic effect and mechanism of *Anemarrhenae rhizoma* on Alzheimer's disease based on multi-platform metabolomics analyses. *Frontiers in Pharmacology, 13*. https://doi.org/10.3389/fphar.2022.940555

Wang, Q., Zhang, N., Liu, S., Jiang, X., & Liu, S. (2021). Saposhnikoviae radix enhanced the angiogenic and anti-inflammatory effects of Huangqi Chifeng Tang in a rat model of cerebral infarction. *Evidence-based Complementary and Alternative Medicine, 2021*, 1–12. https://doi.org/10.1155/2021/4232708

Wang, S., He, F., Wang, H., Fu, X., Zheng, H., Wu, W., & Li, S. (2023). Health-promoting activities and associated mechanisms of Polygonati Rhizoma polysaccharides. *Molecules*, *28*(3), 1350. https://doi.org/10.3390/molecules28031350

Wang, S.-C. (2019). Therapeutic classes of CHEG formulas. In S.-C. Wang, *Clinical herbal prescriptions: Principles and practices of herbal formulations from deep learning health insurance herbal prescription Big Data* (pp. 16–89). World Scientific Publishing. https://doi.org/10.1142/11211

Wang, S.-C. (2020). Modern therapeutic uses of CHEG herbs and herb pairs. In S.-C. Wang, *Veterinary herbal pharmacopoeia* (pp. 35–233). Nova Science Publishers. https://doi.org/10.52305/GHTR1903

Wang, Y., Yang, Y., Xiao, C., Zhang, J., Wan, L., & Du, G. (2019). *Xiao-Xu-Ming* decoction extract regulates differentially expressed proteins in the hippocampus after chronic cerebral hypoperfusion. *Neural Regeneration Research*, *14*(3), 470. https://doi.org/10.4103/1673-5374.245471

Wu, L., Zhang, T., Chen, K., Lu, C., Liu, X. F., Jia, Z., Huang, Y., Yan, H., Chen, Y., Zhang, C. J., Li, J. F., Shi, S. Q., Ren, P., & Huang, X. (2021). Rapid antidepressant-like effect of fructus aurantii depends on cAMP-response element binding protein/Brain-derived neurotrophic factor by mediating synaptic transmission. *Phytotherapy Research*, *35*(1), 404–414. https://doi.org/10.1002/ptr.6812

Wu, X., Zhao, J., Zhang, M., Li, F., & Zhao, T. (2011). Sedative, hypnotic and anticonvulsant activities of the ethanol fraction from Rhizoma Pinelliae Praeparatum. *Journal of Ethnopharmacology*, *135*(2), 325–329. https://doi.org/10.1016/j.jep.2011.03.016

Xian, Y., Mao, Q., Ip, S., Lin, Z., & Che, C. (2011). Comparison on the anti-inflammatory effect of Cortex Phellodendri Chinensis and Cortex Phellodendri Amurensis in 12-O-tetradecanoyl-phorbol-13-acetate-induced ear edema in mice. *Journal of Ethnopharmacology*, *137*(3), 1425–1430. https://doi.org/10.1016/j.jep.2011.08.014

Xie, J., Li, Y., Liang, Y., Kui, H., Wang, C., & Huang, J. (2023). Integration of non-targeted metabolomics with network pharmacology deciphers the anxiolytic mechanisms of Platycladi Semen extracts in CUMS mice. *Journal of Ethnopharmacology*, *315*, 116571. https://doi.org/10.1016/j.jep.2023.116571

Xie, Z., Tian, X., Zheng, Y., Li, Z., Chen, X., Xin, X., Huang, C., & Gao, Z. (2020). Antiepileptic geissoschizine methyl ether is an inhibitor of multiple neuronal channels. *Acta Pharmacologica Sinica*, *41*(5), 629–637. https://doi.org/10.1038/s41401-019-0327-4

Xiong, Z., Yi, P., Zhang, L., Ma, H., Li, W., & Tan, M. (2020). Efficacy and safety of modified Duhuo jisheng decoction in the treatment of lumbar disc herniation: A systematic review and Meta-Analysis, *Evidence-Based Complementary and Alternative Medicine*, *2020*, 1–11. https://doi.org/10.1155/2020/2381462

Yang, X., Liu, L., Ming, S., Fang, J., & Wu, D. (2019). Tian Wang Bu Xin Dan for insomnia: A systematic review of efficacy and safety. *Evidence-Based Complementary and Alternative Medicine*, *2019*, 1–7. https://doi.org/10.1155/2019/4260801

Yang, X., Wang, Y., Ding, X., Ju, S., An, X., Zhang, B., & Lin, Z. (2023). Network pharmacology identification and in vivo validation of key pharmacological pathways of Qin Jiao for gout and arthritis. *Pharmaceutical Biology*, *61*(1), 1525–1535. https://doi.org/10.1080/13880209.2023.2288289

Yang, X., Zhou, S., Ma, A., Xu, H., Guan, H., & Liu, H. (2012). Chemical profiles and identification of key compound caffeine in marine-derived traditional Chinese medicine Ostreae concha. *Marine Drugs*, *10*(12), 1180–1191. https://doi.org/10.3390/md10051180

Ye, K. F. (1999). Treating 86 cases of Ménière's syndrome with Wu Ling San. *J New TCM*, *31*, 43–44.

Yeung, W., Chung, K. F., Ng, K., Yu, B. Y. M., Ziea, E. T. C., & Ng, B. F. L. (2014). A meta-analysis of the efficacy and safety of traditional Chinese medicine formula Ganmai Dazao decoction for depression. *Journal of Ethnopharmacology*, *153*(2), 309–317. https://doi.org/10.1016/j.jep.2014.02.046

Zhang, C., Song, S., Han, J., Zhao, L., Zhang, W., & Ma, X. (2020b). Effect of Sanbi granules on TLR4/MAPKs/NF-κB signal pathway in type II collagen induced arthritis rats. *Chinese Pharmaceutical Journal*, *55*(7), 519–526. http://journal11.magtechjournal.com/Jwk_zgyxzz/EN/abstract/abstract32666.shtml

Zhang, H., Chi, X., Pan, W., Wang, S., Zhang, Z., Zhao, H., Wang, Y., Wu, Z., Zhou, M., Ma, S., Zhao, Q., & Ma, K. (2020c). Antidepressant mechanism of classical herbal formula lily bulb and Rehmannia decoction: Insights from gene expression profile of medial prefrontal cortex of mice with stress-induced depression-like behavior. *Genes, Brain and Behavior*, *19*(5). https://doi.org/10.1111/gbb.12649

Zhang, J., He, S., Wang, J., Wang, C., Ju, W., Wang, W., Fan, L., Li, S., Zhao, C., & Fang, L. (2020a). A review of the traditional uses, botany, phytochemistry, pharmacology, pharmacokinetics, and toxicology of *Corydalis yanhusuo*. *Natural Product Communications*, *15*(9), 1934578X2095775. https://doi.org/10.1177/1934578x20957752

Zhang, N., Zhang, D., Zhang, Q., Zhang, R., & Wang, Y. (2023). Mechanism of Danggui Sini underlying the treatment of peripheral nerve injury based on network pharmacology and molecular docking: A review. *Medicine*, *102*(19), e33528. https://doi.org/10.1097/md.0000000000033528

Zhang, S., Lei, L., Li, W., Zou, B., Cai, Y., Liu, D., Xiao, D., Chen, J., Li, P., Zhong, Y., Liao, Q., & Xie, Z. (2019b). Shen-Ling-Bai-Zhu-San alleviates functional dyspepsia in rats and modulates the composition of the gut microbiota. *Nutrition Research*, *71*, 89–99. https://doi.org/10.1016/j.nutres.2019.10.001

Zhang, W., & Dong, J. (2018). Effectiveness of *Radix astragali* and Salvia miltiorrhiza injection in treatment of skeletal muscle injury of aerobics athletes. *Pak J Pharm Sci*, *31*(4(Special)), 1767–1771. https://pubmed.ncbi.nlm.nih.gov/30203777

Zhang, W., Zhao, Z., Chang, L., Cao, Y., Wang, S., Kang, C., Wang, H., Zhou, L., Huang, L., & Guo, L. (2021). Atractylodis Rhizoma: A review of its traditional uses, phytochemistry, pharmacology, toxicology and quality control. *Journal of Ethnopharmacology*, *266*, 113415. https://doi.org/10.1016/j.jep.2020.113415

Zhang, X., Ding, W., Wang, Z., Gu, X., & Zhu, W. (2019a). The effectiveness and safety of acupuncture for the treatment of myasthenia gravis: A systematic review and meta-analysis of randomized controlled trials. *Annals of Palliative Medicine*, *8*(5), 576–585. https://doi.org/10.21037/apm.2019.10.10

Zhang, Y., Wu, H., Ren, L., Zhang, H., Xu, J., & Zhang, Y. (2010). Study on modified Shengmai Yin injection for prevention and treatment of brain impairment in endotoxin shock rats. *Journal of Traditional Chinese Medicine*, *30*(4), 272–277. https://doi.org/10.1016/s0254-6272(10)60055-6

Zhang, Z., & Shi, L. (2010). Anti-inflammatory and analgesic properties of cis-mulberroside A from *Ramulus mori*. *Fitoterapia*, *81*(3), 214–218. https://doi.org/10.1016/j.fitote.2009.09.005

Zhao, L., Sun, Z., Yang, L., Cui, R., Yang, W., & Li, B. (2020). Neuropharmacological effects of Aconiti Lateralis Radix Praeparata. *Clinical and Experimental Pharmacology & Physiology*, *47*(4), 531–542. https://doi.org/10.1111/1440-1681.13228

Zhao, Q., Chen, X., & Martin, C. (2016). Scutellaria baicalensis, the golden herb from the garden of Chinese medicinal plants. *Science Bulletin*, *61*(18), 1391–1398. https://doi.org/10.1007/s11434-016-1136-5

Zhao, Y., Xu, D., Wang, J., Zhou, D., Liu, A., Sun, Y., Yuan, Y., Li, J., & Guo, W. (2023). The pharmacological mechanism of chaihu-jia-longgu-muli-tang for treating depression: Integrated meta-analysis and network pharmacology analysis. *Frontiers in Pharmacology*, *14*. https://doi.org/10.3389/fphar.2023.1257617

Zheng, F., Wei, P., Huo, H., Xing, X., Chen, F., Tan, X., & Jia-Bo, L. (2015). Neuroprotective effect of Gui Zhi (Ramulus Cinnamomi) on Ma Huang- (Herb Ephedra-) induced toxicity in rats treated with a Ma Huang-Gui Zhi herb pair. *Evidence-Based Complementary and Alternative Medicine*, *2015*, 1–9. https://doi.org/10.1155/2015/913461

Zheng, G.-Q. (2009). Therapeutic history of Parkinson's disease in Chinese medical treatises. *Journal of Alternative and Complementary Medicine*, *15*(11), 1223–1230. https://doi.org/10.1089/acm.2009.0101

Zheng, M., Liu, C., Fan, Y., Shi, D., & Jian, W. (2019). Total glucosides of paeony (TGP) extracted from Radix Paeoniae Alba exerts neuroprotective effects in MPTP-induced experimental parkinsonism by regulating the cAMP/PKA/CREB signaling pathway. *Journal of Ethnopharmacology*, *245*, 112182. https://doi.org/10.1016/j.jep.2019.112182

Zhong, Y., Lee, K. H., Deng, Y., Ma, Y., Chen, Y., Li, X., Wei, C., Yang, S., Wang, T., Wong, N. J., Muwonge, A. N., Azeloglu, E. U., Zhang, W., Das, B., He, J. C., & Liu, R. (2019). Arctigenin attenuates diabetic kidney disease through the activation of PP2A in podocytes. *Nature Communications*, *10*(1). https://doi.org/10.1038/s41467-019-12433-w

Zhou, X., Zhang, H., Li, S., Jiang, Y., Kang, L., Deng, J., Yang, C., Zhao, X., Zhao, J., Jiang, L., & Chen, X. (2023). The effects of fermented feedstuff derived from Citri Sarcodactylis Fructus by-products on growth performance, intestinal digestive enzyme activity, nutrient utilization, meat quality, gut microbiota, and metabolites of broiler chicken. *Frontiers in Veterinary Science*, *10*. https://doi.org/10.3389/fvets.2023.1231996

Zhu, S.-J., Wang, R.-T., Yu, Z.-Y., Zheng, R.-X., Liang, C.-H., Zheng, Y.-Y., Fang, M., Han, M., & Liu, J.-P. (2022). Chinese Herbal medicine for myasthenia gravis: A systematic review and meta-analysis of randomized clinical trials. *Integrative Medicine Research*, *11*(2), 100806. https://doi.org/10.1016/j.imr.2021.100806

Zulfugarova, P., Zivari-Ghader, T., Maharramova, S., Ahmadian, E., Eftekhari, A., Khalilov, R., Türksoy, V. A., Rosić, G., & Selaković, D. (2023). A mechanistic review of pharmacological activities of homeopathic medicine licorice against neural diseases. *Frontiers in Neuroscience*, *17*. https://doi.org/10.3389/fnins.2023.1148258

3 GMP Herbal Medicine for Rare Systemic or Rheumatologic Diseases

Systemic diseases affect a number of organs or even the whole body. Lupus is an example of a systemic disease. Rheumatologic diseases are problems of the soft tissues related to the musculoskeletal system. Rheumatoid arthritis, osteoarthritis, and gout are common rheumatologic diseases. Systemic or rheumatologic diseases can be painful and disabling. Although one-third of the rare systemic or rheumatologic diseases of this chapter involve genes, the etiology of most systemic or rheumatologic diseases is complex, involving genetics, behaviors (e.g., diet and smoking), environment (e.g., coldness and humidity), and their interactions. The majority of the disease onsets are adolescent or later.

The herbs and formulas that are frequently discussed for the clinical manifestations of the common rare systemic or rheumatologic diseases are Rhubarb Root and Rhizome (Dàhuáng), Licorice Root (Gāncǎo), Scutellaria Root (Huángqín), Cardamon Seed (Shārén), Dahurian Angelica Root (Báizhǐ), Poria (Fúlíng), Aconite Accessory Root (Fùzǐ), White Peony Root (Báisháo), Dried Ginger Rhizome (Gānjiāng), White Atractylodis (Báizhú), Chinese Wild Ginger (Xìxīn), Salvia Root (Dānshēn), Five Ingredient Formula with Poria (Wǔlíngsǎn), Polyporus Decoction (Zhūlíngtāng), Free and Easy Wanderer Plus (Augmented Rambling Powder; Jiāwèixiāoyáosǎn), Achyranthes and Plantago Formula (Jìshēngshènqìwán), Prepared Licorice Decoction (Zhìgāncǎotāng), Relax the Channels and Invigorate the Blood Decoction (Shūjīnghuóxuètāng), Cinnamon and Angelica Gout Formula (Shàngzhōngxiàtōngyòngtòngfēngwán), Pulse Generating Decoction (Shēngmàiyǐn), Tonify the Middle and Augment the Qi Decoction (Bǔzhōngyìqìtāng), Wind Reducing Formula (Xiāofēngsǎn), and Sweet Dew Decoction (Gānlùyǐn). Wǔlíngsǎn, Zhūlíngtāng, Jiāwèixiāoyáosǎn, Jìshēngshènqìwán, and Shūjīnghuóxuètāng all contain Fúlíng, which "clears dampness and promotes diuresis." Wǔlíngsǎn (Zhūlíngtāng) "removes excessive water retention in the (lower) body." High humidity is known to aggravate pain and stiffness of rheumatic joints. The usage pattern of herbs and formulas follows features of disease manifestations.

Acupuncture is commonly co-prescribed to manage the symptoms of the systemic or rheumatologic diseases of this chapter.

3.1 PRIMARY SJÖGREN SYNDROME

Patients with primary Sjögren syndrome present with dryness because their immune system mistakenly attacks the exocrine glands, including the lacrimal and salivary glands. The cause of primary Sjögren syndrome is unknown but is believed to involve genetic, hormonal, and environmental factors as the onset can follow a viral or bacterial infection. Table 3.1 gives the prescriptions for a 55-year-old woman who most likely suffers from the condition.

Gǒuqǐzǐ and Júhuā were introduced in Section 1.2 for the eye. Báizhǐ, first annotated in Section 1.4, is anti-inflammatory, analgesic and beneficial for the skin and joint as summarized in Section 1.7. Huángqín (cf. Section 2.1) extract was shown to protect against ultraviolet radiation in human keratinocytes (Seok et al., 2016). Huángliánjiědútāng contains Huángqín, while Zhēnrénhuómìngyǐn contains Báizhǐ. Jiāwèixiāoyáosǎn was originally formulated to "soothe a depressed Liver" and is nowadays known for its hepatoprotective and neuropsychological effects (Chien et al., 2014; Xie et al., 2023). The prescriptions in the table are believed to alleviate the eye, skin, hematologic, hepatic, and neuropsychologic symptoms of the patients with primary Sjögren syndrome.

DOI: 10.1201/9781032726625-3

TABLE 3.1

GMP Herbal Medicines for a 55-Year-Old Woman with Primary Sjögren Syndrome

Primary Sjögren syndrome (OrphaCode: 289390)

A disease with a prevalence of ~5 in 10,000

Not applicable

Xerostomia, Keratoconjunctivitis sicca

Abnormality of the kidney, Abnormality of the nervous system, Anxiety, Abnormality of the skin, Tubulointerstitial nephritis, Arthralgia, Abnormality of the musculature, Complement deficiency, Polyarticular arthropathy, Parotitis, Fatigue, Chronic pain, Usual interstitial pneumonia

Renal insufficiency, Glomerulonephritis, Behavioral abnormality, Depression, Dry skin, Cutis marmorata, Purpura, Vitiligo, Seizure, Meningitis, Abnormal cerebellum morphology, Muscle weakness, Arthritis, Abnormality of blood and blood-forming tissues, Thrombocytopenia, Leukopenia, Lymphopenia, Normochromic anemia, Normocytic anemia, Morphological abnormality of the central nervous system, Biliary cirrhosis, Vasculitis, Lymphoma, Lymphadenopathy, Myalgia, Sensory impairment, Functional motor deficit, Decreased antibody level in blood, Decreased proportion of CD4-positive T cells, Decreased serum complement C3, Lymphoproliferative disorder, Lymphoid interstitial pneumonia, Interstitial pulmonary abnormality, Airway obstruction, Increased antibody level in blood, Arteritis, Erythema nodosum, Bronchitis, Raynaud phenomenon, Vaginal dryness, Nonproductive cough, Lichenoid skin lesion, Abnormal pulmonary thoracic imaging finding, Decreased serum complement C4, Myositis, Thyroiditis, Optic neuritis, Cryoglobulinemia, Skin ulcer, Chronic hepatitis, Abnormality of the peripheral nervous system

Keratoconjunctivitis sicca (375.15):

Qǐjúdìhuángwán 5g + zīshènmíngmùtāng 5-0g + xǐgānmíngmùtāng 5-0g + juémíngzǐ 2-1g + shíhú 1-0g + xiàkūcǎo 1-0g + júhuā 1-0g.

Jiāwèixiāoyáosǎn 5g + xiāngshāliùjūnzǐtāng 5g + bànxiàxièxīntāng 2-0g + gāncǎoxiǎomàidàzǎotāng 2-0g + shānzhā 1g + héhuānpí 1g.

Zīshènmíngmùtāng 5g + xǐgānmíngmùtāng 2g + juémíngzǐ 1g.

Gǒuqǐzǐ 5g + júhuā 5g + niúbàngzǐ 4g + shègān 4g + xìxīn 1g + huánglián 1g.

Gǒuqǐzǐ 5g + júhuā 5g + dìhuáng 4-2g + dāngguī 4-2g + fángfēng 4-2g + xìxīn 2-1g + huánglián 2-1g.

Abnormality of the skin (702), Arthralgia (D018771), Fatigue (D005221), Chronic pain (D059350):

Huángliánjiědútāng 5g + lóngdǎnxiègāntāng 5g + jīnyínhuā 1g + liánqiáo 1-0g + dàqīngyè 1-0g + bǎnlángēn 1-0g.

Huángliánjiědútāng 5g + jīnyínhuā 2-1g + púgōngyīng 2-0g + liánqiáo 1-0g + zǐhuādìdīng 1-0g.

Xiāofēngsǎn 5g + huángliánjiědútāng 4g + dàhuáng 0g.

Zhēnrénhuómìngyǐn 5g + jīngfángbàidúsǎn 5g + tǔfúlíng 1g + jīnyínhuā 1g + liánqiáo 1g.

Dāngguīsìnìtāng 5g + fùzǐ 2g + shēngjiāng 1g + wúzhūyú 1g.

Báizhǐ 5g + gāncǎo 5-4g + huángqín 5-0g + shārén 4-3g + tiānhuā 2-0g + dàhuáng 1-0g.

Huángqín 5-4g + báizhǐ 5-4g + zhìgāncǎo 4-3g + shārén 4-3g + tiānhuā 2-0g + xìxīn 1-0g + dàhuáng 0g.

Renal insufficiency (586), Purpura (D011693), Vitiligo (709.01), Seizure (345.9), Meningitis (322.9), Muscle weakness (D018908), Abnormality of blood and blood-forming tissues (289.9), Thrombocytopenia (287.5), Leukopenia (288.50), Lymphopenia (288.51), Biliary cirrhosis (571.6), Myalgia (D063806), Sensory impairment (D006987), Decreased antibody level in blood (279.00), Increased antibody level in blood (D006942), Bronchitis (466.0, 490, 491), Thyroiditis (245), Optic neuritis (377.3), Chronic hepatitis (570, 571.4, 571.41):

Jiāwèixiāoyáosǎn 5g + guīpítāng 5g + nǚzhēnzǐ 2g + hànliáncǎo 2g + dānshēn 2-0g + ējiāo 2-0g + jīxuèténg 2-0g.

Guīpítāng 5g + jīxuèténg 1-0g.

Tiānmágōuténgyǐn 5g + guīpítāng 5g + xiānhècǎo 2g + ǒujié 2g.

Bǔzhōngyìqìtāng 5g + guīpítāng 5-3g + jiāwèixiāoyáosǎn 4-0g + hànliáncǎo 2-1g + xiānhècǎo 2-0g + nǚzhēnzǐ 1g + jīxuèténg 1g + dānshēn 1-0g.

Báizhú 5g + fùzǐ 5g + báisháo 4g + fúlíng 4g + gāncǎo 4-2g + máhuáng 4-0g + huángqí 4-0g + máhuáng 4-0g + dǎngshēn 2-0g + báijièzǐ 2-0g.

Báizhú 5g + fùzǐ 5g + dàzǎo 2g + shēngjiāng 2g + báisháo 2g + guìzhī 2g + fúlíng 2g + huángqí 2g + dǎngshēn 2g + dàhuáng 1g + gāncǎo 1g + mǔlì 1g + gānjiāng 1g.

Báizhú 5g + fùzǐ 5g + cháihú 5g + bàijiàngcǎo 5-0g + yìyǐrén 5-0g + báisháo 4-0g + fúlíng 4-0g + tiānhuā 2g + guìzhī 2g + huángqín 2g + gāncǎo 2-1g + dǎngshēn 2-0g + mǔlì 1g + gānjiāng 1g.

3.2 SARCOIDOSIS

Sarcoidosis, also known as Boeck sarcoid, is characterized by the formation of lumps or nodules, called granulomas, in the parts of the body such as the lungs, lymph nodes, skin, eyes, and muscles. Severity of sarcoidosis depends on the body part the overacting immune system attacks; nevertheless, many cases of sarcoidosis resolve on their own or recover after treatment.

Báizhú, which makes up Wǔlíngsǎn, is not only neuroprotective (cf. Sections 1.21 and 2.2) but also antitumor and antihepatotoxic (Ruqiao et al., 2020). Cháihú (cf. Section 1.45) is the major

---

TABLE 3.2

GMP Herbal Medicines for a 30-Year-Old Adult with Sarcoidosis

Sarcoidosis (OrphaCode: 797)

A disease with a prevalence of ~3 in 10,000

Major susceptibility factor: butyrophilin like 2 (*BTNL2* / Entrez: 56244) at 6p21.32

Major susceptibility factor: major histocompatibility complex, class II, DR beta 1 (*HLA-DRB1* / Entrez: 3123) at 6p21.32

Multigenic/multifactorial

Uveitis, Joint swelling, Decreased liver function, Weight loss, Thrombocytopenia, Leukopenia, Fever, Abnormal lung morphology, Dyspnea, Abnormality of the pleura, Pleural effusion, Abnormality of the musculature, Abnormality of skin morphology, Erythema nodosum, Fatigue, Cough, Chest pain, Increased T cell count, Skin nodule

Renal insufficiency, Nephrocalcinosis, Abnormality of the nasal mucosa, Glaucoma, Abnormal conjunctiva morphology, Cataract, Blindness, Dacryocystitis, Nephrolithiasis, Diabetes insipidus, Hyperpigmentation of the skin, Hypopigmentation of the skin, Keratoconjunctivitis sicca, Hepatic failure, Portal hypertension, Subcutaneous nodule, Alopecia, Anemia, Tubulointerstitial nephritis, Emphysema, Pneumothorax, Bronchiectasis, Hypercalciuria, Pulmonary fibrosis, Hepatomegaly, Lymphadenopathy, Abnormality of the lymph nodes, Upper airway obstruction, Abnormality of the cerebrospinal fluid, Increased CSF protein, Hypercalcemia, Proximal muscle weakness, Ventricular tachycardia, Enlarged lacrimal glands, Peripheral neuropathy, Chylothorax, Facial palsy, Abnormality of the gastrointestinal tract, Arrhythmia, Enlargement of parotid gland, Parotitis, Bone cyst, Abnormal reproductive system morphology, Heart block, Abnormal liver parenchyma morphology, Abnormal cardiac ventricular function, Maculopapular exanthema, Scarring, Skin plaque

Childhood, Adolescent, Adult, Elderly

Decreased liver function (573.9), Weight loss (D015431), Thrombocytopenia (287.5), Leukopenia (288.50), Fever (D005334), Dyspnea (D004417), Fatigue (D005221), Cough (D003371), Chest pain (D002637):

Wǔlíngsǎn 5g + yīnchén 2-1g.	Báizhú 5g + fùzǐ 5g + cháihú 5g + báisháo 4g + fúlíng 4g + tiānhuā 2g + dǎngshēn 2g + guìzhī 2g + huángqín 2g + wǔwèizǐ 2-0g + xìxīn 2-0g + gāncǎo 1g + mǔlì 1g + gānjiāng 1g + dàhuáng 1-0g.
Lóngdǎnxiègāntāng 5g + yīnchén 0g.	
Yīnchénhāotāng 5g + lóngdǎnxiègāntāng 5g.	
Xiǎocháihútāng 5g + lóngdǎnxiègāntāng 5g + yīnchén 1g.	Huángqí 5g + báizhú 3g + báisháo 3g + báibiǎndòu 3g + fúlíng 3g + gāncǎo 2g + dàzǎo 2g + shēngjiāng 2g.
	Yīnchén 5g + báizhú 4-3g + mǔdānpí 4-2g + zhǐqiào 4-2g + huángqín 4-2g + zéxiè 4-2g + chēqiánzǐ 3-0g + fùzǐ 2-0g.

Renal insufficiency (586), Glaucoma (365), Cataract (366.8), Blindness (D001766), Dacryocystitis (375.0, 375.30), Nephrolithiasis (592), Diabetes insipidus (253.5), Keratoconjunctivitis sicca (375.15), Portal hypertension (572.3), Alopecia (704.0), Anemia (285.9), Emphysema (492.8), Bronchiectasis (494), Hypercalciuria (D053565), Hypercalcemia (275.42), Facial palsy (351.0), Abnormality of the gastrointestinal tract (520-579.99):

Zhūlíngtāng 5g + jìshēngshènqìwán 5g + xiānhècǎo 2-0g + báimáogēn 2-0g + chēqiánzǐ 2-0g + jīnqiáncǎo 2-0g + báimáogēn 2-0g + dōngguāzǐ 2-0g + yìyǐrén 2-0g.	Dàhuáng 5g + gāncǎo 5g + dìhuáng 5g + chēqiánzǐ 5g + zéxiè 5g + huángqín 5g + jīnyínhuā 5-0g + fúlíng 5-0g + zhīzǐ 5-0g + dāngguī 5-0g + liánqiáo 5-0g + cháihú 5-0g + lóngdǎncǎo 5-0g.
Zhūlíngtāng 5g + chēqiánzǐ 2-0g + tínglìzǐ 2-0g + huángqí 1-0g + gāncǎo 1-0g.	Huǒmárén 5g + dìhuáng 5g + hòupò 5g + zhǐshí 5g + yīnchén 5g + chuānxiōng 4g + běishāshēn 4g + fùzǐ 2g + dāngguī 2g + dàhuáng 1g.
Dìngchuǎntāng 5g + wēndǎntāng 5g + dānshēn 1g + bèimǔ 1g + fúshén 1g.	Dìhuáng 5g + zhǐqiào 5g + yīnchén 5g + huángjīng 5g + chuānxiōng 4g + dǎodìwúgōng 4g + bǔgǔzhī 4g + fùzǐ 2g + huángqín 2g.
	Zhǐqiào 5g + chántuì 5g.

herb in many multi-herb formulas, including Xiǎocháihútāng and Lóngdǎnxiègāntāng, for the protection of the TCM liver; its bioactive compounds exhibit such pharmacological effects as anti-inflammatory, anticancer, antipyretic, antimicrobial, antiviral, hepatoprotective, neuroprotective, and immunomodulatory activities (Yang et al., 2017). Zéxiè, or Rhizoma Alismatis, "discharges water, removes dampness, lets off heat" and is used for edema, sleep disturbances, essential hypertension, and functional disorder of the intestine (Wang, 2020). Zhūlíngtāng encloses Zéxiè and is used for symptoms involving the urinary system (cf. Section 1.39). Some prescriptions in the table focus on the liver and kidney symptoms, while others on the lung and gastrointestinal system of sarcoidosis patients.

3.3 GIANT CELL ARTERITIS

Giant cell arteritis, also known as temporal arteritis or Horton disease, is inflammation of the blood vessels on each side of the head called the temples. The most common symptom of giant cell arteritis is a headache, especially pain over the temples. If the inflammation spreads to the arteries of the eye, vision can be impaired. The cause of giant cell arteritis is unknown but involves autoimmunity.

TABLE 3.3

GMP Herbal Medicines for a 50-Year-Old Adult with Giant Cell Arteritis

Giant cell arteritis (OrphaCode: 397)

A disease with a prevalence of ~3 in 10,000

Major susceptibility factor: protein tyrosine phosphatase non-receptor type 22 (*PTPN22* / Entrez: 26191) at 1p13.2

Major susceptibility factor: major histocompatibility complex, class II, DR beta 1 (*HLA-DRB1* / Entrez: 3123) at 6p21.32

Major susceptibility factor: major histocompatibility complex, class I, B (*HLA-B* / Entrez: 3106) at 6p21.33

Major susceptibility factor: prolyl 4-hydroxylase subunit alpha 2 (*P4HA2* / Entrez: 8974) at 5q31.1

Multigenic/multifactorial

Joint stiffness, Weight loss, Fever, Anorexia, Headache, Vasculitis, Cerebral ischemia, Impaired mastication, Fatigue

Visual impairment, Ophthalmoparesis, Depression, Arthritis, Alopecia, Elevated erythrocyte sedimentation rate

Renal insufficiency, Glossitis, Hearing impairment, Conductive hearing impairment, Epistaxis, Ptosis, Visual loss, Nystagmus, Optic atrophy, Diplopia, Hematuria, Diabetes insipidus, Hyperhidrosis, Visual field defect, Ataxia, Meningitis, Muscle weakness, Hepatic failure, Sudden cardiac death, Pericarditis, Abnormality of thrombocytes, Abdominal pain, Abnormality of the pleura, Vertigo, Aortic dissection, Arthralgia, Myalgia, Paresthesia, Arterial thrombosis, Dilatation of abdominal aorta, Gastrointestinal infarctions, Peripheral neuropathy, Double outlet right ventricle with subpulmonary ventricular septal defect without pulmonary stenosis, Arrhythmia, Cough, Amaurosis fugax, Mediastinal lymphadenopathy, Gangrene, Recurrent pharyngitis, Skin ulcer

Adult

Weight loss (D015431), Fever (D005334), Anorexia (D000855), Headache (D006261), Fatigue (D005221):

Wǔlíngsǎn 5g + hòupò 1-0g + zhǐshí 1-0g + bànxià 1-0g + fùzǐ 1-0g + báisháo 1-0g + huángqín 1-0g + dǐdāngtāng 0g + dàhuáng 0g.	Gāncǎo 5g + báisháo 5g + shíhú 5g + bǎihé 5g + chēqiánzǐ 5g + fúlíng 5g + màiméndōng 5g.
	Gāncǎo 5g + báizhú 5g + fúlíng 5g + gānjiāng 5g.
Guìzhītāng 5g + xìngrén 1-0g + hòupò 1-0g + báisháo 1-0g + dàhuáng 0g.	Gāncǎo 5g + báizhǐ 5g + shārén 3g + huángqín 3g + guālóugēn 2g + dàhuáng 1g.
	Gāncǎo 5g + hòupò 5-2g + zhǐshí 5-2g + dàhuáng 1-0g.
	Zhìgāncǎo 5g + hòupò 5g + zhǐshí 5g + dàhuáng 1g.

Visual impairment (D014786), Ophthalmoparesis (378.56), Alopecia (704.0):

Jiāwèixiāoyáosǎn 5g + chántuì 1g + júhuā 1-0g + zhǐqiào 1-0g + júhóng 0g.	Zhǐqiào 5g + jílí 5g + júhuā 5-4g + chántuì 5-4g + sīguāluò 1-0g.
Jiāwèixiāoyáosǎn 5g + jílí 2-1g + chántuì 1-0g + zhǐqiào 1-0g.	Huángqín 5g + báizhǐ 3g + shārén 2g + gāncǎo 2-1g + tiānhuā 1g + dàhuáng 0g.
	Chántuì 5g + jílí 4g + júhóng 3g.

(Continued)

TABLE 3.3 *(Continued)*

GMP Herbal Medicines for a 50-Year-Old Adult with Giant Cell Arteritis

Renal insufficiency (586), Glossitis (529.0), Hearing impairment (D003638), Conductive hearing impairment (D006314), Ptosis (374.3), Nystagmus (379.53, 379.55, 379.50), Optic atrophy (377.1), Diplopia (D004172), Diabetes insipidus (253.5), Ataxia (D002524), Meningitis (322.9), Muscle weakness (D018908), Abdominal pain (D015746), Vertigo (386.2), Arthralgia (D018771), Myalgia (D063806), Paresthesia (D010292), Cough (D003371), Amaurosis fugax (D020757):

Zhūlíngtāng 5g + dàhuáng 2g + niúxī 2g + báimáogēn 2g + chēqiánzǐ 2g + jīnqiáncǎo 2g + dǎodìwúgōng 2g + liánqiáo 2g.

Jìshēngshènqìwán 5g + zhūlíngtāng 5-2g + dàhuáng 2-0g + niúxī 2-0g + báimáogēn 2-0g + chēqiánzǐ 2-0g + jīnqiáncǎo 2-0g + bèimǔ 2-0g + hǎipiāoxiāo 2-0g + hòupò 2-0g + zhǐshí 2-0g + yìmǔcǎo 2-0g.

Língguìshùgāntāng 5g + zhūlíngtāng 5g + zhēnwǔtāng 5-0g + mázǐrénwán 5-0g + jìshēngshènqìwán 5-0g + xiānhècǎo 2-0g + báimáogēn 2-0g + chēqiánzǐ 2-0g + púhuáng 2-0g + yuǎnzhì 2-0g.

Wǔlíngsǎn 5g + jìshēngshènqìwán 5g.

Gāncǎo 5g + júhuā 5-4g + jílí 5-4g + chántuì 5-4g + huángqí 5-0g + júhóng 5-0g + zhǐqiào 4-0g + zéxiè 3-0g + bīngláng 2-0g.

Jílí 5g + júhóng 5-2g + chántuì 5-2g + bīngláng 1-0g.

Júhuā 5g + shānyào 4g + jílí 4g + chántuì 4g.

Gāncǎo is anti-inflammatory, as mentioned in Section 1.1. The compounds in Zhǐqiào (cf. Sections 1.31, 1.54, and 2.8) were reviewed to have such pharmacological effects as immunomodulation and anti-vascular damage (Gao et al., 2021). Both Júhuā and Jílí benefit the eye, as revealed earlier. A compound isolated from Fúlíng (cf. Sections 1.21, 1.66, 2.37, and 2.52) was shown to be anti-inflammatory and antitumor in monocyte/macrophage-like cells derived from mice (Liu et al., 2019). Wǔlíngsǎn, Jiāwèixiāoyáosǎn, Zhūlíngtāng, Língguìshùgāntāng, and Zhēnwǔtāng all contain Fúlíng.

3.4 FAMILIAL MEDITERRANEAN FEVER

Familial Mediterranean fever, also known as familial paroxysmal polyserositis, is characterized by recurrent episodes of fever accompanied with abdominal, pleural, or arthritic pain. Familial Mediterranean fever is caused by mutations in a gene whose products are believed to help control innate immune response. Familial Mediterranean fever is not uncommon in people originating from around the Mediterranean Sea.

Today, Shānyào (cf. Section 1.62) and Shānyào-containing formulas are extensively used for diabetes (Sun et al., 2020; Wang, 2020), with which patients can manifest proteinuria. Xiāofēngsǎn

TABLE 3.4

GMP Herbal Medicines for a 17-Year-Old Adolescent with Familial Mediterranean Fever

Familial Mediterranean fever (OrphaCode: 342)

A disease with a prevalence of ~3 in 10,000

Disease-causing germline mutation(s): MEFV innate immunity regulator, pyrin (*MEFV* / Entrez: 4210) at 16p13.3

Autosomal dominant, Autosomal recessive

Fever, Nausea and vomiting, Constipation, Abdominal pain, Arthralgia, Myalgia

Proteinuria, Erysipelas, Seizure, Arthritis, Diarrhea, Pleuritis, Oral leukoplakia, Erythema, Chest pain

Nephrotic syndrome, Nephropathy, Nephrocalcinosis, Skin rash, Meningitis, Ascites, Myocardial infarction, Pericarditis, Pancreatitis, Splenomegaly, Malabsorption, Peritonitis, Vasculitis, Lymphadenopathy, Osteoarthritis, Elevated erythrocyte sedimentation rate, Intestinal obstruction, Gastrointestinal infarctions, Acute hepatic failure, Pedal edema, Arrhythmia, Orchitis

Infancy, Childhood, Adolescent, Adult

(Continued)

TABLE 3.4 *(Continued)*

GMP Herbal Medicines for a 17-Year-Old Adolescent with Familial Mediterranean Fever

Fever (D005334), Constipation (564.0), Abdominal pain (D015746), Arthralgia (D018771), Myalgia (D063806):

Wǔlíngsǎn 5g + fùzǐ 1g + xìxīn 1g + huángqín 1g + dǐdāngtāng 0g.

Gāncǎo 5g + dàhuáng 1g.

Wǔlíngsǎn 5g + xìxīn 1g + huángqín 1g + tiáowèichéngqìtāng 1-0g + xiǎochéngqìtāng 1-0g + dǐdāngtāng 0g + dàhuáng 0g.

Gāncǎo 5g + hòupò 5-2g + zhǐshí 5-2g + dàhuáng 1-0g.

Gāncǎo 5g + báizhǐ 5g + shārén 5-3g + huángqín 5-0g + tiānhuā 3-0g + dàhuáng 1-0g.

Proteinuria (791.0), Erysipelas (035), Seizure (345.9), Diarrhea (D003967), Erythema (D005483), Chest pain (D002637):

Wǔlíngsǎn 5g + jìshēngshènqìwán 5g.

Wǔlíngsǎn 5g + yuèbìjiāshùtāng 5g + niúxī 1-0g.

Qīngxīnliánzǐyǐn 5g + zhūlíngtāng 5g + jīnyínhuā 1-0g + liánqiáo 1-0g + báimáogēn 1-0g.

Zhēnwǔtāng 5g + huángqí 2g + báizhú 1g + fùzǐ 1g.

Zhūlíngtāng 5g + jìshēngshènqìwán 3-0g + niúxī 1-0g + báimáogēn 1-0g + chēqiánzǐ 1-0g.

Shānyào 5g + tiānhuā 5g + fùzǐ 5g + fúlíng 5g + jùmài 5g.

Shānyào 5g + dìhuáng 5g + mǔdānpí 5g + fúlíng 5g + zéxiè 5g + shānzhūyú 4-0g + fùzǐ 4-0g + guìzhī 4-0g.

Fùzǐ 5g + fúlíng 5g + gāncǎo 3g + dǎngshēn 3g + gānjiāng 2g.

Dìhuáng 5g + fúlíng 5-4g + zéxiè 5-4g + qínpí 5-0g + huángbò 5-0g + shānzhūyú 4-0g + shānyào 4-0g + mǔdānpí 3-0g + fùzǐ 3-0g + guìzhī 3-0g.

Báimáogēn 5g + chēqiánzǐ 5g + niúxī 2g + jīnqiáncǎo 1g.

Nephrotic syndrome (581), Skin rash (782.1), Meningitis (322.9), Pancreatitis (577.0), Osteoarthritis (715.3), Intestinal obstruction (560.9):

Xiāofēngsǎn 5g + qīngxīnliánzǐyǐn 5-0g + tǔfúlíng 1g + báixiānpí 1-0g + jīnyínhuā 1-0g + dìfūzǐ 1-0g + liánqiáo 1-0g + chìsháo 1-0g.

Zhūlíngtāng 5g + dāngguīniāntòngtāng 5-0g + gānlùxiāodúdān 5-0g + tǔfúlíng 1g + báixiānpí 1g + dìfūzǐ 1g.

Zhūlíngtāng 5g + jìshēngshènqìwán 5-0g + tǔfúlíng 1g + yìyǐrén 1g + báimáogēn 1-0g + jīnyínhuā 1-0g + liánqiáo 1-0g + huòxiāng 1-0g + púgōngyīng 1-0g.

Jiāwèixiāoyáosǎn 5g + xiāofēngsǎn 5g + tǔfúlíng 1g + jīnyínhuā 1g + liánqiáo 1g + yìyǐrén 1g.

Báizhǐ 5g + gāncǎo 5-4g + shārén 5-4g + jīnyínhuā 5-0g + liánqiáo 5-0g + báixiānpí 5-0g + dàhuáng 1-0g.

Báizhǐ 5g + zhìgāncǎo 5-4g + shārén 5-4g + huángqín 4-0g + tiānhuā 2-0g + xìxīn 0g + dàhuáng 0g.

Chìxiǎodòu 5g + chēqiánzǐ 5g + yìmǔcǎo 5g + dāngguī 2g + dàhuáng 0g.

(cf. Section 1.23) has traditionally been used for skin rashes resulting from "fighting between external pathogens and internal damp-heat." The herbal medicines in this section address the digestive, nephrotic, and skin symptoms of the patients.

3.5 OLIGOARTICULAR JUVENILE IDIOPATHIC ARTHRITIS

Juvenile idiopathic arthritis (JIA) is the most common chronic arthritis in children. Oligoarticular JIA is the most common type of JIA, presenting with four or less swelling and painful joints when the symptoms first occur. JIA is considered an autoinflammatory disease without a known cause.

TABLE 3.5

GMP Herbal Medicines for a Four-Year-Old Child with Oligoarticular Juvenile Idiopathic Arthritis

Oligoarticular juvenile idiopathic arthritis (OrphaCode: 85410)

A disease with a prevalence of ~2 in 10,000

Major susceptibility factor: protein tyrosine phosphatase non-receptor type 22 (*PTPN22* / Entrez: 26191) at 1p13.2

Major susceptibility factor: signal transducer and activator of transcription 4 (*STAT4* / Entrez: 6775) at 2q32.2-q32.3

Major susceptibility factor: interleukin 2 receptor subunit alpha (*IL2RA* / Entrez: 3559) at 10p15.1

Major susceptibility factor: CD247 molecule (*CD247* / Entrez: 919) at 1q24.2

(Continued)

TABLE 3.5 *(Continued)*

GMP Herbal Medicines for a Four-Year-Old Child with Oligoarticular Juvenile Idiopathic Arthritis

Major susceptibility factor: protein tyrosine phosphatase non-receptor type 2 (*PTPN2* / Entrez: 5771) at 18p11.21

Major susceptibility factor: ankyrin repeat domain 55 (*ANKRD55* / Entrez: 79722) at 5q11.2

Major susceptibility factor: interleukin 2 receptor subunit beta (*IL2RB* / Entrez: 3560) at 22q12.3

Multigenic/multifactorial

Antinuclear antibody positivity, Oligoarthritis

Uveitis, Joint hypermobility, Failure to thrive, Autoimmunity, Abnormality of the ankles, Elevated erythrocyte
  sedimentation rate, Knee osteoarthritis, Increased serum interferon-gamma level, Abnormal serum interleukin level

Visual loss, Band keratopathy, Rheumatoid arthritis, Reduced visual acuity, Anterior chamber synechiae, Severe postnatal
  growth retardation

Childhood

Rheumatoid arthritis (714.0), Band keratopathy (371.43):

Guìzhīsháoyàozhīmǔtāng 5g + yìyǐréntāng 5g + dānshēn 1-0g + niúxī 1-0g.	Jīnyínhuā 5g + xuánshēn 4-2g + dìhuáng 4-0g + màiméndōng 4-0g + gāncǎo 3-0g + běishāshēn 2-0g + yùzhú 2-0g + dāngguī 1-0g.
Guìzhīsháoyàozhīmǔtāng 5g + niúxī 1g + huángbò 1g + cāngzhú 1g + yìyǐrén 1g + chìsháo 1-0g.	Jīnyínhuā 5g + liánqiáo 5-0g + gāncǎo 3-2g + báizhǐ 3-0g + shārén 3-0g + dàhuáng 1-0g.
Dāngguīniántòngtāng 5g + guìzhīsháoyàozhīmǔtāng 5-0g + niúxī 1g + huángbò 1g + cāngzhú 1g + yìyǐrén 1-0g + wēilíngxiān 1-0g.	Rěndōngténg 5g + liánqiáo 5g + dìhuáng 4g + mǔdānpí 4g + chìsháo 4g + sāngzhī 4g + zéxiè 4g + gāncǎo 2g.
	Báizhǐ 5g + zhìgāncǎo 5g + shārén 5g + dàhuáng 0g.

Jīnyínhuā (Flos Lonicerae Japonicae) is anti-inflammatory (Zheng et al., 2022). Rěndōngténg (Caulis Lonicerae Japonicae) "clears heat, neutralizes pathogens, opens collaterals" and is used today for Klippel-Feil syndrome, myalgia and myositis, and rheumatoid arthritis (Wang, 2020). Sāngzhī, introduced in Section 2.4, is also antirheumatic. Guìzhīsháoyàozhīmǔtāng was introduced in Section 1.37 for rheumatoid arthritis and gout.

3.6   TENOSYNOVIAL GIANT CELL TUMOR

Tenosynovial giant cell tumor, also called pigmented villonodular synovitis, is a benign tumor of the lining of the joint. Some of the tenosynovial giant cell tumor cells contain chromosomal translocations in specific regions on chromosomes 1 and 2. The altered DNA leads to recruitment of white blood cells to joint linings, causing inflammation. However, it is not known what drives the chromosomal translocation.

Niúxī (Achyranthis Bidentatae) "promotes circulation, stimulates menstruation, replenishes the Liver and Kidney, strengthens muscles and bones, relieves stranguria, induces diuresis, draws fire and blood

TABLE 3.6

GMP Herbal Medicines for a 30-Year-Old Adult with Tenosynovial Giant Cell Tumor

Tenosynovial giant cell tumor (OrphaCode: 66627)

A disease with a prevalence of ~2 in 10,000

Not applicable

Arthralgia

Limitation of joint mobility, Joint swelling, Joint stiffness, Osteolysis, Abnormality of the knee

Abnormality of the auditory canal, Conductive hearing impairment, Multiple lentigines, Lymphedema, Abnormality of the
  hip joint, Abnormality of the wrist, Abnormality of the ankles, Abnormality of the shoulder, Abnormality of the elbow,
  Abnormal temporal bone morphology, Groin pain, Abnormality of the tympanic membrane

Childhood, Adolescent, Adult

(Continued)

TABLE 3.6 *(Continued)*
GMP Herbal Medicines for a 30-Year-Old Adult with Tenosynovial Giant Cell Tumor

Arthralgia (D018771):

Shàngzhōngxiàtōngyòngtòngfēngwán 5g + guìzhīsháoyàozhīmǔtāng 5g + niúxī 1g + huángbò 1g + cāngzhú 1g + yìyǐrén 1g.

Shàngzhōngxiàtōngyòngtòngfēngwán 5g + dúhuójìshēngtāng 5g + dāngguīniántòngtāng 5-0g + niúxī 1-0g + huángbò 1-0g + cāngzhú 1-0g + yìyǐrén 1-0g.

Shàngzhōngxiàtōngyòngtòngfēngwán 5g + shūjīnghuóxuètāng 5g + dāngguīniántòngtāng 5-0g + acupuncture.

Niúxī 5g + chìsháo 5g + zhìgāncǎo 5g + huángqí 5g + fùzǐ 3g + máhuáng 3g.

Niúxī 5g + huángbò 5g + cāngzhú 5g + yìyǐrén 5-0g + bīngláng 4-0g + dàhuáng 0g.

Conductive hearing impairment (D006314):

Yìqìcōngmíngtāng 5g + jìshēngshènqìwán 5-0g + xuèfǔzhúyūtāng 4-0g + shíchāngpú 1g + yuǎnzhì 1g + tiānmá 1-0g + suānzǎorén 1-0g + dānshēn 1-0g.

Zīshèntōngěrtāng 5g + jìshēngshènqìwán 5g + dānshēn 1g + shíchāngpú 1g + yuǎnzhì 1g.

Cōngbái 5g + tiānhuā 2g + fùzǐ 2g + júhuā 2g + bànxià 1g + xìxīn 1g + ròuguì 1g + wúzhūyú 1g.

Cōngbái 5g + fùzǐ 3-2g + rénshēn 2-1g + gānjiāng 2-1g + ròuguì 1g + wúzhūyú 1g + xìxīn 1g + bànxià 1-0g.

downwards" and is used for musculoskeletal conditions, as we will see its predominant use in Chapter 10 on rare bone diseases. Cōngbái (cf. Section 2.34) "conducts yang Qi throughout the body" and is supposed to treat hearing impairment due to "ascending phlegm that jams the ear orifice." The same idea that proper functioning of our sense organs requires refreshing yang Qi is behind the formulation of Yìqìcōngmíngtāng. Zīshèntōngěrtāng (cf. Section 2.34) is said to treat "deafness due to Gallbladder fire induced by anger." It is used today for disorders of the ear and neurotic disorders (Wang, 2019).

3.7 BUERGER DISEASE

Buerger disease, also known as thromboangiitis obliterans, is swelling and clotting of the small and medium arteries and veins of the feet and hands. The cause of Buerger disease is unknown; however, since it is strongly associated with tobacco product use, immune response of the blood vessel walls to chemicals in tobacco is suggested.

TABLE 3.7
GMP Herbal Medicines for a 30-Year-Old Man with Buerger Disease

Buerger disease (OrphaCode: 36258)

A disease with a prevalence of ~2 in 10,000

Not applicable

Sensory neuropathy, Vasculitis, Arterial thrombosis, Gangrene, Skin ulcer

Acrocyanosis, Arthralgia, Paresthesia

Hyperhidrosis, Insomnia

Adult

Gangrene (D005734) [Gangrene (785.4)]:

Zhìgāncǎotāng 5g + shēngmàiyǐn 4g + dānshēn 1g + yùjīn 1-0g.

Jiāwèixiāoyáosàn 5g + zhìgāncǎotāng 5g + bózǐrén 1g + yuǎnzhì 1g + yùjīn 1g + shíchāngpú 1-0g + dānshēn 1-0g.

Língguìshùgāntāng 5g + bànxià 1g + shārén 1g + dàhuáng 0g.

Tiānwángbǔxīndān 5g + zhìgāncǎotāng 5g + língguìshùgāntāng 5g + zīshèntōngěrtāng 5g + yǎngxīntāng 5g.

Rénshēn 5g + zhìgāncǎo 5g + gānjiāng 5g + fùzǐ 5-3g.

Zhìgāncǎo 5g + guìzhī 5-0g + táorén 5-0g + gānjiāng 5-0g + fùzǐ 3-0g + zhǐqiào 3-0g + hónghuā 0g + dàhuáng 0g.

Fúlíng 5g + gāncǎo 4g + fùzǐ 4g + dǎngshēn 4g + gānjiāng 1g.

Huángqí 5g + chìsháo 0g + fángfēng 0g + xìxīn 0g + huánglián 0g.

(Continued)

TABLE 3.7 *(Continued)*

GMP Herbal Medicines for a 30-Year-Old Man with Buerger Disease

Arthralgia (D018771), Paresthesia (D010292):

Shàngzhōngxiàtōngyòngtòngfēngwán 5g + dāngguīniàntòngtāng 5g.	Niúxī 5g + huángbò 5g + cāngzhú 5g + yìyǐrén 5g.
Shàngzhōngxiàtōngyòngtòngfēngwán 5g + dúhuójìshēngtāng 5g + yánhúsuǒ 1g + acupuncture.	Niúxī 5g + báisháo 5g + guìzhī 5g + gǔsuìbǔ 5g + xùduàn 5g + mùguā 4g + dāngguī 4g + mòyào 2g + rǔxiāng 2g.
Shàngzhōngxiàtōngyòngtòngfēngwán 5g + juānbìtāng 5g + yánhúsuǒ 1g + acupuncture.	Niúxī 5g + chìsháo 5g + chēqiánzǐ 5g + zhìgāncǎo 5g + huángqí 5g + fùzǐ 4g + máhuáng 4g + dàhuáng 1g.
Shàngzhōngxiàtōngyòngtòngfēngwán 5g + shūjīnghuóxuètāng 5g + niúxī 1-0g + chēqiánzǐ 1-0g + acupuncture.	Fúlíng 5g + fùzǐ 3g + báisháo 2g + dǎngshēn 2g + báizhú 2g.

Rénshēn (cf. Sections 1.15 and 2.33) is adaptogenic as it has been used in traditional medicine to restore body homeostasis after a long illness or aging. The compounds in it were summarized to be vasorelaxing (angio-modulating), antioxidant, anti-inflammatory, anticancer, and antidiabetic (He et al., 2018). Língguìshùgāntāng, combined with conventional antiarrhythmic drugs, was concluded to be more effective than conventional antiarrhythmic drugs alone in the treatment of premature contraction in patients with coronary heart disease in a systematic review and meta-analysis of randomized controlled trials (Liu et al., 2022a). Shàngzhōngxiàtōngyòngtòngfēngwán "dispels Wind, eliminates dampness, activates Blood and clears heat." It was formulated for numbness and pain all over the body.

3.8 SYSTEMIC SCLEROSIS

Systemic sclerosis, or systemic scleroderma, is an autoimmune condition characterized by buildup of scar tissue in the skin and internal organs including the esophagus, heart, lungs, and kidneys. Some variants of the HLA complex, which helps the immune system differentiate self from nonself proteins, increase the risk of developing systemic sclerosis.

TABLE 3.8

GMP Herbal Medicines for a 35-Year-Old Woman with Systemic Sclerosis

Systemic sclerosis (OrphaCode: 90291)

A disease with a prevalence of ~2 in 10,000

Major susceptibility factor: major histocompatibility complex, class II, DR beta 1 (*HLA-DRB1* / Entrez: 3123) at 6p21.32

Multigenic/multifactorial, Not applicable

Thickened skin, Arthralgia, Myalgia, Antinuclear antibody positivity, Abnormality of the gastrointestinal tract, Raynaud phenomenon, Cutaneous sclerotic plaque

Abnormality of the kidney, Narrow mouth, Telangiectasia, Nail bed telangiectasia, Muscle weakness, Joint swelling, Abnormal esophagus morphology, Pulmonary fibrosis, Elevated circulating creatine kinase concentration, Spotty hypopigmentation, Acral ulceration, Abnormal phalangeal joint morphology of the hand, Interstitial pulmonary abnormality, Irregular hyperpigmentation, Sclerodactyly, Pain, Finger swelling, Calcinosis cutis, Topoisomerase I antibody positivity, Anticentromere antibody positivity, Digital pitting scar, Digital ulcer

Renal insufficiency, Proteinuria, Glomerulonephritis, Hypohidrosis, Pruritus, Syncope, Arthritis, Flexion contracture, Recurrent skin infections, Alopecia, Pericarditis, Right ventricular failure, Acute kidney injury, Dysphagia, Gastroesophageal reflux, Pulmonary arterial hypertension, Dyspnea, Abnormality of the small intestine, Abnormal large intestine morphology, Abnormality of the stomach, Gastroparesis, Intestinal bleeding, Gastrointestinal telangiectasia, Bowel incontinence, Dilatation, Osteomyelitis, Osteolytic defects of the phalanges of the hand, Abnormality of facial soft tissue, Constrictive median neuropathy, Albuminuria, Chronic kidney disease, Myocarditis, Interstitial cardiac fibrosis, Barrett esophagus

Adult

(Continued)

TABLE 3.8 *(Continued)*

GMP Herbal Medicines for a 35-Year-Old Woman with Systemic Sclerosis

Arthralgia (D018771), Myalgia (D063806), Abnormality of the gastrointestinal tract (520-579.99):

Wǔlíngsǎn 5g + gānlùyǐn 5g + píngwèisǎn 5-0g.

Wǔlíngsǎn 5g + gānlùyǐn 5g + qīngwèisǎn 5-0g.

Wǔlíngsǎn 5g + báizhǐ 2-0g + shārén 2-0g + báisháo 1-0g + fùzǐ 1-0g + gānjiāng 1-0g + dàhuáng 0g.

Niúxī 5g + huángbò 5g + cāngzhú 5g + yìyǐrén 5-0g.

Báizhǐ 5g + gāncǎo 4g + shārén 4g + huángqín 4g + xìxīn 1g + dàhuáng 0g.

Fúlíng 5g + fùzǐ 4-3g + dǎngshēn 4-0g + báisháo 3-0g + bànxià 3-0g + xìxīn 2-0g + báizhú 2-0g + dàhuáng 1-0g.

Muscle weakness (D018908), Pulmonary fibrosis (D011658) [Idiopathic pulmonary fibrosis (516.31)], Pain (D010146):

Zhēnwǔtāng 5g + wǔwèizǐ 1-0g + bànxià 1-0g + gānjiāng 1-0g + xìxīn 1-0g + fùzǐ 1-0g.

Dāngguīsìnìtāng 5g + báizhú 2g + fùzǐ 2g + báisháo 2g + fúlíng 2g + dǎngshēn 1g + shēngjiāng 1g + wúzhūyú 1g.

Língguìshùgāntāng 5g + bànxià 1g + fùzǐ 1g + shārén 1g + dàhuáng 0g.

Báizhú 5g + fùzǐ 5g + cháihú 5g + báisháo 4g + fúlíng 4g + tiānhuā 2g + dǎngshēn 2g + guìzhī 2g + huángqín 2g + shēngjiāng 2-0g + wǔwèizǐ 2-0g + xìxīn 2-0g + gāncǎo 1g + mǔlì 1g + gānjiāng 1g + máhuáng 1-0g.

Báizhú 5g + fúlíng 5g + zhìgāncǎo 3g + zhǐshí 3g + niúxī 2g + fùzǐ 2g + guìzhī 2g + dàhuáng 0g.

Renal insufficiency (586), Proteinuria (791.0), Hypohidrosis (705.0), Pruritus (D011537), Syncope (D013575), Alopecia (704.0), Right ventricular failure (428, 428.0), Gastroesophageal reflux (530.81), Dyspnea (D004417), Gastroparesis (536.3), Dilatation (442.9), Albuminuria (D000419), Myocarditis (429.0), Barrett esophagus (530.85):

Shēngmàiyǐn 5g + zhūlíngtāng 5g + jìshēngshènqìwán 5g + xiānhècǎo 2g + báimáogēn 2g + hànliáncǎo 2-0g + ējiāo 2-0g + jīxuèténg 2-0g + chēqiánzǐ 2-0g + jīnqiáncǎo 2-0g.

Shēngmàiyǐn 5g + xiāngshāliùjūnzǐtāng 5g + bìxièfēnqīngyǐn 4g + bèimǔ 1g + hǎipiāoxiāo 1g.

Zhūlíngtāng 5g + shēngmàiyǐn 5-4g + báimáogēn 1g + chēqiánzǐ 1-0g + jīnqiáncǎo 1-0g + hǎipiāoxiāo 1-0g.

Yùzhú 5g + chēqiánzǐ 5g + suǒyáng 5-0g + fúxiǎomài 5-0g + fúlíng 5-0g + huángqí 5-0g.

Shānzhīzǐ 5g + zhīmǔ 3g + gōuténg 3g + dàhuáng 0g + huánglián 0g.

Gāncǎo 5g + zhīmǔ 5-3g + huángqín 5-3g + huángbò 5-0g + yìyǐrén 5-0g + dàhuáng 1-0g + huánglián 0g.

Wǔlíngsǎn is a popular formula for exacerbated pain due to swelling (Sunagawa et al., 2021). Báizhú (cf. Section 1.21) "replenishes Qi, benefits the Spleen" and was shown to prevent skeletal muscle atrophy in obese mice (Song et al., 2018). Zhēnwǔtāng (cf. Sections 2.49 and 3.3) "warms Kidney yang and helps draining." The TCM kidney is in charge of growth and development after birth. Both Zhēnwǔtāng and Língguìshùgāntāng contains Báizhú. Yùzhú was introduced in Section 1.5 to nourish yin. Chēqiánzǐ (Semen Plantaginis) "promotes urination, relieves stranguria" and is used today for oliguria and anuria (Wang, 2020). Shēngmàiyǐn is used for heart diseases, as we will see in Chapter 14 on rare cardiac diseases.

3.9 MARFAN SYNDROME

Marfan syndrome (MFS) is a genetic condition affecting the connective tissue which provides support for the heart, blood vessels, nerves, bones, joints, and eyes. Mutations in the genes that instruct production of large proteins for the elastic fibers of the connective tissue cause Marfan syndrome.

Jīnyínhuā (cf. Section 3.5) regulates immunity, inhibits inflammation, pyrexia, viruses, and bacteria (Zhao et al., 2021) and is used for contact dermatitis (Wang, 2020). Zhènggǔzǐjīndān contains Érchá (Acacia catechu (L.) Willd.), which is known in the Ayurveda for the treatment of skin diseases (Adhikari et al., 2021), has been used in TCM for aphthous sores, skin ulcers, eczema, chancre and so on. Dāngguī (cf. Section 2.43) was shown to prevent bone loss in ovariectomized rats via estrogen-independent mechanisms (Lim & Kim, 2014). Lìzhīhé (cf. Section 1.8) "moves Qi, dissolves congelation, disperses coldness, stops pain" and is used today for prolapse (Wang, 2020).

TABLE 3.9

GMP Herbal Medicines for a 19-Year-Old Adult with Marfan Syndrome

Marfan syndrome (OrphaCode: 558)

A disease with a prevalence of ~1 in 10,000

Disease-causing germline mutation(s): fibrillin 1 (*FBN1* / Entrez: 2200) at 15q21.1

Disease-causing germline mutation(s): transforming growth factor beta receptor 2 (*TGFBR2* / Entrez: 7048) at 3p24.1

Autosomal dominant

Pectus carinatum, Striae distensae, Arachnodactyly, Disproportionate tall stature, Slender build, Pes planus, Spontaneous pneumothorax, Dilatation of the ascending aorta, Chronic fatigue

Narrow face, Visual impairment, Myopia, Dental crowding, Pectus excavatum, Ectopia lentis, Lens subluxation, Joint hypermobility, Mitral valve prolapse, Sleep disturbance, Scoliosis, High, narrow palate, Protrusio acetabuli, Arthralgia/arthritis, Increased axial length of the globe, Lens luxation, Malar anomaly, Dural ectasia

Inguinal hernia, Cleft palate, Dolichocephaly, Retrognathia, Micrognathia, Downslanted palpebral fissures, Glaucoma, Retinal detachment, Osteopenia, Osteoporosis, Hypotonia, Congestive heart failure, Emphysema, Hemoptysis, Meningocele, Aneurysm of an abdominal artery, Kyphosis, Limited elbow movement, Skeletal muscle atrophy, Spondylolisthesis, Myalgia, Cachexia, Mitral valve calcification, Pulmonary artery dilatation, Ascending aortic dissection, Arterial dissection, Aortic tortuosity, Attention deficit hyperactivity disorder, Hypoplasia of the iris, Flat cornea, Open bite, Descending aortic dissection

All ages

Striae distensae (D057896):

Zhènggǔzǐjīndān 5g + shūjīnghuóxuètāng 5-0g + acupuncture.

Zhènggǔzǐjīndān 5g + sháoyàogāncǎotāng 5-0g + acupuncture.

Fùyuánhuóxuètāng 5g + dānshēn 1-0g + yánhúsuǒ 1-0g + yùjīn 1-0g + mùxiāng 0g + gāncǎo 0g + hòupò 0g + cāngzhú 0g + acupuncture.

Zhènggǔzǐjīndān 5g + sháoyàogāncǎotāng 5g + dāngguīniántòngtāng 5g + sānqī 2g + dānshēn 2g + mùguā 2g + niúxī 2g + gégēn 2g + sūmù 2g + xùduàn 2g + acupuncture.

Jīnyínhuā 5g + dāngguī 5g + niúxī 3-2g + xuánshēn 3-2g + gāncǎo 3-2g + chìsháo 3-2g + dǎodìwúgōng 3-2g + huángqí 3-2g.

Jīnyínhuā 5g + dāngguī 5g + niúxī 2g + xuánshēn 2g + chìsháo 2g + zhìgāncǎo 2g + dǎodìwúgōng 2g + huángqí 2g.

Visual impairment (D014786), Myopia (367.1), Lens subluxation (379.32):

Qǐjúdìhuángwán 5g + yìqìcōngmíngtāng 5g.

Qǐjúdìhuángwán 5g + zīshènmíngmùtāng 5g + mùzéicǎo 2-0g + gǔjīngcǎo 2-0g + mìménghuā 2-0g + juémíngzǐ 1-0g.

Jiāwèixiāoyáosàn 5g + zīshènmíngmùtāng 5g + juémíngzǐ 1g + gǒuqǐzǐ 1g + júhuā 1g + gǔjīngcǎo 1g.

Hángjú 5g + gǒuqǐzǐ 5g + shíchāngpú 4-2g + yuǎnzhì 4-2g + nǚzhēnzǐ 2-0g + gāncǎo 2-0g.

Chántuì 5g + jílí 4g.

Inguinal hernia (550), Cleft palate (749.0), Glaucoma (365), Retinal detachment (361.9), Osteoporosis (733.0), Hypotonia (D009123), Congestive heart failure (428, 428.0), Emphysema (492.8), Hemoptysis (D006469), Skeletal muscle atrophy (D009133), Myalgia (D063806), Cachexia (D002100):

Wǔlíngsǎn 5g + xiǎohuíxiāng 1g + chuānliànzǐ 1g + mùxiāng 1g + wúzhūyú 1g + wūyào 1g + lìzhīhé 1-0g.

Júhéwán 5g + chuānliànzǐ 1g + gāncǎo 1g + báisháo 1g + yánhúsuǒ 1g.

Lìzhīhé 5g + shǎofùzhúyūtāng 5g + chuānliànzǐ 1g + wūyào 1g + júhé 1-0g + yánhúsuǒ 1-0g + xiāngfù 1-0g.

Dāngguī 5g + báijièzǐ 2g + mòyào 2g + rǔxiāng 2g + chìsháo 2-0g + dàhuáng 1-0g.

Cháihú 5g + chuānliànzǐ 3g + báisháo 3g + zhǐshí 3g + bànxià 2g + shēngjiāng 2g.

Jílí 5g + chántuì 5g.

Huángqí 5g + dāngguī 3g + báijièzǐ 2g + dìlóng 2g + mòyào 2g + rǔxiāng 2g.

3.10   HYPERMOBILE EHLERS-DANLOS SYNDROME

Hypermobile Ehlers-Danlos syndrome (hEDS), also known as Ehlers-Danlos syndrome type 3, is a connective tissue disease characterized by loose and unstable joints, leading to frequent joint dislocations. Although EDS is known to involve faulty or inadequate collagen production in the body, the causal genes for hEDS have not been identified.

TABLE 3.10
GMP Herbal Medicines for a 15-Year-Old Adolescent with Hypermobile Ehlers-Danlos Syndrome

Hypermobile Ehlers-Danlos syndrome (OrphaCode: 285)

A disease with a prevalence of ~1 in 10,000

Autosomal dominant, Autosomal recessive

Hyperextensible skin, Acrocyanosis, Joint dislocation, Abnormality of the foot, Vertigo, Sleep disturbance, Wormian bones, Hip dislocation, Arthralgia, Elbow dislocation, Myalgia, Joint hyperflexibility, Fatigue

Depression, Decreased nerve conduction velocity, Thin skin, Soft skin, Pes planus, Nausea and vomiting, Constipation, Malabsorption, Migraine, Osteoarthritis, Arrhythmia

Inguinal hernia, Abnormality of the menstrual cycle, Decreased fertility, Abnormality of the dentition, Abnormality of the gingiva, Abnormal palate morphology, Gingival overgrowth, Gingivitis, Epicanthus, Ptosis, Keratoconus, Microdontia, Atypical scarring of skin, Keratoconjunctivitis sicca, Limitation of joint mobility, Subcutaneous nodule, Umbilical hernia, Gastroesophageal reflux, Apnea, Gastrointestinal dysmotility, Scoliosis, Osteolysis, Abnormality of the wrist, Paresthesia, Dilatation of the ascending aorta, Venous insufficiency, Arterial dissection, Aplasia/Hypoplasia of the abdominal wall musculature, Anorectal anomaly, Tendon rupture, Cystocele, Genital hernia

All ages

Vertigo (386.2), Arthralgia (D018771), Myalgia (D063806), Fatigue (D005221):

Língguìshùgāntāng 5g + fùzǐ 1g + gānjiāng 1g + xìxīn 1-0g + tiáowèichéngqìtāng 0g.

Língguìshùgāntāng 5g + zhēnwǔtāng 5g.

Língguìshùgāntāng 5g + bànxiàbáizhútiānmátāng 4-3g + tiānmá 1-0g + gōuténg 1-0g.

Rénshēn 5g + bànxià 5g + gānjiāng 5g + dàhuáng 0g.

Gāncǎo 5g + fùzǐ 5g + fúlíng 5g + gānjiāng 5g + dǎngshēn 5g.

Gāncǎo 5g + báisháo 5g + shúdìhuáng 5g + biējiǎ 5g + màiméndōng 4g + ējiāo 3g + huǒmárén 2g.

Gāncǎo 5g + báizhǐ 5g + shārén 5g + huángqín 5g + xìxīn 2-1g + tiānhuā 2-0g + dàhuáng 1-0g.

Constipation (564.0), Migraine (346), Osteoarthritis (715.3):

Jiāwèixiāoyáosǎn 5g + zhībódìhuángwán 5g + shēnlíngbáizhúsǎn 5g + báizhú 1g + pípáyè 1g + fúlíng 1g.

Jiāwèixiāoyáosǎn 5g + zhībódìhuángwán 5g + mázǐrénwán 5g + nǔzhēnzǐ 2-0g + dānshēn 2-0g + hànliáncǎo 2-0g + tùsīzǐ 2-0g + chuānxiōng 2-0g + gāncǎo 1-0g.

Bǔzhōngyìqìtāng 5g + rùnchángwán 5g + gāncǎo 1g.

Gānlùyǐn 5g + rùnchángwán 3g + xuánshēn 1g + dìhuáng 1g + màiméndōng 1g.

Mǔlì 5g + jílí 5g + dàfùpí 4g + gāncǎo 4g + sāngbáipí 4g + sāngzhī 4g + hǎipiāoxiāo 4g + gǔsuìbǔ 4g + bīngláng 4g + dàhuáng 2g.

Dàfùpí 5g + jílí 5g + yánhúsuǒ 3g + sānléng 2g + wǔlíngzhī 2g + qiánhú 2g + éshù 2g + dàhuáng 1g + xīnyí 1g + cāngěrzǐ 1g.

Inguinal hernia (550), Gingivitis (523.0, 523.1), Ptosis (374.3), Keratoconus (371.6), Keratoconjunctivitis sicca (375.15), Gastroesophageal reflux (530.81), Apnea (D001049), Paresthesia (D010292), Venous insufficiency (459.81):

Bǔzhōngyìqìtāng 5g + xiǎohuíxiāng 1g + chuānliànzǐ 1g + wūyào 1g + lìzhīhé 1-0g + dānshēn 1-0g.

Dāngguīsìnìtāng 5g + xiǎohuíxiāng 1g + chuānliànzǐ 1g + wúzhūyú 1g + yánhúsuǒ 1g + wūyào 1g.

Wúzhūyú 5g + xiǎohuíxiāng 5-2g + chuānliànzǐ 5-2g + mùxiāng 5-2g + wūyào 5-2g + lìzhīhé 5-2g + júhé 5-2g + yánhúsuǒ 2-0g + qīngpí 2-0g.

Shēngmá 5g + dāngguī 3g + mǔdānpí 2g + guìzhī 2g + táorén 2g + dàhuáng 0g.

Lìzhīhé 5g + chuānliànzǐ 3g + mùxiāng 3g + zhǐqiào 3g + júhé 3g + kǔshēngēn 1g + lóngdǎncǎo 0g.

Báisháo (cf. Section 2.15) "nourishes Blood, modulates menstruation, soothes the Liver, stops pain, conserves yin, arrests sweating" and is used for hypertension, abdominal pain, Ménière's disease, dysmenorrhea, and so on (Wang, 2020). Dàfùpí (cf. Section 2.45) "lowers Qi, widens interior, moves fluid, reduces swelling" and is used for flatulence, eructation, gas pain, and constipation (Wang, 2020). Zhībódìhuángwán (cf. Section 1.4) "nourishes yin, quells fires" and has been used for "yin-deficiency-heat" TCM syndrome manifesting oral ulcers, dry mouth, and constipation.

(Yi et al., 2020). Wúzhūyú (Fructus Evodiae) "disperses coldness, stops pain, warms interior, stops vomiting, helps yang, stops diarrhea" and has traditionally been used for "cold hernia" TCM syndrome manifesting periumbilical colic, cold sweats, abnormal limbs, heavy and tight pulse, and chills over the body.

3.11 GRANULOMATOSIS WITH POLYANGIITIS

Granulomatosis with polyangiitis (GPA) is characterized by inflammation of the blood vessel walls of the small and medium blood vessels of the upper respiratory tract, lungs, and kidneys. The exact cause of GPA is unknown, although infections and autoimmunity are implicated.

Jīngjièliánqiáotāng "dispels Wind, clears heat, reduces swelling, stops pain" and has been used for swelling and pain around the ear caused by "wind-heat." Báimáogēn (cf. Section 1.66) "cools

---

TABLE 3.11

GMP Herbal Medicines for a 45-Year-Old Adult with Granulomatosis with Polyangiitis

Granulomatosis with polyangiitis (OrphaCode: 900)

A disease with a prevalence of ~9 in 100,000

Major susceptibility factor: major histocompatibility complex, class II, DP alpha 1 (*HLA-DPA1* / Entrez: 3113) at 6p21.32

Major susceptibility factor: major histocompatibility complex, class II, DP beta 1 (*HLA-DPB1* / Entrez: 3115) at 6p21.32

Major susceptibility factor: cytotoxic T-lymphocyte associated protein 4 (*CTLA4* / Entrez: 1493) at 2q33.2

Major susceptibility factor: protein tyrosine phosphatase non-receptor type 22 (*PTPN22* / Entrez: 26191) at 1p13.2

Major susceptibility factor: proteinase 3 (*PRTN3* / Entrez: 5657) at 19p13.3

Not applicable

Abnormal oral cavity morphology, Sinusitis, Abnormality of the nose, Otitis media, Epistaxis, Hematuria, Weight loss, Fever, Pulmonary infiltrates, Recurrent respiratory infections, Vasculitis, Cerebral ischemia, Arthralgia, Granulomatosis, Autoimmunity, Fatigue, Glomerulopathy

Proteinuria, Abnormality of the hypothalamus-pituitary axis, Skin rash, Nausea and vomiting, Abdominal pain, Respiratory insufficiency, Hemoptysis, Pulmonary fibrosis, Elevated erythrocyte sedimentation rate, Chronic obstructive pulmonary disease, Recurrent intrapulmonary hemorrhage, Peripheral neuropathy, Elevated C-reactive protein level, Increased inflammatory response, Cough, Inflammatory abnormality of the eye, Periorbital edema, Chest pain, Papule

Prostatitis, Ureteral stenosis, Renal insufficiency, Hydronephrosis, Chronic otitis media, Sensorineural hearing impairment, Retinopathy, Visual impairment, Proptosis, Sensory neuropathy, Hypertension, Diabetes insipidus, Purpura, Seizure, Meningitis, Angina pectoris, Pericarditis, Pancreatitis, Restrictive ventilatory defect, Pleuritis, Gastrointestinal hemorrhage, Hemiplegia, Headache, Myalgia, Venous thrombosis, Intestinal obstruction, Cranial nerve paralysis, Arrhythmia, Gangrene, Skin ulcer

Childhood, Adolescent, Adult, Elderly

Otitis media (382.9), Epistaxis (D004844) [Epistaxis (784.7)], Hematuria (D006417) [Hematuria, unspecified (599.70)], Weight loss (D015431), Fever (D005334), Arthralgia (D018771), Fatigue (D005221):

Xīnyíqīngfèitāng 5g + lóngdǎnxiègāntāng 5g + xiānhècǎo 1g + báimáogēn 1g + dìhuáng 1g.	Chántuì 5g + jílí 5-3g + zhǐqiào 5-0g.
	Júhuā 5g + jílí 5g + chántuì 4g.
Jīngjièliánqiáotāng 5g + xīnyíqīngfèitāng 5-0g + xiānhècǎo 2-0g + báimáogēn 2-0g.	Báizhǐ 5g + zhìgāncǎo 3g + shārén 3g + huángqín 3g + liánqiáo 2g + zhīzǐ 1g + dàhuáng 0g.
Jīngjièliánqiáotāng 5g + lóngdǎnxiègāntāng 4-0g + xiānhècǎo 1-0g.	

Proteinuria (791.0), Skin rash (782.1), Abdominal pain (D015746), Hemoptysis (D006469), Cough (D003371), Chest pain (D002637):

Qīngxīnliánzǐyǐn 5g + zhūlíngtāng 5g.	Báimáogēn 5g + chēqiánzǐ 4-2g + báizhú 2g + fúlíng 2g + dàzǎo 2-1g + shēngjiāng 2-1g + shígāo 2-1g + zhìgāncǎo 2-1g + máhuáng 2-1g + chìxiǎodòu 2-0g + dàhuáng 1-0g + dāngguī 0g.
Qīngxīnliánzǐyǐn 5g + bìxièfēnqīngyǐn 5g + báimáogēn 1g.	
Wǔlíngsǎn 5g + yuèbìjiāshùtāng 5g + niúxī 1g + chìsháo 1g + chēqiánzǐ 1g.	Chìxiǎodòu 5g + báimáogēn 5-2g + chēqiánzǐ 5-2g + yìmǔcǎo 5-0g + dāngguī 2-1g + huáshí 2-0g + púhuáng 2-0g.

(Continued)

TABLE 3.11 *(Continued)*
GMP Herbal Medicines for a 45-Year-Old Adult with Granulomatosis with Polyangiitis

Prostatitis (601.9), Renal insufficiency (586), Hydronephrosis (591), Sensorineural hearing impairment (389.1), Retinopathy (362.9), Proptosis (376.30), Hypertension (401-405.99), Diabetes insipidus (253.5), Purpura (D011693), Seizure (345.9), Meningitis (322.9), Angina pectoris (D000787), Pancreatitis (577.0), Hemiplegia (343.4), Headache (D006261), Myalgia (D063806), Intestinal obstruction (560.9), Cranial nerve paralysis (352.9):

Zhúyèshígāotāng 5g.	Shíchāngpú 5g + yuǎnzhì 5g + dǎngshēn 5g.
Xìngsūyǐnyòukē 5g.	Huángbò 5g + shúdìhuáng 5g + dìhuáng 2g + zhīmǔ 2g + ējiāo 2g + dāngguī 2g + dǎngshēn 2g + shēngmá 1g + cháihú 1g.
Xìngsūyǐn 5g + xīnyíqīngfèitāng 5-0g.	
Xìngsūyǐn 5g + zhúyèshígāotāng 4-0g.	Huángbò 5g + shārén 4g + dìhuáng 2g + fángfēng 2g + zhìgāncǎo 2g + gǒuqǐzǐ 2g + júhuā 2g + dāngguī 2g + jílí 2g + xìxīn 1g + huánglián 1g + dàhuáng 0g.

Blood, stops bleeding, clears heat, induces urination" and is used for diabetes, hematuria, and epistaxis (Wang, 2020). Qīngxīnliánzǐyǐn has traditionally been used for the syndrome resulting from "damp-heat diffusing downward" and is used today for nephritis and nephropathy (Wang, 2019). Zhúyèshígāotāng (cf. Section 1.52) was shown to have hypoglycemic, hypolipidemic, and antioxidant effects in type 2 diabetic rats (Pei & Zheng, 2017).

3.12 RHEUMATOID FACTOR-NEGATIVE POLYARTICULAR JUVENILE IDIOPATHIC ARTHRITIS

Rheumatoid factor-negative polyarticular juvenile idiopathic arthritis, or juvenile polyarthritis without rheumatoid factor, is chronic pain and swelling of five or more joints at disease onset without rheumatoid factor IgM in the blood. Genetic predispositions and environmental factors are believed to trigger an autoimmune attack on the joints in patients with rheumatoid factor-negative polyarticular JIA.

Oral administration of Shūjīnghuóxuètāng was shown to suppress neuropathic pain in rats with chronic constriction injury of the sciatic nerve (Shu et al., 2010). Màiyá (Fructus Hordei Germinatus)

TABLE 3.12
GMP Herbal Medicines for a Three-Year-Old Child with Rheumatoid Factor-Negative Polyarticular Juvenile Idiopathic Arthritis

Rheumatoid factor-negative polyarticular juvenile idiopathic arthritis (OrphaCode: 85408)

A disease with a prevalence of ~8 in 100,000

Major susceptibility factor: protein tyrosine phosphatase non-receptor type 22 (*PTPN22* / Entrez: 26191) at 1p13.2

Major susceptibility factor: signal transducer and activator of transcription 4 (*STAT4* / Entrez: 6775) at 2q32.2-q32.3

Major susceptibility factor: interleukin 2 receptor subunit alpha (*IL2RA* / Entrez: 3559) at 10p15.1

Major susceptibility factor: CD247 molecule (*CD247* / Entrez: 919) at 1q24.2

Major susceptibility factor: protein tyrosine phosphatase non-receptor type 2 (*PTPN2* / Entrez: 5771) at 18p11.21

Major susceptibility factor: ankyrin repeat domain 55 (*ANKRD55* / Entrez: 79722) at 5q11.2

Major susceptibility factor: interleukin 2 receptor subunit beta (*IL2RB* / Entrez: 3560) at 22q12.3

Multigenic/multifactorial

Arthritis, Joint swelling, Joint stiffness, Ankle swelling, Arthralgia, Abnormality of the wrist, Elevated erythrocyte sedimentation rate, Knee osteoarthritis, Synovial hypertrophy, Enthesitis, Synovitis

Uveitis, Abnormality of the hand, Flexion contracture, Abnormality of the hip joint, Mild postnatal growth retardation, Weight loss, Abnormal metatarsal morphology, Anemia, Lymphadenopathy, Abnormality of the shoulder, Abnormality of the cervical spine, Myalgia, Antinuclear antibody positivity, Hip osteoarthritis, Abnormality of the temporomandibular joint, Low-grade fever, Abnormality of metacarpophalangeal joint, Oligoarthritis

Childhood

(Continued)

TABLE 3.12 *(Continued)*
GMP Herbal Medicines for a Three-Year-Old Child with Rheumatoid Factor-Negative Polyarticular Juvenile Idiopathic Arthritis

Arthralgia (D018771), Synovial hypertrophy (727.83):

Shūjīnghuóxuètāng 5g.	Jīnyínhuā 5g + dāngguī 5-2g + xuánshēn
Guìzhīsháoyàozhīmǔtāng 5g.	3-2g + gāncǎo 3-1g + chìsháo 2g +
Zhènggǔzǐjīndān 5g + sháoyàogāncǎotāng 5-0g.	dǎodìwúgōng 2-1g + huángqí 2-1g + niúxī
	2-0g + acupuncture.
	Gāncǎo 5g + báizhǐ 5g + shārén 5-3g +
	dàhuáng 0g + acupuncture.

Weight loss (D015431), Anemia (285.9), Myalgia (D063806):

Sìjūnzǐtāng 5g + bǎohéwán 5-0g.	Màiyá 5g + shénqū 5-0g.
Liùjūnzǐtāng 5g + shānzhā 0g + shénqū 0g + màiyá 0g.	Zhìgāncǎo 5g + báizhǐ 4g + shārén 4g +
Xiǎojiànzhōngtāng 5g + shānzhā 1g + shénqū 1g + màiyá 1g.	dàhuáng 0g.
Xiāngshāliùjūnzǐtāng 5g + shānzhā 1g + shénqū 1g + màiyá 1g + jīnèijīn 1g.	Gāncǎo 5g + hòupò 5-0g + zhǐshí 5-0g +
	dàhuáng 0g.

was shown to be antihyperglycemic and antioxidant in diabetic rats (Wei et al., 2015). Hypoglycemia makes one feel hungry, leading to weight gain. Shénqū (cf. Section 1.40) "aids digestion, harmonizes the Stomach" and is used to relieve peptic ulcer, dyspepsia, and functional disorder of intestine (Wang, 2020). Sìjūnzǐtāng was introduced in Sections 1.17 and 1.56 to improve digestion.

3.13 POLYMYOSITIS

Polymyositis is chronic inflammation of many muscles. The cause of polymyositis is unknown but cytotoxic T cells of the immune system against the loose connective tissue around the muscle fibers are suggested to play a role.

TABLE 3.13
GMP Herbal Medicines for a 45-Year-Old Woman with Polymyositis

Polymyositis (OrphaCode: 732)

A disease with a prevalence of ~7 in 100,000

Not applicable

Hypotonia, Arthralgia, Autoimmunity, Elevated circulating creatine kinase concentration, EMG abnormality, Proximal muscle weakness, Abnormal muscle fiber morphology, Elevated aldolase level, Cough

Arthritis, Weight loss, Fever, Constipation, Anorexia, Respiratory insufficiency, Exertional dyspnea, Myalgia, Interstitial pulmonary abnormality, Fatigue

Abnormal renal tubule morphology, Chondrocalcinosis, Gait disturbance, Reduced tendon reflexes, Abnormality of the voice, Dysphonia, Abnormal mitral valve morphology, Congestive heart failure, Hypertrophic cardiomyopathy, Dilated cardiomyopathy, Myocardial infarction, Pericarditis, Gastroesophageal reflux, Abdominal pain, Pulmonary fibrosis, Gastrointestinal hemorrhage, Hepatomegaly, Vasculitis, Breast carcinoma, Venous thrombosis, Abnormal atrioventricular conduction, Arrhythmia

Adult, Elderly

Hypotonia (D009123), Arthralgia (D018771), Cough (D003371):

Huángqíwǔwùtāng 5g + dāngguīsìnìtāng 5-0g + chuānxiōng	Huángqí 5g + chìsháo 1-0g + fángfēng 1-0g + xìxīn 0g +
1-0g + dāngguī 1-0g + jīxuèténg 1-0g + dānshēn 1-0g +	huánglián 0g + dàhuáng 0g.
zhúrú 1-0g + sāngzhī 1-0g + jiānghuáng 1-0g + acupuncture.	
Dāngguīsìnìtāng 5g + shēngjiāng 1g + wúzhūyú 1g + fùzǐ 1g.	
Guìzhītāng 5g + báisháo 1g + dàhuáng 0g.	

(Continued)

TABLE 3.13 *(Continued)*

GMP Herbal Medicines for a 45-Year-Old Woman with Polymyositis

Weight loss (D015431), Fever (D005334), Constipation (564.0), Anorexia (D000855), Myalgia (D063806), Fatigue (D005221):

Wǔlíngsǎn 5g + fùzǐ 1g + huángqín 1g + tiáowèichéngqìtāng 1-0g + xiǎochéngqìtāng 1-0g + dàhuáng 0g.

Wǔlíngsǎn 5g + huángqín 1g + fùzǐ 1-0g + xìxīn 1-0g + dǐdāngtāng 0g + dàhuáng 0g.

Guìzhītāng 5g + xìngrén 1g + hòupò 1g + dàhuáng 0g.

Gāncǎo 5g + hòupò 5-2g + zhǐshí 5-2g + dàhuáng 2-0g.

Zhìgāncǎo 5g + hòupò 5-3g + zhǐshí 5-3g + dàhuáng 0g.

Dysphonia (D055154), Congestive heart failure (428, 428.0), Hypertrophic cardiomyopathy (425.1), Gastroesophageal reflux (530.81), Abdominal pain (D015746):

Shēngmàiyǐn 5g + xiāngshāliùjūnzǐtāng 5-2g + bǔzhōngyìqìtāng 3-0g + báijí 2g + hǎipiāoxiāo 2g + huángqí 2-0g + bèimǔ 2-0g.

Xiāngshāliùjūnzǐtāng 5g + sìnìtāng 4g + dānshēn 1g + yùjīn 1g + huánglián 0g.

Bànxiàxièxīntāng 5g + sìnìtāng 5g + gānlùyǐn 5g + hǎipiāoxiāo 2g + bèimǔ 1g.

Fúlíng 5g + mǔlì 4g + dàfùpí 3g + wǔlíngzhī 3g + gāncǎo 3g + sāngbáipí 3g + hǎipiāoxiāo 3g + jīlí 3g + sānléng 2g + éshù 2g + zǐsūyè 2-0g + mùtōng 1g + bǎibù 1g.

Bànxià 5g + fúlíng 5g + fùzǐ 5-4g + xìxīn 2g + dàhuáng 2-1g.

Zhìgāncǎo 5g + jiégěng 5g + xuánshēn 3g + mǔlì 3g + bèimǔ 3g + liánqiáo 3g + shānzhīzǐ 2g + jīnyínhuā 1g.

Hòupò (Cortex Magnoliae Officinalis) "moves Qi, dries dampness, reduces stagnation, stops asthma" and is used for cough, chest pain, dyspepsia, and so on (Wang, 2020). In particular, a Hòupò and Zhǐshí (Fructus Aurantii Immaturus) combination is commonly used for constipation (Wang, 2020). Fúlíng (cf. Sections 2.37 and 3.3) was shown to improve the cardiac function of rats with chronic heart failure through its diuretic effect (Wu et al., 2014). Shēngmàiyǐn is a TCM formula commonly used for heart diseases (cf. Chapter 14).

3.14 DERMATOMYOSITIS

Dermatomyositis is chronic inflammation of the skin and muscles. The cause of dermatomyositis is unknown but autoantibodies of the immune system against the blood vessels and sheaths that group muscle fibers into bundles are suspected.

Huòxiāng (Herba Pogostemonis) "transforms dampness, resolves summer heat, and stops vomiting." It was shown to be anti-inflammatory in mouse monocyte/macrophage-like cells (Xian et al., 2011) and

TABLE 3.14

GMP Herbal Medicines for a 55-Year-Old Woman with Dermatomyositis

Dermatomyositis (OrphaCode: 221)

A disease with a prevalence of ~6 in 100,000

Not applicable

Abnormal eyelid morphology, Edema, Autoimmunity, Myalgia, EMG abnormality, Proximal muscle weakness, Inflammatory myopathy, Erythema, Periorbital edema

Chondrocalcinosis, Dry skin, Pruritus, Acrocyanosis, Hypotonia, Arthritis, Abnormality of the nail, Weight loss, Respiratory insufficiency, Recurrent respiratory infections, Pulmonary fibrosis, Diffuse reticular or finely nodular infiltrations, Arthralgia, Interstitial pulmonary abnormality, Abnormal hair quantity, Fatigue, Papule, Skin ulcer

Cutaneous photosensitivity, Abnormality of the voice, Dysphonia, Myocardial infarction, Pericarditis, Abnormality of eosinophils, Fever, Pulmonary arterial hypertension, Vasculitis, Neoplasm, Lymphoma, Breast carcinoma, Aplasia/Hypoplasia of the skin, Feeding difficulties in infancy, Arrhythmia, Sinus tachycardia, Myocarditis, Lung adenocarcinoma, Telangiectasia of the skin, Cellulitis, Gastrointestinal stroma tumor, Gangrene

All ages

(Continued)

TABLE 3.14 *(Continued)*
GMP Herbal Medicines for a 55-Year-Old Woman with Dermatomyositis

Edema (D004487), Myalgia (D063806), Erythema (D005483):

Lǐzhōngtāng 5g + bǔzhōngyìqìtāng 5g + qīngyānlìgétāng 3g + chuānxiōngchádiàosǎn 3-0g + xiǎojiànzhōngtāng 3-0g + fángfēng 2g + zhǐqiào 2g + jiégěng 2g + gānjiāng 2g + ējiāo 2-0g + zǐwǎn 2-0g.

Lǐzhōngtāng 5g + bànxià 1g + shārén 1g + fúlíng 1g + dàhuáng 0g.

Báizhú 5g + fùzǐ 5g + cháihú 5g + báisháo 4g + fúlíng 4g + tiānhuā 2g + dǎngshēn 2g + wúzhūyú 2g + guìzhī 2g + huángqín 2g + gāncǎo 1g + mǔlì 1g + gānjiāng 1g + huánglián 1g.

Báizhú 5g + fúlíng 5g + huòxiāng 5-0g + zhǐshí 4g + xiāngfù 4-0g + shānzhā 4-0g + cháihú 4-0g + mùxiāng 4-0g + chénpí 4-0g + shénqū 4-0g + púgōngyīng 4-0g + shēngmá 2-0g + báizhǐ 2-0g.

Pruritus (D011537), Hypotonia (D009123), Abnormality of the nail (703), Weight loss (D015431), Pulmonary fibrosis (D011658) [Idiopathic pulmonary fibrosis (516.31)], Arthralgia (D018771), Fatigue (D005221):

Wǔlíngsǎn 5g + báisháo 1-0g + fùzǐ 1-0g + huángqín 1-0g + guìzhī 1-0g + dǐdāngtāng 0g.

Gāncǎo 5g + báizhǐ 5g + shārén 5-3g + huángqín 5-0g + tiānhuā 4-0g + xìxīn 2-0g + dàhuáng 1-0g.

Dysphonia (D055154), Fever (D005334), Neoplasm (199), Myocarditis (429.0), Cellulitis (D002481) [Cellulitis and abscess of unspecified sites (682.9)]:

Gānlùyǐn 5g + sìnìtāng 5-4g + xiāngshāliùjūnzǐtāng 4-2g + bǎihé 2-0g.

Gānlùyǐn 5g + sìnìtāng 4g + lóngdǎnxiègāntāng 4g.

Sìnìtāng 5g + gānlùyǐn 5g + yùzhú 3-0g + shēngmàiyǐn 2-0g.

Báizhǐ 5g + huángqín 5g + tiānhuā 2g + gāncǎo 2g + shārén 2g + dàhuáng 0g.

Huángqín 5g + báizhǐ 5-4g + zhìgāncǎo 3-2g + shārén 3-2g + guālóugēn 2g + dàhuáng 1-0g + xìxīn 1-0g.

is used today for skin, digestive, and respiratory conditions (Wang, 2020). Lǐzhōngtāng (cf. Section 2.48), containing Báizhú (cf. Sections 1.21, 1.63, 2.2, 3.2 and 3.8) as the major herb, "warms interior, dispels coldness, benefits Qi, strengthens the Spleen" and was shown to affect gastrointestinal motility by modulating pacemaker activity in mouse small intestine interstitial cells of Cajal (Hwang et al., 2013).

3.15 ENTHESITIS-RELATED JUVENILE IDIOPATHIC ARTHRITIS

Enthesitis-related juvenile idiopathic arthritis, also called juvenile enthesitis-related arthritis, is inflammation of the entheses where tendons or ligaments attach to the bone of a joint. Malfunction of the immune system that mistakenly attacks the joint is believed to cause enthesitis-related juvenile idiopathic arthritis.

TABLE 3.15
GMP Herbal Medicines for a 12-Year-Old Boy with Enthesitis-Related Juvenile Idiopathic Arthritis

Enthesitis-related juvenile idiopathic arthritis (OrphaCode: 85438)

A disease with a prevalence of ~6 in 100,000

Unknown

Arthritis, Arthralgia, Enthesitis

Abnormality of the vertebral column, Abnormality of the hip joint, Abnormality of the ankles, Back pain, Thickened Achilles tendon, Knee osteoarthritis, Abnormality of the calcaneus, Hip osteoarthritis, Sacroiliac arthritis, Oligoarthritis, Abnormality of the fascia, Abnormality of the lumbar spine

Abnormal heart morphology, Abnormality of the foot, Abnormal metatarsal morphology, Abnormality of the wrist, Abnormality of the shoulder, Abnormality of the cervical spine, Abnormality of the femoral neck or head region, Limited mobility of proximal interphalangeal joint, Abnormality of the elbow, Abnormality of skeletal morphology, Abnormality of metacarpophalangeal joint, Anterior uveitis, Finger dactylitis, Abnormality of the thoracic spine

Childhood, Adolescent

(Continued)

TABLE 3.15 *(Continued)*

GMP Herbal Medicines for a 12-Year-Old Boy with Enthesitis-Related Juvenile Idiopathic Arthritis

Arthralgia (D018771):

Shàngzhōngxiàtōngyòngtòngfēngwán 5g + shūjīnghuóxuètāng 5g + dāngguīniántòngtāng 5-0g + acupuncture.

Shàngzhōngxiàtōngyòngtòngfēngwán 5g + niúxī 2-1g + gǔsuìbǔ 2-1g + sāngjìshēng 2-0g + xùduàn 2-0g + wàndiǎnjīn 2-0g + yánhúsuǒ 1-0g.

Back pain (D001416):

Liùwèidìhuángwán 5g + bǔzhōngyìqìtāng 5g.

Liùwèidìhuángwán 5g + shūjīnghuóxuètāng 5g + gǔsuìbǔ 1g + xùduàn 1g.

Dúhuójìshēngtāng 5g + liùwèidìhuángwán 4-0g + dùzhòng 1g + gǔsuìbǔ 1-0g + jīxuèténg 1-0g + xùduàn 1-0g.

Abnormal heart morphology (746.9):

Tiānwángbǔxīndān 5g + jiāwèixiāoyáosǎn 5g + xīnyíqīngfèitāng 5g.

Tiānwángbǔxīndān 5g + shēnlíngbáizhúsǎn 5g + bǔzhōngyìqìtāng 5g.

Zhìgāncǎotāng 5g + bǔzhōngyìqìtāng 5g + dānshēn 1g + shíchāngpú 1g + yuǎnzhì 1g.

Xīnyíqīngfèitāng 5g + máxìnggānshítāng 5-0g + yínqiàosǎn 5-0g + gāncǎo 1-0g + báizhǐ 1-0g + yúxīngcǎo 1-0g.

Niúxī 5g + huángbò 5g + cāngzhú 5g + yìyǐrén 5-0g.

Niúxī 5g + chìsháo 5g + chēqiánzǐ 5g + zhìgāncǎo 5g + huángqí 5g + fùzǐ 4g + máhuáng 4g + dàhuáng 0g.

Niúxī 5g + báisháo 5g + guìzhī 5g + gǔsuìbǔ 5g + dāngguī 5-4g + xùduàn 5-4g + mùguā 4g + mòyào 2g + rǔxiāng 2g.

Báizhú 5g + fúlíng 5g + zhìgāncǎo 3g + gānjiāng 3g + niúxī 2-0g + fùzǐ 2-0g + guìzhī 2-0g + ròuguì 2-0g.

Gāncǎo 5g + báisháo 5g + shíhú 5g + bǎihé 5g + chēqiánzǐ 5g + fúlíng 5g + màiméndōng 5g.

Gāncǎo 5g + báizhǐ 5g + shārén 5-2g + tiānhuā 3-0g + huángqín 3-0g + dàhuáng 0g.

Dānshēn 5g + tiānhuā 5g + gāncǎo 5g + báisháo 5g + shíhú 5g + chēqiánzǐ 5g + fúlíng 5g + chénpí 5g + huángqí 5g + dǎngshēn 5g + bǎihé 5-0g.

Běishāshēn 5g + xuánshēn 5g + yùzhú 5g + dìhuáng 5g + màiméndōng 5g + hòupò 5-2g + zhǐshí 5-2g + dàhuáng 0g.

Báizhú 5g + fùzǐ 5g + cháihú 5g + báisháo 4g + fúlíng 4g + tiānhuā 2g + shēngjiāng 2g + dǎngshēn 2g + guìzhī 2g + huángqín 2g + gāncǎo 1g + mǔlì 1g + gānjiāng 1g.

Dānshēn (cf. Sections 1.61 and 2.53) is one of the most popular single herbs to promote blood circulation, remove blood stasis, and clear away heat (Pang et al., 2016). Specifically, it was reviewed to be microcirculation-improving, blood vessel-dilating, atherosclerosis-preventing, anti-inflammatory, antitumor, and blood pressure- and blood lipid-lowering (Shan et al., 2021). Tiānwángbǔxīndān is used not only for neurotic disorders (cf. Section 2.24) but also for cardiac dysrhythmias (Wang, 2019). Xīnyíqīngfèitāng contains two herbs that are cardioprotective (cf. Section 1.6).

3.16 AL AMYLOIDOSIS

AL amyloidosis, also known as light-chain amyloidosis or primary amyloidosis, is characterized by buildup in tissues, nerves, or organs of amyloid fibrils that come from aggregates of a misshapen antibody subunit called light chain produced by the plasma cells. Amyloid fibrils are resistant to degradation and their deposits can damage organs, including the heart and kidneys. Acquired abnormality of the plasma cells in the bone marrow causes AL amyloidosis.

Zhìgāncǎotāng, containing Zhìgāncǎo (cf. Section 1.11), "supplements Qi/Blood, nourishes yin, and restores pulse." Bìxièfēnqīngyǐn was shown to alleviate renal inflammation and fibrosis in mice with hyperuricemic nephropathy (Lin et al., 2024) and is used today for nonspecific findings on examination of urine, nephritis, and nephropathy (Wang, 2019). Rénshēnyǎngróngtāng is translated to "Ginseng nutrient-nourishing decoction" and used today for anemia (Wang, 2019).

TABLE 3.16

GMP Herbal Medicines for a 65-Year-Old Man with AL Amyloidosis

AL amyloidosis (OrphaCode: 85443)

A disease with a prevalence of ~5 in 100,000

Not applicable

Fatigue

Abnormality of the kidney, Proteinuria, Nephrotic syndrome, Abnormal heart morphology, Hypertrophic cardiomyopathy, Weight loss, Abnormal EKG, Interstitial pulmonary abnormality, Increased antibody level in blood, Albuminuria, Increased NT-proBNP level, Monoclonal light chain cardiac amyloidosis, Renal interstitial amyloid deposits, Increased troponin I level in blood, Increased troponin T level in blood

Renal insufficiency, Xerostomia, Bruising susceptibility, Abnormality of the liver, Abnormal cardiac ventricle morphology, Anemia, Dyspnea, Hepatomegaly, Autonomic dysregulation, Obstructive sleep apnea, Hypoalbuminemia, Elevated alkaline phosphatase, Abdominal distention, Abnormal cardiac atrium morphology, Postural hypotension with compensatory tachycardia, Reduced factor X activity, Autonomic erectile dysfunction, Peripheral neuropathy, Abnormal salivary gland morphology, Arrhythmia, Constrictive median neuropathy, Peripheral edema, Pulmonary interstitial high-resolution computed tomography abnormality, Jaw claudication, Nonproductive cough, Abnormal P wave, Howell-Jolly bodies

Adult

Fatigue (D005221):

Zhìgāncǎotāng 5g + língguìshùgāntāng 5-0g + shēngmàiyǐn 4-0g + dānshēn 1-0g + wǔwèizǐ 1-0g + màiméndōng 1-0g + dǎngshēn 1-0g + fùzǐ 1-0g + xiāngfù 0g + yùjīn 0g.

Jiāwèixiāoyáosǎn 5g + língguìshùgāntāng 5g + xiǎoqīnglóngtāng 2g + dùzhòng 1g + tùsīzǐ 1g.

Zhìgāncǎo 5g + jiégěng 5g + xuánshēn 4-3g + bèimǔ 4-3g + mǔlì 4-2g + liánqiáo 4-2g + shānzhīzǐ 2-0g + zhīzǐ 2-0g + jīnyínhuā 1-0g.

Proteinuria (791.0), Nephrotic syndrome (581), Abnormal heart morphology (746.9), Hypertrophic cardiomyopathy (425.1), Weight loss (D015431), Increased antibody level in blood (D006942), Albuminuria (D000419):

Bìxièfēnqīngyǐn 5g + jìshēngshènqìwán 5g + dānshēn 1g + báimáogēn 1-0g + yìmǔcǎo 1-0g + zélán 1-0g + tùsīzǐ 1-0g + jīxuèténg 1-0g + dōngguāzǐ 1-0g + bìxiè 1-0g.

Zhūlíngtāng 5g + jìshēngshènqìwán 5g + dōngguāzǐ 1g + báimáogēn 1g + yìmǔcǎo 1g + yùjīn 1g.

Zhēnwǔtāng 5g + jìshēngshènqìwán 5g + dānshēn 1g + huángqí 1g + dàhuáng 0g.

Shānzhūyú 5g + shānyào 5g + dìhuáng 5g + mǔdānpí 5g + fúlíng 5g + zéxiè 5g + fùzǐ 5-0g + guìzhī 5-0g.

Báimáogēn 5g + chìxiǎodòu 5g + chēqiánzǐ 5g + yìmǔcǎo 5g + dāngguī 2g.

Huángqín 5g + báizhǐ 4g + zhìgāncǎo 2g + shārén 2g + tiānhuā 1g + huánglián 1g + dàhuáng 0g.

Renal insufficiency (586), Bruising susceptibility (D004438), Abnormality of the liver (573.9), Anemia (285.9), Dyspnea (D004417), Obstructive sleep apnea (327.23):

Rénshēnyǎngróngtāng 5g + liùwèidìhuángwán 4g + ējiāo 1g + huángqí 1g + dàhuáng 0g.

Rénshēnyǎngróngtāng 5g + jìshēngshènqìwán 5g + dānshēn 1g + ējiāo 1-0g + jīxuèténg 1-0g + bājǐtiān 1-0g + ròucōngróng 1-0g + yínyánghuò 1-0g + tùsīzǐ 1-0g.

Yòuguīwán 5g + bǔzhōngyìqìtāng 5g + guīpítāng 5g + bājǐtiān 2g + ròucōngróng 2g + yínyánghuò 2g + dàhuáng 0g.

Jìshēngshènqìwán 5g + guīpítāng 4g + zhēnwǔtāng 3g + bǔzhōngyìqìtāng 3g + dānshēn 1g.

Báizhú 5g + fùzǐ 5g + cháihú 5g + báisháo 4g + fúlíng 4g + tiānhuā 2g + dǎngshēn 2g + guìzhī 2g + huángqín 2g + gāncǎo 1g + mǔlì 1g + gānjiāng 1g + dàhuáng 1-0g.

Báizhú 5g + fùzǐ 5g + báisháo 4g + fúlíng 4g + dǎngshēn 2g + wǔwèizǐ 2g + bànxià 2g + gāncǎo 2g + xìngrén 2g + gānjiāng 2g + xìxīn 2g + máhuáng 2g + shēngjiāng 2-0g.

Shúdìhuáng 5g + báizhú 4g + fùzǐ 4g + báisháo 3g + fúlíng 3g + báijièzǐ 2g + dǎngshēn 2g + gāncǎo 1g + shēngjiāng 1g + máhuáng 1g + huánglián 0g.

3.17 CLASSICAL EHLERS-DANLOS SYNDROME

Classical Ehlers-Danlos syndrome (classical EDS) is a hereditary condition of the connective tissues characterized by skin hyperextensibility and joint hypermobility. Different mutated genes give different EDS types and classical EDS is mainly caused by mutations in the *COL5A1* or *COL5A2* genes, each of which instructs the body to make a component of type V collagen, a type of collagen.

TABLE 3.17

GMP Herbal Medicines for a Six-Year-Old Child with Classical Ehlers-Danlos Syndrome

Classical Ehlers-Danlos syndrome (OrphaCode: 287)

A disease with a prevalence of ~5 in 100,000

Disease-causing germline mutation(s): collagen type V alpha 2 chain (*COL5A2* / Entrez: 1290) at 2q32.2

Disease-causing germline mutation(s): collagen type V alpha 1 chain (*COL5A1* / Entrez: 1289) at 9q34.3

Disease-causing germline mutation(s): collagen type I alpha 1 chain (*COL1A1* / Entrez: 1277) at 17q21.33

Autosomal dominant

Hyperextensible skin, Soft, doughy skin, Fragile skin, Striae distensae, Cigarette-paper scars, Atrophic scars, Generalized joint laxity

Osteopenia, Poor wound healing, Hypotonia, Muscle weakness, Vomiting, Nausea, Gastroesophageal reflux, Muscle spasm, Pulp stones, Fatigue, Chronic constipation

Bladder diverticulum, Inguinal hernia, Uterine prolapse, Epicanthus, Abnormal cornea morphology, Bruising susceptibility, Molluscoid pseudotumors, Acrocyanosis, Motor delay, Joint swelling, Umbilical hernia, Premature birth, Abnormality of the foot, Talipes equinovarus, Pes planus, Premature rupture of membranes, Rectal prolapse, Hiatus hernia, Aortic root aneurysm, Scoliosis, Osteoarthritis, Hip dislocation, Arthralgia, Patellar dislocation, Prolonged bleeding time, Dislocated radial head, Shoulder dislocation, Incisional hernia, Dilatation of the cerebral artery, Arteriovenous fistula, Arterial dissection, Phalangeal dislocation, Prematurely aged appearance, Limb pain, Blepharochalasis, Dermatochalasis, Abnormality of the temporomandibular joint, Subcutaneous spheroids, Arterial rupture, Piezogenic pedal papules, Cervical insufficiency, Ecchymosis, Abnormal heart valve physiology

Neonatal, Infancy, Childhood

Striae distensae (D057896):

Xiǎojiànzhōngtāng 5g + shēnlíngbáizhúsǎn 5-0g + shānzhā 1-0g + shénqū 1-0g + màiyá 1-0g + jīnèijīn 1-0g.	Xuánshēn 5g + dìhuáng 5g + màiméndōng 5g + hòupò 5-1g + zhǐshí 5-1g + dàhuáng 1-0g.
Bǎohéwán 5g + xiāngshāliùjūnzǐtāng 5g + shénqū 1g + màiyá 1g + jīnèijīn 1g.	

Hypotonia (D009123), Muscle weakness (D018908), Vomiting (D014839), Nausea (D009325), Gastroesophageal reflux (530.81), Muscle spasm (D009120), Fatigue (D005221):

Guìzhītāng 5g + xìngrén 1g + hòupò 1g + zhǐshí 1-0g + dàhuáng 0g.	Wǔwèizǐ 5g + bànxià 5g + zhìgāncǎo 5g + cháihú 5g + gānjiāng 5g + huángqín 5g.
	Huángqí 5g + zhìgāncǎo 3g + wǔwèizǐ 1g + dāngguī 1g.
	Gāncǎo 5g + báisháo 5g + shíhú 5g + bǎihé 5g + chēqiánzǐ 5g + fúlíng 5g + màiméndōng 5g.

Bladder diverticulum (596.3), Inguinal hernia (550), Bruising susceptibility (D004438), Talipes equinovarus (754.51), Rectal prolapse (569.1), Osteoarthritis (715.3), Arthralgia (D018771), Cervical insufficiency (622.5):

Bǔzhōngyìqìtāng 5g + sāngpiāoxiāosǎn 5-0g + shēngmá 1g + wūyào 1-0g + yìzhìrén 1-0g + huángqí 1-0g.	Zhǐqiào 5g + chántuì 5-2g + jílí 1-0g.
Júhéwán 5g + bǔzhōngyìqìtāng 4g + wūyào 1g + yìzhìrén 1g.	Zhǐqiào 5g + jílí 5g + chántuì 5-0g.

Xuánshēn (cf. Sections 1.3 and 1.25) was shown in mice to inhibit substance P-induced itch-scratch response (Tohda et al., 2000) and alleviate the symptoms of allergic contact dermatitis (Song et al., 2011). Zhǐqiào (cf. Section 1.31) was shown to prevent formation of nephrolithiasis in rats (Li et al., 2015). Sāngpiāoxiāosǎn "regulates and replenishes the Heart and Kidney, astringes semen, arrests spermatorrhea" and is used for symptoms involving the urinary system (Wang, 2019).

3.18 BEHÇET DISEASE

Behçet disease is a chronic and recurrent auto-inflammation of the blood vessels and tissues including the mouth, genitals, eye, skin, and joints. The cause of Behçet disease is unknown and the risk factors include genetic predispositions and environmental exposures.

Chuānxiōngchádiàosǎn was concluded to be effective for the treatment of migraine in a systematic review and meta-analysis of randomized controlled trials (Wang et al., 2019). The formula contains Báizhǐ, Zhìgāncǎo, Xìxīn, and so on. Shúdìhuáng (cf. Section 1.71) is said to tonify TCM Kidney yin and used today for constipation, sleep disturbances, anemia of the mother, benign neoplasm of breasts, and epiphora (Wang, 2020). Xiǎoqīnglóngtāng is anti-inflammatory and was shown to

---

TABLE 3.18

GMP Herbal Medicines for a 35-Year-Old Adult with Behçet Disease

Behçet disease (OrphaCode: 117)

A disease with a prevalence of ~5 in 100,000

Major susceptibility factor: interleukin 10 (*IL10* / Entrez: 3586) at 1q32.1

Major susceptibility factor: major histocompatibility complex, class I, B (*HLA-B* / Entrez: 3106) at 6p21.33

Major susceptibility factor: Fas cell surface death receptor (*FAS* / Entrez: 355) at 10q23.31

Major susceptibility factor: UBA domain containing 2 (*UBAC2* / Entrez: 337867) at 13q32.3

Major susceptibility factor: interleukin 23 receptor (*IL23R* / Entrez: 149233) at 1p31.3

Major susceptibility factor: MEFV innate immunity regulator, pyrin (*MEFV* / Entrez: 4210) at 16p13.3

Major susceptibility factor: signal transducer and activator of transcription 4 (*STAT4* / Entrez: 6775) at 2q32.2-q32.3

Major susceptibility factor: complement C4A (Rodgers blood group) (*C4A* / Entrez: 720) at 6p21.33

Major susceptibility factor: interleukin 12A (*IL12A* / Entrez: 3592) at 3q25.33

Major susceptibility factor: toll like receptor 4 (*TLR4* / Entrez: 7099) at 9q33.1

Major susceptibility factor: C-C motif chemokine receptor 1 (*CCR1* / Entrez: 1230) at 3p21.31

Major susceptibility factor: killer cell lectin like receptor C4 (*KLRC4* / Entrez: 8302) at 12p13.2

Major susceptibility factor: IL12A antisense RNA 1 (*IL12A-AS1* / Entrez: 101928376) at 3q25.33

Major susceptibility factor: endoplasmic reticulum aminopeptidase 1 (*ERAP1* / Entrez: 51752) at 5q15

Major susceptibility factor: interferon gamma receptor 1 (*IFNGR1* / Entrez: 3459) at 6q23.3

Multigenic/multifactorial

Oral ulcer, Photophobia, Arthritis, Subcutaneous nodule, Migraine, Vasculitis, Myalgia, Recurrent aphthous stomatitis, Fatigue, Meningitis, Fever, Nausea and vomiting, Orchitis, Papule

Acne, Hemiparesis, Gastrointestinal hemorrhage, Arthralgia, Venous thrombosis, Increased inflammatory response, Immunologic hypersensitivity, Gait disturbance, Confusion, Abdominal pain, Abnormal blistering of the skin

Renal insufficiency, Retinopathy, Cataract, Behavioral abnormality, Keratoconjunctivitis sicca, Seizure, Ataxia, Hyperreflexia, Abnormal myocardium morphology, Mitral regurgitation, Aortic regurgitation, Pericarditis, Splenomegaly, Weight loss, Anorexia, Pleuritis, Hemoptysis, Pleural effusion, Memory impairment, Encephalitis, Increased intracranial pressure, Paresthesia, Cranial nerve paralysis, Abnormal pyramidal sign, Avascular necrosis, Myositis, Optic neuritis, Retrobulbar optic neuritis, Gangrene, Glomerulopathy, Blindness, Irritability, Myocardial infarction, Pancreatitis, Malabsorption, Pulmonary infiltrates, Pulmonary embolism, Vertigo, Developmental regression, Cerebral ischemia, Lymphadenopathy, Arterial thrombosis, Endocarditis

Childhood, Adolescent, Adult

Photophobia (D020795), Migraine (346), Myalgia (D063806), Recurrent aphthous stomatitis (528.2), Fatigue (D005221), Meningitis (322.9), Fever (D005334):

Chuānxiōngchádiàosǎn 5g + gānlùyǐn 5-3g + qīngwèisǎn 5-0g + jiāwèixiāoyáosǎn 3-0g + yèjiāoténg 2-0g + báizhǐ 1-0g + mànjīngzǐ 1-0g + gǎoběn 1-0g. Wǔlíngsǎn 5g + báisháo 1g + huángqín 1g.

Gāncǎo 5g + báisháo 5g + fùzǐ 5g + fúlíng 5g + gānjiāng 5g + suānzǎorén 5g + mázǐrénwán 5g + dàhuáng 2g.

Huángqín 5g + báizhǐ 5-4g + zhìgāncǎo 3-2g + shārén 3-2g + tiānhuā 2-0g + guālóugēn 2-0g + xìxīn 1-0g + dàhuáng 0g.
Báizhǐ 5g + zhìgāncǎo 4-3g + shārén 4-3g + huángqín 3-0g + tiānhuā 2-0g + xìxīn 1-0g + dàhuáng 0g.

Hemiparesis (D010291), Arthralgia (D018771), Confusion (D003221), Abdominal pain (D015746):

Dúhuójìshēngtāng 5g + shūjīnghuóxuètāng 4-0g + dùzhòng 1-0g + xùduàn 1-0g + acupuncture.
Báizhú 5g + fùzǐ 5g + báisháo 3g + fúlíng 3g + dǎngshēn 3g + xiǎochéngqìtāng 2g + dàhuáng 0g.
Báizhú 5g + fùzǐ 5g + gānjiāng 5g + mázǐrénwán 5g + fúlíng 3g + dàhuáng 1g.

Báizhú 5g + fùzǐ 5g + cháihú 5g + báisháo 4g + fúlíng 4g + tiānhuā 2g + dǎngshēn 2g + guìzhī 2g + huángqín 2g + shēngjiāng 2-0g + wūwèizǐ 2-0g + xìxīn 2-0g + gāncǎo 1g + mǔlì 1g + gānjiāng 1g + dàhuáng 1-0g.
Báizhú 5g + fùzǐ 5g + báisháo 5-4g + fúlíng 5-4g + dǎngshēn 5-2g.

(Continued)

TABLE 3.18 *(Continued)*
GMP Herbal Medicines for a 35-Year-Old Adult with Behçet Disease

Renal insufficiency (586), Retinopathy (362.9), Seizure (345.9), Ataxia (D002524), Hyperreflexia (D012021), Mitral regurgitation (396.3, 746.6), Weight loss (D015431), Anorexia (D000855), Hemoptysis (D006469), Memory impairment (D008569), Paresthesia (D010292), Cranial nerve paralysis (352.9), Avascular necrosis (732.3, 733.41, 733.42, 733.43, 733.44), Optic neuritis (377.3), Blindness (D001766), Pancreatitis (577.0), Vertigo (386.2), Endocarditis (421.9):

Zhìgāncǎotāng 5g + língguìshùgāntāng 5g + tiānmá 2-1g + bànxià 2-1g + shēngjiāng 2-1g + xìngrén 2-0g + hòupò 2-0g + guālóurén 2-0g + xièbái 2-0g.
Xiǎoqīnglóngtāng 5g + máxìnggānshítāng 5g + dàzǎo 1g + tínglìzǐ 1g.

Shúdìhuáng 5g + gāncǎo 2g + báisháo 2g + báijièzǐ 2g + ròuguì 2g + máhuáng 2g + huángbò 2g + dāngguī 2g.
Shúdìhuáng 5g + báizhú 4g + fùzǐ 4g + báisháo 3g + fúlíng 3g + báijièzǐ 2g + dǎngshēn 2g + gāncǎo 1g + shēngjiāng 1g + máhuáng 1g + dàhuáng 1-0g + huánglián 0g.
Bànxià 5g + xuánshēn 5g + dìhuáng 5g + zhīmǔ 5g + jiégěng 5g + zhǐzǐ 5g + huángqín 5g + dāngguī 5g + gāncǎo 2g + cháihú 2g + acupuncture.

prevent cardiomyocyte hypertrophy, fibrosis, and development of heart failure with preserved ejection faction in rats by modulating the composition of gut microbiota (Zhou et al., 2019).

3.19 IMMUNOGLOBULIN A VASCULITIS

Immunoglobulin A vasculitis (IgA vasculitis), also known as Henoch-Schönlein purpura or purpura rheumatica, is inflammation of the small blood vessels of the skin, joints, intestines, and kidneys. Restricted blood flow due to blood vessel inflammation can damage organs. IgA vasculitis can develop after an upper respiratory or gastrointestinal infection.

Zhǐqiào is anti-inflammatory and anti-vascular damage (cf. Section 3.3). Zhūlíngtāng with conventional treatment was shown to be more effective for diuretic resistance in patients with heart failure than conventional treatment alone in a randomized controlled trial (Chen et al., 2022). Dǎochìsǎn

TABLE 3.19
GMP Herbal Medicines for a Six-Year-Old Child with Immunoglobulin A Vasculitis

Immunoglobulin A vasculitis (OrphaCode: 761)

A disease with a prevalence of ~5 in 100,000

Not applicable

Hematuria, Bruising susceptibility, Purpura, Skin rash, Nausea and vomiting, Abdominal pain, Vasculitis, Arthralgia, Gastrointestinal infarctions, Pustule

Arthritis, Fever, Anorexia, Migraine, Encephalitis, Myalgia, Erythema, Vascular skin abnormality, Orchitis, Skin ulcer

Renal insufficiency, Proteinuria, Optic atrophy, Edema, Urticaria, Seizure, Muscle weakness, Restrictive deficit on pulmonary function testing, Gastrointestinal hemorrhage, Hemiplegia/hemiparesis, Macule, Episcleritis, Angioedema, Glomerulopathy

Childhood

Hematuria (D006417) [Hematuria, unspecified (599.70)], Bruising susceptibility (D004438), Purpura (D011693), Skin rash (782.1), Abdominal pain (D015746), Arthralgia (D018771):

Zhūlíngtāng 5g + dǎochìsǎn 5-0g + gāncǎo 2-0g + huángqín 2-0g + báimáogēn 1-0g + báixiānpí 1-0g + dìfūzǐ 1-0g + dàhuáng 0g.
Dǎochìsǎn 5g + xiāofēngsǎn 4g + báimáogēn 1g + jīnyínhuā 1g + gāncǎo 0g.

Zhǐqiào 5g + jílí 5-2g + chántuì 5-0g.
Júhóng 5g + zhǐqiào 1g.

Fever (D005334), Anorexia (D000855), Migraine (346), Myalgia (D063806), Erythema (D005483), Vascular skin abnormality (709.1):

Wǔlíngsǎn 5g + gāncǎo 1-0g + tiáowèichéngqìtāng 1-0g + dàhuáng 0g.

Gāncǎo 5g + báizhǐ 5g + shārén 5-3g + dàhuáng 1-0g.

(Continued)

TABLE 3.19 *(Continued)*

GMP Herbal Medicines for a Six-Year-Old Child with Immunoglobulin A Vasculitis

Renal insufficiency (586), Proteinuria (791.0), Optic atrophy (377.1), Edema (D004487), Seizure (345.9), Muscle weakness (D018908), Episcleritis (379.00):

Liùwèidìhuángwán 5g + xiāngshāliùjūnzǐtāng 4g + shānyào 2g + dānshēn 2g + huángqí 2g + dàhuáng 0g.	Gāncǎo 5g + dàhuáng 0g. Júhuā 5g.
Liùwèidìhuángwán 5g + shēnlíngbáizhúsǎn 5g + dānshēn 2-0g + shíchāngpú 2-0g + yuǎnzhì 2-0g + huángqí 2-0g.	Jílí 5g + júhóng 5-0g + chántuì 4-3g + zhǐqiào 3-0g.
Shēnlíngbáizhúsǎn 5g + mázǐrénwán 2g + tiānmá 1g + shíchāngpú 1g + yuǎnzhì 1g.	Huángqí 5g + chìsháo 1g + fángfēng 1g + xìxīn 1g + huánglián 1g + dàhuáng 0g.
Shēnlíngbáizhúsǎn 5g + jìshēngshènqìwán 5g + huángqí 1g + jīxuèténg 1g + dàhuáng 0g.	

"clears heat, helps urinate" and is used today for chronic glomerulonephritis, and cystitis (Wang, 2019). Liùwèidìhuángwán "nourishes yin, replenishes the Kidney" and is used today for diabetes mellitus (Wang, 2019). A case-control study showed that combined use of Liùwèidìhuángwán and oral antidiabetic drugs is associated with a delayed use of insulin in patients with type 2 diabetes (Chen et al., 2021).

3.20 MICROSCOPIC POLYANGIITIS

Microscopic polyangiitis (MPA), or microscopic polyarteritis, is characterized by inflammation of the small blood vessels of the kidneys and lungs. MPA is caused by anti-neutrophil cytoplasmic antibody (ANCA), an autoantibody, mediated attacks of neutrophils on the blood vessel walls. The reason for ANCA's development is however not fully known.

Jìshēngshènqìwán "nourishes the Kidney, helps yang, induces diuresis, eliminates edema" and is used today for hyperplasia of prostate, symptoms involving the urinary system, and nephritis and nephropathy (Wang, 2019). Water extract of Dàfùpí (cf. Sections 2.45 and 3.10) was shown

TABLE 3.20

GMP Herbal Medicines for a 59-Year-Old Adult with Microscopic Polyangiitis

Microscopic polyangiitis (OrphaCode: 727)

A disease with a prevalence of ~5 in 100,000

Not applicable

Renal insufficiency, Hematuria, Skin rash, Fever, Hemoptysis, Vasculitis, Autoimmunity, Erythema, Increased inflammatory response, Oliguria, Glomerulopathy

Subcutaneous hemorrhage, Diarrhea, Nausea and vomiting, Abdominal pain, Gastrointestinal hemorrhage, Peritonitis, Arthralgia, Myalgia, Venous thrombosis, Gastrointestinal infarctions, Skin ulcer

Sinusitis, Epistaxis, Uveitis, Cutis marmorata, Arthritis, Subcutaneous nodule, Congestive heart failure, Pericarditis, Pancreatitis, Paresthesia, Abnormal retinal vascular morphology, Peripheral neuropathy, Arrhythmia, Episcleritis, Gangrene

Childhood, Adult

Renal insufficiency (586), Skin rash (782.1), Fever (D005334), Hemoptysis (D006469), Erythema (D005483), Oliguria (D009846):

Jìshēngshènqìwán 5g + zhūlíngtāng 5-3g + dānshēn 1g + sāngbáipí 1-0g + báimáogēn 1-0g + yìmǔcǎo 1-0g + zélán 1-0g + jīxuèténg 1-0g + chìsháo 1-0g + huángqí 1-0g + dàhuáng 0g.	Báimáogēn 5g + chìxiǎodòu 5-3g + chēqiánzǐ 5-3g + yìmǔcǎo 5-0g + dāngguī 2g + dàhuáng 1-0g.
Jìshēngshènqìwán 5g + wǔlíngsǎn 4g + tǔfúlíng 1g + báimáogēn 1g + dàhuáng 0g.	Fùzǐ 5g + fúlíng 5g + dàhuáng 2g + gāncǎo 2g + gānjiāng 2g + dǎngshēn 2g.

(Continued)

TABLE 3.20 *(Continued)*

GMP Herbal Medicines for a 59-Year-Old Adult with Microscopic Polyangiitis

Diarrhea (D003967), Abdominal pain (D015746), Arthralgia (D018771), Myalgia (D063806):

Wǔlíngsǎn 5g + gégēnhuángqínhuángliántāng 5-0g + huòxiāngzhèngqìsǎn 5-0g.	Gāncǎo 5g + báizhǐ 5-0g + shārén 4-0g + huángqín 4-0g + guālóugēn 2-0g + huánglián 2-0g.
Wǔlíngsǎn 5g + píngwèisǎn 5-0g + huòxiāngzhèngqìsǎn 5-0g.	Gāncǎo 5g + hòupò 5-0g + zhǐshí 5-0g + dàhuáng 0g.

Epistaxis (D004844), Congestive heart failure (428, 428.0), Pancreatitis (577.0), Paresthesia (D010292), Episcleritis (379.00):

Shēngmàiyǐn 5g + xuèfǔzhúyūtāng 5g + xīnyíqīngfèitāng 5g + xiānhècǎo 1g + báimáogēn 1g.	Dàfùpí 5g + gāncǎo 5g + mǔlì 5g + sāngbáipí 5g + hǎigé 5g + fúlíng 5g + gégēn 5g + jílí 5g + wǔlíngzhī 4g + bèimǔ 4g + xīnyí 4g + cāngěrzǐ 4g + yuánzhì 4-0g + bīngláng 4-0g.
Shēngmàiyǐn 5g + zhūlíngtāng 4g + xiānhècǎo 1g + báimáogēn 1g + ǒujié 1g.	
Shēngmàiyǐn 5g + zhìgāncǎotāng 5g + sānqī 1g + xiānhècǎo 1g + dānshēn 1-0g + báimáogēn 1-0g + ǒujié 1-0g.	Gāncǎo 5g + huángqín 5g + yìyǐrén 5-0g + dàhuáng 1-0g + huánglián 1-0g.

to alleviate chronic pancreatitis in mice (Kweon et al., 2022). Shēngmàiyǐn "benefits Qi, generates saliva, conserves yin, stops sweating" and is used today for cardiac dysrhythmias, symptoms involving cardiovascular system, and heart failure (Wang, 2019).

3.21 TAKAYASU ARTERITIS

Takayasu arteritis refers to inflammation of the aorta and its main branches. As the aorta carries blood away from the heart to the rest of the body, aggregates of macrophages in the inflamed arteries narrow the arteries, leading to weak or no pulses in the arms and legs of the patient with Takayasu arteritis. The cause of Takayasu arteritis is unknown and may involve a combination of genetic and environmental factors.

TABLE 3.21

GMP Herbal Medicines for a 27-Year-Old Woman with Takayasu Arteritis

Takayasu arteritis (OrphaCode: 3287)

A disease with a prevalence of ~5 in 100,000

Major susceptibility factor: major histocompatibility complex, class I, B (*HLA-B* / Entrez: 3106) at 6p21.33

Major susceptibility factor: interleukin 12B (*IL12B* / Entrez: 3593) at 5q33.3

Major susceptibility factor: MAX dimerization protein MLX (*MLX* / Entrez: 6945) at 17q21.2

Not applicable

Hyperhidrosis, Subcutaneous nodule, Abnormal heart valve morphology, Weight loss, Fever, Dilatation, Vasculitis, Fatigue, Arterial stenosis, Hypertensive crisis

Hypertension, Seizure, Muscle weakness, Arthritis, Hypertrophic cardiomyopathy, Abnormal aortic valve morphology, Myocardial infarction, Anemia, Anorexia, Migraine, Pulmonary arterial hypertension, Abnormal pattern of respiration, Myalgia, Dilatation of the ascending aorta, Increased inflammatory response, Inflammatory abnormality of the eye, Chest pain, Gangrene, Skin ulcer

Retinopathy, Hemoptysis, Neurological speech impairment, Cerebral ischemia, Arthralgia, Abnormality of the endocardium, Reduced consciousness/confusion, Gastrointestinal infarctions, Amaurosis fugax

Adolescent, Adult

Weight loss (D015431), Fever (D005334), Dilatation (442.9), Fatigue (D005221):

Lǐzhōngtāng 5g + bànxià 1g + shārén 1g + fúlíng 1g + dàhuáng 0g.	Zhìgāncǎo 5g + hòupò 5-2g + zhǐshí 5-2g + dàhuáng 1-0g.
Gégēnhuángqínhuángliántāng 5g + bànxià 0g + fúlíng 0g + dàhuáng 0g.	Gāncǎo 5g + hòupò 5g + zhǐshí 5g + dàhuáng 1g.
Guìzhītāng 5g + bànxià 1g + dàhuáng 0g.	Gāncǎo 5g + báizhǐ 5g + shārén 5g + dàhuáng 0g.

(Continued)

TABLE 3.21 *(Continued)*

GMP Herbal Medicines for a 27-Year-Old Woman with Takayasu Arteritis

Hypertension (401-405.99), Seizure (345.9), Muscle weakness (D018908), Hypertrophic cardiomyopathy (425.1), Anemia (285.9), Anorexia (D000855), Migraine (346), Myalgia (D063806), Chest pain (D002637):

Tiānmágōuténgyǐn 5g + fángfēngtōngshèngsǎn 5g + zhēnrénhuómìngyǐn 5g.	Bànxià 5g + ējiāo 5g + zǐcǎo 5g + dǎngshēn 5g + fùzǐ 3g + gānjiāng 3g.
Tiānmágōuténgyǐn 5g + sìwùtāng 5g + dānshēn 1g + niúxī 1-0g.	Hòupò 5g + zhǐshí 5g + dàhuáng 1g + huǒmárén 1g.
Tiānmágōuténgyǐn 5g + jiāwèixiāoyáosǎn 5g + shēngmàiyǐn 5g.	Qiānghuó 5g + hòupò 5g + zhǐshí 5g + dàhuáng 1g.
Tiānmágōuténgyǐn 5g + jiāwèixiāoyáosǎn 5g + zhìgāncǎotāng 5g + dānshēn 1-0g.	

Retinopathy (362.9), Hemoptysis (D006469), Neurological speech impairment (D013064), Arthralgia (D018771), Amaurosis fugax (D020757):

Zīshènmíngmùtāng 5g + yìqìcōngmíngtāng 4-3g + xuèfǔzhúyūtāng 3-2g + xiàkūcǎo 1-0g + tùsīzǐ 1-0g.	Júhuā 5g + chántuì 5g + júhóng 2g.
Xǐgānmíngmùtāng 5g + zīshènmíngmùtāng 3g + juémíngzǐ 1g + xiàkūcǎo 1g.	Zhǐqiào 5-4g + chántuì 5-4g + jílí 5-0g + júhuā 5-0g.
Zīshènmíngmùtāng 5g + jiāwèixiāoyáosǎn 3g + xuèfǔzhúyūtāng 3g + dānshēn 1g + juémíngzǐ 1g + mànjīngzǐ 1g + gǎoběn 1g.	Gǒuqǐzǐ 5g + júhuā 5g + niúbàngzǐ 3g + shègān 3g + huánglián 2g + xìxīn 1g.

Ējiāo (Colla Corii Asini) "nourishes Blood, stops bleeding" and was confirmed to be effective for women with blood deficiency by a randomized, double-blind, and placebo-controlled clinical trial (Zhang et al., 2021). Tiānmágōuténgyǐn was shown to significantly alter the development and prevent hypertension in spontaneously hypertensive rats (Zhang et al., 1989) and reverse the hypertension-induced cardiovascular remodeling in AngII-induced hypertensive mice (Deng et al., 2022) although its effectiveness as an adjunctive treatment for essential hypertension in humans was not concluded in a systematic review and meta-analysis of randomized controlled trials (Wang et al., 2013).

3.22   MIXED CONNECTIVE TISSUE DISEASE

Mixed connective tissue disease (MCTD), also known as Sharp syndrome, is characterized by symptoms that overlap with four rheumatic diseases including systemic lupus erythematosus, polymyositis, scleroderma and rheumatoid arthritis, plus an elevated level of anti-RNP antibodies in the blood. RNPs are molecules that help process mRNA in the nucleus. When a cell dies, RNPs leave the nucleus. If the body was infected by a virus with a structure similar to the RNP before, the immune system mistakenly considers RNPs as foreign, triggering an immune response to cause MCTD.

TABLE 3.22

GMP Herbal Medicines for a 37-Year-Old Woman with Mixed Connective Tissue Disease

Mixed connective tissue disease (OrphaCode: 809)

A disease with a prevalence of ~5 in 100,000

Multigenic/multifactorial

Skin rash, Arthritis, Gastroesophageal reflux, Dyspnea, Pulmonary fibrosis, Autoimmunity, Myalgia, Elevated erythrocyte sedimentation rate, Gastritis, Fatigue, Scleroderma, Chest pain

Xerostomia, Psychosis, Keratoconjunctivitis sicca, Joint swelling, Fever, Pleuritis, Arthralgia, Myositis

Nephropathy, Purpura, Seizure, Meningitis, Joint stiffness, Alopecia, Splenomegaly, Hemolytic anemia, Pericarditis, Leukopenia, Pulmonary arterial hypertension, Gastrointestinal hemorrhage, Hepatomegaly, Lymphadenopathy, Osteolysis, Prolonged bleeding time, Interstitial pulmonary abnormality, Peripheral neuropathy, Avascular necrosis, Myocarditis, Mediastinal lymphadenopathy

Childhood, Adolescent, Adult

(Continued)

TABLE 3.22 *(Continued)*

GMP Herbal Medicines for a 37-Year-Old Woman with Mixed Connective Tissue Disease

Skin rash (782.1), Gastroesophageal reflux (530.81), Dyspnea (D004417), Myalgia (D063806), Fatigue (D005221), Scleroderma (701.0), Chest pain (D002637):

Xiāofēngsǎn 5g + dāngguīyǐnzǐ 5g + báijí 2g + hǎipiāoxiāo 2g + báixiānpí 1g + dìfūzǐ 1g.	Báizhǐ 5g + huángqín 5g + zhìgāncǎo 3g + shārén 3g + guālóugēn 2g + xìxīn 2-1g + huángbò 2-0g + dàhuáng 0g.
Xiāofēngsǎn 5g + jiědúsìwùtāng 5g + zhēnrénhuómìngyǐnqùchuānshānjiǎ 5-0g + báijí 2-1g + hǎipiāoxiāo 2-1g.	Huángqín 5g + báizhǐ 4-3g + gāncǎo 3-2g + shārén 2g + guālóugēn 2g + jīnyínhuā 2-0g + dàhuáng 0g.
Sǎnzhǒngkuìjiāntāng 5g + lóngdǎnxiègāntāng 2g + zhībódìhuángwán 2g + zǐhuādìdīng 1g + púgōngyīng 1g.	
Jiědúsìwùtāng 5g + xiāngshāliùjūnzǐtāng 2g + báixiānpí 1g + dìhuáng 1g + dìfūzǐ 1g + mǔdānpí 1g + chìsháo 1g + zǐcǎo 1g.	Huángqín 5g + báizhǐ 3g + zhìgāncǎo 2g + shārén 2g + guālóugēn 2g + dàhuáng 0g.

Psychosis (295.4, 295.7), Keratoconjunctivitis sicca (375.15), Fever (D005334), Arthralgia (D018771):

Jiāwèixiāoyáosǎn 5g + qǐjúdìhuángwán 5g + gāncǎoxiǎomàidàzǎotāng 3g + dānshēn 2g + yuǎnzhì 2g + yùjīn 2g.	Báizhǐ 5g + huángqín 5g + zhìgāncǎo 3g + shārén 3g + guālóugēn 2g + dàhuáng 1g + xìxīn 1g.
Jiāwèixiāoyáosǎn 5g + qǐjúdìhuángwán 5g + dānshēn 2-0g + bǎihé 2-0g + yuǎnzhì 2-0g + yùjīn 2-0g + niúxī 2-0g + shíchāngpú 1-0g + diàoténggōu 1-0g + cāngěrzǐ 1-0g.	Huángqín 5g + báizhǐ 5-4g + shārén 4-3g + gāncǎo 4-0g + tiānhuā 2-1g + dàhuáng 1-0g.

Purpura (D011693), Seizure (345.9), Meningitis (322.9), Alopecia (704.0), Leukopenia (288.50), Avascular necrosis (732.3, 733.41, 733.42, 733.43, 733.44), Myocarditis (429.0):

Jiāwèixiāoyáosǎn 5g + zhībódìhuángwán 5g + nǚzhēnzǐ 1g + dānshēn 1g + héshǒuwū 1g + hànliáncǎo 1g.	Huángqín 5g + báizhǐ 3g + gāncǎo 2g + shārén 2g + dàhuáng 0g.
Jiāwèixiāoyáosǎn 5g + qǐjúdìhuángwán 5g + nǚzhēnzǐ 1g + héshǒuwū 1g + hànliáncǎo 1g + tùsīzǐ 1-0g.	Huángqín 5g + báizhǐ 5-4g + zhìgāncǎo 5-2g + shārén 4-2g + tiānhuā 2-0g + dàhuáng 0g.
Yìgānsǎn 5g + guìzhījiālónggǔmǔlìtāng 5g + héshǒuwū 2g + hànliáncǎo 1g + jīxuèténg 1g.	
Dāngguīsháoyàosǎn 5g + xiǎocháihútāng 4g + máxìnggānshítāng 3g + guìzhī 1g + huángqí 1g + púgōngyīng 1g + fángfēng 1g + yuǎnzhì 1g.	

Jiědúsìwùtāng "nourishes Blood, detoxifies, cleans bowels, stops bleeding" and is used for psoriasis and similar disorders (Wang, 2019). Sǎnzhǒngkuìjiāntāng is translated to "deswelling and de-hardening decoction." The pharmacology of Huángqín (cf. Section 1.6) on the central nervous system was reviewed (Eghbaliferiz et al., 2018). Dāngguīsháoyàosǎn "nourishes Blood, modulates the Liver, enhances the Spleen, helps draining" and was shown to ameliorate leukopenia, thrombocytopenia, and the degression of hematocrit after irradiation in mice undergoing treatment with whole-body single X-irradiation (Hsu & Lin, 1996).

3.23 ADULT-ONSET STILL DISEASE

Adult-onset Still disease (AOSD), also known as Wissler-Fanconi syndrome, is an autoinflammatory arthritis characterized by fever, rash, joint pain, and a high white blood cell count. The cause of AOSD is unknown and a combination of genetic predisposition, over-reactive immunity, and environmental exposure is suspected.

Huáihuāsǎn "cleans bowels, stops bleeding, dispels Wind, descends Qi" and is used today for hemorrhoids (Wang, 2019). Guìzhīfúlíngwán (cf. Section 1.62) "activates circulation, resolves stasis, reduces stagnation, dissipates lumps" and is used for disorders of menstruation and other abnormal bleeding from the female genital tract (Wang, 2019). Báizhú was introduced in Section 1.21 to be central nervous system protective in animal models. The herb contains secondary metabolites that are anti-inflammatory (Hai et al., 2023).

TABLE 3.23

GMP Herbal Medicines for a 38-Year-Old Adult with Adult-Onset Still Disease

Adult-onset Still disease (OrphaCode: 829)

A disease with a prevalence of ~5 in 100,000

Not applicable

Skin rash, Pruritus, Arthritis, Joint swelling, Splenomegaly, Fever, Leukocytosis, Restrictive ventilatory defect, Hepatomegaly, Arthralgia, Elevated erythrocyte sedimentation rate, Erythema, Elevated C-reactive protein level, Neutrophilia, Fatigue

Pericarditis, Abdominal pain, Pleuritis, Myalgia, Generalized lymphadenopathy

Meningitis, Elevated hepatic transaminase, Abnormal circulating lipid concentration, Bone marrow hypocellularity, Hepatitis, Myocarditis, Cartilage destruction, Recurrent pharyngitis

Adult, Elderly

Skin rash (782.1), Pruritus (D011537), Fever (D005334), Leukocytosis (D007964), Arthralgia (D018771), Erythema (D005483), Fatigue (D005221):

Xiāofēngsǎn 5g + dāngguīyǐnzǐ 5g + báixiānpí 1g + dìfūzǐ 1g + mǔdānpí 1-0g + chìsháo 1-0g + yìyǐrén 1-0g + gāncǎo 1-0g.

Jiědúsìwùtāng 5g + xiāofēngsǎn 4g + báixiānpí 1g + dìfūzǐ 1g.

Jīngfángbàidúsǎn 5g + dìfūzǐ 1g + jīnchán 1g + huánglián 1g.

Báizhǐ 5g + gāncǎo 4g + shārén 4g + huángqín 4g + tiānhuā 2g + dàhuáng 1g.

Báizhǐ 5g + gāncǎo 5-4g + shārén 4-3g + huángqín 4-2g + guālóugēn 2g + dàhuáng 1-0g.

Abdominal pain (D015746), Myalgia (D063806):

Wǔlíngsǎn 5g + huáihuāsǎn 5g + xiānhècǎo 1-0g + báimáogēn 1-0g + ǒujié 1-0g.

Wǔlíngsǎn 5g + yǐzìtāng 2g + huáihuāsǎn 2g.

Guìzhīfúlíngwán 5g + sānzhǒngkuìjiāntāng 5g + zhēnrénhuómìngyǐn 5-0g + xiàkūcǎo 1 + dānshēn 1-0g + tiānhuā 1-0g + mǔlì 1-0g + bèimǔ 1-0g.

Xuánshēn 5g + dìhuáng 5g + hòupò 5g + zhǐshí 5g + màiméndōng 5g + běishāshēn 4-0g + yùzhú 4-0g + dàhuáng 2-0g.

Meningitis (322.9), Elevated hepatic transaminase (573.9), Myocarditis (429.0):

Jiāwèixiāoyáosǎn 5g + zhìgāncǎotāng 5g + gānlùyǐn 5-0g + shēngmàiyǐn 5-0g + dānshēn 2-1g.

Sìnìtāng 5g + gānlùyǐn 5g + xiāngshāliùjūnzǐtāng 5-0g + mǔdānpí 2-0g + zhīzǐ 2-0g + huánglián 1-0g.

Báizhú 5g + fùzǐ 5g + cháihú 5-0g + báisháo 4g + fúlíng 4g + dǎngshēn 2g + gāncǎo 2-1g + gānjiāng 2-1g + tiānhuā 2-0g + guìzhī 2-0g + huángqín 2-0g + shēngjiāng 2-0g + mǔlì 1-0g + dàhuáng 1-0g.

Zhìgāncǎo 5g + gānjiāng 5g + mùguā 3g + yánhúsuǒ 3g + fùzǐ 3g.

Báizhǐ 5g + shārén 4g + huángqín 4g + gāncǎo 2g + dàhuáng 0g.

3.24 REACTIVE ARTHRITIS

Reactive arthritis is also known as arthritis urethritica, polyarthritis enterica, venereal arthritis, or Fiessinger-Leroy disease. Reactive arthritis is the development of arthritis about two weeks after a bacterial infection, such as a genital infection or gastrointestinal infection. Reactive arthritis is believed to be caused by immune cross reactivity of bacterial antigens with joint tissues.

Qīngwèisǎn, translated to "Stomach-clearing powder," treats the syndrome due to "fire that originates from the stagnant Stomach and burns upward along the meridians." Yǐzìtāng, containing Huángqín and Dàhuáng, "clears heat, purges stagnation, cools Blood, neutralizes toxins" and is used today for hemorrhoids (Wang, 2019). Suānzǎoréntāng "nourishes Blood, calms the mind, clears heat, and removes upsetting." It was shown to improve sleep quality and sleep efficiency among methadone-maintained patients with sleep complaints in a randomized, double-blind, placebo-controlled trial (Chan et al., 2015) and is used for general symptoms and neurotic disorders (Wang, 2019).

TABLE 3.24

GMP Herbal Medicines for a 30-Year-Old Man with Reactive Arthritis

Reactive arthritis (OrphaCode: 29207)

A disease with a prevalence of ~5 in 100,000

Biomarker tested: major histocompatibility complex, class I, B (*HLA-B* / Entrez: 3106) at 6p21.33

Major susceptibility factor: major histocompatibility complex, class I, B (*HLA-B* / Entrez: 3106) at 6p21.33

Multigenic/multifactorial, Not applicable

Conjunctivitis, Hyperkeratosis, Arthritis, Joint swelling, Joint stiffness, Abnormality of the nail, Diarrhea, Osteomyelitis, Arthralgia, Dystrophic fingernails, Recurrent aphthous stomatitis, Cognitive impairment, Enthesitis, Cartilage destruction, Pustule

Abdominal pain, Inflammation of the large intestine, Abnormality of the pleura

Recurrent urinary tract infections, Photophobia, Aortic regurgitation, Pericarditis, Weight loss, Fever, Respiratory insufficiency, Pulmonary fibrosis

Adolescent, Adult, Elderly

Conjunctivitis (372.30), Abnormality of the nail (703), Diarrhea (D003967), Arthralgia (D018771), Recurrent aphthous stomatitis (528.2):

Gānlùyǐn 5g + xǐgānmíngmùtāng 5g + huángliánjiědútāng 5-0g + qīngwèisǎn 5-0g + lóngdǎnxiègāntāng 5-0g.	Júhuā 5g + jílí 5g + chántuì 5g + zhǐqiào 4-0g. Huángqín 5g + báizhǐ 2g + zhìgāncǎo 2g + shārén 2g + júhuā 1g + dàhuáng 0g.
Zīshènmíngmùtāng 5g + huángliánjiědútāng 2g.	Gǒuqǐzǐ 5g + júhuā 5g + dìhuáng 4g +
Qīngwèisǎn 5g + dǎochìsǎn 5-0g + lóngdǎnxiègāntāng 5-0g + tǔfúlíng 1-0g + jīnyínhuā 1-0g + liánqiáo 1-0g + mùzéicǎo 1-0g + xiàkūcǎo 1-0g.	fángfēng 4g + dāngguī 4g + xìxīn 2g + huánglián 2g + dàhuáng 1g.

Abdominal pain (D015746):

Yǐzìtāng 5g + huáihuāsǎn 5-3g + xiānhècǎo 1g + dìyú 1-0g + báimáogēn 1-0g + ǒujiē 1-0g.	Xuánshēn 5g + dìhuáng 5g + hòupò 5g + zhǐshí 5g + màiméndōng 5g + běishāshēn
Yǐzìtāng 5g + huángliánjiědútāng 2g + huáihuāsǎn 2g.	4-0g + yùzhú 4-0g + dàhuáng 1-0g.
Huáihuāsǎn 5g + lóngdǎnxiègāntāng 5g + xiānhècǎo 1g + dìyú 1g.	

Photophobia (D020795), Aortic regurgitation (395.1, 396.3), Weight loss (D015431), Fever (D005334), Pulmonary fibrosis (D011658):

Jiāwèixiāoyáosǎn 5g + gāncǎoxiǎomàidàzǎotāng 5g + cháihújiālónggǔmǔlìtāng 5g + zhībódìhuángwán 5-0g + suānzǎoréntāng 5-0g.	Huángqín 5-4g + báizhǐ 5-3g + zhìgāncǎo 3-2g + shārén 3-2g + guālóugēn 2-0g + tiānhuā 2-0g + xìxīn 1-0g + dàhuáng 0g.
Xuèfǔzhúyūtāng 5g + zhìgāncǎotāng 5g + dānshēn 1g + héhuānpí 1g + yèjiāoténg 1g + yùjīn 1g.	Huángqín 5g + báizhǐ 3g + gāncǎo 2g + shārén 2g + guālóugēn 2-0g + dàhuáng
Tiānwángbǔxīndān 5g + jiāwèixiāoyáosǎn 5g + dānshēn 1g + bǎihé 1g + mǔlì 1g + yèjiāoténg 1g.	1-0g + zhīzǐ 1-0g + liánqiáo 1-0g.
Shēnlíngbáizhúsǎn 5g.	

3.25 WILD TYPE ABeta2M AMYLOIDOSIS

Wild type ABeta2M amyloidosis, also known as dialysis-related amyloidosis, refers to accumulation of misfolded protein fibers, called amyloid fibrils, in the joints of chronic kidney disease patients who undergo long-term hemodialysis. Wild type ABeta2M amyloidosis is caused by aggregates of beta2-microglobulin, which is filtered and degraded by healthy kidneys but not by dialysis.

Fùzǐ (cf. Section 1.16) was shown to be antirheumatic by inhibiting proliferation of human rheumatoid arthritis synovial cells (Wu et al., 2022). Máhuángfùzǐxìxīntāng (cf. Sections 2.2 and 2.41) is used today for migraines (Wang, 2019). Wēilíngxiān and Shēntòngzhúyūtāng were introduced in Section 2.1 for paresthesia. Xiāoyáosǎn was concluded to improve the symptoms of functional gastrointestinal disorders (FGIDs) and reduce recurrence rates in FGIDs patients in a meta-analysis and trial sequential analysis of randomized controlled trials (Liu et al., 2022b). FGIDs are now called disorders of gut-brain interaction.

TABLE 3.25

GMP Herbal Medicines for a 41-Year-Old Adult with Wild Type ABeta2M Amyloidosis

Wild type ABeta2M amyloidosis (OrphaCode: 85446)

A disease with a prevalence of ~4 in 100,000

Not applicable

Arthritis, Neck pain, Shoulder pain

Decreased nerve conduction velocity, Abnormality of the thenar eminence, Paresthesia, Axonal loss, Decreased amplitude of sensory action potentials, Bone cyst, Constrictive median neuropathy, Pain, Dysesthesia

Macroglossia, Dysphagia, Gastrointestinal hemorrhage, Abnormal intestine morphology, Arthropathy, Abnormality of the vertebral endplates, Abnormality of the intervertebral disk

Adult

Neck pain (D019547), Shoulder pain (D020069):

Máhuángfùzǐxìxīntāng 5g + guìzhī 3g + fùzǐ 3-2g + báizhú 2g + wúzhūyú 2g + gānjiāng 2g + gāncǎo 2-0g.	Fùzǐ 5g + gāncǎo 3g + báizhú 3g + báisháo 3g + fúlíng 3g + gānjiāng 3g + guìzhī 3-0g + suānzǎorén 3-0g + dǎngshēn 3-0g + acupuncture.
Máhuángfùzǐxìxīntāng 5g + fùzǐ 3g + guìzhī 3g + dàzǎo 2g + zhìgāncǎo 2g + gānjiāng 2g + zhìgāncǎotāng 2g	Chuānwū 5g + wǔlíngzhī 2g + tiānnánxīng 2g + mùxiāng 2g + gāncǎo 2g + dìlóng 2g + yánhúsuǒ 2g +
Máhuángfùzǐxìxīntāng 5g + fùzǐ 3-2g + guìzhī 3-2g + gānjiāng 3-1g + dàzǎo 2-1g + zhìgāncǎo 2-1g + wēilíngxiān 2-0g.	táorén 2g + huíxiāng 2g + chénpí 2g + dāngguī 2g + acupuncture.

Paresthesia (D010292), Pain (D010146), Dysesthesia (D010292):

Shēntòngzhúyūtāng 5g + dāngguīniántòngtāng 5-0g + huángbò 1-0g + cāngzhú 1-0g + acupuncture.	Wēilíngxiān 5g + chuānshānlóng 5g + sānqī 4g + mùguā 4g + niúxī 4g + hónghuā 4g + huángbò 4g + dàhuáng 2-0g.
Shēntòngzhúyūtāng 5g + shūjīnghuóxuètāng 5-0g + yánhúsuǒ 1-0g + jiānghuáng 1-0g + acupuncture.	Wēilíngxiān 5g + báizhú 3g + qiānghuó 3g + xiāngfù 3g + huángqín 3g + cāngzhú 3g + tiānnánxīng 2g + bànxià 2g + gāncǎo 2g + shēngjiāng 2g + fúlíng 2g + chénpí 2g.

Gastrointestinal hemorrhage (D006471), Abnormal intestine morphology (569.9), Arthropathy (711, 719.90):

Xiāoyáosǎn 5g + gégēntāng 4g + táohéchéngqìtāng 2-0g.	Báizhú 5g + fùzǐ 5g + fúlíng 5g + gānjiāng 5g.
Xiāoyáosǎn 5g + gégēntāng 5g + yǐzìtāng 4-0g.	Huánglián 5g + gégēn 5-0g + huángqín 4-3g + dàhuáng 1-0g.
Gégēnhuángqínhuángliántāng 5g + mùxiāng 1g + bànxià 1g + fúlíng 1g + gégēn 1-0g.	

3.26 PSORIASIS-RELATED JUVENILE IDIOPATHIC ARTHRITIS

Psoriasis-related juvenile idiopathic arthritis, also known as juvenile psoriatic arthritis, is characterized by arthritis accompanied with psoriasis, which is a skin condition marked by raised areas of scaly skin. The cause of psoriasis-related juvenile idiopathic arthritis is unknown and a combination of genetic and environmental factors is proposed to explain the occurrence.

TABLE 3.26

GMP Herbal Medicines for a Ten-Year-Old Child with Psoriasis-Related Juvenile Idiopathic Arthritis

Psoriasis-related juvenile idiopathic arthritis (OrphaCode: 85436)

A disease with a prevalence of ~4 in 100,000

Unknown

Abnormality of tumor necrosis factor secretion

Pruritus, Nail pits, Arthralgia, Autoimmunity, Antinuclear antibody positivity, Psoriasiform dermatitis, Polyarticular arthritis, Finger dactylitis, Toe dactylitis, Oligoarthritis, Enthesitis

(Continued)

TABLE 3.26 *(Continued)*

GMP Herbal Medicines for a Ten-Year-Old Child with Psoriasis-Related Juvenile Idiopathic Arthritis

Uveitis, Skin rash, Limitation of joint mobility, Abnormality of the knee, Abnormality of the wrist, Abnormality of the shoulder, Generalized morning stiffness, Reduced visual acuity, Anterior uveitis, Malar rash, Psoriasiform lesion
Childhood, Adolescent

Pruritus (D011537), Arthralgia (D018771):

Wǔlíngsǎn 5g + zhēnrénhuómìngyǐn 5-0g + jīngfángbàidúsǎn 5-0g + báizhǐ 2-0g + máhuáng 1-0g + bèimǔ 1-0g + gāncǎo 1-0g.	Gāncǎo 5g + báizhǐ 5g + shārén 5-3g + huángqín 5-0g + tiānhuā 3-0g + dàhuáng 1-0g.

Huángliánjiědútāng plus Wǔlíngsǎn was shown to treat dampness-heat pattern type of atopic dermatitis without adverse effects in a parallel, randomized, double-blinded, active-controlled trial (Choi et al., 2012). Báizhǐ (cf. Section 1.7) was shown to attenuate inflammatory pain in mice (Zhu et al., 2022).

3.27 RHEUMATOID FACTOR-POSITIVE POLYARTICULAR JUVENILE IDIOPATHIC ARTHRITIS

Rheumatoid factor-positive polyarticular juvenile idiopathic arthritis, also known as juvenile polyarthritis with rheumatoid factor, is characterized by inflammation of at least five joints in the first six months of the disease with a positive laboratory test of a protein called rheumatoid factor in the blood. Specific causes of the condition, other than autoimmune response, are not known.

Niúxī (cf. Section 3.6) was shown to protect Schwann cells (Li et al., 2021), which are predominant glial cells of the peripheral nervous system (PNS) and are involved in the pathology of inflammatory, metabolic, and degenerative PNS diseases. Chinese herbal medicine combined with acupuncture was concluded, in a systematic review and meta-analysis, to effectively alleviate knee pain, improve knee function, and increase the quality of life in patients with knee osteoarthritis (Yang et al., 2021).

TABLE 3.27

GMP Herbal Medicines for an 11-Year-Old Child with Rheumatoid Factor-Positive Polyarticular Juvenile Idiopathic Arthritis

Rheumatoid factor-positive polyarticular juvenile idiopathic arthritis (OrphaCode: 85435)

A disease with a prevalence of ~4 in 100,000

Unknown

Arthralgia, Rheumatoid factor positive, Polyarticular arthritis

Limitation of joint mobility, Joint swelling, Abnormality of limb bone morphology, Elevated erythrocyte sedimentation rate, Progressive joint destruction, Abnormality of epiphysis morphology, Interphalangeal joint erosions, Elevated C-reactive protein level, Abnormal serum interleukin level, Symetrical distal arthritis, Synovitis

Osteopenia, Reduced bone mineral density, Premature epimetaphyseal fusion, Asymmetric growth
Childhood

Arthralgia (D018771):

Shàngzhōngxiàtōngyòngtòngfēngwán 5g + shūjīnghuóxuètāng 5g + niúxī 1-0g + yánhúsuǒ 1-0g + acupuncture.	Niúxī 5g + huángbò 5g + cāngzhú 5g + bīngláng 5-0g + yìyǐrén 5-0g + dàhuáng 0g.
Shàngzhōngxiàtōngyòngtòngfēngwán 5g + dāngguīniāntòngtāng 5g.	Niúxī 5g + báisháo 5g + guìzhī 5g + gǔsuìbǔ 5g + xùduàn 5g + mùguā 4g + dānggui 4g + mòyào 2g + rǔxiāng 2g.
Shàngzhōngxiàtōngyòngtòngfēngwán 5g + zhènggǔzǐjīndān 5g + acupuncture.	

(Continued)

TABLE 3.27 *(Continued)*
GMP Herbal Medicines for an 11-Year-Old Child with Rheumatoid Factor-Positive Polyarticular Juvenile Idiopathic Arthritis

Synovitis (727.83):

Zhènggǔzǐjīndān 5g + sháoyàogāncǎotāng 5-0g + shūjīnghuóxuètāng 5-0g + mòyào 0g + rǔxiāng 0g + acupuncture.

Shūjīnghuóxuètāng 5g + sháoyàogāncǎotāng 5-0g + mòyào 1-0g + rǔxiāng 1-0g + acupuncture.

Jīnyínhuā 5g + dāngguī 5g + xuánshēn 3g + gāncǎo 3g + niúxī 3-2g + chìsháo 3-2g + dǎodìwúgōng 3-2g + huángqí 3-2g + acupuncture.

Niúxī 5g + báisháo 5g + guìzhī 5g + gǔsuìbǔ 5g + xùduàn 5g + mùguā 4g + dāngguī 4g + mòyào 2g + rǔxiāng 2g + acupuncture.

Gāncǎo 5g + chìsháo 5g + fángfēng 5g + qiānghuó 5g + zhīzǐ 5g + liánqiáo 5g + dāngguī 5g + dàhuáng 1g.

Dāngguī 5g + shúdìhuáng 5g + báisháo 3g + fángjǐ 3g + fángfēng 3g + qiānghuó 3g + táorén 3g + chénpí 3g + cāngzhú 3g.

3.28 ANTISYNTHETASE SYNDROME

Antisynthetase syndrome, also known as anti-Jo1 syndrome, is a chronic autoimmune condition affecting multiple body systems characterized by muscle inflammation, joint inflammation, and interstitial lung disease. Antisynthetase syndrome is caused by autoantibodies mistakenly targeting aminoacyl-tRNA synthetases, which are enzymes in all body cells for RNA translation. Genetic, immune, and environmental factors may combine to trigger the autoimmune response.

TABLE 3.28
GMP Herbal Medicines for a 55-Year-Old Woman with Antisynthetase Syndrome

Antisynthetase syndrome (OrphaCode: 81)

A disease with a prevalence of ~3 in 100,000

Not applicable

Muscle weakness, Respiratory insufficiency, Pulmonary fibrosis, Autoimmunity, Myalgia, Interstitial pulmonary abnormality, Cough, Myositis, Chest pain

Xerostomia, Edema, Keratoconjunctivitis sicca, Hypotonia, Fever, Elevated circulating creatine kinase concentration, EMG abnormality, Lack of skin elasticity

Skin rash, Pruritus, Joint dislocation, Abnormality of the voice, Aortic regurgitation, Dysphagia, Pulmonary arterial hypertension, Recurrent respiratory infections, Neoplasm, Myocarditis, Telangiectasia of the skin

Adult, Elderly

Muscle weakness (D018908), Pulmonary fibrosis (D011658) [Idiopathic pulmonary fibrosis (516.31)], Myalgia (D063806), Cough (D003371), Chest pain (D002637):

Zhìgāncǎotāng 5g + cháixiàntāng 5-0g + shūjīnghuóxuètāng 5-0g + sānqī 1g + dānshēn 1g + chìsháo 1-0g + jiàngzhēnxiāng 1-0g.

Zhēnwǔtāng 5g + fùzǐ 1g + táorén 1g + dǐdāngtāng 0g.

Cháixiàntāng 5g + wēndǎntāng 5g + sānqī 1g + dānshēn 1g + yùjīn 1g.

Báizhú 5g + fúlíng 4g + zhìgāncǎo 3g + fùzǐ 3g + gānjiāng 3g + niúxī 2g + ròuguì 2g + dàhuáng 0g.

Báizhú 5g + fùzǐ 5g + cháihú 5g + báisháo 4g + fúlíng 4g + tiānhuā 2g + dǎngshēn 2g + guìzhī 2g + huángqín 2g + wǔwèizǐ 2-0g + xìxīn 2-0g + shēngjiāng 2-0g + gāncǎo 1g + mǔlì 1g + gānjiāng 1g.

Edema (D004487), Keratoconjunctivitis sicca (375.15), Hypotonia (D009123), Fever (D005334):

Jiāwèixiāoyáosǎn 5g + xiāngshāliùjūnzǐtāng 5g + gégēntāng 2g + shānzhā 1g + héhuānpí 1g.

Jiāwèixiāoyáosǎn 5g + xiāngshāliùjūnzǐtāng 5-4g + bànxiàxièxīntāng 3-2g + héhuānpí 1g + yánhúsuǒ 1-0g + shānzhā 1-0g.

Gǒuqǐzǐ 5g + júhuā 5g + niúbàngzǐ 3g + shègān 3g + xìxīn 1g + huánglián 1g.

Gǒuqǐzǐ 5g + júhuā 5g + dìhuáng 4-3g + dāngguī 4-3g + fángfēng 4-2g + xìxīn 2-1g + huánglián 2-1g + dàhuáng 1-0g.

(Continued)

TABLE 3.28 *(Continued)*
GMP Herbal Medicines for a 55-Year-Old Woman with Antisynthetase Syndrome

Skin rash (782.1), Pruritus (D011537), Aortic regurgitation (395.1, 396.3), Neoplasm (199), Myocarditis (429.0):

Xiāofēngsǎn 5g + dāngguīyǐnzǐ 5g + báixiānpí 1g + dìfūzǐ
  1g + mǔdānpí 1-0g + chìsháo 1-0g + dānshēn 1-0g + tǔfúlíng
  1-0g + kǔshēngēn 1-0g.

Gānlùyǐn 5g + jiědúsìwùtāng 5g + sìnìtāng 2g + mǔdānpí 1g +
  zǐcǎo 1g.

Zhìgāncǎotāng 5g + dāngguīyǐnzǐ 5g + dānshēn 1g + héshǒuwū
  1g + mǔdānpí 1g.

Huángqín 5g + báizhí 4-3g + gāncǎo 2g + shārén 2g +
  guālóugēn 2g + dàhuáng 1-0g.

Huángqín 5g + báizhí 4-2g + zhìgāncǎo 3-2g + shārén
  3-2g + huánglián 1g + guālóugēn 1-0g + dàhuáng 0g.

Cháixiàntāng "moderates Shaoyang, clears heat, dissolves phlegm, widens chest, loosens conge-lation" and is used today for symptoms involving the respiratory system and other chest symptoms such as bronchitis (Wang, 2019). Use of Jiāwèixiāoyáosǎn or Xiāngshāliùjūnzǐtāng was found to be associated with a lower risk of developing chronic kidney disease (CKD) in patients with chronic hepatitis C (Chang et al., 2019). Patients with CKD often have edema. Dāngguīyǐnzǐ, consisting of Dāngguī, "cultivates Blood, moisturizes dryness, dispels Wind and stops itching."

3.29 SYSTEMIC-ONSET JUVENILE IDIOPATHIC ARTHRITIS

Systemic-onset juvenile idiopathic arthritis, also known as Still disease, is chronic arthritis in kids characterized by fever, rash, joint pain, and inflammation of organs such as the spleen, lymph nodes, and liver. Children with systemic-onset juvenile idiopathic arthritis have high levels of

TABLE 3.29
GMP Herbal Medicines for a Two-Year-Old Child with Systemic-Onset Juvenile Idiopathic Arthritis

Systemic-onset juvenile idiopathic arthritis (OrphaCode: 85414)

A disease with a prevalence of ~3 in 100,000

Major susceptibility factor: major histocompatibility complex, class II, DR beta 1 (*HLA-DRB1* / Entrez: 3123) at 6p21.32

Major susceptibility factor: macrophage migration inhibitory factor (*MIF* / Entrez: 4282) at 22q11.23

Major susceptibility factor: interleukin 6 (*IL6* / Entrez: 3569) at 7p15.3

Disease-causing germline mutation(s): laccase domain containing 1 (*LACC1* / Entrez: 144811) at 13q14.11

Multigenic/multifactorial, Unknown

Skin rash, Joint swelling, Fever, Arthralgia, Autoimmunity, Elevated erythrocyte sedimentation rate, Juvenile rheumatoid arthritis, Elevated C-reactive protein level

Lymphadenopathy

Pericarditis, Splenomegaly, Abdominal pain, Pleural effusion, Hepatomegaly, Anterior uveitis

Childhood

Skin rash (782.1), Fever (D005334), Arthralgia (D018771):

Jīngfángbàidúsǎn 5g + dìfūzǐ 1-0g + shéchuángzǐ 1-0g + huánglián
  1-0g + jílí 1-0g + bǎibù 1-0g.

Xiāofēngsǎn 5g + dāngguīyǐnzǐ 5g + báixiānpí 1g + dìfūzǐ 1g + jílí 1g.

Báizhí 5g + gāncǎo 5-4g + shārén 4-3g +
  huángqín 4-0g + guālóugēn 2-0g + huánglián
  1-0g + dàhuáng 1-0g.

Abdominal pain (D015746):

Xiǎojiànzhōngtāng 5g + yùpíngfēngsǎn 5-0g + shānzhā 1-0g + shénqū
  1-0g + màiyá 1-0g + jīnèijīn 1-0g.

Shēnlíngbáizhúsǎn 5g + shānzhā 1g + shénqū 1g + màiyá 1g.

Bǎohéwán 5g.

Xuánshēn 5g + dìhuáng 5g + màiméndōng 5g +
  hòupò 5-1g + zhǐshí 5-1g + dàhuáng 2-0g.

proinflammatory cytokines (interleukin 1 and interleukin 6) rather than autoantibodies in the blood. It is an autoinflammatory disease.

Huángqín, Gāncǎo, and Báizhǐ (Xiāofēngsǎn and Jīngfángbàidúsǎn) were among the top 10 commonly used GMP-concentrated single herb (muti-herb formulas) extract granules for patients with atopic dermatitis in Taiwan (Lin et al., 2019). The herb pair Xuánshēn and Báisháo was identified to be commonly prescribed to cancer patients for the reduction of primary pain and adverse events (Jo et al., 2022).

3.30 POLYARTERITIS NODOSA

Polyarteritis nodosa (PAN), also referred to as Küssmaul-Maier disease, is inflammation of medium-sized arteries characterized by alternating sections of arterial constriction and dilation. The exact cause of PAN is unknown; however, associations of drug use, hepatitis B, and bacterial infection with PAN were reported.

The use of GMP-concentrated Huángqín extract granules was found to be associated with a lower risk of heart failure in hypertensive patients (Liu et al., 2022c). A meta-analysis of randomized controlled trials concluded Xuèfǔzhúyūtāng to be effective for hyperlipidemia (cf. Section 1.70). Gōuténgsǎn "normalizes the Liver, relieves depression, clears heat, and calms the mind." It was shown to protect against cerebral vascular injury in stroke-prone spontaneously hypertensive rats (Yang et al., 2002) and is used for essential hypertension (Wang, 2019).

TABLE 3.30
GMP Herbal Medicines for a 45-Year-Old Man with Polyarteritis Nodosa

Polyarteritis nodosa (OrphaCode: 767)

A disease with a prevalence of ~3 in 100,000

Not applicable

Abnormality of skin morphology

Abnormality of the kidney, Weight loss, Fever, Arthralgia, Myalgia, Peripheral neuropathy, Elevated C-reactive protein level, Polyneuritis

Abnormality of the nervous system, Hypertension, Cutis marmorata, Subcutaneous nodule, Pericarditis, Morphological abnormality of the central nervous system, Abdominal pain, Abnormal lung morphology, Sensory axonal neuropathy, Erythema, Abnormality of the gastrointestinal tract, Abnormality of cardiovascular system morphology, Raynaud phenomenon, Skin ulcer

All ages

Weight loss (D015431), Fever (D005334), Arthralgia (D018771), Myalgia (D063806):

Wǔlíngsǎn 5g + píngwèisǎn 5g.	Gāncǎo 5g + hòupò 5g + zhǐshí 5g + dàhuáng 1-0g.
Lǐzhōngtāng 5g + wǔlíngsǎn 5-0g + fùzǐ 2-0g + fúlíng 2-0g + bànxià 1-0g + shārén 1-0g.	Gāncǎo 5g + báizhú 5g + fúlíng 5g + gānjiāng 5g.
	Gāncǎo 5g + báizhú 5g + báisháo 5g + báibiǎndòu 5g + fúlíng 5g + huángqí 5g + dàzǎo 2g + shēngjiāng 2g.
	Zhìgāncǎo 5g + hòupò 3g + zhǐshí 3g + dàhuáng 0g.

Hypertension (401-405.99), Abdominal pain (D015746), Erythema (D005483), Abnormality of the gastrointestinal tract (520-579.99):

Tiānmágōuténgyǐn 5g + zhībódìhuángwán 5g + xuèfǔzhúyūtāng 5-0g + lóngdǎnxiègāntāng 5-0g + xiàkūcǎo 2-0g.	Huángqín 5g + dānshēn 3-0g + niúxī 3-0g + chìsháo 3-0g + jīnyínhuā 3-0g + huánglián 2-1g + fùzǐ 2-0g + ròuguì 1-0g + dàhuáng 0g.
Tiānmágōuténgyǐn 5g + gōuténgsǎn 5g + zhībódìhuángwán 5-0g + niúxī 1-0g + xiàkūcǎo 1-0g.	Qiānghuó 5g + hòupò 5-3g + zhǐshí 5-3g + huángqín 1-0g + huánglián 1-0g + dàhuáng 0g.
Tiānmágōuténgyǐn 5g + qǐjúdìhuángwán 5g.	

3.31 CUTANEOUS SMALL VESSEL VASCULITIS

Cutaneous small vessel vasculitis, also known as cutaneous hypersensitivity vasculitis, is inflammation of the small blood vessels in the superficial dermis of the skin. The cause of most cases of cutaneous small vessel vasculitis is not known. Bacterial infections, autoimmune diseases, antibiotics, and anti-inflammatory medications may increase the risk for cutaneous small vessel vasculitis.

TABLE 3.31

GMP Herbal Medicines for a 16-Year-Old Adolescent with Cutaneous Small Vessel Vasculitis

Cutaneous small vessel vasculitis (OrphaCode: 889)

A disease with a prevalence of ~3 in 100,000

Not applicable

Cutis marmorata, Purpura, Urticaria, Recurrent skin infections, Fever, Vasculitis, Myalgia, Erythema, Gangrene, Papule Skin rash, Arthralgia

Abnormal oral cavity morphology, Subcutaneous nodule

All ages

Purpura (D011693), Fever (D005334), Myalgia (D063806), Erythema (D005483), Gangrene (D005734):

Wǔlíngsǎn 5g + gāncǎo 1-0g + báisháo 1-0g + huángqín 1-0g + tiáowèichéngqìtāng 1-0g + mázǐrénwán 1-0g + dàhuáng 0g.	Gāncǎo 5g + báizhǐ 5g + shārén 5-3g + huángqín 5-0g + tiānhuā 2-0g + xìxīn 2-0g + guālóugēn 2-0g + huánglián 1-0g + dàhuáng 0g.

Skin rash (782.1), Arthralgia (D018771):

Jīngjièliánqiáotāng 5g + dāngguīyǐnzǐ 5-0g + dìfūzǐ 1g + jílí 1g + tǔfúlíng 1-0g + báixiānpí 1-0g + yìyǐrén 1-0g + chántuì 1-0g + wǔbèizǐ 1-0g + shéchuángzǐ 1-0g + huánglián 1-0g.	Báizhǐ 5g + gāncǎo 5-4g + shārén 4-3g + huángqín 4-2g + guālóugēn 2g + huánglián 1-0g + dàhuáng 1-0g.
Xiāofēngsǎn 5g + dāngguīyǐnzǐ 5g + báixiānpí 1g + dìfūzǐ 1g + jílí 1g + yìyǐrén 1g + tǔfúlíng 1-0g + dānshēn 1-0g + chántuì 1-0g.	

Gāncǎo was introduced in Section 1.1 to be anti-inflammatory and antiallergenic. Báizhǐ was summarized in Section 1.7 to treat conditions including skin disease. Shārén (cf. Section 1.14) was shown to be anti-allergic/inflammatory in mice (Fan et al., 2022) and is used today for peptic ulcers, allergic rhinitis, and psoriasis (Wang, 2020). Jīngjièliánqiáotāng (cf. Section 3.11) in combination with conventional medicine (i.e., adapalene and topical antibiotics) was shown to be more effective than conventional medicine alone for the treatment of inflammatory acne in a randomized controlled trial (Ito et al., 2018).

3.32 WILD TYPE ATTR AMYLOIDOSIS

Wild type ATTR amyloidosis, i.e., senile systemic amyloidosis, is deposition of amyloid fibrils, mainly in the heart, from the precursor protein transthyretin (TTR) that is made in the liver. Normal or wild type TTR is prone to misfolding. Wild type ATTR amyloidosis is therefore an age-related disorder. The A in ATTR stands for amyloidosis.

Mǔlì (cf. Sections 2.2 and 2.6) was shown to lower lipids by downregulating the expression of lipogenic genes in vitro (Tran et al., 2015). Dàfùpí was introduced in Section 2.45 to be hypotensive in rats. However, habitual chewing of betel nut can cause oral leukoplakia and oral submucous fibrosis, leading to oral cancer (Warnakulasuriya & Chen, 2022). Use of Dàfùpí

TABLE 3.32

GMP Herbal Medicines for a 60-Year-Old Man with Wild Type ATTR Amyloidosis

Wild type ATTR amyloidosis (OrphaCode: 330001)

A disease with a prevalence of ~2 in 100,000

Not applicable

Congestive heart failure, Hypertrophic cardiomyopathy, Myocardial infarction, Pleural effusion, Abnormal EKG, Interstitial pulmonary abnormality, Pedal edema, Pulmonary edema

Hepatomegaly, Chronic diarrhea, Intermittent diarrhea, Autonomic dysregulation, Gastrointestinal dysmotility, Bowel incontinence, Elevated alkaline phosphatase, Arrhythmia, Orthostatic hypotension due to autonomic dysfunction, Autonomic bladder dysfunction

Renal insufficiency, Proteinuria, Nephrotic syndrome, Nephropathy, Bradycardia, Weight loss

Adult, Elderly

Congestive heart failure (428, 428.0), Hypertrophic cardiomyopathy (425.1):

Shēngmàiyǐn 5g + zhìgāncǎotāng 5g + xuèfǔzhúyūtāng 5-0g + dānshēn 1-0g + yùjīn 1-0g.	Mǔlì 5g + dàfùpí 4g + gāncǎo 4g + sāngbáipí 4g + hǎipiāoxiāo 4g + jílí 4g + sānléng 3g + wǔlíngzhī 3g + éshù 3g + zǐsūyè 3g + qiánhú 2g + guìzhī 2-0g + sāngzhī 2-0g + bǎibù 2-0g.
Xuèfǔzhúyūtāng 5g + shēngmàiyǐn 5-4g + dānshēn 1g + yùjīn 1g.	Jílí 5g + gāncǎo 4g + yánhúsuǒ 3g + chántuì 3g.
	Gāncǎo 5g + báizhú 5g + fúlíng 5g + gānjiāng 5g + guìzhī 4g + fùzǐ 2g.
	Gāncǎo 5g + bǎibù 5g + yánhúsuǒ 5g + sāngbáipí 5g + jílí 5g + zéxiè 5g.

Renal insufficiency (586), Proteinuria (791.0), Nephrotic syndrome (581), Bradycardia (D001919) [Other specified cardiac dysrhythmias (427.89)], Weight loss (D015431):

Qīngxīnliánzǐyǐn 5g + bìxièfēnqīngyǐn 5-0g + zhūlíngtāng 5-0g + jìshēngshènqìwán 5-0g + tǔfúlíng 1-0g.	Shānyào 5g + dānshēn 5g + dìhuáng 5g + bǎihé 5g + chēqiánzǐ 5g + fúlíng 5g + màiméndōng 5g + huángqí 5g + huángjīng 5-0g + bìxiè 5-0g + zéxiè 5-0g + dǎngshēn 5-0g.
Jìshēngshènqìwán 5g + bìxièfēnqīngyǐn 4g + dānshēn 1g + yìmǔcǎo 1g + zélán 1g.	Zhīmǔ 5g + huángbò 5-4g + gāncǎo 5-3g + chēqiánzǐ 5-0g + dàhuáng 0g + huánglián 0g.
Bìxièfēnqīngyǐn 5g + liùwèidìhuángwán 4g + tǔfúlíng 1g + bìxiè 1g.	Báimáogēn 5g + chìxiǎodòu 3g + chēqiánzǐ 3g + dāngguī 2g.

should therefore be minimized. Jílí (cf. Sections 1.3 and 1.41) was shown to lower serum cholesterol, high density lipid-cholesterol, low density lipid-cholesterol, triglyceride levels, and decrease abdominal aorta endothelial cellular surface damage and rupture in rabbits fed a cholesterol-rich diet (Tuncer et al., 2009). Complementary use of Zhīmǔ or Liùwèidìhuángwán was found to be associated with a lower risk of end-stage renal disease, mortality, and hospitalization in systemic lupus erythematosus patients with chronic kidney disease in Taiwan (Chen et al., 2024).

3.33   EOSINOPHILIC GRANULOMATOSIS WITH POLYANGIITIS

Eosinophilic granulomatosis with polyangiitis (EGPA), also known as Churg-Strauss syndrome or Granulomatous allergic angiitis, is characterized by inflammation of the airways, elevation in blood eosinophil count, and inflammation within small blood vessels. The cause of EGPA is unknown and the risk factors include asthma and allergic rhinitis.

Wǔlínsǎn's indications include urethritis, cystitis, and gonorrhea, and its combination with Bāzhèngsǎn and Dǐdāngtāng was elucidated to be for cystitis patients with blood stasis (Lee et al., 2020). Qínpí (Cortex Fraxini) "clears heat, eliminates dampness, arrests secretion, and improves eyesight." It was shown to be anti-inflammatory and relieved swelling in rats (Zhao et al., 2018) and protected rat pheochromocytoma cells against oxidative damage (Li et al., 2015).

TABLE 3.33
GMP Herbal Medicines for a 42-Year-Old Adult with Eosinophilic Granulomatosis with Polyangiitis

Eosinophilic granulomatosis with polyangiitis (OrphaCode: 183)

A disease with a prevalence of ~2 in 100,000

Not applicable

Sinusitis, Purpura, Urticaria, Congestive heart failure, Weight loss, Eosinophilia, Asthma, Pulmonary infiltrates, Vasculitis, Autoimmunity, Central nervous system degeneration, Peripheral neuropathy, Increased inflammatory response

Hematuria, Hypertension, Skin rash, Hypopigmented skin patches, Gait disturbance, Hypertrophic cardiomyopathy, Abnormal pericardium morphology, Tubulointerstitial nephritis, Dysphagia, Nausea and vomiting, Abdominal pain, Abnormality of the pleura, Arthralgia, Venous thrombosis, Fatigue

Renal insufficiency, Proteinuria, Cutis marmorata, Acrocyanosis, Arthritis, Subcutaneous nodule, Myocardial infarction, Fever, Gastroesophageal reflux, Malabsorption, Respiratory insufficiency, Hemoptysis, Transient ischemic attack, Myalgia, Hemiplegia/hemiparesis, Intestinal obstruction, Recurrent intrapulmonary hemorrhage, Cranial nerve paralysis, Cough, Myocarditis, Nasal polyposis, Endocarditis, Myositis, Glomerulopathy, Papule

Adolescent, Adult, Elderly

Purpura (D011693), Congestive heart failure (428, 428.0), Weight loss (D015431), Eosinophilia (288.3), Asthma (493):

Zhēnwǔtāng 5g + wǔwèizǐ 1g + bànxià 1g + gāncǎo 1g + xìngrén 1g + fúlíng 1g + gānjiāng 1g + xìxīn 1g + máhuáng 1-0g.

Sūzǐjiàngqìtāng 5g + báisháo 2-1g + shēngjiāng 1g.

Gāncǎo 5g + báizhú 5g + fúlíng 5g + gānjiāng 5g + fùzǐ 5-3g.

Guālóurén 5g + dānshēn 3g + bànxià 3g + zhǐshí 3g + guìzhī 3g + xièbái 3g.

Xìngrén 5g + fùzǐ 5g + guìzhī 5g + máhuáng 5g + wǔwèizǐ 4g + gānjiāng 4g + xìxīn 4g.

Hematuria (D006417), Hypertension (401-405.99), Skin rash (782.1), Hypertrophic cardiomyopathy (425.1), Abdominal pain (D015746), Arthralgia (D018771), Fatigue (D005221):

Bāzhèngsǎn 5g + wǔlínsǎn 5g + dǐdāngtāng 5g.

Zhūlíngtāng 5g + zhībódìhuángwán 5-0g + báimáogēn 1g + chēqiánzǐ 1-0g + púgōngyīng 1-0g + jīnyínhuā 1-0g + liánqiáo 1-0g.

Zhūlíngtāng 5g + dǎochìsǎn 4g + báimáogēn 1g + chēqiánzǐ 1-0g + jīnyínhuā 1-0g + liánqiáo 1-0g.

Báimáogēn 5g + chēqiánzǐ 5g + chìxiǎodòu 5-3g + dānggui 5-2g + niúxī 2-0g.

Huángqín 5g + báizhǐ 3g + gāncǎo 2g + shārén 2g + zhīzǐ 2g + liánqiáo 2g + dàhuáng 1g.

Chìxiǎodòu 5g + báimáogēn 3g + chēqiánzǐ 3g + huáshí 2g + púhuáng 2g + dānggui 1g.

Renal insufficiency (586), Proteinuria (791.0), Fever (D005334), Gastroesophageal reflux (530.81), Myalgia (D063806), Intestinal obstruction (560.9), Cranial nerve paralysis (352.9), Cough (D003371), Myocarditis (429.0), Endocarditis (421.9):

Zhūlíngtāng 5g + jìshēngshènqìwán 5g + báimáogēn 1g + chēqiánzǐ 1g + tǔfúlíng 1-0g + jīnqiáncǎo 1-0g + bìxiè 1-0g + dàhuáng 0g.

Wǔlíngsǎn 5g + jìshēngshènqìwán 5g + dānshēn 1g + yìmǔcǎo 1g + zélán 1g + dàhuáng 0g.

Dìhuáng 5g + fúlíng 5g + huángbò 5g + zéxiè 5-4g + qínpí 5-0g.

Fùzǐ 5g + báizhú 5-4g + cháihú 5-4g + báisháo 4-3g + fúlíng 4-3g + tiānhuā 2g + dǎngshēn 2g + guìzhī 2g + huángqín 2g + shēngjiāng 2-0g + gāncǎo 1g + mǔlì 1g + gānjiāng 1g.

3.34 EOSINOPHILIC FASCIITIS

Eosinophilic fasciitis, also known as diffuse fasciitis with eosinophilia or Shulman syndrome, is characterized by eosinophil-mediated inflammation of the tissue underneath the skin and above the muscle called fascia in the arms and legs. The exact cause of eosinophilic fasciitis is not known; however, allergy, infection, toxin, and medication may trigger the abnormal inflammatory reaction behind the condition.

Gāncǎo (cf. Section 1.1) was shown to reduce ear edema in mice through antiinflammation (Kim et al., 2010). However, cases have been reported that excessive intake of Gāncǎo causes edema (Blanpain, 2023; Celik et al., 2012). Chronic consumption of Gāncǎo should be avoided. Wángbùliúxíng (Semen Vaccariae) "moves Blood, opens meridians, induces lactation, eliminates

TABLE 3.34
GMP Herbal Medicines for a 45-Year-Old Adult with Eosinophilic Fasciitis

Eosinophilic fasciitis (OrphaCode: 3165)

A disease with a prevalence of ~1 in 100,000

Unknown

Edema, Acrocyanosis, Subcutaneous nodule, Abnormality of eosinophils, Eosinophilia, Myalgia, Fatigue, Macule, Cellulitis, Muscular edema

Arthritis, Arthralgia

Weight loss, Paresthesia, Fasciitis, Myositis

Adult

Edema (D004487), Eosinophilia (288.3), Myalgia (D063806), Fatigue (D005221), Cellulitis (D002481) [Cellulitis and abscess of unspecified sites (682.9)]:

Lǐzhōngtāng 5g + bànxià 2-0g + shārén 2-0g + fúlíng 2-0g + báisháo 1-0g + guìzhī 1-0g + fùzǐ 1-0g + tiáowèichéngqìtāng 1-0g + dàhuáng 0g.	Gāncǎo 5g + báizhǐ 5g + shārén 5-3g + huángqín 5-0g + dàhuáng 0g.
	Gāncǎo 5g + hòupò 5g + zhǐshí 5g + dàhuáng 1g.
	Gāncǎo 5g + báizhú 5g + fúlíng 5g + gānjiāng 5g.

Arthralgia (D018771):

Shàngzhōngxiàtōngyòngtòngfēngwán 5g + shūjīnghuóxuètāng 5-0g + sháoyàogāncǎotāng 5-0g + niúxī 1-0g + acupuncture.	Niúxī 5g + huángbò 5g + cāngzhú 5g + yìyǐrén 5-0g.
Shàngzhōngxiàtōngyòngtòngfēngwán 5g + dāngguīniāntòngtāng 5-0g + niúxī 1-0g + huángbò 1-0g + cāngzhú 1-0g + yìyǐrén 1-0g + acupuncture.	Chuānwū 5g + shúdìhuáng 5g + gāncǎo 3g + báisháo 3g + máhuáng 3g + huángqí 3g + báijièzǐ 2g + dàhuáng 1g + shēngjiāng 1g + huánglián 0g.
	Cāngzhú 5g + huángbò 2g + niúxī 2g + fángjǐ 2g + bìxiè 2g + dāngguīwěi 2g + guībǎn 2g.

Weight loss (D015431), Paresthesia (D010292), Fasciitis (729.4):

Guìzhītāng 5g + shūjīnghuóxuètāng 5g + acupuncture.	Wángbùliúxíng 5g + sāngbáipí 5g + xiánfēngcǎo 3g + wūyào 3g + gāncǎo 2g + báisháo 2g + hòupò 2g + gānjiāng 2g + huángqín 2g + acupuncture.
Guìzhītāng 5g + yánhúsuǒ 1g + dàhuáng 0g + acupuncture.	
Guìzhītāng 5g + báizhú 1g + fùzǐ 1g.	Báizhú 5g + dāngguī 5g + dǎngshēn 5g + wǔlíngzhī 2g + mǔdānpí 2g + chìsháo 2g + fángfēng 2g + hónghuā 2g + cháihú 2g + táorén 2g + púhuáng 2g.
Guìzhītāng 5g + gégēn 2-1g + dàhuáng 0g.	

carbuncle, promotes urination, and relieves stranguria." It was shown to stimulate mammary development and promote lactation in rats (Shi & Shan, 2011) and is used today for coughs, dyspepsia, absence of menstruation, and so on (Wang, 2020). Sāngbáipí (cf. Section 2.45) "purges the Lung, quells asthma, promotes urination, reduces swelling" and is used for diabetes and skin conditions (Wang, 2020). Xiánfēngcǎo (Herba Bidentis) "reduces inflammation, clears heat, promotes urination" and is used for rhinitis and functional disorder of intestine (Wang, 2020). Wūyào (Radix Linderae) "moves Qi, stops pain, warms the Kidney, dissipates coldness" and is used for gastritis and urinary frequency (Wang, 2020).

3.35   PEDIATRIC SYSTEMIC LUPUS ERYTHEMATOSUS

Pediatric systemic lupus erythematosus is a lifelong, autoantibody-mediated autoimmune condition characterized by joint pain, fever, rash, fatigue, and organ damage that starts in one's childhood. The exact cause of pediatric systemic lupus erythematosus is unknown. Mutations in immune response–related genes such as *STAT4*, *SPP1*, and *IRAK1* increase one's susceptibility to the condition.

Zhūlíngtāng, together with two other formulas, was found to significantly improve bilateral lower-limbs edema and urinary total protein in a patient with lupus nephritis (Wu et al., 2018). Dīngshùxiù (Herba Elephantopus) "clears heat, neutralizes pathogens" and is used for hypertensive heart disease and chronic renal failure (Wang, 2020). Shuǐdīngxiāng (Herba Ludwigiae) "promotes

TABLE 3.35

GMP Herbal Medicines for a 12-Year-Old Child with Pediatric Systemic Lupus Erythematosus

Pediatric systemic lupus erythematosus (OrphaCode: 93552)

A disease with a prevalence of ~1 in 100,000

Major susceptibility factor: signal transducer and activator of transcription 4 (*STAT4* / Entrez: 6775) at 2q32.2-q32.3

Major susceptibility factor: secreted phosphoprotein 1 (*SPP1* / Entrez: 6696) at 4q22.1

Major susceptibility factor: interleukin 1 receptor associated kinase 1 (*IRAK1* / Entrez: 3654) at Xq28

Not applicable

Elevated erythrocyte sedimentation rate, Decreased serum complement C3, Decreased serum complement C4

Abnormality of the urinary system, Renal insufficiency, Proteinuria, Nephrotic syndrome, Nephritis, Hematuria, Abnormality of the skin, Edema, Skin rash, Pericardial effusion, Thrombocytopenia, Leukopenia, Lymphopenia, Microangiopathic hemolytic anemia, Fever, Pleural effusion, Lymphadenopathy, Antinuclear antibody positivity, Antiphospholipid antibody positivity, Abnormality of the gastrointestinal tract, Increased lactate dehydrogenase activity

Oral ulcer, Abnormality of the nervous system, Psychosis, Seizure, Muscle weakness, Arthritis, Ascites, Vomiting, Abdominal pain, Abnormality of the respiratory system, Dyspnea, Hemiplegia, Headache, Systemic lupus erythematosus, Arthralgia, Abdominal distention, Reduced consciousness/confusion, Discoid lupus rash, Malar rash, Lupus anticoagulant, Dark urine

Neonatal, Infancy, Childhood, Adolescent

Renal insufficiency (586), Proteinuria (791.0), Nephrotic syndrome (581), Edema (D004487), Skin rash (782.1), Pericardial effusion (423.0), Thrombocytopenia (287.5), Leukopenia (288.50), Lymphopenia (288.51), Fever (D005334):

Zhūlíngtāng 5g + jìshēngshènqìwán 5-0g + dīngshùxiù 1-0g + báimáogēn 1-0g + yìmǔcǎo 1-0g + zélán 1-0g + shuǐdīngxiāng 1-0g + dōngguāzǐ 1-0g + xiānhècǎo 1-0g + dàhuáng 1-0g.	Chēqiánzǐ 5g + yìmǔcǎo 5g + fúlíng 5g + huángqí 5g + zéxiè 5g + báimáogēn 5-0g + yìyǐrén 5-0g. Gāncǎo 5g + huángbǎ 5g + dàhuáng 0g + huánglián 0g. Báimáogēn 5g + chēqiánzǐ 3g + niúxī 2-0g + dàhuáng 1-0g + huánglián 0g.

Psychosis (295.4, 295.7), Seizure (345.9), Muscle weakness (D018908), Vomiting (D014839), Abdominal pain (D015746), Dyspnea (D004417), Hemiplegia (343.4), Headache (D006261), Systemic lupus erythematosus (710.0), Arthralgia (D018771):

Gāncǎoxiǎomàidàzǎotāng 5g + yìgānsǎn 5g + cháihújiālónggǔmǔlìtāng 5g. Gāncǎoxiǎomàidàzǎotāng 5g + cháihújiālónggǔmǔlìtāng 5-3g + yuǎnzhì 1g + shíchāngpú 1-0g + fúshén 1-0g. Gāncǎoxiǎomàidàzǎotāng 5g + wēndǎntāng 5g + shíchāngpú 1g + mǔlì 1g + yuǎnzhì 1g + lónggǔ 1g.	Gāncǎo 5g + hòupò 5-0g + zhǐshí 5-0g + dàhuáng 1g. Gāncǎo 5g + báizhǐ 5-0g + shārén 5-0g + dàhuáng 1g. Dàhuáng 5g + gāncǎo 5-2g. Xuánshēn 5g + yùzhú 5g + dìhuáng 5g + shāshēn 5g + hòupò 5g + zhǐshí 5g + màiméndōng 5g + dàhuáng 1g.

urination, reduces swelling, clears heat, neutralizes pathogens" and is used for chronic renal failure, hypertensive heart disease, and proteinuria (Wang, 2020). Dōngguāzǐ (Semen Benincasae) "cleans the Lung, dissolves phlegm, reduces carbuncle, removes pus, dries dampness" and is used for chronic rhinitis, coughs, and pruritic disorder (Wang, 2020).

REFERENCES

Adhikari, B., Aryal, B., & Bhattarai, B. R. (2021). A comprehensive review on the chemical composition and pharmacological activities of *Acacia catechu* (L.f.) Willd. *Journal of Chemistry, 2021*, 1–11. https://doi.org/10.1155/2021/2575598

Blanpain, J. (2023). A Licorice-flavored edema: A case report of glycyrrhizic acid toxicity from chronic Licorice root consumption. *Cureus, 15*(1), e34425. https://doi.org/10.7759/cureus.34425

Celik, M. M., Karakuş, A., Zeren, C., Demir, M., Bayaroğulları, H., Duru, M. E., & Al, M. (2012). Licorice induced hypokalemia, edema, and thrombocytopenia. *Human & Experimental Toxicology, 31*(12), 1295–1298. https://doi.org/10.1177/0960327112446843

Chan, Y., Chen, Y., Yang, S., Lo, W., & Lin, J. (2015). Clinical efficacy of traditional Chinese medicine, Suan Zao Ren Tang, for sleep disturbance during methadone maintenance: A randomized, double-blind, placebo-controlled trial. *Evidence-Based Complementary and Alternative Medicine, 2015*, 1–9. https://doi.org/10.1155/2015/710895

Chang, C., Su, Y., Lin, M., & Huang, S. (2019). Chinese herbal medicine ameliorated the development of chronic kidney disease in patients with chronic hepatitis C: A retrospective population-based cohort study. *Evidence-Based Complementary and Alternative Medicine, 2019*, 1–11. https://doi.org/10.1155/2019/5319456

Chen, H., Tung, C., Yu, B., Chang, C., & Chen, Y. (2024). Renal and survival benefits of seventeen prescribed Chinese herbal medicines against oxidative-inflammatory stress in systemic lupus erythematosus patients with chronic kidney disease: A real-world longitudinal study. *Frontiers in Pharmacology, 14*. https://doi.org/10.3389/fphar.2023.1309582

Chen, H., Wu, C., Tsai, Y. Y., Ho, C., Hsieh, M., & Lai, J. (2021). Liu Wei Di Huang Wan and the delay of insulin use in patients with type 2 diabetes in Taiwan: A nationwide study. *Evidence-Based Complementary and Alternative Medicine, 2021*, 1–8. https://doi.org/10.1155/2021/1298487

Chen, Y., Fan, L., Zhang, T., & Liu, X. (2022). Effectiveness of Zhuling decoction on diuretic resistance in patients with heart failure: A randomized, controlled trial. *Journal of Traditional Chinese Medicine, 42*(3), 439–445. https://doi.org/10.19852/j.cnki.jtcm.20220311.003

Chien, S., Chang, W. C., Lin, P. H., Chang, W. P., Hsu, S. C., Chang, J., Wu, Y., Pei, J. K., & Lin, C. H. (2014). A Chinese herbal medicine, Jia-Wei-Xiao-Yao-San, prevents dimethylnitrosamine-induced hepatic fibrosis in rats. *The Scientific World Journal, 2014*, 1–7. https://doi.org/10.1155/2014/217525

Choi, I., Kim, S., Kim, Y., & Yun, Y. (2012). The effect of TJ-15 plus TJ-17 on atopic dermatitis: A pilot study based on the principle of pattern identification. *Journal of Alternative and Complementary Medicine, 18*(6), 576–582. https://doi.org/10.1089/acm.2011.0208

Deng, L., Liu, W., Chen, N., Guo, R., Zhang, D., Ni, J., Li, L., Cai, X., Fan, G., & Zhao, Y. (2022). Tianma Gouteng Decoction regulates oxidative stress and inflammation in AngII-induced hypertensive mice via transcription factor EB to exert anti-hypertension effect. *Biomedicine & Pharmacotherapy, 145*, 112383. https://doi.org/10.1016/j.biopha.2021.112383

Eghbaliferiz, S., Taleghani, A., & Tayarani-Najaran, Z. (2018). Central nervous system diseases and Scutellaria: A review of current mechanism studies. *Biomedicine & Pharmacotherapy, 102*, 185–195. https://doi.org/10.1016/j.biopha.2018.03.021

Fan, Y., Nguyen, T., Piao, C. H., Shin, H. S., Song, C. H., & Chai, O. H. (2022). *Fructus Amomi* extract attenuates nasal inflammation by restoring Th1/Th2 balance and down-regulation of NF-κB phosphorylation in OVA-induced allergic rhinitis. *Bioscience Reports, 42*(3). https://doi.org/10.1042/bsr20212681

Gao, T., Jiang, M., Deng, B., Zhang, Z., Fu, Q., & Fu, C. (2021). Aurantii Fructus: A systematic review of ethnopharmacology, phytochemistry and pharmacology. *Phytochemistry Reviews, 20*(5), 909–944. https://doi.org/10.1007/s11101-020-09725-1

Hai, C. T., Luyen, N. T., Giang, D. H., Minh, B. Q., Trung, N. Q., Chinh, P. T., Hau, D. V., & Dat, N. T. (2023). *Atractylodes macrocephala* rhizomes contain anti-inflammatory sesquiterpenes. *Chemical & Pharmaceutical Bulletin, 71*(6), 451–453. https://doi.org/10.1248/cpb.c22-00779

He, M., Huang, X., Liu, S., Guo, C., Xie, Y., Meijer, A. H., & Wang, M. (2018). The difference between white and red Ginseng: Variations in Ginsenosides and immunomodulation. *Planta Medica, 84*(12/13), 845–854. https://doi.org/10.1055/a-0641-6240

Hsu, H., & Lin, C. (1996). A preliminary study on the radioprotection of mouse hematopoiesis by Dang-Gui-Shao-Yao-San. *Journal of Ethnopharmacology, 55*(1), 43–48. https://doi.org/10.1016/s0378-8741(96)01472-9

Hwang, M., Kim, J. N., Song, H., Lim, B., Kwon, Y. K., & Kim, B. J. (2013). Effects of Lizhong Tang on cultured mouse small intestine interstitial cells of Cajal. *World Journal of Gastroenterology, 19*(14), 2249. https://doi.org/10.3748/wjg.v19.i14.2249

Ito, K., Masaki, S., Hamada, M., Tokunaga, T., Kokuba, H., Tashiro, K., Yano, I., Yasumoto, S., & Imafuku, S. (2018). Efficacy and safety of the traditional Japanese medicine Keigairengyoto in the treatment of acne vulgaris. *Dermatology Research and Practice, 2018*, 1–7. https://doi.org/10.1155/2018/4127303

Jo, H., Seo, J., Choi, S. K., & Lee, D. (2022). East Asian herbal medicine to reduce primary pain and adverse events in cancer patients: A systematic review and meta-analysis with association rule mining to identify core herb combination. *Frontiers in Pharmacology, 12*. https://doi.org/10.3389/fphar.2021.800571

Kim, K. R., Jeong, C., Park, K., Jh, C., Park, J. H. Y., Lim, S. S., & Chung, W. Y. (2010). Anti-inflammatory effects of licorice and roasted licorice extracts on TPA-induced acute inflammation and collagen-induced arthritis in mice. *Journal of Biomedicine and Biotechnology, 2010*, 1–8. https://doi.org/10.1155/2010/709378

Kweon, B., Kim, D., Oh, J., Oh, H., Kim, Y., Mun, Y., Bae, G., & Park, S. (2022). Arecae pericarpium water extract alleviates chronic pancreatitis by deactivating pancreatic stellate cells. *Frontiers in Pharmacology, 13*. https://doi.org/10.3389/fphar.2022.941955

Lee, C., Huan, S. K., Lee, Y., Yeh, Y., Lin, I., & Wang, C. (2020). Prescription patterns of Wu Lin San concentrated extract product for cystitis in Taiwan: A population-based study. *Evidence-Based Complementary and Alternative Medicine, 2020*, 1–9. https://doi.org/10.1155/2020/2605462

Li, J., Zhou, S., Zhang, H., Lam, K. H., Lee, S. M., Yu, P. H., & Chan, S. (2015). Cortex Fraxini (Qingpi) protects rat pheochromocytoma cells against 6-hydroxydopamine-induced apoptosis. *Parkinson's Disease, 2015*, 1–11. https://doi.org/10.1155/2015/532849

Li, M., Zhu, Y., Tang, L., Xu, H., Zhong, J., Peng, W., Yuan, Y., Gu, X., & Wang, H. (2021). Protective effects and molecular mechanisms of *Achyranthes bidentata* polypeptide k on Schwann cells. *Annals of Translational Medicine, 9*(5), 381. https://doi.org/10.21037/atm-20-2900

Li, X., Liang, Q., Sun, Y., Diao, L., Qin, Z., Wang, W., Lü, J., Fu, S., Ma, B., & Yue, Z. (2015). Potential mechanisms responsible for the antinephrolithic effects of an aqueous extract of fructus aurantii. *Evidence-Based Complementary and Alternative Medicine, 2015*, 1–11. https://doi.org/10.1155/2015/491409

Lim, D. W., & Kim, Y. T. (2014). Anti-osteoporotic effects of *Angelica sinensis* (Oliv.) Diels extract on ovariectomized rats and its oral toxicity in rats. *Nutrients, 6*(10), 4362–4372. https://doi.org/10.3390/nu6104362

Lin, P., Chu, C., Chang, F., Huang, Y., Tsai, H., & Yao, T. (2019). Trends and prescription patterns of traditional Chinese medicine use among subjects with allergic diseases: A nationwide population-based study. *World Allergy Organization Journal, 12*(2), 100001. https://doi.org/10.1016/j.waojou.2018.11.001

Lin, X., Zou, X., Hu, H., Sheng, D., Zhu, T., Yin, M., Xia, H., Hu, H., & Hu, H. (2024). Bi Xie Fen Qing Yin decoction alleviates potassium oxonate and adenine induced-hyperuricemic nephropathy in mice by modulating gut microbiota and intestinal metabolites. *Biomedicine & Pharmacotherapy, 170*, 116022. https://doi.org/10.1016/j.biopha.2023.116022

Liu, C., Hung, I., Hsu, C. Y., Hu, K., Chen, Y., & Tsai, M. (2022c). Chinese herbal medicine reduces the risk of heart failure in hypertensive patients: A nationwide, retrospective, cohort study. *Frontiers in Cardiovascular Medicine, 9*. https://doi.org/10.3389/fcvm.2022.922728

Liu, Q., Shi, Z., Zhang, T., Jiang, T., Luo, X., Xiaolan, S., Yang, Y., & Wei, W. (2022b). Efficacy and safety of Chinese herbal medicine Xiao Yao San in functional gastrointestinal disorders: A meta-analysis and trial sequential analysis of randomized controlled trials. *Frontiers in Pharmacology, 12*. https://doi.org/10.3389/fphar.2021.821802

Liu, L., Zhao, Y., Birling, Y., Sun, Y., Shang, Q., Hu, Z., Liu, J., & Liu, Z. (2022a). Effectiveness and safety of Linggui Zhugan decoction for the treatment of premature contraction in patients with coronary heart disease: A systematic review and meta-analysis. *Frontiers in Cardiovascular Medicine, 9*. https://doi.org/10.3389/fcvm.2022.1002378

Liu, X., Wang, X., Xu, X., & Zhang, X. (2019). Purification, antitumor and anti-inflammation activities of an alkali-soluble and carboxymethyl polysaccharide CMP33 from *Poria cocos*. *International Journal of Biological Macromolecules, 127*, 39–47. https://doi.org/10.1016/j.ijbiomac.2019.01.029

Pang, H., Wu, L., Tang, Y., Zhou, G., Qu, C., & Duan, J. (2016). Chemical analysis of the herbal medicine *Salviae miltiorrhizae* Radix et Rhizoma (Danshen). *Molecules, 21*(1), 51. https://doi.org/10.3390/molecules21010051

Pei, J., & Zheng, S. (2017). Hypoglycemic, hypolipidemic and antioxidant effects of Zhuye Shigao Decoction on type 2 diabetes mellitus rats. *Journal of Guangzhou University of Traditional Chinese Medicine*, (6), 729–733. https://pesquisa.bvsalud.org/portal/resource/pt/wpr-611195

Ruqiao, L., Yueli, C., Xuelan, Z., Huifen, L., Xin, Z., Danjie, Z., Le, S., & Yanxue, Z. (2020). Rhizoma *Atractylodis macrocephalae*: A review of photochemistry, pharmacokinetics and pharmacology. *Pharmazie, 75*(2), 42–55. https://pubmed.ncbi.nlm.nih.gov/32213234

Seok, J. K., Kwak, J. Y., Choi, G. W., An, S. M., Kwak, J., Seo, H., Suh, H., & Boo, Y. C. (2016). Scutellaria radix extract as a natural UV protectant for human skin. *Phytotherapy Research, 30*(3), 374–379. https://doi.org/10.1002/ptr.5534

Shan, X., Hong, B., Liu, J., Wang, G., Chen, W., Yu, N., Peng, D., Wang, L., & Zhang, C. (2021). Review of chemical composition, pharmacological effects, and clinical application of *Salviae Miltiorrhizae* Radix et Rhizoma and prediction of its Q-markers]. *Zhongguo Zhong Yao Za Zhi, 46*(21), 5496–5511. [Article in Chinese] https://doi.org/10.19540/j.cnki.cjcmm.20210630.203

Shi, B., & Shan, A. (2011). Dietary *Semen Vaccariae* enhances mammary development and lactation potential in rats. *Journal of Applied Animal Research, 39*(3), 245–247. https://doi.org/10.1080/09712119.2011.588402

Shu, H., Arita, H., Hayashida, M., Zhang, L., An, K. N., Huang, W., & Hanaoka, K. (2010). Anti-hypersensitivity effects of Shu-jing-huo-xue-tang, a Chinese herbal medicine, in CCI-neuropathic rats. *Journal of Ethnopharmacology, 131*(2), 464–470. https://doi.org/10.1016/j.jep.2010.07.004

Song, J., Lee, J., Choi, J., Kim, J., & Park, S. Y. (2011). Effects of Scrophulariae Radix (SR) on allergic contact dermatitis (ACD) induced by DNCB in mice. *The Journal of Korean Medicine Ophthalmology and Otolaryngology and Dermatology, 24*(3), 1–16. [Article in Korean] https://doi.org/10.6114/jkood.2011.24.3.001

Song, M. J., Lim, S., Wang, J., & Kim, H. (2018). The root of *Atractylodes macrocephala* Koidzumi prevents obesity and glucose intolerance and increases energy metabolism in mice. *International Journal of Molecular Sciences, 19*(1), 278. https://doi.org/10.3390/ijms19010278

Sun, L., Di, Y. M., Lu, C., Guo, X., Tang, X., Zhang, A. L., Xue, C. C., & Fan, G. (2020). Additional benefit of Chinese medicine formulae including *Dioscoreae rhizome* (Shanyao) for diabetes mellitus: Current state of evidence. *Frontiers in Endocrinology, 11*. https://doi.org/10.3389/fendo.2020.553288

Sunagawa, M., Takayama, Y., Kato, M., Tanaka, M., Okumo, T., Fukuoka, S., Yamaguchi, K., & Tsukada, M. (2021). Kampo formulae for the treatment of neuropathic pain ~ especially the mechanism of action of *Yokukansan* ~. *Frontiers in Molecular Neuroscience, 14*. https://doi.org/10.3389/fnmol.2021.705023

Tohda, C., Kakihara, Y., Komatsu, K., & Kuraishi, Y. (2000). Inhibitory effects of methanol extracts of herbal medicines on substance P-induced itch-scratch response. *Biological & Pharmaceutical Bulletin, 23*(5), 599–601. https://doi.org/10.1248/bpb.23.599

Tran, N. K. S., Kwon, J. E., Kang, S. C., Shim, S., & Park, T. (2015). *Crassaostrea gigas* oyster shell extract inhibits lipogenesis via suppression of serine palmitoyltransferase. *Natural Product Communications, 10*(2), 1934578X1501000. https://doi.org/10.1177/1934578x1501000236

Tuncer, M., Yaymaci, B., Sati, L., Çayli, S., Acar, G., Altug, T., & Demir, R. (2009). Influence of *Tribulus terrestris* extract on lipid profile and endothelial structure in developing atherosclerotic lesions in the aorta of rabbits on a high-cholesterol diet. *Acta Histochemica, 111*(6), 488–500. https://doi.org/10.1016/j.acthis.2008.06.004

Wang, J., Feng, B., Yang, X., Liu, W., Liu, Y., Zhang, Y., Gui, Y., Li, S., Zhang, Y., & Xiong, X. (2013). Tianma Gouteng Yin as adjunctive treatment for essential hypertension: A systematic review of randomized controlled trials. *Evidence-Based Complementary and Alternative Medicine, 2013*, 1–18. https://doi.org/10.1155/2013/706125

Wang, S.-C. (2019). Therapeutic classes of CHEG formulas. In S.-C. Wang (Ed.), *Clinical herbal prescriptions: Principles and practices of herbal formulations from deep learning health insurance herbal prescription big data* (pp. 16–89). World Scientific Publishing. https://doi.org/10.1142/11211

Wang, S.-C. (2020). Modern therapeutic uses of CHEG herbs and herb pairs. In S.-C. Wang (Ed.), *Veterinary herbal pharmacopoeia* (pp. 35–233). Nova Science Publishers. https://doi.org/10.52305/GHTR1903

Wang, Y., Shi, Y., Zhang, X., Zou, J., Liang, Y., Tai, J., Wang, M., Cui, C., & Guo, D. (2019). A Chinese prescription Chuanxiong Chatiao San for migraine: A systematic review and meta-analysis of randomized controlled trials. *Evidence-Based Complementary and Alternative Medicine, 2019*, 1–17. https://doi.org/10.1155/2019/2301680

Warnakulasuriya, S., & Chen, T. H. H. (2022). Areca nut and oral cancer: Evidence from studies conducted in humans. *Journal of Dental Research, 101*(10), 1139–1146. https://doi.org/10.1177/00220345221092751

Wei, H., Liang, X., Wu, B., Zhang, J., Qin, Y., Luo, G. Q., & Luo, Z. (2015). Antihyperglycemic and antioxidant activity of Fructus hordei Germinatus extract on streptozotocin-induced diabetic rats. *Tropical Journal of Pharmaceutical Research, 14*(9), 1651–1657. https://doi.org/10.4314/tjpr.v14i9.15

Wu, Y., Liu, Y., Zhang, L., Li, W., & Xie, Y. (2022). Aconiti lateralis radix praeparata total alkaloids exert anti-RA effects by regulating NF-κB and JAK/STAT signaling pathways and promoting apoptosis. *Frontiers in Pharmacology, 13*. https://doi.org/10.3389/fphar.2022.980229

Wu, P., Shih, P. H., Kung, Y. Y., Chen, F. P., & Chang, C. (2018). Integrated therapy improve urinary total protein in patients with lupus nephritis: A case report. *Complementary Therapies in Medicine, 39*, 87–91. https://doi.org/10.1016/j.ctim.2018.05.016

Wu, Z., Ren, H., Lai, W., Lin, S., Jiang, R., Ye, T., Shen, Q., Zeng, Q., & Xu, D. (2014). Sclederma of Poria cocos exerts its diuretic effect via suppression of renal aquaporin-2 expression in rats with chronic heart failure. *Journal of Ethnopharmacology, 155*(1), 563–571. https://doi.org/10.1016/j.jep.2014.05.054

Xian, Y., Li, Y., Ip, S., Lin, Z., Lai, X., & Su, Z. (2011). Anti-inflammatory effect of patchouli alcohol isolated from Pogostemonis Herba in LPS-stimulated RAW264.7 macrophages. *Experimental and Therapeutic Medicine, 2*(3), 545–550. https://doi.org/10.3892/etm.2011.233

Xie, J., Xu, D., Wang, C., & Huang, J. (2023). Jiawei Xiaoyao San in treatment of anxiety disorder and anxiety: A review. *Chinese Herbal Medicines, 15*(2), 214–221. https://doi.org/10.1016/j.chmed.2022.12.007

Yang, F., Chen, Y., Lu, Z., Xie, W., Shan, Y. S., Yang, J., & Li, Y. (2021). Treatment of knee osteoarthritis with acupuncture combined with Chinese herbal medicine: A systematic review and meta-analysis. *Annals of Palliative Medicine*, *10*(11), 11430–11444. https://doi.org/10.21037/apm-21-2565

Yang, F., Dong, X., Yin, X., Wang, W., You, L., & Ni, J. (2017). Radix Bupleuri: A review of traditional uses, botany, phytochemistry, pharmacology, and toxicology. *BioMed Research International*, *2017*, 1–22. https://doi.org/10.1155/2017/7597596

Yang, Q., Goto, H., Shimada, Y., Kita, T., Shibahara, N., & Terasawa, K. (2002). Effects of Choto-san on hemorheological factors and vascular function in stroke-prone spontaneously hypertensive rats. *Phytomedicine*, *9*(2), 93–98. https://doi.org/10.1078/0944-7113-00088

Yi, W., Chen, J., Li, Z., Jiang, T., Bi, D., Liu, C., Yang, S., Hu, Y., Gan, L., Tu, H., Huang, H., & Li, J. (2020). Screening of potential biomarkers for Yin-deficiency-heat syndrome based on UHPLC–MS method and the mechanism of Zhibai Dihuang granule therapeutic effect. *Anatomical Record*, *303*(8), 2095–2108. https://doi.org/10.1002/ar.24352

Zhang, L., Xu, Z., Jiang, T., Zhang, J., Huang, P., Tan, J., Chen, G., Yuan, M., Li, Z., Liu, H., Gao, D., Xiao, L., Feng, H., Xu, J., & Xu, H. (2021). Efficacy and safety of Ejiao (Asini Corii Colla) in women with blood deficient symptoms: A randomized, double-blind, and placebo-controlled clinical trial. *Frontiers in Pharmacology*, *12*. https://doi.org/10.3389/fphar.2021.718154

Zhang, T., Wang, Y., & Ciriello, J. (1989). The herbal medicine Tian Ma Gou Teng Yen alters the development of high blood pressure in the spontaneously hypertensive rat. *American Journal of Chinese Medicine*, *17*(03n04), 211–219. https://doi.org/10.1142/s0192415x89000309

Zhao, C., Wang, J., Zou, J., Wu, J.-H., Li, X., Shi, Y., & Wang, C. (2018). Effect of integration of habitat processing and pieces processing on anti-inflammatory of Cortex Fraxini. *World Science and Technology - Modernization of Traditional Chinese Medicine*, (12), 1040–1046. https://pesquisa.bvsalud.org/portal/resource/pt/wpr-752078

Zhao, H., Zeng, S., Chen, L., Sun, Q., Liu, M., Yang, H., Ren, S., Ming, T., Meng, X., & Xu, H. (2021). Updated pharmacological effects of *Lonicerae japonicae flos*, with a focus on its potential efficacy on coronavirus disease–2019 (COVID-19). *Current Opinion in Pharmacology*, *60*, 200–207. https://doi.org/10.1016/j.coph.2021.07.019

Zheng, S., Liu, S., Hou, A., Wang, S., Na, Y., Hu, J., Jiang, H., & Liu, Y. (2022). Systematic review of *Lonicerae japonicae flos*: A significant food and traditional Chinese medicine. *Frontiers in Pharmacology*, *13*. https://doi.org/10.3389/fphar.2022.1013992

Zhou, G., Jiang, Y., Ma, D., Wang, Y., Yang, J., Chen, J., Chi, C., Han, X., Li, Z., & Li, X. (2019). Xiao-Qing-Long Tang prevents cardiomyocyte hypertrophy, fibrosis, and the development of heart failure with preserved ejection faction in rats by modulating the composition of the gut microbiota. *BioMed Research International*, *2019*, 1–17. https://doi.org/10.1155/2019/9637479

Zhu, C., Wang, M., Guo, J., Su, S., Yu, G., Yang, Y., Zhou, Y., & Tang, Z. (2022). *Angelica dahurica* extracts attenuate CFA-induced inflammatory pain via TRPV1 in mice. *Evidence-Based Complementary and Alternative Medicine*, *2022*, 1–12. https://doi.org/10.1155/2022/4684830

4 GMP Herbal Medicine for Rare Neoplastic Diseases

A neoplasm results from an uncoordinated proliferation of cells, manifesting a mass called a tumor. The abnormal tissue growth is driven by altered DNA, at multiple sites of the genome. The alterations can be caused chemically by agents such as tobacco smoke; biologically by infections such as hepatitis viruses; and physically by radiation such as ultraviolet light. If the chemical, biological, and/or physical assault on the body takes place constantly, the affected cells eventually evolve limitless replicative potential in response to the chronic assault, giving rise to cancer. As the DNA alterations occur gradually and accumulate over time, adult-onset cancers are acquired. Childhood neoplasms are, however, usually inherited, predisposing one to early-onset cancers.

The GMP herbal products that are frequently discussed for the rare neoplastic diseases are Rhubarb Root and Rhizome (Dàhuáng), Licorice Root (Gāncǎo), Magnolia Bark (Hòupò), Scutellaria Root (Huángqín), Immature Bitter Orange (Zhǐshí), Processed Licorice Root (Zhìgāncǎo), Cardamon Seed (Shārén), Figwort Root (Xuánshēn), Dahurian Angelica Root (Báizhǐ), White Peony Root (Báisháo), Poria (Fúlíng), Aconite Accessory Root (Fùzǐ), Oyster Shell (Mǔlì), Salvia Root (Dānshēn), Five Ingredient Formula with Poria (Wǔlíngsǎn), Earth Restoring Decoction (Guīpítāng), Cinnamon Twig Decoction (Guìzhītāng), Free and Easy Wanderer Plus (Augmented Rambling Powder; Jiāwèixiāoyáosǎn), Disperse the Swelling and Break the Hardness Decoction (Sǎnzhǒngkuìjiāntāng), Aucklandia, Cardamon and the Six Gentlemen Decoction (Xiāngshāliùjūnzǐtāng), Tonify the Middle and Augment the Qi Decoction (Bǔzhōngyìqìtāng), Lycium, Chrysanthemum and Rehmannia Pill (Qǐjúdìhuángwán), Enrich the Kidneys and Improve Vision Decoction (Zīshènmíngmùtāng), Pogostemon Correct the Qi Powder (Huòxiāngzhèngqìsǎn), Ginseng, Poria and Atractylodes Powder (Shēnlíngbáizhúsǎn), Drive Out Stasis from the Mansion of Blood Decoction (Xuèfǔzhúyūtāng), and Prepared Licorice Decoction (Zhìgāncǎotāng), many of which are known to address complications of cancer or adverse effects of cancer therapy. For example, Wǔlíngsǎn has been used for lymphedema in gynecologic cancer patients after lymphadenectomy (Komiyama et al., 2015; Yoshikawa et al., 2020).

4.1 FOLLICULAR LYMPHOMA

Follicular lymphoma, a cancer of the lymphatic system, is thought to be caused by chromosome abnormalities, such as translocation of *BCL2* oncogene, or gene mutations during division of the lymphocytes called B cells. The abnormal B cells form follicles in lymph nodes. As they grow and spread slowly, it is considered a chronic condition; however, a small percent of the follicular lymphoma cases can transform into a type of fast-growing and aggressive B-cell cancer.

Hòupò (cf. Section 3.13) has traditionally been used to "move Qi" and "dry dampness" over the spleen, stomach, lung, and large intestine meridians. It has pharmacological effects on the digestive system, nervous system, cardiovascular, and cerebrovascular systems (Luo et al., 2019). Zhìgāncǎo is tonifying, as annotated in Section 1.11. Guìzhītāng was formulated for "wind cold damage" characterized by headache, fever, and "exterior deficiency." Bǔzhōngyìqìtāng, containing Huángqí (cf. Section 1.9) and Zhìgāncǎo, benefits Qi and suppresses inflammation (Yang & Yu, 2008). The herbal prescriptions in the table help digestion and immunity of follicular lymphoma patients.

DOI: 10.1201/9781032726625-4

TABLE 4.1

GMP Herbal Medicines for a 60-Year-Old Adult with Follicular Lymphoma

Follicular lymphoma (OrphaCode: 545)

A disease with a prevalence of ~4 in 10,000

Part of a fusion gene: BCL2 apoptosis regulator (*BCL2* / Entrez: 596) at 18q21.33

Major susceptibility factor: major histocompatibility complex, class II, DR beta 1 (*HLA-DRB1* / Entrez: 3123) at 6p21.32

Part of a fusion gene: BCL6 transcription repressor (*BCL6* / Entrez: 604) at 3q27.3

Part of a fusion gene: immunoglobulin heavy locus (*IGH* / Entrez: 3492) at 14q32.33

Multigenic/multifactorial, Not applicable

Weight loss, Fever, Lymphoma, Lymphadenopathy, Night sweats, Mediastinal lymphadenopathy

Splenomegaly, Fatigue

Lymphedema, Meningitis, Pleural effusion, Abnormality of the peritoneum, Skin nodule

Adult

Weight loss (D015431), Fever (D005334):

Guìzhītāng 5g + báisháo 2-0g + gégēn 1-0g + xìngrén 1-0g + hòupò 1-0g + dàhuáng 0g.

Wǔlíngsǎn 5g + báisháo 1-0g + huángqín 1-0g + xiǎochéngqìtāng 1-0g + bànxià 1-0g + shēngjiāng 1-0g.

Wǔlíngsǎn 5g + hòupò 1g + zhǐshí 1g + dàhuáng 0g.

Gāncǎo 5g + hòupò 5-2g + zhǐshí 5-2g + běishāshēn 3-0g + yùzhú 3-0g + dàhuáng 2-0g.

Zhìgāncǎo 5g + hòupò 5g + zhǐshí 5g + xuánshēn 4-0g + dìhuáng 4-0g + màiméndōng 4-0g + dàhuáng 1-0g.

Fatigue (D005221):

Jiāwèixiāoyáosǎn 5g + zhìgāncǎotāng 5g + dānshēn 1g + xiāngfù 1g + yùjīn 1g.

Zhìgāncǎotāng 5g + shēngmàiyǐn 4-0g + bǔzhōngyìqìtāng 3-0g + fùzǐ 1-0g + dānshēn 1-0g.

Zhìgāncǎotāng 5g + língguìshùgāntāng 5g + suānzǎoréntāng 5g + jiāwèixiāoyáosǎn 3g + gégēn 2g + zhǐqiào 1g + guālóurén 1g + màiméndōng 1g + huángqín 1g.

Zhìgāncǎotāng 5g + língguìshùgāntāng 5g + dānshēn 1g + wǔwèizǐ 1-0g + màiméndōng 1-0g + dǎngshēn 1-0g + fùzǐ 1-0g + niúxī 1-0g + chēqiánzǐ 1-0g.

Zhìgāncǎotāng 5g + língguìshùgāntāng 5g + wēndǎntāng 5g + suānzǎoréntāng 5g.

Zhìgāncǎotāng 5g + língguìshùgāntāng 5g + jìshēngshènqìwán 5g + dùzhòng 2g + xùduàn 2g.

Zhìgāncǎo 5g + jiégěng 5g + tiānméndōng 4g + xìngrén 4g + sāngbáipí 4g + màiméndōng 4g + dìgǔpí 2g + huángqín 2g.

Zhìgāncǎo 5g + jiégěng 5-3g + xuánshēn 4-3g + mǔlì 4-3g + bèimǔ 4-3g + liánqiáo 4-2g + shānzhīzǐ 2-0g + zhīzǐ 2-0g + jīnyínhuā 1-0g.

Zhìgāncǎo 5g + xuánshēn 4g + dìhuáng 4g + màiméndōng 4g + dàhuáng 0g.

Zhìgāncǎo 5g + hòupò 5g + zhǐshí 5-3g + dàhuáng 0g.

Meningitis (322.9):

Bǔzhōngyìqìtāng 5g + guīpítāng 5g + sānqī 1-0g + xiānhècǎo 1-0g + dùzhòng 1-0g.

Bǔzhōngyìqìtāng 5g + jìshēngshènqìwán 5g + dānshēn 1g + tiānmá 1g + shíchāngpú 1g + yuǎnzhì 1g.

Bǔzhōngyìqìtāng 5g + dúhuójìshēngtāng 5g + dānshēn 1g + niúxī 1g + dùzhòng 1g.

Liùwèidìhuángwán 5g + shēnlíngbáizhúsǎn 5g + bǔzhōngyìqìtāng 5g + báizhú 1g + huángqí 1g + dǎngshēn 1g.

Xiāngshāliùjūnzǐtāng 5g + shūjīnghuóxuètāng 5g + huòxiāngzhèngqìsǎn 5g + báizhú 1g + fúlíng 1g + yuǎnzhì 1g.

Bànxiàbáizhútiānmátāng 5g + bǔzhōngyìqìtāng 5g + jìshēngshènqìwán 5g + báizhú 1g + fúlíng 1g + zéxiè 1g.

Báizhǐ 5g + zhìgāncǎo 5-4g + shārén 5-4g + huángqín 5-1g + tiānhuā 2-1g + xìxīn 2-0g + dàhuáng 1-0g.

Huángbò 5g + shārén 3g + guībǎn 3g + zhìgāncǎo 2g + fùzǐ 2g.

Mùguā 5g + niúxī 5g + huángbò 5g + cāngzhú 5g + yìyǐrén 5g.

Báisháo 5g + dìhuáng 5g + mǔdānpí 5g + ējiāo 5g + dāngguī 5g + dàzǎo 3-2g + niúxī 3-2g + xiāngfù 3-2g + huángbò 3-2g.

Niúxī 5g + báisháo 5g + guìzhī 5g + gǔsuìbǔ 5g + xùduàn 5-4g + dāngguī 5-4g + mùguā 4g + mòyào 2g + rǔxiāng 2g.

4.2 CLASSIC HODGKIN LYMPHOMA

Classic Hodgkin lymphoma (cHL; classic Hodgkin disease) is characterized by the presence of crippled B lymphocytes, called Reed-Sternberg cells, in the lymph node. The cause of cHL is unknown; however, damage to the B-cell DNA by Epstein-Barr virus or HIV infection is suspected. Table 4.2 shows the prescriptions for cHL patients at age 28, which is the median age of patients with cHL.

Zhìgāncǎotāng contains Zhìgāncǎo and was introduced in Section 3.16 for fatigue. Comparing the prescriptions for fatigue in Tables 4.1 and 4.2, we observe variations in the constituent herbs in the prescriptions. This is because TCM prescriptions are age specific (Wang, 2019). Báizhǐ is used for the skin and pain (cf. Sections 1.4 and 3.1); it is also an antitumor (cf. Section 1.7). The herbal prescriptions in the table are seen to improve the various symptoms of cHL patients.

TABLE 4.2
GMP Herbal Medicines for a 28-Year-Old Adult with Classic Hodgkin Lymphoma

Classic Hodgkin lymphoma (OrphaCode: 391)

A disease with a prevalence of ~3 in 10,000

Candidate gene tested: kelch domain containing 8B (*KLHDC8B* / Entrez: 200942) at 3p21.31

Unknown

Lymphoma, Lymphadenopathy, Cellular immunodeficiency, Fatigue

Hyperhidrosis, Pruritus, Weight loss, Fever, Anorexia, Poor appetite, Cough, Chest pain

Skin rash, Ataxia, Splenomegaly, Migraine, Respiratory insufficiency, Hemoptysis, Hepatomegaly, Bone pain, Neoplasm, Osteolysis, Bone marrow hypocellularity, Peripheral neuropathy

All ages

Fatigue (D005221):

Jiāwèixiāoyáosǎn 5g + zhìgāncǎotāng 5g + wēndǎntāng 5g + fúshén 1g + yuǎnzhì 1g.

Jiāwèixiāoyáosǎn 5g + zhìgāncǎotāng 5g + dānshēn 1g + yùjīn 1g + bǎihé 1-0g + bózǐrén 1-0g + yuǎnzhì 1-0g + xiāngfù 1-0g + yìmǔcǎo 1-0g.

Zhìgāncǎotāng 5g + cháihújiālónggǔmǔlìtāng 4g + dānshēn 1g + yùjīn 1g.

Zhìgāncǎotāng 5g + shēngmàiyǐn 4g + bǔzhōngyìqìtāng 4-0g + dānshēn 1g + xiāngfù 1-0g.

Zhìgāncǎotāng 5g + línggùishùgāntāng 5g + dānshēn 1g + fùzǐ 1g.

Zhìgāncǎotāng 5g + sìnìtāng 3g + mǔdānpí 1g + zhīzǐ 1g.

Zhìgāncǎo 5g + jiégěng 5-3g + xuánshēn 4-2g + bèimǔ 4-2g + liánqiáo 4-2g + mǔlì 4-1g + shègān 2-0g + zhīzǐ 2-0g + shānzhīzǐ 2-0g + jīnyínhuā 1-0g + niúbàngzǐ 1-0g.

Pruritus (D011537), Weight loss (D015431), Fever (D005334), Anorexia (D000855), Cough (D003371), Chest pain (D002637):

Wǔlíngsǎn 5g + báisháo 1g + tiáowèichéngqìtāng 1-0g + huángqín 1-0g + gāncǎo 1-0g + dǐdāngtāng 0g + dàhuáng 0g.

Wǔlíngsǎn 5g + fùzǐ 1g + huángqín 1g + tiáowèichéngqìtāng 0g + dǐdāngtāng 0g.

Gāncǎo 5g + báizhǐ 5g + shārén 5-0g + huángqín 5-0g + guālóugēn 2-0g + tiānhuā 2-0g + xìxīn 2-0g + dàhuáng 1-0g.

Skin rash (782.1), Ataxia (D002524), Migraine (346), Hemoptysis (D006469), Neoplasm (199):

Dāngguīyǐnzǐ 5g + jīngfángbàidúsǎn 5-0g + xiāofēngsǎn 4-0g + báixiānpí 1g + dìfūzǐ 1g + tǔfúlíng 1-0g + mǔdānpí 1-0g + chìsháo 1-0g + liánqiáo 1-0g + jīnchán 1-0g + yìyǐrén 1-0g + zǐcǎogēn 1-0g + acupuncture.

Yuèbìjiāshùtāng 5g + báixiānpí 1g + dìfūzǐ 1g + jīnchán 1g + jílí 1g.

Báizhǐ 5g + gāncǎo 4g + shārén 4g + huángqín 4-0g + tiānhuā 2-0g + dàhuáng 1-0g.

Huángqín 5g + báizhǐ 4g + gāncǎo 3-2g + shārén 3-2g + tiānhuā 2-0g + dàhuáng 0g.

4.3 INDOLENT SYSTEMIC MASTOCYTOSIS

Systemic mastocytosis means there is an excessive number of abnormal mast cells throughout the body, including the skin, bone marrow, liver, spleen, gastrointestinal tract, and lungs. Normal mast cells defend our body by setting off inflammatory reactions to such intruders as allergens and bacteria. Systemic mastocytosis overreacts to such events without a stop, resulting in episodes of persistent allergic reactions. In indolent systemic mastocytosis, the most common and mildest form of systemic mastocytosis, the abnormal mast cells increase slowly.

TABLE 4.3

GMP Herbal Medicines for an 18-Year-Old Adult with Indolent Systemic Mastocytosis

Indolent systemic mastocytosis (OrphaCode: 98848)

A disease with a prevalence of ~3 in 10,000

Not applicable

Abnormality of bone marrow cell morphology, Abnormality of skin morphology, Increased proportion of CD25⁺ mast cells, Abnormal mast cell morphology, Mastocytosis

Osteoporosis, Skin rash, Pruritus, Urticaria, Generalized abnormality of skin, Allergy, Darier's sign, Flushing, Increased serum mast cell beta-tryptase concentration, Abdominal cramps, Maculopapular exanthema

Anaphylactic shock

Adult, Elderly

Osteoporosis (733.0), Skin rash (782.1), Pruritus (D011537):

Qīngshàngfángfēngtāng 5g + jiāwèixiāoyáosǎn 5-4g + zhībódìhuángwán 5-0g + dānshēn 1-0g + báizhǐ 1-0g + chìsháo 1-0g + jīnyínhuā 1-0g + liánqiáo 1-0g + púgōngyīng 1-0g + yìyǐrén 1-0g + sāngbáipí 1-0g.	Báizhǐ 5g + zhìgāncǎo 4g + shārén 4g + tiānhuā 3-0g + huángqín 3-0g + dàhuáng 0g.
	Báizhǐ 5g + shārén 5-4g + gāncǎo 5-3g + huángqín 5-0g + tiānhuā 2-0g + guālóugēn 2-0g + dàhuáng 1-0g.

Jiāwèixiāoyáosǎn and Zhībódìhuángwán were among the most commonly prescribed GMP herbal formulas for osteoporosis in Taiwan (Shih et al., 2012). Qīngshàngfángfēngtāng, whose component herbs include Báizhǐ, Huángqín, and Gāncǎo, "clears heat pathogens affecting the upper body" and is used today for diseases of the sebaceous glands (Wang, 2019). The multi-herb formula prescriptions in the table improve both the bone and skin conditions of the patient.

4.4 HEREDITARY BREAST AND OVARIAN CANCER SYNDROME

Hereditary breast and ovarian cancer syndrome is an inherited condition, with which a person has an increased risk of developing breast or ovarian cancer before the age of 50, and so do his or her family members. The cause of hereditary breast and ovarian cancer syndrome is usually either *BRCA2* or *BRCA1* gene mutations.

TABLE 4.4

GMP Herbal Medicines for a 45-Year-Old Adult with Hereditary Breast and Ovarian Cancer Syndrome

Hereditary breast and ovarian cancer syndrome (OrphaCode: 145)

A disease with a prevalence of ~2 in 10,000

Candidate gene tested: phosphatase and tensin homolog (*PTEN* / Entrez: 5728) at 10q23.31

Candidate gene tested: RAD51 recombinase (*RAD51* / Entrez: 5888) at 15q15.1

Disease-causing germline mutation(s) (loss of function): BRCA2 DNA repair associated (*BRCA2* / Entrez: 675) at 13q13.1

(Continued)

TABLE 4.4 *(Continued)*

GMP Herbal Medicines for a 45-Year-Old Adult with Hereditary Breast and Ovarian Cancer Syndrome

Candidate gene tested: BRCA1 interacting helicase 1 (*BRIP1* / Entrez: 83990) at 17q23.2

Candidate gene tested: checkpoint kinase 2 (*CHEK2* / Entrez: 11200) at 22q12.1

Candidate gene tested: tumor protein p53 (*TP53* / Entrez: 7157) at 17p13.1

Candidate gene tested: MRE11 homolog, double strand break repair nuclease (*MRE11* / Entrez: 4361) at 11q21

Candidate gene tested: nibrin (*NBN* / Entrez: 4683) at 8q21.3

Candidate gene tested: partner and localizer of BRCA2 (*PALB2* / Entrez: 79728) at 16p12.2

Candidate gene tested: BRCA1 associated RING domain 1 (*BARD1* / Entrez: 580) at 2q35

Disease-causing germline mutation(s): RAD51 paralog C (*RAD51C* / Entrez: 5889) at 17q22

Candidate gene tested: RAD50 double strand break repair protein (*RAD50* / Entrez: 10111) at 5q31.1

Disease-causing germline mutation(s): RAD51 paralog D (*RAD51D* / Entrez: 5892) at 17q12

Disease-causing germline mutation(s) (loss of function): BRCA1 DNA repair associated (*BRCA1* / Entrez: 672) at 17q21.31

Autosomal dominant

Abnormality of the fallopian tube, Primary peritoneal carcinoma, Ovarian neoplasm

Breast carcinoma

Melanoma, Neoplasm of the pancreas, Prostate cancer

All ages

Ovarian neoplasm (183.0):

Xiāngshāliùjūnzǐtāng 5g + huòxiāngzhèngqìsǎn 5g + Jiāwèixiāoyáosǎn 5-0g + nǚzhēnzǐ 1g + báizhú 1-0g + fúshén 1-0g + bànzhīlián 1-0g + báihuāshéshécǎo 1-0g + xiàkūcǎo 1-0g.

Xiāngshāliùjūnzǐtāng 5g + cháihúshūgāntāng 5g + huòxiāngzhèngqìsǎn 5g + nǚzhēnzǐ 1g + zhǐqiào 1g + xiàkūcǎo 1g.

Xiāngshāliùjūnzǐtāng 5g + bǔzhōngyìqìtāng 5g + huòxiāngzhèngqìsǎn 5g + nǚzhēnzǐ 1g + báizhú 1g + fúshén 1g.

Xiāngshāliùjūnzǐtāng 5g + shēnlíngbáizhúsǎn 5g + huòxiāngzhèngqìsǎn 5g + nǚzhēnzǐ 1-0g + báihuāshéshécǎo 1-0g + xiàkūcǎo 1-0g + báizhú 1-0g + huángqí 1-0g + fúshén 1-0g + dǎngshēn 1-0g.

Bànzhīlián 5g + báihuāshéshécǎo 5g.

Báisháo 5g + cháihú 5-3g + fúlíng 5-0g + zhìgāncǎo 2g + bànxià 2-0g + xiāngfù 2-0g + yùjīn 2-0g + zhǐshí 1-0g.

Chìxiǎodòu 5g + chēqiánzǐ 5g + yìmǔcǎo 5g + dāngguī 2g + dàhuáng 0g.

Dǎngshēn 5-0g + gégēn 5-0g + zhìgāncǎo 2g + huángqín 2-1g + huánglián 1g + gānjiāng 1-0g.

Neoplasm of the pancreas (157.0, 157.1, 157.2, 157.8), Prostate cancer (185):

Bànzhīlián 5g + báihuāshéshécǎo 5g + xiāngshāliùjūnzǐtāng 5g + zhēnrénhuómìngyǐnqùchuānshānjiǎ 5g.

Sǎnzhǒngkuìjiāntāng 5g + guīpítāng 5g + jīxuèténg 2g.

Sǎnzhǒngkuìjiāntāng 5g + bànzhīlián 2-1g + báihuāshéshécǎo 2-0g + cāngzhú 1-0g + jīxuèténg 1-0g.

Sǎnzhǒngkuìjiāntāng 5g + shíliùwèiliúqìyǐn 4-0g + huáihuā 2-1g + cāngzhú 2-0g.

Bànzhīlián 5g + báihuāshéshécǎo 5-0g + huángqí 1-0g.

Hòupò 5g + zhǐshí 5g + dàhuáng 1g.

Gāncǎo 5g + dàhuáng 0g.

Bànzhīlián, i.e., Herba Scutellariae Barbatae, was shown to induce apoptosis in 11 ovarian cancer cell lines (Powell et al., 2003). Báihuāshéshécǎo, or Herba Hedyotidis, is the most commonly prescribed single herb for colon cancer and breast cancer in Taiwan (Chen et al., 2016). Xiāngshāliùjūnzǐtāng (cf. Section 1.27) relieves dyspepsia (Wang, 2019; Xiao et al., 2012) and has been suggested to be used as an adjunct for cancer patients receiving chemotherapy (Shiah et al., 2023). The prescriptions in the table target cancer and/or cancer-medication side-effects.

4.5   GASTROINTESTINAL STROMAL TUMOR

Gastrointestinal stromal tumor, or gastrointestinal stromal sarcoma, is a tumor of the interstitial cells in the digestive tract, such as the stomach, small intestine, and esophagus. Gastrointestinal stromal tumor can be inherited or sporadic. Its malignancy varies, depending on the site of origin and size of the tumor.

TABLE 4.5
GMP Herbal Medicines for a 12-Year-Old Child with Gastrointestinal Stromal Tumor

Gastrointestinal stromal tumor (OrphaCode: 44890)

A disease with a prevalence of ~1 in 10,000

Disease-causing germline mutation(s) (loss of function): succinate dehydrogenase complex flavoprotein subunit A (*SDHA* / Entrez: 6389) at 5p15.33

Candidate gene tested: succinate dehydrogenase complex iron sulfur subunit B (*SDHB* / Entrez: 6390) at 1p36.13

Candidate gene tested: succinate dehydrogenase complex subunit C (*SDHC* / Entrez: 6391) at 1q23.3

Disease-causing somatic mutation(s): KIT proto-oncogene, receptor tyrosine kinase (*KIT* / Entrez: 3815) at 4q12

Disease-causing germline mutation(s) (gain of function): KIT proto-oncogene, receptor tyrosine kinase (*KIT* / Entrez: 3815) at 4q12

Disease-causing somatic mutation(s): platelet derived growth factor receptor alpha (*PDGFRA* / Entrez: 5156) at 4q12

Autosomal dominant, Not applicable

Neoplasm of the stomach, Sarcoma, Gastrointestinal stroma tumor

Dysphagia, Nausea and vomiting, Constipation, Gastrointestinal hemorrhage, Intestinal obstruction, Fatigue

Skin rash, Abnormality of the liver, Anemia, Neoplasm of the gastrointestinal tract, Irregular hyperpigmentation, Neoplasm of the colon, Neoplasm of the rectum, Esophageal neoplasm, Neoplasm of the small intestine

Childhood, Adolescent, Adult

Neoplasm of the stomach (151, 151.4, 151.5, 151.6):

Xiāngshāliùjūnzǐtāng 5g + shānzhā 1g + shénqū 1g + màiyá 1g.	Hòupò 5g + zhǐshí 5g + xuánshēn 4-0g + dìhuáng 4-0g + màiméndōng 4-0g + běishāshēn 4-0g + yùzhú 4-0g + dàhuáng 1-0g.
Xiāngshāliùjūnzǐtāng 5g + shēnlíngbáizhúsǎn 5g + huòxiāngzhèngqìsǎn 5g + báizhú 1g + dǎngshēn 1g + mùxiāng 1-0g + huángqí 1-0g + pípáyè 1-0g + fúlíng 1-0g.	Xuánshēn 5g + dìhuáng 5g + màiméndōng 5g + hòupò 2-1g + zhǐshí 2-1g + dàhuáng 0g.

Constipation (564.0), Intestinal obstruction (560.9), Fatigue (D005221):

Dàchéngqìtāng 5g.	Gāncǎo 5g + dàhuáng 1g.
Fángfēngtōngshèngsǎn 5g + hòupò 2-0g + zhǐshí 2-0g.	Xuánshēn 5g + dìhuáng 5g + màiméndōng 5g + hòupò 5-2g + zhǐshí 5-2g + yùzhú 5-0g + shāshēn 5-0g + dàhuáng 1-0g.
Rùnchángwán 5g.	
Xiǎojiànzhōngtāng 5g + gāncǎo 2g + dàhuáng 0g.	
Dàcháihútāng 5g + xuánshēn 2g + dìhuáng 2g + màiméndōng 2g + dàhuáng 0g.	

Skin rash (782.1), Abnormality of the liver (573.9), Anemia (285.9), Neoplasm of the gastrointestinal tract (239.0):

Liùwèidìhuángwán 5g + shēnlíngbáizhúsǎn 5g + bǔzhōngyìqìtāng 5g.	Gāncǎo 5g + báizhú 5g + fùzǐ 5g + fúlíng 5g + gānjiāng 5g.
Shēnlíngbáizhúsǎn 5g + bǔzhōngyìqìtāng 5g + guīpítāng 5g + báixiānpí 1g + dìfūzǐ 1g.	Huángqín 5-3g + báizhǐ 5-2g + gāncǎo 5-2g + shārén 5-2g + tiānhuā 3-0g + dàhuáng 0g.
Dāngguīyǐnzǐ 5g + bǔzhōngyìqìtāng 5g + guīpítāng 5g + ējiāo 1g.	Báizhú 5g + fùzǐ 5g + cháihú 5g + báisháo 4g + fúlíng 4g + dǎngshēn 2g + tiānhuā 2g + shēngjiāng 2g + guìzhī 2g + huángqín 2g + gāncǎo 1g + mǔlì 1g + gānjiāng 1g.
Bǔzhōngyìqìtāng 5g + liùwèidìhuángwán 5-4g + guīpítāng 5-4g + ējiāo 1-0g + jīxuèténg 1-0g.	

Hòupò's modern uses include peptic ulcers and disorders in the stomach's function (Wang, 2020). A compound isolated from Hòupò was reviewed and summarized to prevent or inhibit the growth of cancers originating from different organs, including the brain, breast, cervical, colon, liver, lung, prostate, and skin (Ranaware et al., 2018). Dàchéngqìtāng, containing Hòupò, Zhǐshí (cf. Section 3.13), and Dàhuáng (cf. Section 2.17), "purges heat-accumulation" and is used today for disorders of the function of the stomach (Wang, 2019). Liùwèidìhuángwán "nourishes yin of the Liver and Kidney."

4.6 MULTIPLE MYELOMA

Multiple myeloma, also known as plasma cell myeloma, is a cancer of plasma cells, which originate from B cells in the bone marrow to produce antibodies. Overgrowth of plasma cells in the bone marrow disrupts the normal hematopoiesis, bone remodeling and immunity, leading to anemia,

TABLE 4.6

GMP Herbal Medicines for a 60-Year-Old Man with Multiple Myeloma

Multiple myeloma (OrphaCode: 29073)

A disease with a prevalence of ~1 in 10,000

Major susceptibility factor: cyclin D1 (*CCND1* / Entrez: 595) at 11q13.3

Not applicable

Osteopenia, Pathologic fracture

Nephrotic syndrome, Nephropathy, Anemia, Acute kidney injury, Hyperproteinemia, Bone pain, Increased circulating IgG level, Elevated serum creatinine, Generalized muscle weakness, Decreased antibody level in blood, Fatigue

Abnormality of the bladder, Tall stature, Weight loss, Spinal cord compression, Vertebral compression fractures, Hypercalcemia, Increased circulating IgA level, Paresthesia, Abnormality of vitamin B12 metabolism, Functional abnormality of the gastrointestinal tract

Adult

Nephrotic syndrome (581), Anemia (285.9), Decreased antibody level in blood (279.00), Fatigue (D005221):

Jìshēngshènqìwán 5g + guīpítāng 5g + dānshēn 1g + huángqí 1g + jīxuèténg 1-0g.	Shúdìhuáng 5g + shānzhūyú 4g + shānyào 4g + mǔdānpí 4g + fúlíng 4g + zéxiè 4g + ròuguì 2-0g + fùzǐ 2-0g.
Rénshēnyǎngróngtāng 5g + yòuguīwán 5g + dānshēn 1g + ējiāo 1g + tùsīzǐ 1g + jīxuèténg 1g.	Shānzhūyú 5g + shānyào 5g + dānshēn 5g + niúxī 5g + dìhuáng 5g + mǔdānpí 5g + chēqiánzǐ 5g + fúlíng 5g + zéxiè 5g.
Zhēnwǔtāng 5g + guīpítāng 4g + dānshēn 1g + héshǒuwū 1g.	Shānzhūyú 5g + shānyào 5g + niúxī 5g + báizhú 5g + báisháo 5g + sāngjìshēng 5g + fúlíng 5g + tùsīzǐ 5g + huángqí 5g + dǎngshēn 5g.
Qǐjúdìhuángwán 5g + zhūlíngtāng 5g + nǚzhēnzǐ 1g + dānshēn 1g + hànliáncǎo 1g.	Shānzhūyú 5g + shānyào 5g + bājǐtiān 5g + báizhú 5g + ròucōngróng 5g + gǒuqǐzǐ 5g + tùsīzǐ 5g + huángqí 5g + shúdìhuáng 5g + dǎngshēn 5g.

Weight loss (D015431), Hypercalcemia (275.42), Paresthesia (D010292):

Guìzhītāng 5g + xìngrén 1g + hòupò 1g + dàhuáng 0g.	Zhìgāncǎo 5g + hòupò 5g + zhǐshí 5g + dàhuáng 1-0g.
Guìzhītāng 5g + báizhú 2g + fùzǐ 2g + báisháo 2g + fúlíng 2g + dǎngshēn 1g + shēngjiāng 1g + wúzhūyú 1g.	Běishāshēn 5g + hòupò 5g + zhǐshí 5g + yùzhú 5g + xuánshēn 5-0g + dìhuáng 5-0g + màiméndōng 5-0g + dàhuáng 0g.
	Jīnyínhuā 5g + dāngguī 5g + niúxī 2g + xuánshēn 2g + chìsháo 2g + zhìgāncǎo 2g + dǎodìwúgōng 2g + huángqí 2g.

bone pain, and infection. The cause of multiple myeloma is unknown; however, occupations that work with organic solvents, herbicides, and pesticides, such as firefighters, hairdressers, and farmers, have an increased risk of developing multiple myeloma.

Shúdìhuáng wass introduced in Section 1.71 for renal failure and in Section 3.18 for anemia of the mother. Shānzhūyú was introduced in Section 2.18 to be nephroprotective and Shānyào was introduced in Section 3.4 to be antidiabetic. Jìshēngshènqìwán translates to "prosperous life and Kidney Qi pill." It is thus meant for individuals with compromised kidney functions (cf. Sections 1.61 and 3.20).

4.7   DERMATOFIBROSARCOMA PROTUBERANS

Dermatofibrosarcoma protuberans (DFSP) is a tumor in the deep layers of the skin on the torso, arms, legs, head, and neck. DFSP is caused by the fusion of the two genes *COL1A1* and *PDGFB* in the affected skin cells, turning the cells into cancerous cells. DFSP is acquired, not inherited.

Fúxiǎomài, introduced in Section 2.24 to "arrest sweating and clear heat," is used today for generalized hyperhidrosis (Wang, 2020). Residual sweat left on the surface of the skin can cause erythema. For example, idiopathic craniofacial erythema is associated with focal hyperhidrosis. Yùpíngfēngsǎn "benefits Qi, fortifies surface and stops sweating" in order to prevent a common cold.

TABLE 4.7
GMP Herbal Medicines for a 30-Year-Old Adult with Dermatofibrosarcoma protuberans

Dermatofibrosarcoma protuberans (OrphaCode: 31112)

A disease with a prevalence of ~1 in 10,000

Part of a fusion gene: collagen type I alpha 1 chain (*COL1A1* / Entrez: 1277) at 17q21.33

Part of a fusion gene: platelet derived growth factor subunit B (*PDGFB* / Entrez: 5155) at 22q13.1

Not applicable

Thickened skin, Subcutaneous nodule, Neoplasm of the skin, Erythema, Fibrosarcoma

Skin ulcer

All ages

Erythema (D005483):

Yùpíngfēngsǎn 5g + bǔzhōngyìqìtāng 5g + guìzhītāng 5-0g.

Yùpíngfēngsǎn 5g + cāngěrsǎn 5g + shíhúsuī 1g.

Yùpíngfēngsǎn 5g + xiāngshāliùjūnzǐtāng 3g + xīnyí 1g + cāngěrzǐ 1g.

Yùpíngfēngsǎn 5g + guìzhītāng 5g + mǔlì 1g + máhuánggēn 1g.

Fúxiǎomài 5g + dàzǎo 2g + gāncǎo 2-1g + báisháo 2-1g + gānjiāng 2-1g + huángqín 2-0g.

4.8 BENIGN SCHWANNOMA

Benign schwannoma, also known as neurilemmoma or peripheral fibroblastoma, is a benign tumor of the nerve sheath covering peripheral nerves. Benign schwannomas occur sporadically and grow slowly.

Báizhú was introduced in Section 1.21 to be neuroprotective and in Section 3.2 to be anti-hepatotoxic. It "supplements Qi, strengthens the Spleen, dries dampness, helps draining, arrests sweating, and prevents preterm birth." Together with its use patterns from the health insurance claims data, we summarize applications of GMP Báizhú extract granules for the following clinical conditions: heart disease, dermatoses, disorders of intestine, disorders of the nervous system, disorders of function of stomach, chronic liver disease and cirrhosis, conditions of the brain, myoneural disorders, cerebrovascular disease, disorders of joints, diseases of the esophagus, endocrine disorders,

TABLE 4.8
GMP Herbal Medicines for a 55-Year-Old Adult with Benign Schwannoma

Benign schwannoma (OrphaCode: 252164)

A disease with a prevalence of ~6 in 100,000

Not applicable

Abnormal cranial nerve morphology, Vestibular schwannoma, Peripheral schwannoma, Abnormal temporal bone morphology, Abnormality of peripheral nervous system electrophysiology, Schwannoma, Scleral schwannoma

Hearing abnormality, Vertigo, Facial palsy, Allodynia

Abnormal parotid gland morphology, Abnormality of the breast, Abnormality of the adrenal glands, Abnormality of the liver, Abnormality of the larynx, Morphological abnormality of the central nervous system, Abnormal esophagus morphology, Abnormality of fibula morphology, Acute episodes of neuropathic symptoms, Abnormality of the twelfth cranial nerve, Pain, Nasal polyposis, Intestinal polyposis

Adult, Elderly

Vertigo (386.2), Facial palsy (351.0), Allodynia (D006930):

Bǔyánghuánwǔtāng 5g + fùzǐ 3-2g + báizhú 2g + báisháo 2g + fúlíng 2g + dǎngshēn 1g + gānjiāng 1g + guìzhī 1-0g + shēngjiāng 1-0g + gāncǎo 1-0g + dàhuáng 0g.

Báizhú 5g + fùzǐ 5g + cháihú 5g + báisháo 4g + fúlíng 4g + tiānhuā 2g + dǎngshēn 2g + guìzhī 2g + huángqín 2g + wǔwèizǐ 2-0g + xìxīn 2-0g + shēngjiāng 2-0g + gāncǎo 1g + mǔlì 1g + gānjiāng 1g.

Huángbò 5g + shārén 4g + shānzhīzǐ 2g + dìhuáng 2g + bǎihé 2g + dàndòuchǐ 2g + gāncǎo 2g + chìsháo 2g + ējiāo 2g + huángqín 2g + jiānghuáng 2g + jiāngcán 2g + chántuì 2g + dàhuáng 0g + huánglián 0g.

(Continued)

TABLE 4.8 (Continued)
GMP Herbal Medicines for a 55-Year-Old Adult with Benign Schwannoma

Abnormality of the adrenal glands (255.9), Abnormality of the liver (573.9), Pain (D010146):

Jiāwèixiāoyáosǎn 5g + cháihúshūgāntāng 5g + jìshēngshènqìwán 5g.

Jiāwèixiāoyáosǎn 5g + xiāngshāliùjūnzǐtāng 5g + bǔzhōngyìqìtāng 5g + dānshēn 1g + yùjīn 1g.

Jiāwèixiāoyáosǎn 5g + zuǒguīwán 5g + bǔzhōngyìqìtāng 5g + dānshēn 1g.

Bāwèidìhuángwán 5g + jiāwèixiāoyáosǎn 5g + xiāngshāliùjūnzǐtāng 5g + wǔwèizǐ 1g + shíhú 1g + màiméndōng 1g.

Báizhú 5g + báisháo 5g + fúlíng 5g + dǎngshēn 5g + fùzǐ 5-2g. Zhìgāncǎo 5g + gānjiāng 5g + fùzǐ 3g + gǒuqǐzǐ 3g + júhuā 3g.

Zhìgāncǎo 5g + guìzhī 5g + táorén 5g + zhǐqiào 3g + dàhuáng 0g + hónghuā 0g.

Xuánshēn 5g + yùzhú 5g + dìhuáng 5g + hòupò 5g + zhǐshí 5g + màiméndōng 5g + dàhuáng 0g.

Gégēn 5g + báisháo 2g + shígāo 2g + dàzǎo 2g + shēngjiāng 2g + zhìgāncǎo 2g + jīnyínhuā 2g + bòhé 2g + máhuáng 0g.

and intestinal malabsorption. In addition, the symptoms and anatomies Báizhú addresses include back pain, edema, body weight, bone marrow, diarrhea, postoperative pain, bone and bones, lumbar vertebrae, pain, hypoxia, fever, and fatigue. Multiple bioactive compounds in the herb account for the multiple indications of the herb, which is common in TCM phytochemistry and pharmacology. Note that Jiāwèixiāoyáosǎn contains Báizhú, Báisháo, Cháihú, Fúlíng, Zhìgāncǎo, Gānjiāng, and so on.

4.9 CHRONIC MYELOID LEUKEMIA

Chronic myeloid leukemia (CML), also called chronic granulocytic leukemia, is a cancer of the myeloid cells in the bone marrow. CML progresses slowly. Fusion of the two genes *BCR* and *ABL1* in the myeloid stem cells in the bone marrow turns the fused gene products into oncogenic, causing CML. Exposure to radiation increases the risk for CML.

TABLE 4.9
GMP Herbal Medicines for a 63-Year-Old Adult with Chronic Myeloid Leukemia

Chronic myeloid leukemia (OrphaCode: 521)

A disease with a prevalence of ~6 in 100,000

Part of a fusion gene: BCR activator of RhoGEF and GTPase (*BCR* / Entrez: 613) at 22q11.23

Part of a fusion gene: ABL proto-oncogene 1, non-receptor tyrosine kinase (*ABL1* / Entrez: 25) at 9q34.12

Biomarker tested: RUNX family transcription factor 1 (*RUNX1* / Entrez: 861) at 21q22.12

Not applicable

Myeloproliferative disorder

Splenomegaly, Abnormality of blood and blood-forming tissues, Thrombocytopenia, Thrombocytosis, Abnormality of granulocytes, Abnormality of basophils, Fever, Leukocytosis, Poor appetite, Fatigue

Infancy, Childhood, Adolescent, Adult

Abnormality of blood and blood-forming tissues (289.9), Thrombocytopenia (287.5), Fever (D005334), Fatigue (D005221):

Xiōngguījiāoàitāng 5g + guīpítāng 5g + nǚzhēnzǐ 1-0g + dìyú 1-0g + hànliáncǎo 1-0g + xiānhècǎo 1-0g + báimáogēn 1-0g + dìhuáng 1-0g.

Rénshēnyǎngróngtāng 5g + bǔzhōngyìqìtāng 5g + dānshēn 1g + jīxuèténg 1g.

Guīpítāng 5g + xuèfǔzhúyūtāng 4g + dānshēn 1g + jīxuèténg 1g.

Xiānhècǎo 5g + dìhuáng 5g + mǔdānpí 5g + chìsháo 5g + jīnyínhuā 5-0g + liánqiáo 5-0g + zǐcǎo 5-0g + dānguī 5-0g + jīxuèténg 5-0g + gāncǎo 3-0g.

Shúdìhuáng 5g + báizhú 4g + fùzǐ 4g + báisháo 3g + fúlíng 3g + báijièzǐ 2g + dǎngshēn 2g + shēngjiāng 1g + máhuáng 1g + gāncǎo 1-0g + dàhuáng 1-0g + huánglián 0g.

Mǔdānpí 5g + huángbò 5g + shārén 3g + guībǎn 3g + zhìgāncǎo 2g + fùzǐ 2g.

Xiānhècǎo (cf. Section 1.2) "stops bleeding, replenishes deficiency, eliminates stagnation, stops diarrhea, expels parasites" and was demonstrated to have an effect on blood coagulation in humans (Fei et al., 2017). Xiōngguījiāoàitāng "nourishes Blood, stops bleeding, regulates menstruation, prevents miscarriage" and was shown to improve an unstable early pregnancy with uterine bleeding in women diagnosed with threatened abortion (Ushiroyama et al., 2006).

4.10 VON HIPPEL-LINDAU DISEASE

Von Hippel-Lindau disease (VHL), also known as familial cerebelloretinal angiomatosis, is a genetic multisystem disease characterized by the formation of tumors called *hemangioblastomas* in the central nervous system and retina. VHL also develops fluid-filled sacs called *cysts* in such organs as the kidneys and pancreas. VHL is caused by mutations in the *VHL* gene, which functions as a tumor suppressor.

Lóngdǎnxiègāntāng (cf. Section 1.4) was shown to efficiently alleviate the symptoms of auto-immune uveitis in rats through its immunomodulatory effects (Tang et al., 2016). Qiānghuó

TABLE 4.10

GMP Herbal Medicines for a 26-Year-Old Adult with von Hippel-Lindau Disease

Von Hippel-Lindau disease (OrphaCode: 892)

A disease with a prevalence of ~5 in 100,000

Modifying germline mutation: cyclin D1 (*CCND1* / Entrez: 595) at 11q13.3

Disease-causing germline mutation(s): von Hippel-Lindau tumor suppressor (*VHL* / Entrez: 7428) at 3p25.3
Autosomal dominant

Abnormality of the eye

Hypertension, Renal cell carcinoma, Adrenal pheochromocytoma, Cerebellar hemangioblastoma, Retinal capillary hemangioma, Elevated urinary catecholamines

Visual loss, Anxiety, Hyperhidrosis, Pallor, Papilledema, Hypertensive retinopathy, Stroke, Cardiomyopathy, Pancreatic cysts, Palpitations, Abdominal pain, Headache, Vertigo, Elevated circulating catecholamine level, Back pain, Upper limb muscle weakness, Left ventricular dysfunction, Multiple renal cysts, Pancreatic islet cell adenoma, Distal lower limb muscle weakness, Papillary cystadenoma of the epididymis, Limb pain, Arrhythmia, Endolymphatic sac tumor, Pancreatic endocrine tumor, Macular edema

Childhood, Adolescent, Adult

Abnormality of the eye (379.90):

Xǐgānmíngmùtāng 5g + zǐshènmíngmùtāng 5-4g + qǐjúdìhuángwán 5-4g + lóngdǎnxiègāntāng 4-0g + mìmēnghuā 1-0g.

Gǒuqǐzǐ 5g + júhuā 5g + niúbàngzǐ 4g + shègān 4g + xìxīn 1g + huánglián 1g.

Xǐgānmíngmùtāng 5g + zǐshènmíngmùtāng 5g + xiàkūcǎo 1g + mìmēnghuā 1g + gǔjīngcǎo 1g.

Gǒuqǐzǐ 5g + júhuā 5g + dāngguī 5-2g + dìhuáng 4-2g + fángfēng 4-2g + xìxīn 2-1g + huánglián 2-1g.

Xǐgānmíngmùtāng 5g + qǐjúdìhuángwán 4g + mùzéicǎo 1g + chōngwèizǐ 1g + mìmēnghuā 1g + gǔjīngcǎo 1g.

Hypertension (401-405.99):

Tiānmágōuténgyǐn 5g + xuèfǔzhúyūtāng 5-2g + zhǐbódìhuángwán 5-0g + dānshēn 1-0g + xiàkūcǎo 1-0g + gōuténg 1-0g + niúxī 1-0g.

Qiānghuó 5g + hòupò 5-3g + zhǐshí 5-3g + fángfēng 4-0g + huángqín 1-0g + huánglián 1-0g + dàhuáng 1-0g.

Pallor (D010167), Papilledema (362.83, 377.0, 377.01), Hypertensive retinopathy (362.11), Cardiomyopathy (425, 425.9), Abdominal pain (D015746), Headache (D006261), Vertigo (386.2), Back pain (D001416), Left ventricular dysfunction (428, 428.0):

Bǔyánghuánwǔtāng 5g + dúhuójìshēngtāng 5g + mùguā 1g + niúxī 1g + acupuncture.

Júhuā 5g + júhóng 5g + chántuì 4g + bīngláng 2g.

Bǔyánghuánwǔtāng 5-4g + bànxiàbáizhútiānmátāng 5-0g + dānshēn 1g + shíchāngpú 1g + yuǎnzhì 1g + dìlóng 1-0g + sānqī 1-0g + acupuncture.

Júhuā 5g + chántuì 5-3g + jílí 5-0g + zhǐqiào 4-0g + zéxiè 4-0g.

(cf. Section 2.14) was shown to have a vasorelaxant effect on rat aortic rings (Lee et al., 2013). Bǔyánghuánwǔtāng, introduced in Sections 1.71 and 2.36 for brain protection, is used today for late effects of cerebrovascular disease (Wang, 2019). Note that acupuncture is a component of the prescriptions for conditions including pain.

4.11   LI-FRAUMENI SYNDROME

Li-Fraumeni syndrome is characterized by the development of cancer before the age of 45 and multiple cancers throughout the patient's lifetime. Li-Fraumeni syndrome is caused by mutations in the *TP53* gene, dubbed "the guardian of the genome," which is a tumor suppressor gene.

TABLE 4.11

GMP Herbal Medicines for a 17-Year-Old Adolescent with Li-Fraumeni Syndrome

Li-Fraumeni syndrome (OrphaCode: 524)

A disease with a prevalence of ~5 in 100,000

Candidate gene tested: cyclin-dependent kinase inhibitor 2A (*CDKN2A* / Entrez: 1029) at 9p21.3

Modifying germline mutation: MDM2 proto-oncogene (*MDM2* / Entrez: 4193) at 12q15

Disease-causing germline mutation(s): tumor protein p53 (*TP53* / Entrez: 7157) at 17p13.1

Candidate gene tested: checkpoint kinase 2 (*CHEK2* / Entrez: 11200) at 22q12.1

Autosomal dominant

Neoplasm

Breast carcinoma

Leukemia, Lymphoma, Osteosarcoma, Rhabdomyosarcoma, Ependymoma, Adrenocortical carcinoma, Neoplasm of the gastrointestinal tract, Astrocytoma, Stomach cancer, Glioblastoma multiforme, Central primitive neuroectodermal tumor, Choroid plexus carcinoma, Neoplasm of the central nervous system, Colorectal polyposis

All ages

Neoplasm (199):

Gānlùyǐn 5g + qīngwèisǎn 5g + lóngdǎnxiègāntāng 5-0g + tiānhuā 1-0g + xuánshēn 1-0g + shíhú 1-0g.

Xiāngshāliùjūnzǐtāng 5g + shēnlíngbáizhúsǎn 5g + huòxiāngzhèngqìsǎn 5g + báizhú 1g + pípáyè 1g + fúshén 1g.

Lǐzhōngtāng 5g + bǔzhōngyìqìtāng 5-0g + xiǎojiànzhōngtāng 3-0g + qínjiāobiējiǎsǎn 3-0g + fángfēng 2-0g + zhǐqiào 2-0g + jiégěng 2-0g + gānjiāng 2-0g + bànxià 1-0g + shārén 1-0g + fúlíng 1-0g + fùzǐ 1-0g.

Běishāshēn 5g + yùzhú 5g + xuánshēn 5-4g + dìhuáng 5-4g + màiméndōng 5-4g + hòupò 5-2g + zhǐshí 5-2g + dàhuáng 2-0g.

Leukemia (208), Neoplasm of the gastrointestinal tract (239.0):

Sǎnzhǒngkuìjiāntāng 5g + guīpítāng 5g + jīxuèténg 2-0g.

Xiāngshāliùjūnzǐtāng 5g + shēnlíngbáizhúsǎn 5g + huòxiāngzhèngqìsǎn 5g + báizhú 1g + huángqí 1g + dǎngshēn 1-0g + xiàkūcǎo 1-0g.

Xuánshēn 5g + dìhuáng 5g + màiméndōng 5g + zhìgāncǎo 2g + dàhuáng 0g.

Xuánshēn 5g + dìhuáng 5g + màiméndōng 5g + hòupò 5-1g + zhǐshí 5-1g + dàhuáng 0g.

Běishāshēn and Gānlùyǐn were introduced in Section 1.63 for neoplasm. Compounds in Xuánshēn (cf. Sections 1.25 and 3.29) were shown to be cytotoxic to three tumor cell lines: human liver cancer cell line, human non-small-cell lung cancer cell line, and murine mammary carcinoma cell line (Zhou et al., 2022). Use of Xuánshēn or Gānlùyǐn increased the survival of patients with oral cancer compared to non-TCM users (Ben-Arie et al., 2022). Sǎnzhǒngkuìjiāntāng was shown to inhibit proliferation of human breast cancer cells (Hsu et al., 2006), exhibit antitumor effects on colon cancer in mice (Cheng et al., 2010), inhibit proliferation of human pancreatic cancer cells (Su, 2014), and exert antitumor effects on oral cavity squamous cell carcinoma in mice (Hsu et al., 2022).

4.12 MALIGNANT PERITONEAL MESOTHELIOMA

Malignant peritoneal mesothelioma is an aggressive cancer that arises in the lining of the abdomen. Asbestos exposure is known to cause malignant peritoneal mesothelioma in people who are susceptible to developing different cancers after being exposed to mineral fibers.

TABLE 4.12

GMP Herbal Medicines for a 68-Year-Old Adult with Malignant Peritoneal Mesothelioma

Malignant peritoneal mesothelioma (OrphaCode: 168811)

A disease with a prevalence of ~5 in 100,000

Multigenic/multifactorial, Not applicable

Ascites, Abdominal pain, Peritonitis, Neoplasm, Abdominal distention

Weight loss

Abnormality of coagulation, Dyspnea, Ileus, Pedal edema

Adult

Ascites (D001201) [Ascites (789.5)], Abdominal pain (D015746), Neoplasm (199):

Wǔlíngsǎn 5g + dǎoshuǐfúlíngtāng 5g + chēqiánzǐ 1-0g.	Chìxiǎodòu 5g + chēqiánzǐ 5g + yìmǔcǎo 5g + báimáogēn 5-0g + dāngguī 2g + dàhuáng 0g.
Wǔlíngsǎn 5g + píngwèisǎn 5g.	Hòupò 5g + zhǐshí 5g + dàhuáng 0g.
Wǔlíngsǎn 5g + sìnìtāng 5g.	Fùzǐ 5g + bànxià 4g + fúlíng 4g + xìxīn 2g + dàhuáng 0g.
Dǎoshuǐfúlíngtāng 5g + yīnchénwǔlíngsǎn 5-0g + chēqiánzǐ 1g.	

Weight loss (D015431):

Guìzhītāng 5g + shēngjiāng 1-0g + guìzhī 1-0g + báisháo 1-0g + bànxià 1-0g + xìngrén 1-0g + hòupò 1-0g + dàhuáng 0g.	Zhìgāncǎo 5g + hòupò 5-3g + zhǐshí 5-3g + dàhuáng 1-0g.

Abnormality of coagulation (286), Dyspnea (D004417):

Xuèfǔzhúyūtāng 5g + shūjīnghuóxuètāng 5g + dānshēn 1g + mòyào 1g + rǔxiāng 1g + acupuncture.	Hóngqū 5g.
Xuèfǔzhúyūtāng 5g + shūjīnghuóxuètāng 5g + sháoyàogāncǎotāng 3-0g + acupuncture.	Dānshēn 5g + báisháo 5g + dìhuáng 5g + fúlíng 5g + huángjīng 5g + kuǎndōnghuā 3g + báibiǎndòu 3g + qiàncǎo 3g + dāngguī 3g.
Xuèfǔzhúyūtāng 5g + zhìgāncǎotāng 5-0g + dānshēn 1-0g.	Guālóurén 5g + bànxià 4g + xiāngfù 4g + cháihú 4g + shēngjiāng 2g + zhǐshí 2g + chénpí 2g + huángqín 2g + huánglián 2g + gāncǎo 1g.
	Fùzǐ 5g + bànxià 3g + xìxīn 1g + dàhuáng 0g.

Chìxiǎodòu (cf. Section 1.66) "eliminates fluid, dries dampness, soothes blood, drains pus, deswells, de-toxifies" and is used today for skin conditions, leukorrhea, urethral abscess, and so on (Wang, 2020). Dǎoshuǐfúlíngtāng "moves Qi, transforms dampness, induces urination, reduces swelling" and is used today for nephritis and nephropathy (Wang, 2019). Hóngqū (Fermentum Rubrum) was shown to be anti-atherosclerotic in atherosclerotic rats (Gou et al., 2018) and is used for hypercholesterolemia (Wang, 2020). Xuèfǔzhúyūtāng was introduced in Sections 1.70 and 2.45 for disorders of lipoid metabolism.

4.13 NEPHROBLASTOMA

Nephroblastoma, also known as Wilms tumor, is the most common tumor of the kidney in children. Nephroblastoma is usually unilateral. Several nephroblastoma cases are associated with mutations in the *WT1* gene, whose products are a transcription factor regulating growth, differentiation, and death of the cells in the kidney filters.

TABLE 4.13

GMP Herbal Medicines for a Three-Year-Old Child with Nephroblastoma

Nephroblastoma (OrphaCode: 654)

A disease with a prevalence of ~5 in 100,000

Candidate gene tested: BRCA2 DNA repair associated (*BRCA2* / Entrez: 675) at 13q13.1

Biomarker tested: glypican 3 (*GPC3* / Entrez: 2719) at Xq26.2

Disease-causing germline mutation(s): tripartite motif containing 28 (*TRIM28* / Entrez: 10155) at 19q13.43

Disease-causing somatic mutation(s): tripartite motif containing 28 (*TRIM28* / Entrez: 10155) at 19q13.43

Major susceptibility factor: RE1 silencing transcription factor (*REST* / Entrez: 5978) at 4q12

Disease-causing germline mutation(s) (loss of function): thyroid hormone receptor interactor 13 (*TRIP13* / Entrez: 9319) at
    5p15.33

Major susceptibility factor: POU class 6 homeobox 2 (*POU6F2* / Entrez: 11281) at 7p14.1

Disease-causing somatic mutation(s): WT1 transcription factor (*WT1* / Entrez: 7490) at 11p13

Major susceptibility factor: WT1 transcription factor (*WT1* / Entrez: 7490) at 11p13

Role: the phenotype of H19 imprinted maternally expressed transcript (*H19* / Entrez: 283120) at 11p15.5

Major susceptibility factor: DIS3 like 3′-5′ exoribonuclease 2 (*DIS3L2* / Entrez: 129563) at 2q37.1

Autosomal dominant, Not applicable

Abdominal pain, Neoplasm, Nephroblastoma

Aniridia, Hematuria, Hypertension, Weight loss, Fever, Lymphadenopathy, Neoplasm of the liver, Neoplasm of the lung

Childhood

Abdominal pain (D015746), Neoplasm (199):

Wǔlíngsǎn 5g + píngwèisǎn 5-0g + gāncǎo 1-0g.	Gāncǎo 5g + hòupò 5-0g + zhǐshí 5-0g + dàhuáng 1-0g.
Wǔlíngsǎn 5g + báisháo 1-0g + gāncǎo 1-0g + tiáowèichéngqìtāng 0g.	Xuánshēn 5g + dìhuáng 5g + hòupò 5g + zhǐshí 5g + màiméndōng 5g + dàhuáng 1-0g.
Wǔlíngsǎn 5g + bǎohéwán 2-0g + mázǐrénwán 1-0g + gāncǎo 1-0g.	

Aniridia (743.45), Hypertension (401-405.99), Weight loss (D015431), Fever (D005334), Neoplasm of the liver (155.0, 155.2):

Shēnlíngbáizhúsǎn 5g + shānzhā 1g + shénqū 1g + màiyá 1g + huǒmárén 1-0g + jīnèijīn 1-0g.	Hòupò 5g + zhǐshí 5-4g + xuánshēn 4-0g + yùzhú 4-0g + dìhuáng 4-0g + shāshēn 4-0g + màiméndōng 4-0g + dàhuáng 2-0g
Xiǎojiànzhōngtāng 5g + shānzhā 1g + shénqū 1g + màiyá 1g.	
Sìjūnzǐtāng 5g + shānzhā 1g + shénqū 1g + màiyá 1g.	Dàhuáng 5g + gāncǎo 5g + huángqín 5g + huánglián 5g

Píngwèisǎn, containing Hòupò (cf. Sections 3.13, 4.1, and 4.5), "dries dampness, strengthens the Spleen, moves Qi, harmonizes the Stomach" and is often prescribed to middle-aged patients with gastritis, duodenitis, or functional digestive disorders (Wang, 2019). Bǎohéwán (cf. Section 1.39) "digests food, conducts stagnation, strengthens the Spleen, harmonizes the Stomach" and is prescribed to pediatric patients with functional digestive disorders (Wang, 2019).

4.14 UNDIFFERENTIATED PLEOMORPHIC SARCOMA

Undifferentiated pleomorphic sarcoma (UPS) is a connective tissue cancer whose cell type is uncertain and tumor morphology is variable. UPS is aggressive and can occur in any part of the body, including the arms, thighs, and back of the abdomen. The cause of UPS is unknown.

Xīnyísǎn "dispels wind and cold, clears the nose and orifice" and is used today for allergic rhinitis (cf. Section 1.33). The TCM syndrome that Wǔlíngsǎn treats is due to "unresolved external pathogens in the body causing dysregulation of water metabolism and thus storage of water in the lower body." Patients with this so-called "internal water retention syndrome" can manifest headache, fever, thirst, fatigue, dizziness, vomiting, dysuria, and edema. Wǔlíngsǎn is formulated to help "urinate by enhancing the bladder Qi; regulate water metabolism by strengthening the Spleen yang; and transport fluid to the mouth for thirst quenching and to the skin for perspiration induction."

TABLE 4.14

GMP Herbal Medicines for a 60-Year-Old Adult with Undifferentiated Pleomorphic Sarcoma

Undifferentiated pleomorphic sarcoma (OrphaCode: 2023)

A disease with a prevalence of ~5 in 100,000

Not applicable

Abnormality of the peritoneum, Abnormality of the lower limb, Soft tissue sarcoma, Abnormal test result

Fever, Abnormality of the musculature

Weight loss, Anorexia, Abnormality of the upper limb, Fatigue

Childhood, Adolescent, Adult, Elderly

Fever (D005334):	
Wǔlíngsǎn 5g + xīnyíqīngfèitāng 5g + jīngfángbàidúsǎn 5-0g + bèimǔ 1-0g. Wǔlíngsǎn 5g + xīnyísǎn 5g + jīngfángbàidúsǎn 5-0g + bèimǔ 1-0g. Wǔlíngsǎn 5g + píngwèisǎn 5g.	Gāncǎo 5g + báizhǐ 5g + shārén 5-3g + huángqín 5-0g + tiānhuā 2-0g + xìxīn 2-0g + guālóugēn 2-0g + dàhuáng 1-0g.
Weight loss (D015431), Anorexia (D000855), Fatigue (D005221):	
Wǔlíngsǎn 5g + bànxià 1-0g. Guìzhītāng 5g + xìngrén 1-0g + hòupò 1-0g + shēngjiāng 1-0g + báisháo 1-0g + dàhuáng 0g.	Gāncǎo 5g + hòupò 5-0g + zhǐshí 5-0g + dàhuáng 1-0g. Zhìgāncǎo 5g + hòupò 5-3g + zhǐshí 5-3g + dàhuáng 1-0g.

4.15 OSTEOSARCOMA

Osteosarcoma, also called osteogenic sarcoma, is cancer of the bone. Osteosarcoma usually occurs in the end of the bone around the knee, hip, shoulder, and jaw where new bone grows. Osteosarcoma is caused by mutations in the *TP53* gene, which encodes a tumor suppressor.

TABLE 4.15

GMP Herbal Medicines for a 17-Year-Old Adolescent with Osteosarcoma

Osteosarcoma (OrphaCode: 668)

A disease with a prevalence of ~5 in 100,000

Candidate gene tested: checkpoint kinase 2 (*CHEK2* / Entrez: 11200) at 22q12.1

Candidate gene tested: RB transcriptional corepressor 1 (*RB1* / Entrez: 5925) at 13q14.2

Disease-causing somatic mutation(s): tumor protein p53 (*TP53* / Entrez: 7157) at 17p13.1

Disease-causing germline mutation(s): tumor protein p53 (*TP53* / Entrez: 7157) at 17p13.1

Not applicable

Osteolysis, Abnormality of the femoral metaphysis

Abnormality of the metaphysis, Joint swelling, Elevated alkaline phosphatase, Abnormality of the tibial metaphysis, Pain, Increased lactate dehydrogenase activity, Abnormal lactate dehydrogenase activity

Childhood

Pain (D010146):	
Wǔlíngsǎn 5g + shūjīnghuóxuètāng 5g + acupuncture. Shūjīnghuóxuètāng 5g + acupuncture. Wǔlíngsǎn 5g + zhènggǔzǐjīndān 5g + sǎnzhǒngkuìjiāntāng 5-0g + yánhúsuǒ 1-0g.	Gāncǎo 5g + jīnyínhuā 5g + dāngguī 3g + chìsháo 2g + dǎodìwúgōng 2g + huángqí 2g + xuánshēn 2g + acupuncture. Gāncǎo 5g + báizhǐ 5g + shārén 5g + huángqín 5g + dàhuáng 0g + acupuncture. Gāncǎo 5g + báisháo 5g + shíhú 5g + chēqiánzǐ 5g + fúlíng 5g + màiméndōng 5g + huángqí 5g + dǎngshēn 5g. Gāncǎo 5g + chìsháo 5g + fángfēng 5g + qiānghuó 5g + zhīzǐ 5g + liánqiáo 5g + dāngguī 5g + dàhuáng 1g. Niúxī 5g + báisháo 5g + guìzhī 5g + gǔsuìbǔ 5g + xùduàn 5g + mùguā 4g + dāngguī 4g + mòyào 2g + rǔxiāng 2g.

Shíhú (Caulis Dendrobii) "nourishes yin, clears heat, benefits the Stomach, generates saliva" and was summarized to be anti-inflammatory, antibacterial, antioxidant, antitumor, immune regulating, blood pressure lowering, and blood sugar regulating (Zhao et al., 2022). Acupuncture was concluded to be effective, compared to sham or no acupuncture control, for the relief of chronic pain, including back and neck pain, osteoarthritis, chronic headache, and shoulder pain (Vickers et al., 2012). The pain relief effect of acupuncture was also shown to be immediate, i.e., within 30 minutes of first acupuncture treatment, without serious adverse effects (Xiang et al., 2017).

4.16 MEDULLARY THYROID CARCINOMA

Medullary thyroid carcinoma (MTC) is a neuroendocrine tumor originating from the so-called C cells in the medulla of the thyroid gland. MTC can spread to lymph nodes and other organs. Most MTC cases occur sporadically.

TABLE 4.16

GMP Herbal Medicines for a 45-Year-Old Woman with Medullary Thyroid Carcinoma

Medullary thyroid carcinoma (OrphaCode: 1332)

A disease with a prevalence of ~5 in 100,000

Not applicable

Medullary thyroid carcinoma

Elevated calcitonin, Nodular goiter

Hyperhidrosis, Diarrhea, Dysphagia, Lymphadenopathy

Dysphonia, Weight loss, Pheochromocytoma, Primary hyperparathyroidism, Neoplasm of the skeletal system, Abnormal liver parenchyma morphology, Neoplasm of the lung

Adult

Diarrhea (D003967):

Gégēnhuángqínhuángliántāng 5g + mùxiāng 1-0g + bànxià 1-0g + fúlíng 1-0g + dàhuáng 0g.

Gégēn 5g + bànxià 2g + zhìgāncǎo 2g + fúlíng 2g + huángqín 2g + huánglián 2g + dàhuáng 0g.
Gégēn 5g + huánglián 3-2g + huángqín 2g + dàhuáng 0g.
Huánglián 5g.

Dysphonia (D055154), Weight loss (D015431), Primary hyperparathyroidism (252.01):

Guìzhītāng 5g + bànxià 1-0g + báisháo 1-0g + jiégěng 1-0g + dàhuáng 0g.
Sānzhǒngkuìjiāntāng 5g + shíliùwèiliúqìyǐn 4g + xuánshēn 1g + mǔlì 1g + bèimǔ 1g + xiàkūcǎo 1g.
Jiégěngtāng 5g + xuánshēn 1g + mǔlì 1g + bèimǔ 1g + dàzǎo 1g + shēngjiāng 1g + zhīzǐ 1g + liánqiáo 1g + dàhuáng 0g.

Xuánshēn 5g + mǔlì 5g + bèimǔ 5g + zhìgāncǎo 5g + jiégěng 5g + liánqiáo 4g + shānzhīzǐ 2-0g + xìngrén 2-0g + zhīzǐ 2-0g.
Gāncǎo 5g + jiégěng 5g + xuánshēn 3-2g + mǔlì 3-2g + bèimǔ 3-2g + liánqiáo 3-2g + zhīzǐ 2g + dàhuáng 0g.

Gégēn (Radix Puerariae Lobatae) "releases muscles, reduces fever, lets out skin eruptions, generates saliva, arrests thirst, lifts yang, and stops diarrhea." Gégēnhuángqínhuángliántāng "resolves exterior and interior, clears heat, stops diarrhea" and is used for gastritis and duodenitis (Wang, 2019). Jiégěngtāng, introduced in Section 2.57 for symptoms involving head and neck, was shown to protect against acute lung injury in mice (Liu et al., 2019).

4.17 UVEAL MELANOMA

Uveal melanoma, also known as choroidal melanoma or iris melanoma, is an intraocular malignancy arising from the melanocytes in the choroid, ciliary body, or iris. The cause of uveal melanoma is unknown; however, ultraviolet light exposure and mutations in the *BAP1* gene, whose products form part of a tumor suppressor, increase the risk of uveal melanoma.

TABLE 4.17
GMP Herbal Medicines for a 55-Year-Old Adult with Uveal Melanoma

Uveal melanoma (OrphaCode: 39044)

A disease with a prevalence of ~5 in 100,000

Disease-causing somatic mutation(s): cysteinyl leukotriene receptor 2 (*CYSLTR2* / Entrez: 57105) at 13q14.2

Disease-causing germline mutation(s): BRCA1 associated protein 1 (*BAP1* / Entrez: 8314) at 3p21.1

Disease-causing somatic mutation(s): BRCA1 associated protein 1 (*BAP1* / Entrez: 8314) at 3p21.1

Disease-causing somatic mutation(s): G protein subunit alpha q (*GNAQ* / Entrez: 2776) at 9q21.2

Disease-causing somatic mutation(s): G protein subunit alpha 11 (*GNA11* / Entrez: 2767) at 19p13.3

Biomarker tested: splicing factor 3b subunit 1 (*SF3B1* / Entrez: 23451) at 2q33.1

Not applicable

Visual loss, Abnormal fundus morphology, Choroidal melanoma

Retinal detachment, Iris melanoma, Ciliary body melanoma

Abnormality of refraction, Vitreous hemorrhage, Ocular hypertension, Inferior lens subluxation, Zonular cataract, Mydriasis, Metamorphopsia, Photopsia, Abnormal visual accommodation

Adult

Retinal detachment (361.9):

Zīshènmíngmùtāng 5g + qǐjúdìhuángwán 4g + xǐgānmíngmùtāng 4-0g + mùzéicǎo 1-0g + juémíngzǐ 1-0g + mìménghuā 1-0g + gǔjīngcǎo 1-0g.	Júhuā 5g + jílí 5-4g + chántuì 5-4g + zhǐqiào 4g.
Zīshènmíngmùtāng 5g + jiāwèixiāoyáosǎn 4-3g + qǐjúdìhuángwán 4-0g + xuèfǔzhúyūtāng 3-0g + yèjiāoténg 2-0g + mùxiāng 1-0g + xiàkūcǎo 1-0g + dānshēn 1-0g.	Gǒuqǐzǐ 5g + júhuā 5g + niúbàngzǐ 4-3g + shègān 4-3g + xìxīn 1g + huánglián 1g.

Vitreous hemorrhage (D014823), Metamorphopsia (D014786):

Zīshènmíngmùtāng 5g + xǐgānmíngmùtāng 4g + qǐjúdìhuángwán 4-0g + chēqiánzǐ 1-0g + juémíngzǐ 1-0g + mìménghuā 1-0g.	Chántuì 5g + zhǐqiào 4-0g + jílí 4-0g + júhóng 4-0g.
Zīshènmíngmùtāng 5g + língguìshùgāntāng 4g + chēqiánzǐ 1g + tùsīzǐ 1g.	Jílí 5g + chántuì 5g + zhǐqiào 4-0g.

Niúbàngzǐ (cf. Section 2.23) "dispels wind-heat, lets out skin eruptions, benefits throat, neutralizes pathogens, reduces swelling" and was demonstrated to have a preventive and therapeutic effect on diabetic retinopathy in rats (Zhang et al., 2020). Mùzéicǎo (Herba Equiseti Hiemalis) was reported to have been employed topically to the inner surface of the eyelid for trachoma since the disease spread into China around the time of the Tang dynasty (Chen, 1981).

4.18 KAPOSI SARCOMA

Kaposi sarcoma is an endothelial cancer arising in the cells that line the blood vessels or lymphatic vessels. Depending on the affected part of the body, Kaposi sarcoma can result in severe health problems or no symptoms. Kaposi sarcoma is caused by infection with an oncogenic virus called *human gammaherpesvirus 8*, which is also known as Kaposi's sarcoma–associated herpesvirus.

TABLE 4.18
GMP Herbal Medicines for a 60-Year-Old Man with Kaposi Sarcoma

Kaposi sarcoma (OrphaCode: 33276)

A disease with a prevalence of ~5 in 100,000

Not applicable

Recurrent herpes

Hypermelanotic macule, Abnormality of the lower limb, Neoplasm of the skin, Macule

Abnormal retinal morphology, Hemangioma, Encephalopathy, Abnormality of the spleen, Immunodeficiency, Lymphoproliferative disorder, Generalized lymphadenopathy, Abnormality of the gastrointestinal tract, Papule, Skin nodule

(Continued)

TABLE 4.18 *(Continued)*

GMP Herbal Medicines for a 60-Year-Old Man with Kaposi Sarcoma

Skin rash, Lymphedema, Abnormality of the liver, Weight loss, Fever, Diarrhea, Abnormal lung morphology, Venous insufficiency, Neoplasm by anatomical site, Fatigue, Skin plaque

Adult

Abnormal retinal morphology (362.9), Hemangioma (228.00), Encephalopathy (348.30, 348.9), Immunodeficiency (279.3), Abnormality of the gastrointestinal tract (520-579.99):

Qǐjúdìhuángwán 5g + jiāwèixiāoyáosǎn 5-4g + dānshēn 1g + nǚzhēnzǐ 1-0g + hànliáncǎo 1-0g + tiānmá 1-0g + shíchāngpú 1-0g + yuǎnzhì 1-0g.

Qǐjúdìhuángwán 5g + bǔyánghuánwǔtāng 5g + nǚzhēnzǐ 1g + dānshēn 1g + hànliáncǎo 1g + cǎojuémíng 1g + acupuncture.

Qǐjúdìhuángwán 5g + zīshènmíngmùtāng 5g + dānshēn 1g + tiānmá 1g + shíchāngpú 1-0g + yuǎnzhì 1-0g + chōngwèizǐ 1-0g + nǚzhēnzǐ 1-0g + hànliáncǎo 1-0g + juémíngzǐ 1-0g.

Dāngguī 5g + báijièzǐ 1-0g + mòyào 1-0g + rǔxiāng 1-0g + jīngjiè 1-0g + jīnèijīn 1-0g + biējiǎ 1-0g.

Báizhú 5g + fùzǐ 5g + cháihú 5g + báisháo 4g + fúlíng 4g + tiānhuā 2g + shēngjiāng 2g + dǎngshēn 2g + guìzhī 2g + yīnchén 2g + huángqín 2g + gāncǎo 1g + mǔlì 1g + gānjiāng 1g.

Huángqí 5g + chìsháo 1g + fángfēng 1g.

Skin rash (782.1), Abnormality of the liver (573.9), Weight loss (D015431), Fever (D005334), Diarrhea (D003967), Venous insufficiency (459.81), Fatigue (D005221):

Xuèfǔzhúyūtāng 5g + xiāofēngsǎn 5g + lóngdǎnxiègāntāng 5g + báixiānpí 2-1g + dìfūzǐ 2-1g + mǔdānpí 1-0g.

Xuèfǔzhúyūtāng 5g + sǎnzhǒngkuìjiāntāng 5g + zhēnrénhuómìngyǐn 5-0g + xiàkūcǎo 1g + dānshēn 1-0g + liánqiáo 1-0g + púgōngyīng 1-0g.

Wǔwèixiāodúyǐn 5g + xiāofēngsǎn 5g + lóngdǎnxiègāntāng 5g + jīnyínhuā 1g + liánqiáo 1g.

Huángqín 5g + báizhǐ 4-3g + zhìgāncǎo 2g + shārén 2g + guālóugēn 2-0g + tiānhuā 2-0g + xìxīn 1-0g + dàhuáng 1-0g.

Huángqín 5g + báizhǐ 4g + gāncǎo 3g + shārén 3g + tiānhuā 2g + dàhuáng 0g.

Jiāwèixiāoyáosǎn, containing Dāngguī as the major herb, "soothes the Liver, resolves depression, clears heat, nourishes Blood" and is used for menopausal/postmenopausal disorders, neurotic disorders, and general symptoms (Wang, 2019). The formula was reviewed to be effective for anxiety disorders, such as depression and anxiety, by regulating the central nervous system (cf. Section 3.1). Báijièzǐ "dissolves nodules" and is used for lipoma (cf. Section 1.20).

4.19 WALDENSTRÖM MACROGLOBULINEMIA

Waldenström macroglobulinemia is an overgrowth of abnormal B cells and plasma cells in the bone marrow with excessive immunoglobulin M (IgM) antibodies in the blood. Waldenström macroglobulinemia is associated with somatic mutations in the *MYD88* gene, whose products function in signaling pathways for the activation of numerous proinflammatory genes.

Huángbò (cf. Section 1.61) was summarized to be an antitumor in cell lines and mice, including two leukemic cell lines (Sun et al., 2019). Guīpítāng "replenishes Qi-Blood, benefits the Spleen, nourishes

---

TABLE 4.19

GMP Herbal Medicines for a 65-Year-Old Man with Waldenström Macroglobulinemia

Waldenström macroglobulinemia (OrphaCode: 33226)

A disease with a prevalence of ~5 in 100,000

Disease-causing somatic mutation(s): MYD88 innate immune signal transduction adaptor (*MYD88* / Entrez: 4615) at 3p22.2

Multigenic/multifactorial

Leukemia, Lymphoma, Monoclonal immunoglobulin M proteinemia

Gingival bleeding, Pallor, Abnormality of neutrophils, Normocytic anemia, Respiratory insufficiency, Vertigo, Hypercoagulability

(Continued)

TABLE 4.19 *(Continued)*

GMP Herbal Medicines for a 65-Year-Old Man with Waldenström Macroglobulinemia

Renal insufficiency, Hearing impairment, Epistaxis, Proptosis, Retinal hemorrhage, Cutis marmorata, Purpura, Urticaria, Ataxia, Stroke, Congestive heart failure, Splenomegaly, Fever, Diarrhea, Malabsorption, Anorexia, Migraine, Pulmonary infiltrates, Pleural effusion, Gastrointestinal hemorrhage, Hepatomegaly, Memory impairment, Vasculitis, Lymphadenopathy, Recurrent infections, Elevated erythrocyte sedimentation rate, Reduced consciousness/confusion, Cranial nerve paralysis, Abnormal retinal vascular morphology, Peripheral neuropathy, Pedal edema, Multifocal epileptiform discharges, Fatigue, Periorbital edema, Cryoglobulinemia
Elderly

Leukemia (208), Monoclonal immunoglobulin M proteinemia (273.3):

Guīpítāng 5-4g + sǎnzhǒngkuìjiāntāng 5-0g + jīxuèténg 2-1g + hànliáncǎo 1-0g.

Huángbò 5g + shārén 3g + guībǎn 3-0g + zhìgāncǎo 2g + fùzǐ 2-0g.
Shúdìhuáng 5g + shānyào 2g + zhìgāncǎo 2g + chénpí 2g + dāngguī 2g + rénshēn 1g + shēngmá 1g + shēngjiāng 1g + cháihú 1g.
Huángqí 5g + dǎngshēn 5g + shúdìhuáng 5-3g + shānyào 3-2g + zhìgāncǎo 2g + chénpí 2g + shēngjiāng 2-1g + cháihú 2-1g + dāngguī 1g + shēngmá 1-0g.

Gingival bleeding (D005884), Pallor (D010167), Vertigo (386.2):

Tiānmágōuténgyǐn 5g + xuèfǔzhúyūtāng 3g + qǐjúdìhuángwán 3g + dānshēn 1-0g.
Tiānmágōuténgyǐn 5g + xuèfǔzhúyūtāng 5g + zhǐbódìhuángwán 5g.
Bǔyánghuánwǔtāng 5g + dānshēn 1g + shíchāngpú 1g + yuǎnzhì 1g.
Zhǐbódìhuángwán 5g + bànxiàbáizhútiānmátāng 4g + dānshēn 1g + shíchāngpú 1g + yùjīn 1g.

Dānshēn 5g + gāncǎo 5g + báisháo 5g + bǎihé 5g + màiméndōng 5g + huángqí 5g + dǎngshēn 5g.
Dānshēn 5g + tiānmá 5g + niúxī 5g + gāncǎo 5g + báisháo 5g + dìhuáng 5g + xìngrén 5g + chénpí 5g + màiméndōng 5g + shúdìhuáng 5g.
Huángbò 5g + zhìgāncǎo 3g + shārén 3g + ròuguì 1g + wúzhūyú 1g + xìxīn 1g.
Rénshēn 5g + zhìgāncǎo 5g + fùzǐ 3g + gānjiāng 3g.

Renal insufficiency (586), Hearing impairment (D003638), Proptosis (376.30), Retinal hemorrhage (D012166), Purpura (D011693), Ataxia (D002524), Congestive heart failure (428, 428.0), Fever (D005334), Diarrhea (D003967), Anorexia (D000855), Migraine (346), Memory impairment (D008569), Cranial nerve paralysis (352.9), Fatigue (D005221):

Wǔlíngsǎn 5g + zhēnwǔtāng 5g + jìshēngshènqìwán 5-0g.
Wǔlíngsǎn 5g + jìshēngshènqìwán 5g + dānshēn 1-0g + huángqí 1-0g + dǎngshēn 1-0g + dàhuáng 0g.
Zhēnwǔtāng 5g + lǐzhōngtāng 5g + fùzǐ 1g.

Fùzǐ 5g + báizhú 5-3g + cháihú 5-3g + báisháo 4-2g + fúlíng 4-2g + tiānhuā 2g + dǎngshēn 2g + guìzhī 2-1g + huángqín 2-1g + wūwèizǐ 2-0g + xìxīn 2-0g + shēngjiāng 2-0g + gāncǎo 1g + mǔlì 1g + gānjiāng 1g.

the mind" and is used today for anemia and general symptoms (Wang, 2019). Zhǐbódìhuángwán (cf. Section 3.10) treats "yin deficiency and fire excess" TCM syndrome that manifests hectic fever, night sweats, lower back pain, sore knees, sore throat, insomnia, chronic swelling of the gums, ringing in the ears, and nocturnal seminal emission. Zhǐbódìhuángwán contains Huángbò. Adjunctive use of GMP Dānshēn, Huángqí, Jīxuèténg, Báihuāshéshécǎo, Màiméndōng, Gāncǎo, Dùzhòng, Jiāwèixiāoyáosǎn, Guīpítāng, Qǐjúdìhuángwán, Zhǐbódìhuángwán, Xiāngshāliùjūnzǐtāng, Shūjīnghuóxuètāng, or Shēnlíngbáizhúsǎn concentrated extract granules was found to be associated with an improved survival in patients with acute myeloid leukemia in Taiwan (Fleischer et al., 2016).

4.20 SYSTEMIC MASTOCYTOSIS WITH ASSOCIATED HEMATOLOGIC NEOPLASM

Systemic mastocytosis with associated hematologic neoplasm, also called systemic mastocytosis with an associated clonal hematologic non-mast-cell lineage disease, refers to excessive buildup of neoplastic mast cells in one or multiple tissues, such as the bone marrow and lymph nodes, together with another blood cancer. Systemic mastocytosis with certain associated hematologic neoplasm is caused by acquired mutations

TABLE 4.20
GMP Herbal Medicines for a 55-Year-Old Adult with Systemic Mastocytosis with Associated Hematologic Neoplasm

Systemic mastocytosis with associated hematologic neoplasm (OrphaCode: 98849)

A disease with a prevalence of ~5 in 100,000

Disease-causing somatic mutation(s): KIT proto-oncogene, receptor tyrosine kinase (*KIT* / Entrez: 3815) at 4q12

Disease-causing somatic mutation(s): tet methylcytosine dioxygenase 2 (*TET2* / Entrez: 54790) at 4q24

Disease-causing somatic mutation(s): serine and arginine rich splicing factor 2 (*SRSF2* / Entrez: 6427) at 17q25.2

Disease-causing somatic mutation(s): ASXL transcriptional regulator 1 (*ASXL1* / Entrez: 171023) at 20q11.21

Not applicable

Hematological neoplasm, Myeloid leukemia, Increased serum mast cell beta-tryptase concentration, Abnormal mast cell morphology

Pallor, Pruritus, Weight loss, Thrombocytopenia, Eosinophilia, Normochromic anemia, Normocytic anemia, Fever, Leukocytosis, Headache, Myeloproliferative disorder, Fatigue, Bone marrow hypercellularity

Osteoporosis, Urticaria, Syncope, Tachycardia, Splenomegaly, Diarrhea, Nausea, Abdominal pain, Abnormality of the respiratory system, Hepatomegaly, Hypotension, Bone pain, Increased susceptibility to fractures, Lymphoma, Lymphadenopathy, Arthralgia, Myelodysplasia, Myalgia, Peptic ulcer, Acute myeloid leukemia, Neutrophilia, Granulocytic hyperplasia, Chronic myelomonocytic leukemia, Flushing, Increased basophil count

Adult, Elderly

Myeloid leukemia (206.1, 205):

Guīlùèrxiānjiāo 5g.

Guīpítáng 5g + bànzhīlián 2-0g + jīxuèténg 2-0g + xiānhècǎo 1-0g + hànliáncǎo 1-0g + zhīmǔ 1-0g.

Jiāwèixiāoyáosǎn 5g + shēnlíngbáizhúsǎn 5g + huòxiāngzhèngqìsǎn 5g + nǚzhēnzǐ 1g + dānshēn 1g + huángqí 1g.

Bànzhīlián 5g + báihuāshéshécǎo 5g.

Xuánshēn 5g + dìhuáng 5g + hòupò 5g + zhǐshí 5g + màiméndōng 5g + yùzhú 5-3g + shāshēn 3-0g + dàhuáng 1-0g.

Mǔdānpí 5g + zhīmǔ 5-0g + huángbò 5-0g + jīnyínhuā 5-0g + qiàncǎo 5-0g + dànzhúyè 5-0g + yùjīn 5-0g + báimáogēn 4-0g + chìsháo 2-0g.

Pallor (D010167), Pruritus (D011537), Weight loss (D015431), Thrombocytopenia (287.5), Eosinophilia (288.3), Fever (D005334), Headache (D006261), Fatigue (D005221):

Wǔlíngsǎn 5g + shēnlíngbáizhúsǎn 5g.

Wǔlíngsǎn 5g + bǔzhōngyìqìtāng 5g.

Wǔlíngsǎn 5g + guīpítáng 5g + xiānhècǎo 1-0g + báimáogēn 1-0g + ējiāo 1-0g.

Wǔlíngsǎn 5g + píngwèisǎn 5g + huòxiāngzhèngqìsǎn 5g + bànzhīlián 1g + báihuāshéshécǎo 1g.

Lǐzhōngtāng 5g + bǔzhōngyìqìtāng 5g + chuānxiōngchádiàosǎn 3g + qīngyānlìgétāng 3g + báizhǐ 2g + fángfēng 2g + zhǐqiào 2g + jiégěng 2g + gānjiāng 2g.

Dǎngshēn 5g + bànxià 3g + gānjiāng 2g.

Gāncǎo 5g + báizhú 5g + báisháo 5g + báibiǎndòu 5g + fúlíng 5g + huángqí 5g + dàzǎo 2g + shēngjiāng 2g.

Osteoporosis (733.0), Syncope (D013575), Diarrhea (D003967), Nausea (D009325), Abdominal pain (D015746), Arthralgia (D018771), Myalgia (D063806), Peptic ulcer (533), Acute myeloid leukemia (205.0):

Hǔqiánwánqùhǔgǔ 5g + guīlùèrxiānjiāo 5g.

Hǔqiánwánqùhǔgǔ 5g + dāngguīniántòngtāng 2g + dúhuójìshēngtāng 2g + niúxī 1g + dùzhòng 1g + gǔsuìbǔ 1g + gāncǎo 0g.

Hǔqiánwánqùhǔgǔ 5g + dúhuójìshēngtāng 5g + shūjīnghuóxuètāng 4g + xiāngshāliùjūnzǐtāng 1g.

Guìzhīsháoyàozhīmǔtāng 5g + dúhuójìshēngtāng 5g + mùguā 1g + niúxī 1g + wēilíngxiān 1g + qínjiāo 1g + jīxuèténg 1g.

Shúdìhuáng 5g + báizhú 4g + fùzǐ 4g + báisháo 3g + fúlíng 3g + báijièzǐ 2g + dǎngshēn 2g + shēngjiāng 1g + máhuáng 1g + gāncǎo 1-0g + dàhuáng 1-0g + huánglián 0g.

Shúdìhuáng 5g + báizhú 3-2g + qiànshí 3-2g + yìyǐrén 3-2g + shānzhūyú 2g + báijièzǐ 2-1g + dùzhòng 2-1g + dǎngshēn 2-1g + wǔwèizǐ 2-0g + guìzhī 2-0g + fúlíng 2-0g + rénshēn 2-0g + ròuguì 1-0g + júhóng 1-0g + yìzhìrén 1-0g + shārén 1-0g.

in the *KIT* gene, whose products activate transduction in multiple signaling pathways for the control of growth, division, and migration of cells, including hematopoietic stem cells and mast cells. Additional mutated genes are required for systemic mastocytosis with other associated hematologic neoplasms.

Mǔdānpí (Cortex Moutan) "clears heat, cools Blood, activates circulation, removes stasis" and is anticancer (Deng et al., 2019). Guīlùèrxiānjiāo "replenishes marrow, benefits Qi, nourishes the mind" and is used today for disorders of the back and joints (Wang, 2019). Dǎngshēn (cf. Sections 1.65 and 1.68) "benefits Qi, generates saliva, nourishes Blood" and its current clinical uses include syncope and collapse, and anemia (Wang, 2020). Hǔqiánwánqùhǔgǔ, containing Shúdìhuáng, "nourishes yin, lowers fire, strengthens muscles and bones" and is used for disorders of the joints and arthropathies (Wang, 2019). Herbal products for acute myeloid leukemia were introduced in Section 4.19.

4.21 KLATSKIN TUMOR

Klatskin tumor, also known as hilar cholangiocarcinoma, is a cancer of the biliary tree, originating in the region where the left and right bile ducts meet and leave the liver. The cause of Klatskin tumor is unknown and may involve genetic, environmental, and lifestyle factors.

TABLE 4.21

GMP Herbal Medicines for a 60-Year-Old Adult with Klatskin Tumor

Klatskin tumor (OrphaCode: 99978)

A disease with a prevalence of ~5 in 100,000

Not applicable

Jaundice, Extrahepatic cholestasis, Cholangiocarcinoma

Hepatomegaly, Lymphadenopathy

Weight loss, Fever, Abdominal pain, Venous thrombosis, Fatigue

Adult

Jaundice (D007565):

Yīnchénwǔlíngsǎn 5g + huòxiāngzhèngqìsǎn 5g + yèjiāoténg 3g + hǎipiāoxiāo 3g + dānshēn 2g + bózǐrén 2g + cāngzhú 2g.	Yīnchén 5g + tōngcǎo 1-0g.
	Yīnchén 5g + bànxià 3-0g + fùzǐ 2-0g + xìxīn 2-0g + dàhuáng 1-0g.
Yīnchénwǔlíngsǎn 5g + lóngdǎnxiègāntāng 5g + yīnchén 1-0g + huángshuǐqié 1-0g.	Yīnchén 5g + shānzhīzǐ 4-0g + dàhuáng 2-0g + huángqín 2-0g + huǒmárén 1-0g.
Yīnchénwǔlíngsǎn 5g + huángliánjiědútāng 5g + lóngdǎnxiègāntāng 5-0g + dàqīngyè 1-0g + jīnyínhuā 1-0g + púgōngyīng 1-0g.	

Weight loss (D015431), Fever (D005334), Abdominal pain (D015746), Fatigue (D005221):

Wǔlíngsǎn 5g + bànxià 1-0g + gāncǎo 1-0g + báisháo 1-0g.	Gāncǎo 5g + hòupò 5-2g + zhǐshí 5-2g + dàhuáng 1-0g.
Guìzhītāng 5g + bànxià 1-0g + báisháo 1-0g + dàhuáng 0g.	Zhìgāncǎo 5g + hòupò 3g + zhǐshí 3g + dàhuáng 0g.

Yīnchén (cf. Section 1.57) has long been used to protect the gallbladder and is used today for fetal and neonatal jaundice (Wang, 2020); indeed, its compounds were isolated and summarized to be choleretic, antioxidant, anti-inflammatory, antifibrotic, and hepatoprotective (Cai et al., 2020). Yīnchénwǔlíngsǎn, containing Yīnchén, was shown to alleviate cholestasis in mice with cholestatic liver disease (You et al., 2023).

4.22 SQUAMOUS CELL CARCINOMA OF THE ESOPHAGUS

Squamous cell carcinoma of the esophagus, also known as esophageal epidermoid carcinoma, is cancer arising from the epithelial cells in the upper two-thirds of the esophagus. Squamous cell carcinoma of the esophagus is thought to be caused by the exposure of esophageal mucosa to toxic stimuli as it is linked to alcohol drinking and tobacco smoking.

TABLE 4.22

GMP Herbal Medicines for a 60-Year-Old Adult with Squamous Cell Carcinoma of the Esophagus

Squamous cell carcinoma of the esophagus (OrphaCode: 99977)

A disease with a prevalence of ~5 in 100,000

Major susceptibility factor: WW domain containing oxidoreductase (*WWOX* / Entrez: 51741) at 16q23.1-q23.2

Candidate gene tested: ring finger protein 6 (*RNF6* / Entrez: 6049) at 13q12.13

Candidate gene tested: transforming growth factor beta receptor 2 (*TGFBR2* / Entrez: 7048) at 3p24.1

Candidate gene tested: DLEC1 cilia and flagella associated protein (*DLEC1* / Entrez: 9940) at 3p22.2

Multigenic/multifactorial, Not applicable

Clinodactyly of the 5th toe, Feeding difficulties in infancy, Esophageal carcinoma

Abnormality of the voice, Nausea and vomiting, Cough, Chest pain

Lymphadenopathy

Adult, Elderly

Cough (D003371), Chest pain (D002637):	
Dàqīnglóngtāng 5g + jīngfángbàidúsǎn 3g + pǔjìxiāodúyǐn 3g + mǔlì 1g + lónggǔ 1g + hǎipiāoxiāo 1-0g.	Gāncǎo 5g + yúxīngcǎo 5g + tǔfúlíng 4g + báijiāngcán 4g + dìlóng 4g + fángfēng 4g + jiégěng 4g + jīngjiè 4g + bòhé 4g.
Máhuángtāng 5g + bànxià 1g + shēngjiāng 1g + xìxīn 1g + dàhuáng 0g.	Gāncǎo 5g + dìlóng 5-4g + fángfēng 5-4g + jiégěng 5-4g + jīngjiè 5-4g + yúxīngcǎo 5-4g + bòhé 5-4g + jiāngcán 5-4g + púgōngyīng 4-0g.

Yúxīngcǎo (Herba Houttuyniae) was demonstrated to relieve airway hyperresponsiveness and inflammation in asthmatic mice (Yang et al., 2022) and is used for coughs (Wang, 2020). Máhuángtāng, being pungent and warm, "induces perspiration, frees the Lung, quells asthma" and is used today for asthma and rhinitis (Wang, 2019). Dàqīnglóngtāng, a derivative of Máhuángtāng, "induces sweating, releases exterior, clears internal heat" and is used for rhinitis and asthma (Wang, 2019).

4.23　ADENOCARCINOMA OF THE ESOPHAGUS

Adenocarcinoma of the esophagus, or esophageal adenocarcinoma, is cancer arising from the glandular cells in the lower one-third of the esophagus. Adenocarcinoma of the esophagus is believed to be caused by the long-term erosive effects of acid reflux. Its risk factors also include tobacco use and abdominal obesity.

Hóngqū (cf. Section 4.12) was shown to be anti-atherosclerotic in mice (Wu et al., 2017) and is used for disorders of lipoid metabolism including pure hypercholesterolemia, mixed hyperlipidemia, pure hyperglyceridemia, and other unspecified hyperlipidemia (Wang, 2020). Zhīmǔ and Huánglián mixture was shown to be anticolitic in mice (Jang et al., 2013). Modified Bànxiàxièxīntāng was

TABLE 4.23

GMP Herbal Medicines for a 60-Year-Old Man with Adenocarcinoma of the Esophagus

Adenocarcinoma of the esophagus (OrphaCode: 99976)

A disease with a prevalence of ~5 in 100,000

Not applicable

Obesity, Clinodactyly of the 5th toe, Gastroesophageal reflux, Feeding difficulties in infancy, Esophageal carcinoma, Barrett esophagus

Nausea and vomiting, Cough, Chest pain

Lymphadenopathy

Adult, Elderly

(Continued)

TABLE 4.23 *(Continued)*

GMP Herbal Medicines for a 60-Year-Old Man with Adenocarcinoma of the Esophagus

Obesity (278.00), Gastroesophageal reflux (530.81), Barrett esophagus (530.85):

Bànxiàxièxīntāng 5g + xiāngshāliùjūnzǐtāng 5g + píngwèisǎn 5-0g + hǎipiāoxiāo 3-0g + báijí 2-0g + bèimǔ 2-0g + mǔlì 1-0g.

Hóngqū 5g.

Zhīmǔ 5g + gāncǎo 5-3g + huángqín 5-3g + huángbò 5-0g + huánglián 1-0g + dàhuáng 0g.

Bànxiàxièxīntāng 5g + wēndǎntāng 5g + báijí 1g + bèimǔ 1g + hǎipiāoxiāo 1g.

Cough (D003371), Chest pain (D002637):

Dàqīnglóngtāng 5g + dàqīngyè 0g + niúbàngzǐ 0g + bǎnlángēn 0g + shègān 0g.

Gāncǎo 5g + púgōngyīng 5g + niúbàngzǐ 4g + báijiāngcán 4g + xìngrén 4g + fángfēng 4g + jiégěng 4g + jīngjiè 4g + bòhé 4g.

Dàqīnglóngtāng 5g + jīngfángbàidúsǎn 3-2g + pǔjìxiāodúyǐn 3-2g + hǎipiāoxiāo 1-0g + mǔlì 1-0g + lónggǔ 1-0g.

Gāncǎo 5g + dìlóng 5g + fángfēng 5g + jiégěng 5g + jīngjiè 5g + yúxīngcǎo 5g + bòhé 5g + jiāngcán 5g.

Gāncǎo 5g + yúxīngcǎo 5-3g + tǔfúlíng 4-3g + báijiāngcán 4-3g + dìlóng 4-3g + fángfēng 4-3g + jiégěng 4-3g + jīngjiè 4-3g + bòhé 4-3g.

concluded to be safe and effective for gastroesophageal reflux disease in adults in a systematic review and meta-analysis of randomized controlled trials (Dai et al., 2017). Note that Hǎipiāoxiāo, i.e., Endoconcha Sepiae or cuttlefish bone, contains calcium carbonate as a key ingredient that is basic and thus neutralizes acidic gastric secretion.

4.24 CUTANEOUS NEUROENDOCRINE CARCINOMA

Cutaneous neuroendocrine carcinoma, also known as Merkel cell carcinoma, is cancer arising from the precursors of a subset of cells in the epidermis for touch sensation. It often occurs on the skin of the head, neck, and extremities that have been exposed to sunlight. The risk factors of cutaneous neuroendocrine carcinoma include ultraviolet light exposure and weakened immunity.

Jīxuèténg (cf. Sections 2.4, 2.44, and 4.19) "moves Blood, replenishes Blood, modulates menstruation, relaxes tendons, activates collaterals" and was reviewed and summarized to be antitumor, hematopoietic, anti-inflammatory, antidiabetic, antioxidant, antiviral, and antibacterial (Pan et al.,

TABLE 4.24

GMP Herbal Medicines for a 72-Year-Old Man with Cutaneous Neuroendocrine Carcinoma

Cutaneous neuroendocrine carcinoma (OrphaCode: 79140)

A disease with a prevalence of ~4 in 100,000

Not applicable

Merkel cell skin cancer

Cutaneous photosensitivity, Chronic noninfectious lymphadenopathy, Cellular immunodeficiency, Regional abnormality of skin, Erythematous plaque, Erythematous macule, Skin nodule

Basal cell carcinoma, Lymphoid leukemia, Squamous cell carcinoma of the skin, Multiple myeloma, Carcinoid tumor

Adult, Elderly

Lymphoid leukemia (204), Multiple myeloma (203.0):

Sǎnzhǒngkuìjiāntāng 5g + guīpítāng 5-4g + jīxuèténg 2-1g + hànliáncǎo 2-0g.

Huángbò 5g + guībǎn 5-0g + shārén 3-2g + zhìgāncǎo 2g + fùzǐ 2-0g.

Gāncǎo 5g + báisháo 5g + shíhú 5g + bǎihé 5g + chēqiánzǐ 5g + fúlíng 5g + màiméndōng 5g.

Shānyào 5g + huángqí 3g + shúdìhuáng 3g + dǎngshēn 3g + shēngmá 2g + zhìgāncǎo 2g + cháihú 2g + chénpí 2g + shēngjiāng 1g + dāngguī 1g.

2023). Adjunctive use of Huángqí, Shānyào, Gāncǎo, Jīxuèténg, or Màiméndōng was found to be associated with improved survival in patients with chronic myeloid leukemia in Taiwan (Fleischer et al., 2016).

4.25 MALT LYMPHOMA

MALT lymphoma, also known as extranodal marginal zone B-cell lymphoma or mucosa-associated lymphatic tissue lymphoma, is a slow-growing cancer of the B cells starting from the lymphatic tissues that line some organs and body cavities such as the stomach, lung, and thyroid. Chronic immune stimulation is suspected to cause MALT lymphoma. For example, many patients with gastric MALT lymphoma have a history of chronic gastric mucosa inflammation resulting from a *Helicobacter pylori* infection.

Hòupò, together with Zhǐshí, was introduced in Section 3.13 for constipation. Mázirénwán, containing Fructus Cannabis, Hòupò, Zhǐshí, and Dàhuáng, "moistens intestines, moisturizes dryness, smoothly passes stools" and is used today for functional digestive disorders

---

TABLE 4.25

GMP Herbal Medicines for a 65-Year-Old Adult with MALT Lymphoma

MALT lymphoma (OrphaCode: 52417)

A disease with a prevalence of ~4 in 100,000

Part of a fusion gene: MALT1 paracaspase (*MALT1* / Entrez: 10892) at 18q21.32

Part of a fusion gene: baculoviral IAP repeat containing 3 (*BIRC3* / Entrez: 330) at 11q22.2

Part of a fusion gene: immunoglobulin heavy locus (*IGH* / Entrez: 3492) at 14q32.33

Part of a fusion gene: forkhead box P1 (*FOXP1* / Entrez: 27086) at 3p13

Part of a fusion gene: BCL10 immune signaling adaptor (*BCL10* / Entrez: 8915) at 1p22.3

Multigenic/multifactorial, Not applicable

Weight loss, Anemia, Fever, Nausea and vomiting, Pulmonary infiltrates, B-cell lymphoma, Fatigue, Hyperhidrosis

Constipation

Visual impairment, Abnormal nasolacrimal system morphology, Abnormality of the thyroid gland, Abdominal pain, Recurrent respiratory infections, Lymphadenopathy, Mediastinal lymphadenopathy, Posterior uveitis

Adult

Weight loss (D015431), Anemia (285.9), Fever (D005334), Fatigue (D005221):

Bǔzhōngyìqìtāng 5g + guīpítāng 5-0g.

Lǐzhōngtāng 5g + bǔzhōngyìqìtāng 5-0g + chuānxiōngchádiàosǎn 2-0g + fúlíng 1g + fùzǐ 1-0g + bànxià 1-0g + shārén 1-0g.

Sìjūnzǐtāng 5g + sìwùtāng 5g + dānshēn 1g + huángqí 1g.

Gāncǎo 5g + báizhú 5g + báisháo 5g + báibiǎndòu 5g + fúlíng 5g + huángqí 5g + dàzǎo 2g + shēngjiāng 2g.

Màiyá 5g + báizhú 4g + zhǐshí 4g + fúlíng 4g + gāncǎo 3g + báibiǎndòu 3g + qiànshí 2g.

Zhìgāncǎo 5g + hòupò 3g + zhǐshí 3g + dàhuáng 0g.

Gāncǎo 5g + hòupò 5g + zhǐshí 5g + dàhuáng 1g.

Constipation (564.0):

Mázirénwán 5g + rùnchángwán 5g + xuánshēn 1-0g + dìhuáng 1-0g + màiméndōng 1-0g + huángqí 1-0g + dàhuáng 1-0g.

Dàchéngqìtāng 5g + mázirénwán 5g + dàhuáng 1g.

Hòupò 5g + zhǐshí 5g + běishāshēn 5-0g + xuánshēn 5-0g + yùzhú 5-0g + dìhuáng 5-0g + màiméndōng 5-0g + dàhuáng 1g.

Xuánshēn 5g + dìhuáng 5g + màiméndōng 5g + hòupò 5-4g + zhǐshí 5-4g + yùzhú 5-0g + dàhuáng 1g.

Visual impairment (D014786), Abnormality of the thyroid gland (246.9), Abdominal pain (D015746):

Zīshènmíngmùtāng 5g + jiāwèixiāoyáosǎn 4-0g + qǐjúdìhuángwán 4-0g + yèjiāoténg 2-0g + juémíngzǐ 1-0g + xiàkūcǎo 1-0g + júhuā 1-0g + suānzǎorén 1-0g.

Zīshènmíngmùtāng 5g + qǐjúdìhuángwán 5-0g + juémíngzǐ 1-0g + xiàkūcǎo 1-0g + gǔjīngcǎo 1-0g + mànjīngzǐ 1-0g.

Gāncǎo 5g + báizhú 5g + shārén 5g + huángqín 5g + tiānhuā 2g + xìxīn 2-1g + dàhuáng 1-0g.

Gǒuqǐzǐ 5g + júhuā 5g + niúbàngzǐ 4g + shègān 4g + bèimǔ 4-0g + hǎipiāoxiāo 4-0g + xìxīn 1g + huánglián 1g.

Jílí 5g + chántuì 5g.

(Wang, 2019). Rùnchángwán, containing Fructus Cannabis and Dàhuáng, "moistens intestines, passes stools, increases bowel movements" and is also used for functional digestive disorders (Wang, 2019).

4.26 MANTLE CELL LYMPHOMA

Mantle cell lymphoma, also called mantle zone lymphoma, is an aggressive cancer of the lymphatic system arising from the B cells in a region called the mantle zone surrounding a transient structure where B cells proliferate and differentiate in a lymph node. Mantle cell lymphoma is caused by acquired DNA changes in the mantel zone B cells, such as mutations in the *CCND1* gene, whose products regulate cell cycle and cell proliferation. Mutations in other genes, such as a tumor suppressor gene, may also be required for the malignancy transformation.

TABLE 4.26

GMP Herbal Medicines for a 65-Year-Old Man with Mantle Cell Lymphoma

Mantle cell lymphoma (OrphaCode: 52416)

A disease with a prevalence of ~3 in 100,000

Disease-causing somatic mutation(s): cyclin D1 (*CCND1* / Entrez: 595) at 11q13.3

Disease-causing somatic mutation(s): ATM serine/threonine kinase (*ATM* / Entrez: 472) at 11q22.3

Disease-causing somatic mutation(s): immunoglobulin heavy locus (*IGH* / Entrez: 3492) at 14q32.33

Multigenic/multifactorial, Not applicable

Lymphadenopathy, B-cell lymphoma

Splenomegaly, Weight loss, Anorexia, Abnormality of bone marrow cell morphology, Fatigue, Fever

Abnormality of the gastrointestinal tract

Adult

Weight loss (D015431), Anorexia (D000855), Fatigue (D005221), Fever (D005334):

Guìzhītāng 5g + xìngrén 2-1g + hòupò 2-1g + dàhuáng 0g.	Zhìgāncǎo 5g + hòupò 5-3g + zhǐshí 5-3g + dàhuáng 1-0g.
	Gāncǎo 5g + hòupò 5-3g + zhǐshí 5-3g + dàhuáng 1-0g.

Abnormality of the gastrointestinal tract (520-579.99):

Xiāngshāliùjūnzǐtāng 5g + píngwèisǎn 5-0g.	Hòupò 5g + zhǐshí 5g + dàhuáng 1g.
Xiāngshāliùjūnzǐtāng 5g + shēnlíngbáizhúsǎn 5-0g.	Huánglián 5g + huángqín 4-0g + dàhuáng 1-0g.
Bǔzhōngyìqìtāng 5g + wēilíngtāng 5-0g + báijí 1g + shārén 1g.	Báizhú 5g + fùzǐ 3g + gānjiāng 3g + zǐwǎn 3g + gāncǎo 2g.
Bǔzhōngyìqìtāng 5g + bǎohéwán 5-0g + báijí 1g + shārén 1g.	

Hòupò (cf. Section 3.13) was reviewed to exert rich, local, and distal pharmacological effects in the digestive, respiratory, cardiovascular, and cerebrovascular systems through its effects on the gastrointestinal tract (Niu et al., 2021). Wèilíngtāng is a combination of two formulas: Píngwèisǎn and Wǔlíngsǎn. Wèilíngtāng "dries dampness, strengthens the Spleen, transforms Qi, helps draining, regulates Qi, guides stagnation" and is used today for gastritis and duodenitis, and functional digestive disorders (Wang, 2019).

4.27 MULTIPLE ENDOCRINE NEOPLASIA TYPE 1

Multiple endocrine neoplasia type 1 (MEN1), also known as Wermer syndrome, is two or more tumors of the parathyroid glands, the pituitary gland, and the pancreas. MEN1 is clinically characterized by overactivity of the parathyroid glands, resulting in abnormally high levels of calcium in the blood. MEN1 is caused by mutations in the *MEN1* gene, which is a tumor suppressor gene.

TABLE 4.27

GMP Herbal Medicines for a 20-Year-Old Adult with Multiple Endocrine Neoplasia Type 1

Multiple endocrine neoplasia type 1 (OrphaCode: 652)

A disease with a prevalence of ~3 in 100,000

Candidate gene tested: cyclin-dependent kinase inhibitor 1B (*CDKN1B* / Entrez: 1027) at 12p13.1

Candidate gene tested: cyclin-dependent kinase inhibitor 1A (*CDKN1A* / Entrez: 1026) at 6p21.2

Candidate gene tested: cyclin-dependent kinase inhibitor 2B (*CDKN2B* / Entrez: 1030) at 9p21.3

Candidate gene tested: cyclin-dependent kinase inhibitor 2C (*CDKN2C* / Entrez: 1031) at 1p32.3

Disease-causing germline mutation(s): menin 1 (*MEN1* / HGNC:7010) at 11q13

Autosomal dominant, Not applicable

Hypercalcemia, Primary hyperparathyroidism, Parathyroid hyperplasia, Angiofibromas, Impairment of activities of daily living

Impotence, Adrenocortical abnormality, Multiple lipomas, Weight loss, Diarrhea, Gastroesophageal reflux, Abdominal pain, Zollinger-Ellison syndrome, Hypercalciuria, Pituitary adenoma, Neoplasm of the pancreas, Reduced bone mineral density, Peptic ulcer, Large cafe-au-lait macules with irregular margins, Pituitary prolactin cell adenoma, Decreased male libido, Galactorrhea, Hypergastrinemia

Amenorrhea, Gingival fibromatosis, Depression, Short attention span, Nephrolithiasis, Hypertension, Growth hormone excess, Goiter, Lethargy, Confusion, Cranial nerve compression, Primary hypercortisolism, Dehydration, Vomiting, Nausea, Constipation, Anorexia, Hematemesis, Melena, Headache, Duodenal ulcer, Increased susceptibility to fractures, Osteolysis, Meningioma, Thyroid carcinoma, Increased circulating cortisol level, Intestinal carcinoid, Adrenocortical carcinoma, Confetti-like hypopigmented macules, Proportionate tall stature, Pituitary growth hormone cell adenoma, Insulinoma, Shortened QT interval, Pancreatic endocrine tumor, Decreased vigilance, Abnormal circulating aldosterone, Carcinoid tumor

All ages

Hypercalcemia (275.42), Primary hyperparathyroidism (252.01):

Jiāwèixiāoyáosǎn 5g + zhēnrénhuómìngyǐn 5g + xuánshēn 2-0g + mǔlì 2-0g + bèimǔ 2-0g + xiàkūcǎo 2-0g + acupuncture.

Sǎnzhǒngkuìjiāntāng 5g + xuánshēn 0g + mǔlì 0g + bèimǔ 0g + xiàkūcǎo 0g.

Jiāwèixiāoyáosǎn 5g + zhībódìhuángwán 5g + xuánshēn 1g + mǔlì 1g + bèimǔ 1g + xiàkūcǎo 1g.

Xuánshēn 5g + yùzhú 5g + dìhuáng 5g + shāshēn 5g + hòupò 5g + zhǐshí 5g + màiméndōng 5g + dàhuáng 0g.

Zhìgāncǎo 5g + jiégěng 5g + xuánshēn 5-3g + mǔlì 5-3g + bèimǔ 5-3g + liánqiáo 5-2g + zhīzǐ 2-0g + shānzhīzǐ 2-0g + xìngrén 2-0g + dàhuáng 1-0g.

Multiple lipomas (214), Weight loss (D015431), Diarrhea (D003967), Gastroesophageal reflux (530.81), Abdominal pain (D015746), Hypercalciuria (D053565), Neoplasm of the pancreas (157.0, 157.1, 157.2, 157.8), Peptic ulcer (533):

Sǎnzhǒngkuìjiāntāng 5g + guīlùèrxiānjiāo 5g + zhēnrénhuómìngyǐnqùchuānshānjiǎ 2-0g + bànxiàxièxīntāng 1-0g + xiāngshāliùjūnzǐtāng 1-0g.

Sǎnzhǒngkuìjiāntāng 5g + bèimǔ 2-1g + xiàkūcǎo 2-1g + xuánshēn 2-0g + mǔlì 2-0g + sānléng 1-0g + éshù 1-0g + púgōngyīng 1-0g + táohéchéngqìtāng 1-0g.

Bèimǔ 5g + xuánshēn 5-4g + zhìgāncǎo 5-4g + jiégěng 5-4g + liánqiáo 5-2g + mǔlì 4g + zhīzǐ 2-1g + dàzǎo 2-0g + shēngjiāng 2-0g + dàhuáng 1-0g.

Xuánshēn 5g + dìhuáng 5g + hòupò 5g + màiméndōng 5g + zhǐshí 5-1g + dàhuáng 0g.

Nephrolithiasis (592), Hypertension (401-405.99), Goiter (240.9), Lethargy (D053609), Confusion (D003221), Vomiting (D014839), Nausea (D009325), Constipation (564.0), Anorexia (D000855), Hematemesis (D006396), Headache (D006261), Duodenal ulcer (532), Thyroid carcinoma (193):

Zhūlíngtāng 5g + huàshícǎo 5-1g + jīnqiáncǎo 2-0g + jīnèijīn 2-0g + dàhuáng 1-0g.

Wǔlínsǎn 5g + huàshícǎo 5-2g + jīnqiáncǎo 5-0g + bāzhèngsǎn 5-0g + jīnèijīn 5-0g + yùjīn 5-0g + huángqín 1-0g + dàhuáng 0g.

Chēqiánzǐ 5g + báimáogēn 3g + jīnqiáncǎo 3g + jùmài 3-2g + niúxī 2g + dàhuáng 0g.

Fúlíng 5g + zhūlíng 5g + zéxiè 5g.

Tiānhuā 5g + chēqiánzǐ 5g + fúlíng 5g + jùmài 5g + shānyào 3g + fùzǐ 3g.

Fúlíng 5g + bànxià 3g + fùzǐ 3g + xìxīn 2g + dàhuáng 1g.

Xuánshēn was introduced in Section 4.11 as an antitumor. Bèimǔ (Bulbus Fritillariae Cirrhosae) was reviewed and summarized to be a potential anticancer agent with high bioactivity and low toxicity for cancers, including lung cancer, colorectal cancer, liver cancer, endometrial cancer, oral cancer, ovarian cancer, and myelogenous leukemia (Chen et al., 2020). Huàshícǎo (Herba Orthosiphonae) is translated to "stone-dissolving herb." Its ethanol extract was shown to treat neph-rolithiasis in mice (Chao et al., 2020) and it is used today for calculus in the kidney, gallbladder, ureter, and urethra (Wang, 2020). Jīnqiáncǎo (Herba Lysimachiae) "removes dampness, eliminates jaundice, promotes urination, relieves stranguria, detoxifies, de-swells" and is used today for calcu-lus of the kidneys and so on (Wang, 2020).

4.28 NEUROENDOCRINE TUMOR OF STOMACH

Neuroendocrine tumor of the stomach, also called gastric neuroendocrine tumor, is a tumor starting in the neuroendocrine cells in the lining of the stomach. A neuroendocrine tumor of the stomach is associated with chronic inflammation and thinning of the stomach lining.

TABLE 4.28

GMP Herbal Medicines for a 60-Year-Old Adult with Neuroendocrine Tumor of Stomach

Neuroendocrine tumor of stomach (OrphaCode: 100075)

A disease with a prevalence of ~3 in 100,000

Candidate gene tested: ATRX chromatin remodeler (*ATRX* / Entrez: 546) at Xq21.1

Candidate gene tested: death domain associated protein (*DAXX* / Entrez: 1616) at 6p21.32
Not applicable

Carcinoid tumor

Weight loss, Iron deficiency anemia, Nausea and vomiting, Anorexia, Intermittent diarrhea, Episodic abdominal pain, Poor appetite

Dermatological manifestations of systemic disorders, Zollinger-Ellison syndrome, Hepatomegaly, Hematemesis, Melena, Chronic noninfectious lymphadenopathy, Elevated hepatic transaminase, Bloody diarrhea, Lack of bowel sounds, Atypical pulmonary carcinoid tumor

Adult, Elderly

Weight loss (D015431), Anorexia (D000855):

Guìzhītāng 5g + xìngrén 1-0g + hòupò 1-0g + shēngjiāng 1-0g + dàhuáng 0g.	Gāncǎo 5g + hòupò 5-3g + zhǐshí 5-3g + dàhuáng 1-0g.
Wǔlíngsǎn 5g + hòupò 1g + zhǐshí 1g + dàhuáng 0g.	Zhìgāncǎo 5g + hòupò 5-3g + zhǐshí 5-3g + dàhuáng 1-0g.

Hematemesis (D006396), Melena (D008551) [Blood in stool (578.1)], Elevated hepatic transaminase (573.9):

Bànxiàxièxīntāng 5g + xiāngshāliùjūnzǐtāng 5g + cháihúshūgāntāng 5-0g + píngwèisǎn 5-0g + báijí 2-0g + bèimǔ 2-0g + hǎipiāoxiāo 2-0g.	Báijí 5g + chuānqī 3-2g + huángqín 3-1g + huánglián 2-1g + dàhuáng 0g.
Xiǎocháihútāng 5g + yīnchénwǔlíngsǎn 5g + huángliánjiědútāng 5-0g + hǔzhàng 3-0g + zhīzǐ 2-0g + huángbò 2-0g + dàqīngyè 2-0g + jīnyínhuā 2-0g + zhǐqiào 2-0g + púgōngyīng 2-0g.	Huángqín 5g + huánglián 2g + dàhuáng 0g.
Píngwèisǎn 5g + cháihúshūgāntāng 4g + báijí 1g.	

Báijí (Rhizoma Bletillae) "stops bleeding, reduces swelling, promotes muscle growth" and is used today for acute as well as chronic gastric ulcer (Wang, 2020). Bànxiàxièxīntāng (cf. Sections 1.12 and 4.23) was concluded, in a systematic review and meta-analysis of randomized controlled trials, to be effective and safe for the treatment of chronic atrophic gastritis by improving stomach distend-ing pain and belching; inhibiting *Helicobacter pylori*–related inflammation; and relieving glandular atrophy, intestinal metaplasia, and gastric mucosa dysplasia (Cao et al., 2020).

4.29 PLEURAL MESOTHELIOMA

Pleural mesothelioma is a cancer affecting the lining of the lung called the *pleura*. Pleural mesothelioma is almost always caused by inhalation of asbestos fibers. Inhaled asbestos fibers travel and lodge themselves in the pleura, causing inflammation and scarring of the pleura. Additionally, mutations in the *BAP1* gene, which is a tumor suppressor gene, increase susceptibility to cancers including mesothelioma.

TABLE 4.29

GMP Herbal Medicines for a 72-Year-Old Adult with Pleural Mesothelioma

Pleural mesothelioma (OrphaCode: 50251)

A disease with a prevalence of ~3 in 100,000

Disease-causing germline mutation(s): BRCA1 associated protein 1 (*BAP1* / Entrez: 8314) at 3p21.1

Not applicable

Pleural effusion

Abnormality of the thorax, Weight loss, Dyspnea, Respiratory distress, Abnormality of the pleura, Cough, Constitutional symptom, Chest pain

Dysphagia, Abnormal lung morphology, Hepatomegaly, Lymphadenopathy, Functional respiratory abnormality, Fourth cranial nerve palsy, Abnormality of cardiovascular system physiology, Obstruction of the superior vena cava

All ages

Weight loss (D015431), Respiratory distress (D004417), Cough (D003371), Chest pain (D002637):

Guìzhītāng 5g + xìngrén 2-1g + hòupò 1g + dàhuáng 0g. Gāncǎo 5g + hòupò 5-0g + zhǐshí 5-0g + dàhuáng 1-0g.

Lǐzhōngtāng 5g + bànxià 1g + shārén 1g + fúlíng 1g.

Fourth cranial nerve palsy (378.53):

Zīshènmíngmùtāng 5g + qǐjúdìhuángwán 4g + xǐgānmíngmùtāng 4-0g + juémíngzǐ 1g + mùzéicǎo 1-0g + mìmēnghuā 1-0g + gǔjīngcǎo 1-0g + tùsīzǐ 1-0g.

Báizhú 5g + báisháo 5g + fúlíng 5g + dǎngshēn 5g + fùzǐ 3g.
Huángqí 5g + chìsháo 0g + fángfēng 0g + dàhuáng 0g.
Cháihú 5g + tiānhuā 2g + guìzhī 2g + huángqín 2g + gāncǎo 1g + mǔlì 1g + gānjiāng 1g + bànxià 1g + báizhú 1g + fúlíng 1g.

Zīshènmíngmùtāng 5g + jìshēngshènqìwán 5g + mùzéicǎo 1g + juémíngzǐ 1g + chēqiánzǐ 1g.

Màiyá 5g + báizhú 4g + zhǐshí 4g + chénpí 4g + báibiǎndòu 3g + qiànshí 2g.

Xìngrén was introduced in Sections 1.12 and 1.47 for chest pain and coughs. Its active compound was proposed as a therapeutical agent for the treatment of COVID-19 (coronavirus disease 2019) (Wang et al., 2021). Hòupò, introduced previously for digestive conditions, was shown in mice to alleviate loss of body mass, skeletal muscle weight, and grip strength by increasing the number of anti-inflammatory macrophages that play a role in muscle repair (Hong et al., 2021). The fourth cranial nerve is one of the ocular motor nerves that control eye movement. Báizhú was introduced in Section 1.21 for neuroprotection.

4.30 PRIMARY MYELOFIBROSIS

Primary myelofibrosis, also known as agnogenic myeloid metaplasia or osteomyelofibrosis, is a bone marrow disease characterized by abnormal blood cell production and fibrous tissue formation in the bone marrow. Other features include hardening of the bone marrow and development of too many small blood vessels in the bone marrow. Many cases of primary myelofibrosis are associated with acquired mutations of the *JAK2* gene in the hematopoietic stem cells in the bone marrow.

Mǔdānpí (cf. Section 4.20) is hemostatic, and the active ingredients in Mǔdānpí and their targets for hemorrhagic diseases were identified (Li et al., 2019). Zhīmǔ (cf. Section 2.35) "clears

TABLE 4.30

GMP Herbal Medicines for a 65-Year-Old Adult with Primary Myelofibrosis

Primary myelofibrosis (OrphaCode: 824)

A disease with a prevalence of ~3 in 100,000

Disease-causing somatic mutation(s): Janus kinase 2 (*JAK2* / Entrez: 3717) at 9p24.1

Disease-causing somatic mutation(s): MPL proto-oncogene, thrombopoietin receptor (*MPL* / Entrez: 4352) at 1p34.2

Disease-causing somatic mutation(s): tet methylcytosine dioxygenase 2 (*TET2* / Entrez: 54790) at 4q24

Disease-causing somatic mutation(s): calreticulin (*CALR* / Entrez: 811) at 19p13.13

Not applicable

Abnormality of bone marrow cell morphology

Pallor, Hepatosplenomegaly, Splenomegaly, Abnormality of blood and blood-forming tissues, Thrombocytopenia, Anemia, Hepatomegaly, Abnormal megakaryocyte morphology, Fatigue, Constitutional symptom

Petechiae, Purpura, Portal hypertension, Pancytopenia, Abnormal bleeding, Thrombocytosis, Fever, Leukocytosis, Abnormal thrombosis, Extramedullary hematopoiesis, Anorexia, Lymphadenopathy, Easy fatigability, Arterial thrombosis, Poikilocytosis, Venous thrombosis, Low-grade fever, Flank pain, Bone marrow hypercellularity, Ecchymosis

Adult

Pallor (D010167), Abnormality of blood and blood-forming tissues (289.9), Thrombocytopenia (287.5), Anemia (285.9), Fatigue (D005221):

Guīpítāng 5g + xiānhècǎo 2g + ējiāo 2g + jīxuèténg 2g.	Mǔdānpí 5g + zhīmǔ 5g + huángbò 5-0g.
Rénshēnyǎngróngtāng 5g + guīpítāng 5g + bǔzhōngyìqìtāng 5-0g.	Báizhú 5g + fúlíng 5-4g + fùzǐ 5-0g + cháihú 5-0g + báisháo 4-0g + tiānhuā 2-0g + dǎngshēn 2-0g + guìzhī 2-0g + huángqín 2-0g + shēngjiāng 2-0g + gāncǎo 1-0g + mǔlì 1-0g + gānjiāng 1-0g.
Guīpítāng 5g + bǔzhōngyìqìtāng 5-0g + jiāwèixiāoyáosǎn 4-0g + dānshēn 1g + ējiāo 1g + jīxuèténg 1g + xiānhècǎo 1-0g + huángqí 1-0g.	
	Bànzhīlián 5g + báihuāshéshécǎo 5g + huángqí 5g.

Petechiae (D011693), Portal hypertension (572.3), Pancytopenia (284.1), Fever (D005334), Anorexia (D000855), Flank pain (D021501):

Xiāofēngsǎn 5g + dāngguīyǐnzǐ 5g + báixiānpí 1-0g + dìfūzǐ 1-0g + tǔfúlíng 1-0g + mǔdānpí 1-0g + jīnyínhuā 1-0g + liánqiáo 1-0g.	Gāncǎo 5g + báizhǐ 5g + shārén 5-3g + jīnyínhuā 5-0g + huángqín 5-0g + tiānhuā 2-0g + xìxīn 2-0g + dàhuáng 0g.
Guìzhītāng 5g + xìngrén 1g + máhuáng 1g.	Dǎngshēn 5g + báixiānpí 4g + wūméi 4g + mǔdānpí 2g + chìsháo 2g + kǔshēn 1g + guìzhī 1g + dānguī 1g.

heat, quenches fire, nourishes yin, moisturizes dryness" and was found to inhibit platelet aggregation in human blood (Zhang et al., 1999). Dǎngshēn (cf. Section 1.65) extract was shown to protect melanocytes against oxidative stress in melanocyte cells derived from embryonic mouse skin (Cho, 2021).

4.31 MULTIPLE ENDOCRINE NEOPLASIA TYPE 2

Multiple endocrine neoplasia type 2 (MEN2) is characterized by the presence of a tumor that forms inside the thyroid gland, together with a tumor of the inner part of the adrenal gland or tumor of the parathyroid gland. MEN2 is caused by mutations in the *RET* gene, which is an oncogene. Specific mutations in the *RET* gene determine clinical features and subtypes of MEN2.

Gāncǎo (cf. Section 1.1) was shown to cure diarrhea in piglets inoculated with porcine rotavirus,] through coordinating antiviral and anti-inflammatory effects (Alfajaro et al., 2012). It was also shown to reduce diarrhea in castor oil–induced diarrheal mice (Wen et al., 2023). Jīnèijīn (Endothelium Corneum Gigeriae Galli) "decumulates foods, strengthens the Stomach, conserves semen, arrests spermatorrhea" and was shown to reduce the number of kidney stones and kidney damage in rats with renal calculi (Wang et al., 2019).

TABLE 4.31
GMP Herbal Medicines for a 12-Year-Old Child with Multiple Endocrine Neoplasia Type 2

Multiple endocrine neoplasia type 2 (OrphaCode: 653)

A disease with a prevalence of ~3 in 100,000

Disease-causing germline mutation(s): ret proto-oncogene (*RET* / Entrez: 5979) at 10q11.21

Autosomal dominant

Medullary thyroid carcinoma

Anxiety, Hyperhidrosis, Pallor, Palpitations, Diarrhea, Headache, Hypertension associated with pheochromocytoma, Pheochromocytoma, Elevated urinary norepinephrine, Elevated calcitonin, Elevated urinary epinephrine, Parathyroid hyperplasia, Thyroid C cell hyperplasia, Elevated urinary catecholamines, Elevated urinary vanillylmandelic acid, Thyroid nodule, Cervical neoplasm, Hypertensive crisis

Nephrolithiasis, Muscle weakness, Disproportionate tall stature, Constipation, Hypercalciuria, Aganglionic megacolon, Kyphoscoliosis, Paraganglioma of head and neck, Neoplasm of the liver, Parathyroid adenoma, Hypercalcemia, Elevated circulating parathyroid hormone level, Abdominal distention, Hyperlordosis, Primary hyperparathyroidism, Neoplasm of the skeletal system, Prominent corneal nerve fibers, Thick vermilion border, Ganglioneuromatosis, Cervical lymphadenopathy, Neuroma, Abnormal tongue morphology, Neck pain, Multiple mucosal neuromas, Cutaneous lichen amyloidosis, Neoplasm of the lung

Infancy, Childhood, Adolescent, Adult

Pallor (D010167), Diarrhea (D003967), Headache (D006261):

Wǔlíngsǎn 5g + lǐzhōngtāng 5-0g + gāncǎo 0g.	Gāncǎo 5g + báizhǐ 5-0g + shārén 5-0g + dàhuáng 1-0g.
Wǔlíngsǎn 5g + píngwèisǎn 5-0g + bànxià 1-0g + gāncǎo 0g.	Gāncǎo 5g + hòupò 3-0g + zhǐshí 3-0g + dàhuáng 1-0g.

Nephrolithiasis (592), Muscle weakness (D018908), Constipation (564.0), Hypercalciuria (D053565), Neoplasm of the liver (155.0, 155.2), Parathyroid adenoma (194.1), Hypercalcemia (275.42), Primary hyperparathyroidism (252.01), Neck pain (D019547):

Zhūlíngtāng 5g + huàshícǎo 5-2g + jīnèijīn 2-1g + jīnqiáncǎo 2-0g + dàhuáng 1-0g.	Chìxiǎodòu 5g + dāngguī 5g + chēqiánzǐ 3-2g + niúxī 2g + dàhuáng 1-0g.
Bāzhèngsǎn 5g + huàshícǎo 3g + táohéchéngqìtāng 2g + dàhuáng 1g.	Báimáogēn 5g + niúxī 2g + chēqiánzǐ 2g + jīnqiáncǎo 2g + dàhuáng 1-0g.
	Fúlíng 5g + fùzǐ 4g + bànxià 3g + xìxīn 2g + dàhuáng 1g.

4.32   CHOLANGIOCARCINOMA

Cholangiocarcinoma, also known as bile duct cancer, is cancer that begins in the bile ducts. Acquired genetic mutations in the bile duct cells cause cholangiocarcinoma. The mutated genes include the tumor suppressor genes *BRCA1* and *BRCA2*.

Hǔzhàng (Rhizoma et Radix Polygoni Cuspidati), "being choleric and anti-jaundice," was shown in rats to improve non-alcoholic fatty liver disease via regulating lipid metabolism (Zhang et al., 2023) and

TABLE 4.32
GMP Herbal Medicines for a 65-Year-Old Adult with Cholangiocarcinoma

Cholangiocarcinoma (OrphaCode: 70567)

A disease with a prevalence of ~2 in 100,000

Disease-causing somatic mutation(s): BRCA1 DNA repair associated (*BRCA1* / Entrez: 672) at 17q21.31

Disease-causing somatic mutation(s): BRCA2 DNA repair associated (*BRCA2* / Entrez: 675) at 13q13.1

Disease-causing somatic mutation(s): protein tyrosine phosphatase non-receptor type 3 (*PTPN3* / HGNC:9655) at 9q31

Not applicable

Jaundice, Acholic stools, Biliary tract neoplasm

Pruritus, Fatigue

Fever, Abdominal pain, Anorexia

Adult

(Continued)

TABLE 4.32 *(Continued)*

GMP Herbal Medicines for a 65-Year-Old Adult with Cholangiocarcinoma

Jaundice (D007565), Biliary tract neoplasm (156.9):

Yīnchénwǔlíngsǎn 5g + huángliánjiědútāng 5-2g + jīnyínhuā 2-1g + púgōngyīng 2-1g + dàqīngyè 2-0g.

Fúlíng 5g + yīnchén 5-0g + bànxià 4-3g + fùzǐ 4-3g + xìxīn 2g + dàhuáng 1-0g.

Hǔzhàng 5g + nǚzhēnzǐ 2g + tiānhuā·2g + shíhú 2g + hànliáncǎo 2g + shāshēn 2g + zhìgāncǎo 2g + chuānliànzǐ 1g + héshǒuwū 1g + gǒuqǐzǐ 1g + màiméndōng 1g + júhuā 1g + huángjīng 1g.

Cháihú 5g + bànxià 4g + báisháo 4g + zhǐshí 4g + huángqín 4g + dàzǎo 2g + shēngjiāng 2g + dàhuáng 0g.

Bànzhīlián 5g + báihuāshéshécǎo 5g.

Pruritus (D011537), Fatigue (D005221):

Wǔlíngsǎn 5g + gāncǎo 1g + báisháo 1g + tiáowèichéngqìtāng 1g + dàhuáng 0g.

Wǔlíngsǎn 5g + huángqín 1g + báisháo 1-0g + fùzǐ 1-0g + dǐdāngtāng 0g + dàhuáng 0g.

Gāncǎo 5g + báizhǐ 5g + shārén 5-3g + huángqín 5-0g + tiānhuā 2-0g + xìxīn 2-0g + dàhuáng 1-0g.

Fever (D005334), Abdominal pain (D015746), Anorexia (D000855):

Wǔlíngsǎn 5g + xìxīn 1g + huángqín 1g + dǐdāngtāng 0g + dàhuáng 0g.

Wǔlíngsǎn 5g + xìxīn 1g + huángqín 1g + tiáowèichéngqìtāng 0g.

Gāncǎo 5g + báizhǐ 5g + huángqín 5-4g + shārén 4-3g + guālóugēn 2-0g + dàhuáng 1-0g.

---

is used for pure hypercholesterolemia (Wang, 2020). Huángliánjiědútāng (cf. Section 3.1) "quenches fire, de-toxifies" and was shown to arrest the cell cycle and trigger mitochondrial apoptosis in two human liver cancer cell lines (Hsu et al., 2008). Guālóugēn (Radix Trichosanthis) is bitter and cold in TCM taste and nature; it "treats thirst, hyperthermia, irritability and yin-deficiency resulting from fire."

4.33 PSEUDOMYXOMA PERITONEI

Pseudomyxoma peritonei (PMP), also called adenomucinosis or gelatinous ascites, is a cancer that starts in the appendix as a polyp and migrates through the flow of peritoneal fluid to the lining of the abdominal and pelvic cavity. These tumor cells secrete mucus, filling the cavity to cause the symptoms of the disease. The cause of PMP is not known.

TABLE 4.33

GMP Herbal Medicines for a 50-Year-Old Adult with Pseudomyxoma Peritonei

Pseudomyxoma peritonei (OrphaCode: 26790)

A disease with a prevalence of ~2 in 100,000

Unknown

Ascites, Abnormality of the peritoneum, Abnormality of the abdominal wall

Inflammation of the large intestine

Weight loss, Nausea and vomiting, Constipation, Abdominal pain, Respiratory insufficiency, Lymphadenopathy, Intestinal obstruction, Hernia

Adult

Ascites (D001201):

Dǎoshuǐfúlíngtāng 5g + yīnchénwǔlíngsǎn 5-0g + chēqiánzǐ 1-0g + zéxiè 1-0g.

Dǎoshuǐfúlíngtāng 5g + wǔlíngsǎn 5-0g + chēqiánzǐ 1-0g + zéxiè 1-0g.

Jiāwèixiāoyáosǎn 5g + zhǐqiào 2g + jílí 2g + chántuì 2g.

Báimáogēn 5g + chìxiǎodòu 5g + chēqiánzǐ 5g + yìmǔcǎo 5-0g + dāngguī 2g.

Chìxiǎodòu 5-3g + chēqiánzǐ 5-2g + yìmǔcǎo 5-2g + dāngguī 2-0g + dàhuáng 0g.

(Continued)

TABLE 4.33 *(Continued)*
GMP Herbal Medicines for a 50-Year-Old Adult with Pseudomyxoma Peritonei

Weight loss (D015431), Constipation (564.0), Abdominal pain (D015746), Intestinal obstruction (560.9), Hernia (618.6):

Mázǐrénwán 5g + dàhuáng 1g.	Gāncǎo 5g + dàhuáng 5-0g + huángqín 5-0g +
Dàchéngqìtāng 5g.	huánglián 5-0g + gégēn 5-0g.
Dàhuáng 5g + mùxiāngbīnglángwán 5g + mázǐrénwán 5-0g +	
táohéchéngqìtāng 5-0g.	
Sìnìtāng 5g + hòupò 1g + zhǐshí 1g + dàhuáng 0g.	

The term dǎoshuǐ in Dǎoshuǐfúlíngtāng (cf. Section 4.12) means "fluid guiding." The formula contains the major herb Fúlíng (cf. Section 1.66), which was shown to improve proteinuria and ascites in rats with nephrotic syndrome (Lee et al., 2014). Dàhuáng, Hòupò, Zhǐshí, Gāncǎo, Mázǐrénwán, Mùxiāngbīnglángwán, and Táohéchéngqìtāng were among the most commonly prescribed single herbs and formulas to constipation patients in Taiwan (Jong et al., 2010).

REFERENCES

Alfajaro, M. M., Kim, H., Park, J., Ryu, E., Kim, J., Jeong, Y., Kim, D., Hosmillo, M., Son, K., Lee, J., Kwon, H. J., Ryu, Y. B., Park, S., Park, S., Lee, W. S., & Cho, K. (2012). Anti-rotaviral effects of *Glycyrrhiza uralensis* extract in piglets with rotavirus diarrhea. *Virology Journal, 9*(1). https://doi.org/10.1186/1743-422x-9-310

Ben-Arie, E., Lottering, B., Inprasit, C., Yip, H., Ho, W., Ton, G., Lee, Y., & Kao, P. (2022). Traditional Chinese medicine use in patients with oral cancer: A retrospective longitudinal cohort study in Taiwan. *Medicine, 101*(38), e30716. https://doi.org/10.1097/md.0000000000030716

Cai, Y., Zheng, Q., Sun, R., Wu, J., Li, X., & Liu, R. (2020). Recent progress in the study of Artemisiae Scopariae Herba (Yin Chen), a promising medicinal herb for liver diseases. *Biomedicine & Pharmacotherapy, 130*, 110513. https://doi.org/10.1016/j.biopha.2020.110513

Cao, Y., Zheng, Y., Niu, J., Zhu, C., Yang, D., Rong, F., & Li, G. (2020). Efficacy of Banxia Xiexin decoction for chronic atrophic gastritis: A systematic review and meta-analysis. *PloS One, 15*(10), e0241202. https://doi.org/10.1371/journal.pone.0241202

Chao, Y., Gao, S., Li, N., Zhao, H., Qian, Y., Zha, H., Chen, W., & Dong, X. (2020). Lipidomics reveals the therapeutic effects of EtOAc extract of *Orthosiphon stamineus* Benth. on nephrolithiasis. *Frontiers in Pharmacology, 11*. https://doi.org/10.3389/fphar.2020.01299

Chen, R., He, J., Tong, X., Tang, L., & Liu, M. (2016). The *Hedyotis diffusa* Willd. (Rubiaceae): A review on phytochemistry, pharmacology, quality control and pharmacokinetics. *Molecules, 21*(6), 710. https://doi.org/10.3390/molecules21060710

Chen, T., Zhong, F., Yao, C., Chen, J., Xiang, Y., Dong, J., Yan, Z., & Ma, Y. (2020). A systematic review on traditional uses, sources, phytochemistry, pharmacology, pharmacokinetics, and toxicity of Fritillariae cirrhosae Bulbus. *Evidence-Based Complementary and Alternative Medicine, 2020*(1), 26. https://doi.org/10.1155/2020/1536534

Chen, Y. (1981). Ramble in Chinese ophthalmology, past and present. *Chinse Medical Journal, 94*(1), 1–4.

Cheng, C., Lin, Y., & Su, C. (2010). Anti-tumor activity of Sann-Joong-Kuey-Jian-Tang alone and in combination with 5-fluorouracil in a human colon cancer colo 205 cell xenograft model. *Molecular Medicine Reports, 3*(2), 227–231. https://pubmed.ncbi.nlm.nih.gov/21472226

Cho, Y. H. (2021). *Codonopsis pilosula* extract protects melanocytes against H_2O_2-induced oxidative stress by activating autophagy. *Cosmetics, 8*(3), 67. https://doi.org/10.3390/cosmetics8030067

Dai, Y., Zhang, Y., Li, D., Ye, J., Chen, W., & Hu, L. (2017). Efficacy and safety of modified Banxia Xiexin decoction (Pinellia decoction for draining the heart) for gastroesophageal reflux disease in adults: A systematic review and meta-analysis. *Evidence-Based Complementary and Alternative Medicine, 2017*, 1–17. https://doi.org/10.1155/2017/9591319

Deng, L., Lei, Y., Chiu, T., Qi, M., Gan, H., Zhang, G., Peng, Z., Zhang, D., Chen, Y., & Chen, J. (2019). The anticancer effects of paeoniflorin and its underlying mechanisms. *Natural Product Communications, 14*(9), 1934578X1987640. https://doi.org/10.1177/1934578x19876409

Fei, X., Yuan, W., Jiang, L., & Wang, H. (2017). Opposite effects of *Agrimonia pilosa* Ledeb aqueous extracts on blood coagulation function. *Annals of Translational Medicine, 5*(7), 157. https://doi.org/10.21037/atm.2017.03.17

Fleischer, T., Chang, T. T., Chiang, J. H., Chang, C., Hsieh, C., & Yen, H. (2016). Adjunctive Chinese herbal medicine therapy improves survival of patients with chronic myeloid leukemia: A nationwide population-based cohort study. *Cancer Medicine, 5*(4), 640–648. https://doi.org/10.1002/cam4.627

Fleischer, T., Chang, T., Chiang, J., Sun, M., & Yen, H. (2016). Improved survival with integration of Chinese herbal medicine therapy in patients with acute myeloid leukemia: A nationwide population-based cohort study. *Integrative Cancer Therapies, 16*(2), 156–164. https://doi.org/10.1177/1534735416664171

Gou, S., Liu, B., Han, X., Wang, L., Zhong, C., Shan, L., Liu, H., Yin, Q., Yun, Z., & Ni, J. (2018). Anti-atherosclerotic effect of Fermentum Rubrum and *Gynostemma pentaphyllum* mixture in high-fat emulsion- and vitamin D_3-induced atherosclerotic rats. *Journal of the Chinese Medical Association, 81*(5), 398–408. https://doi.org/10.1016/j.jcma.2017.08.018

Hong, M., Han, I., Choi, I., Cha, N., Kim, W., Kim, S. K., & Bae, H. (2021). Magnoliae cortex alleviates muscle wasting by modulating M2 macrophages in a cisplatin-induced sarcopenia mouse model. *International Journal of Molecular Sciences, 22*(6), 3188. https://doi.org/10.3390/ijms22063188

Hsu, P., Chen, J., Kuo, S., Wang, W., Jan, F., Yang, S., & Yang, C. Y. (2022). San-Zhong-Kui-Jian-Tang exerts antitumor effects associated with decreased cell proliferation and metastasis by targeting ERK and the epithelial–mesenchymal transition pathway in oral cavity squamous cell carcinoma. *Integrative Cancer Therapies, 21*, 153473542211349. https://doi.org/10.1177/15347354221134921

Hsu, Y. L., Kuo, P. L., Tzeng, T. F., Sung, S. C., Yen, M. H., Lin, L., & Lin, C. (2008). Huang-lian-jie-du-tang, a traditional Chinese medicine prescription, induces cell-cycle arrest and apoptosis in human liver cancer cells in vitro and in vivo. *Journal of Gastroenterology and Hepatology, 23*(7pt2). https://doi.org/10.1111/j.1440-1746.2008.05390.x

Hsu, Y., Yen, M., Kuo, P., Cho, C., Huang, Y., Tseng, C., Lee, J., & Lin, C. (2006). San-Zhong-Kui-Jian-Tang, a traditional Chinese medicine prescription, inhibits the proliferation of human breast cancer cell by blocking cell cycle progression and inducing apoptosis. *Biological & Pharmaceutical Bulletin, 29*(12), 2388–2394. https://doi.org/10.1248/bpb.29.2388

Jang, S., Jeong, J. J., Hyam, S. R., Han, M. J., & Kim, D. H. (2013). Anticolitic effect of the rhizome mixture of *Anemarrhena asphodeloides* and *Coptidis chinensis* (AC-mix) in mice. *Biomolecules & Therapeutics, 21*(5), 398–404. https://doi.org/10.4062/biomolther.2013.048

Jong, M. S., Hwang, S. J., Chen, Y. C., Chen, T. J., Chen, F. J., & Chen, F. P. (2010). Prescriptions of Chinese herbal medicine for constipation under the National Health Insurance in Taiwan. *Journal of the Chinese Medical Association, 73*(7), 375–383. https://doi.org/10.1016/s1726-4901(10)70081-2

Komiyama, S., Takeya, C., Takahashi, R., Yamamoto, Y., & Kubushiro, K. (2015). Feasibility study on the effectiveness of Goreisan-based Kampo therapy for lower abdominal lymphedema after retroperitoneal lymphadenectomy via extraperitoneal approach. *Journal of Obstetrics and Gynaecology Research, 41*(9), 1449–1456. https://doi.org/10.1111/jog.12721

Lee, K., Park, G., Ham, I., Yang, G., M, L., Bu, Y., Kim, H., & Choi, H. (2013). Vasorelaxant effect of Osterici Radix ethanol extract on rat aortic rings. *Evidence-Based Complementary and Alternative Medicine, 2013*, 1–8. https://doi.org/10.1155/2013/350964

Lee, S. M., Lee, Y. J., Yoon, J. J., Kang, D. G., & Lee, H. S. (2014). Effect of *Poria cocos* on puromycin aminonucleoside-induced nephrotic syndrome in rats. *Evidence-Based Complementary and Alternative Medicine, 2014*, 1–12. https://doi.org/10.1155/2014/570420

Li, S., Xue, X., Yang, X., Zhou, S., Wang, S., & Meng, J. (2019). A network pharmacology approach used to estimate the active ingredients of Moutan Cortex charcoal and the potential targets in hemorrhagic diseases. *Biological & Pharmaceutical Bulletin, 42*(3), 432–441. https://doi.org/10.1248/bpb.b18-00756

Liu, Y., Hong, Z., Qian, J., Wang, Y., & Wang, S. (2019). Protective effect of Jie-Geng-Tang against *Staphylococcus aureus* induced acute lung injury in mice and discovery of its effective constituents. *Journal of Ethnopharmacology, 243*, 112076. https://doi.org/10.1016/j.jep.2019.112076

Luo, H., Wu, H., Yu, X., Zhang, X., Lü, Y., Fan, J., Tang, L., & Wang, Z. (2019). A review of the phytochemistry and pharmacological activities of *Magnoliae officinalis* cortex. *Journal of Ethnopharmacology, 236*, 412–442. https://doi.org/10.1016/j.jep.2019.02.041

Niu, L., Hou, Y., Jiang, M., & Bai, G. (2021). The rich pharmacological activities of *Magnolia officinalis* and secondary effects based on significant intestinal contributions. *Journal of Ethnopharmacology, 281*, 114524. https://doi.org/10.1016/j.jep.2021.114524

Pan, Y., Luo, X., & Gong, P. (2023). *Spatholobi caulis*: A systematic review of its traditional uses, chemical constituents, biological activities and clinical applications. *Journal of Ethnopharmacology, 317*, 116854. https://doi.org/10.1016/j.jep.2023.116854

Powell, C. B., Fung, P., Jackson, J. H., Dall'Era, J. E., Lewkowicz, D., Cohen, I., & Smith-McCune, K. (2003). Aqueous extract of herba *Scutellaria barbatae*, a Chinese herb used for ovarian cancer, induces apoptosis of ovarian cancer cell lines. *Gynecologic Oncology*, *91*(2), 332–340. https://doi.org/10.1016/j.ygyno.2003.07.004

Ranaware, A. M., Banik, K., Deshpande, V. A., Padmavathi, G., Roy, N. K., Sethi, G., Fan, L., Kumar, A. P., & Kunnumakkara, A. B. (2018). Magnolol: A neolignan from the Magnolia family for the prevention and treatment of cancer. *International Journal of Molecular Sciences*, *19*(8), 2362. https://doi.org/10.3390/ijms19082362

Shiah, H., Lee, C., Lee, F., Tseng, S., Chen, S., & Wang, C. (2023). Chemopreventive effects of Xiang Sha Liu Jun Zi Tang on paclitaxel-induced leucopenia and neuropathy in animals. *Frontiers in Pharmacology*, *14*. https://doi.org/10.3389/fphar.2023.1106030

Shih, W., Yang, Y., & Chen, P. (2012). Prescription patterns of Chinese herbal products for osteoporosis in Taiwan: A population-based study. *Evidence-Based Complementary and Alternative Medicine*, *2012*, 1–6. https://doi.org/10.1155/2012/752837

Su, C. (2014). Sann-Joong-Kuey-Jian-Tang decreases the protein expression of mammalian target of rapamycin but increases microtubule associated protein II light chain 3 expression to inhibit human BxPC-3 pancreatic carcinoma cells. *Molecular Medicine Reports*, *11*(4), 3160–3166. https://doi.org/10.3892/mmr.2014.3090

Sun, Y., Lenon, G. B., & Yang, A. W. H. (2019). Phellodendri Cortex: A phytochemical, pharmacological, and pharmacokinetic review. *Evidence-Based Complementary and Alternative Medicine*, *2019*, 1–45. https://doi.org/10.1155/2019/7621929

Tang, K., Guo, D., Zhang, L., Guo, D., Zheng, F., & Si, J. (2016). Immunomodulatory effects of Longdan Xiegan Tang on CD4+/CD8+ T cells and associated inflammatory cytokines in rats with experimental autoimmune uveitis. *Molecular Medicine Reports*, *14*(3), 2746–2754. https://doi.org/10.3892/mmr.2016.5558

Ushiroyama, T., Araki, R., Sakuma, K., Nosaka, S., Yamashita, Y., & Kamegai, H. (2006). Efficacy of the Kampo medicine Xiong-Gui-Jiao-Ai-Tang, a traditional herbal medicine, in the treatment of threatened abortion in early pregnancy. *American Journal of Chinese Medicine*, *34*(05), 731–740. https://doi.org/10.1142/s0192415x06004247

Vickers, A. J., Cronin, A. M., Maschino, A. C., Lewith, G., MacPherson, H., Foster, N. E., Sherman, K. J., Witt, C. M., & Linde, K. (2012). Acupuncture for chronic pain. *Archives of Internal Medicine*, *172*(19), 1444. https://doi.org/10.1001/archinternmed.2012.3654

Wang, N., Zhang, D., Zhang, Y., Xu, W., Wang, Y., Zhong, P., Tian-Zhu, J., & Xiu, Y. (2019). Endothelium corneum gigeriae galli extract inhibits calcium oxalate formation and exerts anti-urolithic effects. *Journal of Ethnopharmacology*, *231*, 80–89. https://doi.org/10.1016/j.jep.2018.09.003

Wang, S.-C. (2019). Therapeutic classes of CHEG formulas. In S.-C. Wang (Ed.), *Clinical herbal prescriptions: Principles and practices of herbal formulations from deep learning health insurance herbal prescription big data* (pp. 16–89). World Scientific Publishing. https://doi.org/10.1142/11211

Wang, S.-C. (2020). Modern therapeutic uses of CHEG herbs and herb pairs. In S.-C. Wang (Ed.), *Veterinary herbal pharmacopoeia* (pp. 35–233). Nova Science Publishers. https://doi.org/10.52305/GHTR1903

Wang, Y., Gu, W., Kui, F., Gao, F., Niu, Y., Li, W., Zhang, Y., Guo, Z., & Du, G. (2021). The mechanism and active compounds of semen armeniacae amarum treating coronavirus disease 2019 based on network pharmacology and molecular docking. *Food & Nutrition Research*, *65*. https://doi.org/10.29219/fnr.v65.5623

Wen, J., Zhang, J., Lyu, Y., Zhang, H., Deng, K., Chen, H., & Wang, Y. (2023). Ethanol extract of *Glycyrrhiza uralensis* Fisch: Antidiarrheal activity in mice and contraction effect in isolated rabbit jejunum. *Chinese Journal of Integrative Medicine*, *29*(4), 325–332. https://doi.org/10.1007/s11655-022-3536-5

Wu, M., Zhang, W., & Liu, L. (2017). Red yeast rice prevents atherosclerosis through regulating inflammatory signaling pathways. *Chinese Journal of Integrative Medicine*, *23*(9), 689–695. https://doi.org/10.1007/s11655-017-2416-x

Xiang, A., Cheng, K., Shen, X., Xu, P., & Liu, S. (2017). The immediate analgesic effect of acupuncture for pain: A systematic review and meta-analysis. *Evidence-based Complementary and Alternative Medicine*, *2017*, 1–13. https://doi.org/10.1155/2017/3837194

Xiao, Y., Liu, Y., Yu, K., Ouyang, M., Luo, R., & Zhao, X. (2012). Chinese Herbal medicine Liu Jun Zi Tang and Xiang Sha Liu Jun Zi Tang for functional dyspepsia: Meta-analysis of randomized controlled trials. *Evidence-Based Complementary and Alternative Medicine*, *2012*, 1–7. https://doi.org/10.1155/2012/936459

Yang, S., & Yu, C. (2008). Antiinflammatory effects of Bu-zhong-yi-qi-tang in patients with perennial allergic rhinitis. *Journal of Ethnopharmacology*, *115*(1), 104–109. https://doi.org/10.1016/j.jep.2007.09.011

Yang, Y., Lai, Q., Wang, C., & Zhou, G. (2022). Protective effects of Herba Houttuyniae aqueous extract against OVA-induced airway hyperresponsiveness and inflammation in asthmatic mice. *Evidence-Based Complementary and Alternative Medicine*, *2022*, 1–11. https://doi.org/10.1155/2022/7609785

Yoshikawa, N., Kajiyama, H., Otsuka, N., Tamauchi, S., Ikeda, Y., Nishino, K., Niimi, K., Suzuki, S., Utsumi, F., Shibata, K., & Kikkawa, F. (2020). The therapeutic effects of Goreisan, a traditional Japanese herbal medicine, on lower-limb lymphedema after lymphadenectomy in gynecologic malignancies: A case series study. *Evidence-Based Complementary and Alternative Medicine*, *2020*, 1–6. https://doi.org/10.1155/2020/6298293

You, L., Wang, K., Lin, J., Ren, X., Yu, W., Xu, X., Gao, Y., Kong, X., & Sun, X. (2023). Yin-chen Wu-ling powder alleviate cholestatic liver disease: Network pharmacological analysis and experimental validation. *Gene*, *851*, 146973. https://doi.org/10.1016/j.gene.2022.146973

Zhang, H., Sham, T., Li, C., Hu, X., Li, C., Cheng, K. K., So, C., Huang, Y., Chan, S., & Mok, D. K. (2023). Polygoni Cuspidati Rhizoma et Radix extract attenuates high-fat diet-induced NAFLD in rats: Impact on untargeted serum metabolomics and liver lipidomics. *Pharmacological Research. Modern Chinese Medicine*, *9*, 100335. https://doi.org/10.1016/j.prmcm.2023.100335

Zhang, H., Yingying, G., Zhang, J., Wang, K., Jin, T., Wang, H., Ruan, K., Wu, F., & Xu, Z. (2020). The effect of total lignans from Fructus Arctii on streptozotocin-induced diabetic retinopathy in Wistar rats. *Journal of Ethnopharmacology*, *255*, 112773. https://doi.org/10.1016/j.jep.2020.112773

Zhang, J., Zhang, M., Zhang, M., Ma, D., Xu, S., & Kodama, H. (1999). Effect of six steroidal saponins isolated from anemarrhenae rhizoma on platelet aggregation and hemolysis in human blood. *Clinica Chimica Acta*, *289*(1–2), 79–88. https://doi.org/10.1016/s0009-8981(99)00160-6

Zhao, J., Wang, Y., Jin, Y., Jiang, C., & Zhan, Z. (2022). [Research advances in chemical constituents and pharmacological activities of Dendrobium plants]. *Zhongguo Zhong Yao Za Zhi*, *47*(9), 2358–2372. [Article in Chinese] https://doi.org/10.19540/j.cnki.cjcmm.20220216.601

Zhou, M., Liu, P., Jing, S., Sun, M., Li, X., Zhang, W., & Liu, B. (2022). [Chemical constituents of *Scrophulariae* Radix and their antitumor activities in vitro]. *Zhongguo Zhong Yao Za Zhi*, *47*(1), 111–121. [Article in Chinese] https://doi.org/10.19540/j.cnki.cjcmm.20211126.201

5 GMP Herbal Medicine for Rare Inborn Errors of Metabolism

Inborn errors of metabolism, also called *inherited metabolic disorders*, are caused by defective genes whose protein products are involved in breaking down (or synthesizing) a biomolecule into (from) other biomolecules and energy in cells or organelles within cells. As the cells in our body share the same biochemical pathways of metabolism, accumulation or lack of the resulting biomolecules occur and affect many organ systems of the body. Most of the rare, inborn errors of metabolism of this chapter are autosomal recessive and early onset.

In traditional Chinese medicine (TCM), a functional entity called the Spleen is responsible for transforming food and drink into essence and transporting and distributing the extracted essence, including Qi and blood, to other parts of the body, including the Kidneys, Lungs, and muscles, for further refinement and utilization.

The GMP-concentrated herbal extract granules that are frequently discussed for rare, inborn errors of metabolism include Licorice Root (Gāncǎo), Rhubarb Root and Rhizome (Dàhuáng), Cardamon Seed (Shārén), Dahurian Angelica Root (Báizhǐ), Scutellaria Root (Huángqín), Caltrop Fruit (Puncture-Vine Fruit; Jílí), Chinese Senega Root (Yuǎnzhì), Sweetflag Rhizome (Shíchāngpú), Bitter Orange (Zhǐqiào), Rehmannia Root (Dìhuáng), Cicada Molting (Chántuì), Processed Licorice Root (Zhìgāncǎo), and Magnolia Bark (Hòupò); the GMP-concentrated formular extract granules that are frequently used are Tonify the Middle and Augment the Qi Decoction (Bǔzhōngyìqìtāng), Lycium, Chrysanthemum and Rehmannia Pill (Qǐjúdìhuángwán), Ginseng, Poria and Atractylodes Powder (Shēnlíngbáizhúsǎn), Sweet Dew Decoction (Gānlùyǐn), Jade Windscreen Powder (Yùpíngfēngsǎn), Five Ingredient Formula with Poria (Wǔlíngsǎn), Preserve Harmony Pill (Bǎohéwán), Apricot and Perilla Formula (Pediatrics) (Xìngsūyǐnyòukē), Achyranthes and Plantago Formula (Jìshēngshènqìwán), Mulberry Leaf and Chrysanthemum Drink (Sāngjúyǐn), Coptis and Rehmannia Formula (Clear the Stomach Powder; Qīngwèisǎn), Licorice, Wheat and Jujube Decoction (Gāncǎoxiǎomàidàzǎotāng), Poria, Cinnamon, Atractylodis and Licorice Decoction (Língguìshùgāntāng), and Enrich the Kidneys and Improve Vision Decoction (Zīshènmíngmùtāng). Many of them are known to aid in digestion.

5.1 SYSTEMIC PRIMARY CARNITINE DEFICIENCY

Carnitine is a compound, encoded by *SLC22A5*, that transports long-chain fatty acids across cell membranes into mitochondria for energy production. Carnitine deficiency prevents the body, such as the skeletal muscle and heart, from using fats as energy. Buildup of unoxidized fatty acids can

---

TABLE 5.1

GMP Herbal Medicines for a Two-Year-Old Child with Systemic Primary Carnitine Deficiency

Systemic primary carnitine deficiency (OrphaCode: 158)

A disease with a prevalence of ~4 in 10,000

Disease-causing germline mutation(s): solute carrier family 22 member 5 (*SLC22A5* / Entrez: 6584) at 5q31.1

Autosomal recessive

Neck muscle weakness, Confusion, Muscle weakness, Vomiting, Hepatomegaly, Clumsiness, Elevated hepatic transaminase, Acute encephalopathy, Generalized tonic-clonic seizures with focal onset

Neonatal, Infancy

(Continued)

DOI: 10.1201/9781032726625-5

TABLE 5.1 *(Continued)*

GMP Herbal Medicines for a Two-Year-Old Child with Systemic Primary Carnitine Deficiency

Confusion (D003221), Muscle weakness (D018908), Vomiting (D014839), Elevated hepatic transaminase (573.9):

Dàcháihútāng 5g + tiáowèichéngqìtāng 5-0g.	Zhìgāncǎo 5g + dàhuáng 1-0g.
Dàcháihútāng 5g + guìzhīfúlíngwán 2-0g.	Júhóng 5g + zhǐqiào 5-3g.
Xiǎocháihútāng 5g + wǔlíngsǎn 5g.	Gāncǎo 5g + báizhǐ 5-0g + shārén 5-0g + dàhuáng 1-0g.
Sìnìtāng 5g.	Yīnchén 5g.
Cháihújiālónggǔmǔlìtāng 5g + dǐdāngtāng 3-2g.	

also damage organs. Germline mutations in *SLC22A5* cause systemic primary carnitine deficiency (also called carnitine transporter defect), with varying symptoms ranging from asymptomatic to life-threatening in offspring.

Yīnchén is hepatoprotective (cf. Sections 1.57 and 4.21). Both Dàcháihútāng and Xiǎocháihútāng benefit the TCM liver and gallbladder; however, Dàcháihútāng, a derivative of Xiǎocháihútāng, is suitable for patients with acute liver symptoms, while Xiǎocháihútāng for chronic liver conditions. Both Júhóng (cf. Section 1.3) and Zhǐqiào (cf. Section 1.31) "regulate Qi" and assist in digestion.

5.2 FABRY DISEASE

Fabry disease, also known as Anderson-Fabry disease or Angiokeratoma corporis diffusum, is caused by mutations in the *GLA* gene, which encodes an enzyme called alpha-galactosidase A that breaks down a fatty substance called globotriaosylceramide in the cellular recycling centers called lysosomes within cells. The signs and symptoms of Fabry disease vary, depending on the location and amount of globotriaosylceramide accumulation in the body over time.

Chēqiánzǐ (cf. Section 3.8) was shown to ameliorate renal injury in gouty nephropathy rats by regulating renal inflammation (Zhao et al., 2021). Dīngshùxiǔ was introduced in Section 3.35 for hypertensive heart disease and chronic renal failure. Both Zhēnwǔtāng and Jìshēngshènqìwán

TABLE 5.2

GMP Herbal Medicines for a 16-Year-Old Adolescent with Fabry Disease

Fabry disease (OrphaCode: 324)

A disease with a prevalence of ~3 in 10,000

Disease-causing germline mutation(s): galactosidase alpha (*GLA* / Entrez: 2717) at Xq22.1

X-linked dominant, X-linked recessive

Renal insufficiency, Nephrotic syndrome, Hearing impairment, Conjunctival telangiectasia, Hematuria, Hyperkeratosis, Hypohidrosis, Angiokeratoma, Corneal dystrophy, Arthritis, Subcutaneous nodule, Congestive heart failure, Anemia, Malabsorption, Abdominal pain, Transient ischemic attack, Arthralgia, Myalgia, Corneal opacity, Fatigue, Mucosal telangiectasiae, Telangiectasia of the skin

Abnormal renal tubule morphology, Proteinuria, Nephropathy, Thick lower lip vermilion, Coarse facial features, Cataract, Optic atrophy, Behavioral abnormality, Delayed puberty, Abnormal aortic valve morphology, Mitral regurgitation, Atrioventricular block, Nausea and vomiting, Anorexia, Emphysema, Hyperlipidemia, Abnormal circulating lipid concentration, Short stature, Bundle branch block, Cognitive impairment

Sensorineural hearing impairment, Depression, Anxiety, Hypertension, Diabetes insipidus, Lymphedema, Seizure, Abnormal myocardium morphology, Hypertrophic cardiomyopathy, Angina pectoris, Left ventricular hypertrophy, Fever, Respiratory insufficiency, Dyspnea, Vertigo, Developmental regression, Achalasia, Abnormality of femur morphology, Abnormality of the endocardium, Reduced bone mineral density, Chronic obstructive pulmonary disease, Arrhythmia, Glomerulopathy

Childhood, Adolescent, Adult

(Continued)

TABLE 5.2 *(Continued)*

GMP Herbal Medicines for a 16-Year-Old Adolescent with Fabry Disease

Renal insufficiency (586), Nephrotic syndrome (581), Hearing impairment (D003638), Hypohidrosis (705.0), Congestive heart failure (428, 428.0), Anemia (285.9), Abdominal pain (D015746), Arthralgia (D018771), Myalgia (D063806), Fatigue (D005221):

Wǔlíngsǎn 5g + zhēnwǔtāng 5g + jìshēngshènqìwán 5g + yuèbìjiāshùtāng 5-0g + huángqí 2-0g.

Zhēnwǔtāng 5g + shēngmàiyǐn 4g + huángqí 2g + dàhuáng 0g.

Zhēnwǔtāng 5g + zhūlíngtāng 5g + guīpítāng 5g + dàhuáng 1g.

Zhēnwǔtāng 5g + guīpítāng 5g + dānshēn 1g + yìmǔcǎo 1g + zélán 1g.

Huángqí 5g + chēqiánzǐ 5-2g + fúlíng 5-2g + báimáogēn 5-0g + yìmǔcǎo 5-0g + dǎngshēn 5-0g + zhūlíng 5-0g + zéxiè 5-0g + báizhú 3-0g + báisháo 3-0g + fùzǐ 3-0g + guìzhī 2-0g + dàhuáng 1-0g.

Dīngshùxiǔ 5g + huángqí 4g + báimáogēn 2g + chēqiánzǐ 2g + dàhuáng 1g + jīnyínhuā 1g + gāncǎo 1g.

Huángqí 5g + dìhuáng 5-1g + dāngguī 2-1g + dàhuáng 2-0g + chuānxiōng 2-0g + báisháo 2-0g + fúlíng 2-0g.

Huángqí 5g + báizhú 2g + dìhuáng 2g + ējiāo 2g.

Proteinuria (791.0), Cataract (366.8), Optic atrophy (377.1), Mitral regurgitation (396.3, 746.6), Atrioventricular block (426.10), Anorexia (D000855), Emphysema (492.8):

Zhìgāncǎotāng 5g + zhūlíngtāng 5g + gǒuqǐzǐ 1g + yìmǔcǎo 1g + tùsīzǐ 1g + zélán 1g.

Zhìgāncǎotāng 5g + jìshēngshènqìwán 5g + bǔzhōngyìqìtāng 5-0g + dānshēn 1-0g + shíchāngpú 1-0g + gǒuqǐzǐ 1-0g + yuǎnzhì 1-0g + yùjīn 1-0g + júhuā 1-0g + cāngěrzǐ 1-0g.

Qīngxīnliánzǐyǐn 5g + jìshēngshènqìwán 5g + dānshēn 1g + dìlóng 1g + yùjīn 1g.

Zhūlíngtāng 5g + jìshēngshènqìwán 5g + dōngguāzǐ 1g + báimáogēn 1g + chēqiánzǐ 1g + wūyào 1g.

Jìshēngshènqìwán 5g + shēngmàiyǐn 4g + dānshēn 1g + wǔwèizǐ 1g + chēqiánzǐ 1g + tùsīzǐ 1g + huángqí 1g.

Huángqín 5g + báizhǐ 4-3g + gāncǎo 3-2g + shārén 3-2g + jīnyínhuā 2-0g + zhīzǐ 2-0g + liánqiáo 2-0g + tiānhuā 2-0g + guālóugēn 1-0g + dàhuáng 1-0g.

Gǒuqǐzǐ 5g + júhuā 5g + dìhuáng 4-3g + dāngguī 4-3g + fángfēng 3-2g + niúbàngzǐ 3-0g + shègān 3-0g + xìxīn 1g + huánglián 1g.

Sensorineural hearing impairment (389.1), Hypertension (401-405.99), Diabetes insipidus (253.5), Seizure (345.9), Hypertrophic cardiomyopathy (425.1), Angina pectoris (D000787), Fever (D005334), Dyspnea (D004417), Vertigo (386.2), Achalasia (530.0):

Xìngsūyǐnyòukē 5g + xīnyíqīngfèitāng 5g + máxìnggānshítāng 5g.

Xìngsūyǐnyòukē 5g + xīnyíqīngfèitāng 5g + yínqiàosǎn 5g.

Xìngsūyǐnyòukē 5g + xīnyíqīngfèitāng 5g + cāngěrsǎn 5g.

Yìgānsǎn 5g + yìqìcōngmíngtāng 5-0g + shíchāngpú 1g + yuǎnzhì 1g + acupuncture.

Bǔyánghuánwǔtāng 5g + wēndǎntāng 4-0g + shíchāngpú 1g + yuǎnzhì 1g + acupuncture.

Zīshèntōngěrtāng 5g + tōngqiàohuóxuètāng 4g + shíchāngpú 1g + yuǎnzhì 1g + acupuncture.

Shānzhūyú 5g + shānyào 5g + niúxī 5g + fúlíng 5g + shíchāngpú 5-3g + yuǎnzhì 5-3g + ròucōngróng 5-0g + dùzhòng 5-0g + dānshēn 5-0g + shúdìhuáng 5-0g + bājǐtiān 5-0g + dìhuáng 5-0g + mǔdānpí 5-0g + guībǎn 5-0g + zéxiè 5-0g + dìlóng 3-0g + acupuncture.

Huángbò 5g + guībǎn 4g + zhìgāncǎo 2g + shārén 2g + fùzǐ 1g.

Huángbò 5g + gāncǎo 3g + shārén 3g + ròuguì 1-0g + wúzhūyú 1-0g.

Huángbò 5g + huángqí 5g + tiānmá 2g + dìlóng 2g + chìsháo 2g + xiōngqióng 2g + hónghuā 2g + táorén 2g + dāngguīwěi 2g + gōuténg 2g + acupuncture.

"raise Kidney yang." Zhēnwǔtāng also "strengthens the Spleen," which governs digestion in TCM. Shānzhūyú was introduced in Section 2.18 to be neuro-, hepato-, and nephroprotective. Dānshēn, introduced in Section 3.15 for cardiovascular disease, "activates circulation, regulates menstruation, cools blood, eliminates carbuncle and calms the mind." Huángbò (cf. Sections 1.61 and 4.19) has a bitter flavor and a cold nature. It reduces fever; however, its use in patients with malnutrition should be cautioned. Xìngsūyǐnyòukē is used for fever and headache due to the common cold (Wang, 2019).

5.3 MUCOLIPIDOSIS TYPE III

Mucolipidosis type III, also knowns as pseudo-Hurler polydystrophy, is caused by mutations in genes coding for an enzyme that catalyzes the synthesis of an enzyme complex involved in the degradative activities of the lysosome, causing accumulation of certain fats (mucolipids) and long chains of sugar molecules (mucopolysaccharides) in the cells of various tissues of the body.

TABLE 5.3
GMP Herbal Medicines for a Three-Year-Old Child with Mucolipidosis Type III

Mucolipidosis type III (OrphaCode: 577)

A disease with a prevalence of ~3 in 10,000

Disease-causing germline mutation(s) (loss of function): N-acetylglucosamine-1-phosphate transferase subunits alpha and beta (*GNPTAB* / Entrez: 79158) at 12q23.2

Disease-causing germline mutation(s) (loss of function): N-acetylglucosamine-1-phosphate transferase subunit gamma (*GNPTG* / Entrez: 84572) at 16p13.3

Autosomal recessive

Prominent occiput, Hearing abnormality, Visual impairment, Joint stiffness, Abnormal facial shape, Abnormality of the hip bone, Abnormal form of the vertebral bodies, Short stature, Craniofacial hyperostosis, Large iliac wings, Hypoplastic inferior ilia, Cognitive impairment

Inguinal hernia, Coarse facial features, Acne, Malformation of the heart and great vessels, Hyperlordosis, Corneal opacity

Cleft palate, Abnormal aortic valve morphology, Abnormal heart valve morphology, Reduced bone mineral density, Fatigue

Childhood

Visual impairment (D014786):

Qǐjúdìhuángwán 5g + shēnlíngbáizhúsăn 5-0g + gŏuqǐzǐ 1-0g + shénqū 1-0g + màiyá 1-0g.	Zhǐqiào 5-3g + jílí 5-0g + chántuì 5-0g.
Qǐjúdìhuángwán 5g + xiāngshāliùjūnzǐtāng 5-0g + gāncăo 0g.	Júhuā 5g + jílí 5g + júhóng 5g.
Qǐjúdìhuángwán 5g + bǔzhōngyìqìtāng 5-0g + dàzăo 2-0g.	
Sāngjúyǐn 5g + yínqiàosăn 2-0g + zhǐqiào 1g + jílí 1-0g.	

Inguinal hernia (550):

Júhéwán 5g + băohéwán 2-0g + chuānliànzǐ 1-0g + yánhúsuŏ 1-0g + gāncăo 0g.	Xiǎohuíxiāng 5g + chuānliànzǐ 5g + dānshēn 5g + báizhǐ 5g + báijí 5g + băihé 5g + yánhúsuŏ 5g + wūyào 5g + tánxiāng 5g.
Xiǎojiànzhōngtāng 5g + bǔzhōngyìqìtāng 5g.	
Chuānliànzǐ 5g + hòupò 5g + wūyào 5g + huánglián 5g + ānzhōngsăn 5g + xiāngshāliùjūnzǐtāng 5g.	Xiǎohuíxiāng 5g + mùxiāng 5g + qiānghuó 5g + fūzǐ 5g + gānjiāng 5g + dúhuó 5-0g.
Wúzhūyútāng 5g + qīngxīnliánzǐyǐn 5g + dàhuáng 2g + táorén 2g.	Xiǎohuíxiāng 5g + mùxiāng 5g + shārén 5g + ròudòukòu 3g + hòupò 3g + chénpí 3g + láifúzǐ 3g + gǔyá 3g + zhǐqiào 3-0g.
Bǔzhōngyìqìtāng 5g + chuānliànzǐ 1-0g + yánhúsuŏ 1-0g + xiāngfù 1-0g + xiǎohuíxiāng 0g + wūyào 0g.	Huángqí 5g + shēngmá 1g + zhīmǔ 1g + jiégěng 1g + cháihú 1g.

Cleft palate (749.0), Fatigue (D005221):

Gānlùyǐn 5g + shēnlíngbáizhúsăn 5-0g + gāncăo 1-0g.	Xuánshēn 5g + dìhuáng 5g + màiméndōng 5g + yùzhú 5-0g + shāshēn 5-0g + hòupò 5-0g + zhǐshí 5-0g + dàhuáng 1-0g.
Gānlùyǐn 5g + zhúyèshígāotāng 5-0g + gāncăo 1-0g.	
Gānlùyǐn 5g + xīnyíqīngfèitāng 5-0g + gāncăo 1-0g.	Gāncăo 5g + báizhǐ 5g + shārén 5g + dàhuáng 0g.
Gānlùyǐn 5g + băohéwán 5-0g + gāncăo 2-0g + shénqū 1-0g + màiyá 1-0g.	
Dăochìsăn 5g + gāncăo 0g.	

Chántuì (cf. Sections 1.54 and 2.20) is widely used today for pruritis (Wang, 2020); however, it also treats blurred vision (Choi et al., 2015). Júhéwán, whose components include Chuānliànzǐ, Hòupò, and Mùxiāng (Radix Aucklandiae), has been used for hernia. Xiǎohuíxiāng is also used for inguinal hernia (cf. Section 1.8). Gānlùyǐn, which contains Dìhuáng (cf. Section 1.10), was initially formulated to "eliminate excessive heat arising from the Stomach," and today, it is commonly used to address issues related to oral and dental health (Wang, 2019).

5.4 LONG-CHAIN 3-HYDROXYACYL-CoA DEHYDROGENASE DEFICIENCY

Long-chain 3-hydroxyacyl-CoA dehydrogenase deficiency, or LCHADD, is an inherited condition that prevents the breakdown of long-chain fatty acids from being used as an energy source. LCHADD is caused by mutations in the *HADHA* gene, whose products are a unit of an enzyme complex that catalyzes beta-oxidation of long-chain fatty acids in mitochondria.

TABLE 5.4

GMP Herbal Medicines for a Two-Year-Old Child with Long-Chain 3-hydroxyacyl-CoA Dehydrogenase Deficiency

Long-chain 3-hydroxyacyl-CoA dehydrogenase deficiency (OrphaCode: 5)

A disease with a prevalence of ~8 in 100,000

Disease-causing germline mutation(s): hydroxyacyl-CoA dehydrogenase trifunctional multienzyme complex subunit alpha (*HADHA* / Entrez: 3030) at 2p23.3

Autosomal recessive

Photophobia, Hypoglycemia, Hypoketotic hypoglycemia

Abnormal electroretinogram, Visual loss, Exotropia, Hypotonia, Global developmental delay, Hypertrophic cardiomyopathy, Abnormality of metabolism/homeostasis, Hepatomegaly, Peripheral neuropathy

Retinopathy, Chorioretinal abnormality, Chorioretinal atrophy, Myopia, Nyctalopia, Intellectual disability, Seizure, Generalized hypotonia, Failure to thrive, Cholestatic liver disease, Abnormality of retinal pigmentation, Feeding difficulties, Posterior staphyloma

Neonatal, Infancy

Photophobia (D020795), Hypoglycemia (251.2):	
Yùpíngfēngsǎn 5g + guìzhītāng 5-0g + bǔzhōngyìqìtāng 5-0g + gāncǎo 2-0g.	Chántuì 5g + júhóng 5-0g + júhuā 5-0g + jílí 3-0g.
Bǔzhōngyìqìtāng 5g + yùpíngfēngsǎn 5-0g.	
Sāngjúyǐn 5g + zhǐqiào 1g + jílí 1g.	Sīguāluò 5g + júhuā 5g + jílí 5g.
Rénshēnbàidúsǎn 5g + báihǔtāng 5g + liánggésǎn 5g + xièbáisǎn 5g.	Zhǐqiào 5-3g + jílí 5-2g + júhuā 5-0g.
Exotropia (378.15, 378.1, 378.11), Hypotonia (D009123), Hypertrophic cardiomyopathy (425.1):	
Yùpíngfēngsǎn 5g + bǎohéwán 5g + bǔzhōngyìqìtāng 5-0g + gāncǎo 0g.	Júhuā 5g + jílí 5-3g + chántuì 5-0g + júhóng 5-0g + zhǐqiào 2-0g.
Xiǎojiànzhōngtāng 5-4g + gāncǎoxiǎomàidàzǎotāng 5-0g + língguìshùgāntāng 5-0g + gāncǎo 0g.	Gāncǎo 5g + júhuā 5g + jílí 5g + chántuì 5g.
Shēnlíngbáizhúsǎn 5g + bǎohéwán 5-4g + gāncǎo 1-0g.	Gāncǎo 5g + zhǐqiào 5g + sīguāluò 0g.
	Zhǐqiào 5g + chántuì 5g.
Retinopathy (362.9), Myopia (367.1), Nyctalopia (368.6), Intellectual disability (D008607), Seizure (345.9):	
Sāngjúyǐn 5g + zhǐqiào 2-1g + jílí 2-1g + chántuì 2-0g + sīguāluò 1-0g.	Gǒuqǐzǐ 5g + yuǎnzhì 5-2g + hángjú 5-2g + shíchāngpú 3-2g + huángqí 1-0g.
Qǐjúdìhuángwán 5g + yìqìcōngmíngtāng 5-0g + bǔzhōngyìqìtāng 5-0g + acupuncture.	Zhǐqiào 5-2g + jílí 5-2g + júhuā 5-0g.
Jiāwèixiāoyáosǎn 5g + júhuā 1g + jílí 1g + chántuì 1g.	Yuǎnzhì 5g + jílí 5g + chántuì 3g.

Yùpíngfēngsǎn, introduced in Sections 1.5, 1.29, 1.36, and 4.7, has been used for common infections. Bǔzhōngyìqìtāng, Bǎohéwán, and Shēnlíngbáizhúsǎn improve functions of the digestive system (Wang, 2019). Yuǎnzhì (cf. Sections 1.41 and 1.60) is best known for its tranquilizing and antipsychotic activities. Its beneficial effects and mechanisms of action on the preclinical models of central nervous system diseases including anxiety, depression, learning/memory disorders, Alzheimer's disease, and Parkinson's disease were reviewed (Jiang et al., 2021). Sāngjúyǐn (cf. Sections 1.40 and 2.31), comprising Júhuā (cf. Section 1.2), has been used for early stages of upper respiratory tract infections in the summer. The prescriptions in the table help relieve the visual and metabolic symptoms of LCHADD patients.

5.5 MEDIUM-CHAIN ACYL-CoA DEHYDROGENASE DEFICIENCY

Medium-chain acyl-CoA dehydrogenase deficiency, or MCADD, is characterized by low levels of medium-chain acyl-CoA dehydrogenase (MCAD), which is involved in breaking down fat stores in the body to be used as energy after glucose is used up. MCADD is caused by an alteration in the *ACADM* gene, which codes for the MCAD enzyme. Note that the symptoms of MCADD differ from those of LCHADD, presumably because of variations in the toxicity of the accumulated fatty acids.

TABLE 5.5

GMP Herbal Medicines for a One-Year-Old Infant with Medium-Chain Acyl-CoA Dehydrogenase Deficiency

Medium-chain acyl-CoA dehydrogenase deficiency (OrphaCode: 42)

A disease with a prevalence of ~7 in 100,000

Disease-causing germline mutation(s): acyl-CoA dehydrogenase medium chain (*ACADM* / Entrez: 34) at 1p31.1

Autosomal recessive

Hypotonia, Reduced tendon reflexes, Decreased liver function, Hyperammonemia, Vomiting, Hepatomegaly, Dicarboxylic aciduria, Fatigable weakness, Proximal muscle weakness, Exercise-induced myalgia, Decreased plasma total carnitine, Fatigable weakness of neck muscles

Macrocephaly, Delayed speech and language development, Ataxia, Lethargy, Coma, Hepatic steatosis, Cardiomegaly, Hypoglycemia, Ketosis, Diarrhea, Bilateral tonic-clonic seizure, Febrile seizures, Exertional dyspnea, Elevated hepatic transaminase, Myopathy, Skeletal muscle atrophy, Elevated circulating creatine kinase concentration, Muscle spasm, Cachexia, Distal arthrogryposis, Loss of consciousness, Arrhythmia, Fatigue, Elevated urinary 3-hydroxybutyric acid, Abnormal lactate dehydrogenase activity

Neonatal, Infancy

Hypotonia (D009123), Decreased liver function (573.9), Vomiting (D014839):

Dàcháihútāng 5g.	Zhǐqiào 5g + chántuì 5-0g.
Wǔlíngsǎn 5g + xiǎocháihútāng 5-2g + gāncǎo 0g.	Zhǐqiào 5g + jílí 5-0g.
	Jílí 5g + júhóng 2g.

Delayed speech and language development (D007805), Ataxia (D002524), Lethargy (D053609), Coma (D003128), Hepatic steatosis (571.0), Hypoglycemia (251.2), Diarrhea (D003967), Bilateral tonic-clonic seizure (D012640), Elevated hepatic transaminase (573.9), Myopathy (359.9), Skeletal muscle atrophy (D009133), Muscle spasm (D009120), Cachexia (D002100), Loss of consciousness (D014474), Fatigue (D005221):

Wǔlíngsǎn 5g.	Yīnchén 5g.
Bǔzhōngyìqìtāng 5g + báizhú 4-0g + fùzǐ 2-1g + báisháo 2-0g + fúlíng 2-0g + gānjiāng 1g + dǎngshēn 1-0g + shēngjiāng 1-0g + xìxīn 1-0g + dàhuáng 0g.	Shúdìhuáng 5g + báizhú 4-1g + fùzǐ 4-0g + fúlíng 3g + báijièzǐ 3-2g + báisháo 3-0g + yìyǐrén 3-0g + dǎngshēn 2-1g + gāncǎo 1-0g + shēngjiāng 1-0g + máhuáng 1-0g + wǔwèizǐ 1-0g + júhóng 1-0g + huánglián 0g.
Máhuángtāng 5g + bànxià 1-0g + shēngjiāng 1-0g + xìxīn 1-0g + dàhuáng 0g.	Huángqí 5g + zhīmǔ 2g + shēngmá 1g + jiégěng 1g + cháihú 1g.

Wǔlíngsǎn was shown to alleviate headache and cerebral edema in mice by regulating cerebral blood flow and water distribution (Kurauchi et al., 2024; Shimizu et al., 2023). Máhuáng (Herba Ephedrae) was reviewed to have such pharmacological effects as antipyretic, diaphoretic, anti-asthmatic, anti-inflammatory, anticancer, analgesic, and hepatoprotective (Tang et al., 2023). Máhuángtāng, with Máhuáng as the major herb, was shown to antagonize acute liver failure in mice through regulation of tricarboxylic acid (TCA) cycle and amino acid metabolism (Liao et al., 2021).

5.6 HEREDITARY FRUCTOSE INTOLERANCE

Hereditary fructose intolerance, also known as hereditary fructose-1-phosphate aldolase deficiency, is an inherited condition where a person lacks the enzyme to break down fructose and sucrose, resulting in a buildup of fructose-1-phosphate in the body. Symptoms do not occur until the newborn ingests fructose- or sucrose-containing food during weaning.

TABLE 5.6

GMP Herbal Medicines for a One-Year-Old Infant with Hereditary Fructose Intolerance

Hereditary fructose intolerance (OrphaCode: 469)

A disease with a prevalence of ~5 in 100,000

Disease-causing germline mutation(s): aldolase, fructose-bisphosphate B (*ALDOB* / Entrez: 229) at 9q31.1

Autosomal recessive

Abdominal pain, Reduced aldolase level

Growth delay, Diarrhea, Nausea

Renal insufficiency, Jaundice, Episodic hyperhidrosis, Metabolic acidosis, Vomiting, Constipation, Hypophosphatemia, Hyperuricemia, Hepatomegaly, Hypermagnesemia, Abnormality of the coagulation cascade, Abdominal distention, Reactive hypoglycemia, Chronic kidney disease, Chronic hepatic failure

All ages

Abdominal pain (D015746):

Yǐzìtāng 5g.	Xuánshēn 5g + dìhuáng 5g + màiméndōng 5g +
Bǎohéwán 5g.	hòupò 5-1g + zhǐshí 5-1g + dàhuáng 2-0g.
Xiǎojiànzhōngtāng 5g.	
Shēnlíngbáizhúsǎn 5g + bǎohéwán 2-0g + shānzhā 1-0g + shénqū 1-0g + jīnèijīn 1-0g.	

Diarrhea (D003967), Nausea (D009325):

Wǔlíngsǎn 5g + píngwèisǎn 5-0g + huòxiāngzhèngqìsǎn 5-0g + gāncǎo 0g.	Gāncǎo 5g + báizhǐ 5-0g + shārén 5-0g + dàhuáng 1-0g.

Renal insufficiency (586), Jaundice (D007565), Vomiting (D014839), Constipation (564.0), Abnormality of the coagulation cascade (286), Reactive hypoglycemia (251.2):

Xìngsūyǐnyòukē 5g + mázǐrénwán 5-1g + gāncǎo 0g.	Dàhuáng 5g + gāncǎo 5g.
Xìngsūyǐnyòukē 5g + rùnchángwán 5-3g + dàhuáng 1-0g.	Gāncǎo 5g + báizhǐ 5g + shārén 5g + dàhuáng 1g.
Mázǐrénwán 5g + gāncǎo 2g + dàhuáng 1g.	Zhìgāncǎo 5g + báizhǐ 2g + shārén 2g + dàhuáng 0g.

Yǐzìtāng has been used for anorectal diseases including constipation, hemorrhoids, and abdominal pain (cf. Section 3.24). Xìngsūyǐnyòukē is composed of Xìngrén (cf. Section 1.12) as the major herb, which consists of a compound that was shown to attenuate renal interstitial fibrosis in rats with obstructive nephropathy (Guo et al., 2013). Mázǐrénwán, containing Dàhuáng (cf. Section 2.17) and Xìngrén, was introduced in Section 4.25 for constipation.

5.7 SARCOSINEMIA

Sarcosinemia, also called sarcosine dehydrogenase complex deficiency, is characterized by an increased level of sarcosine, an amino acid, in the blood and urine. Sarcosinemia is caused by mutations in the gene encoding the enzyme that catalyzes sarcosine catabolism in the mitochondrial matrix.

The bioactive compounds, i.e., flavones, in Huángqín (cf. Section 1.6) were shown in mice to pass the blood-brain barrier following oral administration (Fong et al., 2017) and exert antidepressant effects via protecting hippocampal neurons (Zhao et al., 2020). Taking into account the ancient (cf. Section 7.5) and modern medical literature about the effects and health insurance claims data about

TABLE 5.7
GMP Herbal Medicines for a Six-Year-Old Child with Sarcosinemia

Sarcosinemia (OrphaCode: 3129)

A disease with a prevalence of ~5 in 100,000

Disease-causing germline mutation(s): sarcosine dehydrogenase (*SARDH* / Entrez: 1757) at 9q34.2

Autosomal recessive

Hypersarcosinemia

Hypersarcosinuria

Strabismus, Optic atrophy, Emotional lability, Ataxia, Intellectual disability, mild, Global developmental delay, Motor delay, Hypertrophic cardiomyopathy, Pulmonic stenosis, Bilateral tonic-clonic seizure, Tetraparesis, Sleep disturbance, Loss of speech, Poor speech, Congenital blindness, Infantile sensorineural hearing impairment, Infantile muscular hypotonia, Dyslexia, Peroneal muscle weakness, Abnormality of movement

All ages

Strabismus (378.7, 378.6, 378.31), Optic atrophy (377.1), Ataxia (D002524), Hypertrophic cardiomyopathy (425.1), Bilateral tonic-clonic seizure (D012640), Tetraparesis (344.00), Dyslexia (315.01):

Bǔyánghuánwǔtāng 5g + shíchāngpú 1g + yuǎnzhì 1g.	Huángqín 5g + gāncǎo 2g + báizhǐ 2g +
Bǔzhōngyìqìtāng 5g + bǔyánghuánwǔtāng 5-0g + xiǎoqīnglóngtāng 5-0g +	guālóugēn 2g + shārén 1g + dàhuáng 0g.
mázǐrénwán 2-0g + shíchāngpú 1g + yuǎnzhì 1g + acupuncture.	Huángqín 5g + báizhǐ 4g + gāncǎo 2g +
Xiǎoqīnglóngtāng 5g + yùpíngfēngsǎn 5g + shíchāngpú 1g + yuǎnzhì 1g.	shārén 2g + tiānhuā 1-0g + dàhuáng 1-0g.

the uses of GMP Huángqín powder, we summarize that it benefits patients with disorders of the intestine, heart disease, dermatoses, disorders of the eye, disorders of the nervous system, conditions of the brain, cerebrovascular disease, influenza, endocrine disorders, and hypertensive heart and chronic kidney disease through improvement of and effect on body weight, diarrhea, brain, edema, hypoxia, adipose tissue, birth weight, adrenal glands, kidney, and feces. Xiǎoqīnglóngtāng (cf. Section 3.18) was demonstrated to maintain cardiac function during heart failure with reduced ejection fraction in salt-sensitive rats by regulating the imbalance of cardiac sympathetic innervation (Z. Li et al., 2020).

5.8 3-METHYLCROTONYL-CoA CARBOXYLASE DEFICIENCY

3-methylcrotonyl-CoA carboxylase deficiency (MCC deficiency), also called 3-methylcrotonylglycinuria, is caused by mutations in the genes that instruct production of enzymes to break down leucine, an amino acid from the diet, in mitochondria. The buildup of the toxic by-products from improper leucine processing causes variable symptoms.

TABLE 5.8
GMP Herbal Medicines for a Two-Year-Old Child with 3-Methylcrotonyl-CoA Carboxylase Deficiency

3-methylcrotonyl-CoA carboxylase deficiency (OrphaCode: 6)

A disease with a prevalence of ~5 in 100,000

Disease-causing germline mutation(s): methylcrotonyl-CoA carboxylase subunit 1 (*MCCC1* / Entrez: 56922) at 3q27.1

Disease-causing germline mutation(s): methylcrotonyl-CoA carboxylase subunit 2 (*MCCC2* / Entrez: 64087) at 5q13.2

Autosomal recessive

Hypotonia, Hypoglycemia, Organic aciduria, Abnormality of leucine metabolism

Failure to thrive in infancy, Hyperammonemia, Abnormality of movement

Spasticity, Respiratory insufficiency, Abnormality of the cerebral vasculature

All ages

(Continued)

TABLE 5.8 *(Continued)*
GMP Herbal Medicines for a Two-Year-Old Child with 3-Methylcrotonyl-CoA Carboxylase Deficiency

Hypotonia (D009123), Hypoglycemia (251.2):

Yùpíngfēngsǎn 5g + guìzhītāng 5g.	Gāncǎo 5g + báizhǐ 5g + shārén 5-3g + huángqín 3-0g + guālóugēn 2-0g + dàhuáng 1-0g.
Huángqíwǔwùtāng 5g + bǔzhōngyìqìtāng 5-0g + gāncǎo 0g.	
Sìjūnzǐtāng 5g + bǎohéwán 2-0g + gāncǎo 0g.	Gāncǎo 5g + báizhǐ 5g + jīnyínhuā 5g + shārén 5g + dàhuáng 0g.
Sìjūnzǐtāng 5g + yùpíngfēngsǎn 5-0g.	

Spasticity (D009128):

Dāngguīsìnìtāng 5g + dúhuójìshēngtāng 5g + niúxī 1g + dùzhòng 1-0g.	Chuānwū 5g + shúdìhuáng 5g + gāncǎo 3g + báisháo 3g + máhuáng 3g + huángqí 3g + báijièzǐ 2g + dàhuáng 1g + shēngjiāng 1g + huánglián 0g.
Dāngguīsìnìtāng 5g + shēngjiāng 1-0g + wúzhūyú 1-0g + fùzǐ 1-0g + gānjiāng 1-0g.	Chuānwū 5g + yánhúsuǒ 5-2g + wǔlíngzhī 2g + tiānnánxīng 2g + mùxiāng 2g + dìlóng 2g + táorén 2g + huíxiāng 2g + chénpí 2g + dāngguī 2g + gāncǎo 2-0g + acupuncture.

Yùpíngfēngsǎn and Gāncǎo, annotated in Sections 4.7 and 11.3, benefit Qi, which is the vital energy that animates the body in traditional Eastern medicines. Chuānwū was introduced in Section 2.12 for lumbago, myalgia/myositis, and monoplegia. Some compounds in Wǔlíngzhī (cf. Section 2.54), a fecal medicine in TCM, were found to be gastroprotective (Du et al., 2019) and the medicine is used for an assortment of digestive conditions (Wang, 2020). Tiānnánxīng (cf. Section 1.69) "dries dampness, dissolves phlegm, dispels Wind, resolves convulsions" and is used today for coughs, neuralgia, neuritis, radiculitis, myalgia, and myositis (Wang, 2020). Dāngguīsìnìtāng (cf. Sections 2.12 and 2.54) was shown to protect against chemotherapy-induced peripheral neuropathy in rats (Ding et al., 2020).

5.9 HISTIDINEMIA

Histidinemia, also known as HAL deficiency or histidase deficiency, is high levels of amino acid histidine in blood, urine, and cerebrospinal fluid. HAL deficiency is caused by gene mutations rendering the histidine metabolizing enzyme inactive. HAL deficiency rarely presents with a clinical symptom.

TABLE 5.9
GMP Herbal Medicines for a Two-Year-Old Child with Histidinemia

Histidinemia (OrphaCode: 2157)

A disease with a prevalence of ~5 in 100,000

Disease-causing germline mutation(s): histidine ammonia-lyase (*HAL* / Entrez: 3034) at 12q23.1

Autosomal recessive

Histidinuria, Hyperhistidinemia

Hyperactive behavior

Neonatal, Infancy

Hyperactive behavior [Attention deficit disorder with hyperactivity (314.01)]:

Gāncǎoxiǎomàidàzǎotāng 5g + yìgānsǎn 5g.	Gāncǎo 5g + shārén 5g + báizhǐ 5-0g + dàhuáng 1-0g.
Yìgānsǎn 5g + guìzhījiālónggǔmǔlìtāng 5g + shíchāngpú 1g + yuǎnzhì 1g.	Jílí 5g + júhóng 4g + chántuì 4g.
	Zhǐqiào 5g + jílí 5-4g + chántuì 5-0g.
Cháihújiālónggǔmǔlìtāng 5g + gāncǎoxiǎomàidàzǎotāng 5-2g + shíchāngpú 1-0g + yuǎnzhì 1-0g.	

Jílí (cf. Sections 1.3 and 1.41) "normalizes the Liver, soothes the Liver, dispels Wind and improves eyesight." Jílí has long been used in traditional medicines, including TCM, Ayurveda, and traditional Arabic medicine. The pharmacological activities of Jílí were reviewed, including antioxidant, testosterone boosting, antibacterial, antihyperglycemic, anti-inflammatory, and protection of the CNS (Ştefănescu et al., 2020). Gāncǎoxiǎomàidàzǎotāng, containing Gāncǎo, was introduced in Sections 1.3, 1.42, 2.6, and 2.27 for neurotic disorders.

5.10   CYSTATHIONINURIA

Cystathioninuria, also known as cystathionine gamma-lyase deficiency syndrome or gamma-cystathionase deficiency, is excessive accumulation and secretion of cystathionine in the plasma and urine. Cystathioninuria is caused by mutations in the *CTH* gene, whose products convert cystathionine derived from methionine into cysteine.

TABLE 5.10

GMP Herbal Medicines for a Five-Year-Old Child with Cystathioninuria

Cystathioninuria (OrphaCode: 212)

A disease with a prevalence of ~5 in 100,000

Disease-causing germline mutation(s) (loss of function): cystathionine gamma-lyase (*CTH* / Entrez: 1491) at 1p31.1
Autosomal recessive

Cystathioninuria

Intellectual disability, Seizure, Cystathioninemia

Nephrolithiasis, Tremor, Talipes equinovarus, External ear malformation
All ages

Intellectual disability (D008607), Seizure (345.9):	
Cháihújiālónggǔmǔlìtāng 5g + tiānmá 1g + shíchāngpú 1g + yuǎnzhì 1-0g + gōuténg 1-0g.	Xuánshēn 5g + dìhuáng 5g + màiméndōng 5g + hòupò 5-0g + zhǐshí 5-0g + dàhuáng 1-0g.
Sāngjúyǐn 5g + zhǐqiào 1g + chántuì 0g.	
Sāngjúyǐn 5g + júhuā 1g.	Hòupò 5g + zhǐshí 5g + dàhuáng 1g + huǒmárén 1g.
Yìgānsǎn 5g + guìzhījiālónggǔmǔlìtāng 4g + shíchāngpú 1g + yuǎnzhì 1g.	
Nephrolithiasis (592), Tremor (D014202), Talipes equinovarus (754.51):	
Wǔlínsǎn 5g + gāncǎo 1g + báisháo 1g + dàhuáng 0g.	Huáshí 5g + chēqiánzǐ 2-0g + gāncǎo 1g.
Wǔlínsǎn 5g + huàshícǎo 1g + jīnyínhuā 1-0g + huángqín 1-0g.	Huàshícǎo 5g + chēqiáncǎo 5g + hānqiàocǎo 5g.
Zhūlíngtāng 5g + gāncǎo 1-0g + báisháo 1-0g + dàhuáng 0g.	Gāncǎo 5g + báizhǐ 5-0g + shārén 5-0g + hòupò 5-0g + zhǐshí 5-0g + dàhuáng 0g.

Xuánshēn was introduced in Section 1.3 for its potential of benefiting the brain. Huáshí (Talcum) "induces and passes urination, clears summer heat, eliminates dampness, astringes sores" and is used today for polydipsia, headache, digestive (e.g., gastrojejunal ulcer), and skin (e.g., contact dermatitis) conditions (Wang, 2020). Wǔlínsǎn (cf. Section 3.33) was shown to ameliorate substance P–induced bladder inflammation in rats (Chen et al., 2006).

5.11   BUTYRYLCHOLINESTERASE DEFICIENCY

Butyrylcholinesterase deficiency, also called pseudocholinesterase deficiency, is sensitivity to certain anesthetic drugs such as choline esters that relax muscles during general anesthesia. People with butyrylcholinesterase deficiency experience prolonged paralysis of the respiratory muscles after surgery and require mechanical ventilation. Butyrylcholinesterase deficiency is caused by mutations in the *BCHE* gene, whose products are produced in the liver and circulate to break down choline esters.

TABLE 5.11

GMP Herbal Medicines for a 31-Year-Old Adult with Butyrylcholinesterase Deficiency

Butyrylcholinesterase deficiency (OrphaCode: 132)

A disease with a prevalence of ~5 in 100,000

Disease-causing germline mutation(s): butyrylcholinesterase (*BCHE* / Entrez: 590) at 3q26.1

Autosomal recessive

Abnormal enzyme/coenzyme activity

Respiratory failure

Neonatal, Infancy

Acute respiratory failure following trauma and surgery (518.51):

Cháixiàntāng 5g + máxìnggānshítāng 5g + bèimǔ 1-0g + jiégěng 1-0g.   Guālóurén 5g + bànxià 3-2g + huánglián 3-2g.

Cháixiàntāng 5g + wēndǎntāng 5g.   Guālóurén 5g + xièbái 5g + bànxià 4-0g.

Máxìnggānshítāng 5g + dàzǎo 2-0g + tínglìzǐ 2-0g + dàhuáng 1-0g.

Guālóurén (Semen Trichosanthis) "clears heat, transforms phlegm, widens chest, dissolves congelation, moistens bowels, passes stools" and is used for cough, chest pain, rhinitis and bronchitis (Wang, 2020). Cháixiàntāng, introduced in Section 3.28 for symptoms involving the respiratory system and other chest symptoms, was shown to treat chest pain refractory to analgesics in patients with mild to moderate COVID-19 (Arita et al., 2022). Note that Cháixiàntāng contains Bànxià, Guālóurén, and Huánglián.

5.12   VERY LONG-CHAIN ACYL-CoA DEHYDROGENASE DEFICIENCY

Very long-chain acyl-CoA dehydrogenase deficiency, or VLCADD, is a condition in which very long-chain fatty acids, a source of energy from the food for the heart and muscles, cannot be broken down in the body. VLCADD is caused by mutations in the *ACADVL* gene, whose products convert very long-chain fatty acids to energy in mitochondria. Accumulation of partially metabolized fatty acids gives rise to the symptoms of VLCADD.

TABLE 5.12

GMP Herbal Medicines for a One-Year-Old Infant with Very Long-Chain Acyl-CoA Dehydrogenase Deficiency

Very long-chain acyl-CoA dehydrogenase deficiency (OrphaCode: 26793)

A disease with a prevalence of ~5 in 100,000

Disease-causing germline mutation(s): acyl-CoA dehydrogenase very long chain (*ACADVL* / Entrez: 37) at 17p13.1

Autosomal recessive

Increased circulating free fatty acid level

Jaundice, Small for gestational age, Ventricular septal defect, Atrial septal defect, Patent foramen ovale, Hypoketotic hypoglycemia, Hypothermia, Respiratory distress, Hepatomegaly, Episodic tachypnea, Elevated hepatic transaminase, Elevated circulating creatine kinase concentration, Exercise-induced rhabdomyolysis, Feeding difficulties, Overweight

Neonatal, Infancy

Jaundice (D007565), Ventricular septal defect (745.4), Hypothermia (D007035), Respiratory distress (D004417), Elevated hepatic transaminase (573.9):

Zhìgāncǎotāng 5g.   Zhìgāncǎo 5g + gégēn 5-0g + huángqín 2-0g + huánglián

Xiǎocháihútāng 5g + shēnlíngbáizhúsǎn 5g + shānzhā 1g.   2-0g + dàhuáng 1-0g.

Yīnchénwǔlíngsǎn 5g + guīpítāng 5g + wǔwèizǐ 1g.   Gāncǎo 5g.

Shēngmàiyǐn 5g + bǔzhōngyìqìtāng 5g.

Zhìgāncǎo (cf. Section 1.11) is among the top three commonly prescribed single herbs for cardiovascular disease patients (Jin & Li, 2023). Gégēn (cf. Section 4.16) was shown to alleviate alcohol-induced hepatic steatosis in zebrafish larvae through regulation of alcohol and lipid metabolism (Liu et al., 2021). Yīnchénwǔlíngsǎn "clears damp-heat, relieves jaundice" and is used today for both chronic kidney and chronic liver diseases (Wang, 2019).

5.13 BIOTINIDASE DEFICIENCY

Biotinidase deficiency, also known as juvenile-onset multiple carboxylase deficiency, affects how the body processes biotin, i.e., vitamin B7, which helps metabolize carbohydrates, fats, and protein. Biotinidase deficiency is caused by mutations in the *BTD* gene, whose products help recycle biotin for reuse in the body. Symptoms and onset age of biotinidase deficiency depend on how much of the biotinidase enzyme is working.

TABLE 5.13

GMP Herbal Medicines for a Three-Year-Old Child with Biotinidase Deficiency

Biotinidase deficiency (OrphaCode: 79241)

A disease with a prevalence of ~5 in 100,000

Disease-causing germline mutation(s): biotinidase (*BTD* / Entrez: 686) at 3p25.1

Autosomal recessive

Organic aciduria, Metabolic ketoacidosis, Decreased biotinidase activity

Sensorineural hearing impairment, Abnormality of the nervous system, Skin rash, Seizure, Hypotonia, Hyperammonemia, Abnormality of the immune system, Brain imaging abnormality

Hearing impairment, Abnormality of the eye, Conjunctivitis, Scotoma, Optic atrophy, Eczematoid dermatitis, Optic neuropathy, Intellectual disability, Ataxia, Lethargy, Alopecia, Bilateral tonic-clonic seizure, Respiratory distress, Apnea, Generalized myoclonic seizures, Myelopathy, Spastic paraparesis, Recurrent fungal infections, Hyperventilation, Limb muscle weakness, Recurrent viral infections, Recurrent candida infections, Laryngeal stridor, Focal motor seizure, Infantile spasms, Psychomotor retardation, Nonprogressive visual loss

Neonatal, Infancy, Childhood, Adolescent, Adult

Sensorineural hearing impairment (389.1), Skin rash (782.1), Seizure (345.9), Hypotonia (D009123), Hyperammonemia (D022124) [Disorders of urea cycle metabolism (270.6)]:

Xiǎofēngsǎn 5g + yínqiàosǎn 4g + báixiānpí 1g + dìfūzǐ 1g. Xìngsūyǐnyòukē 5g + jīngfángbàidúsǎn 5g.

Gāncǎo 5-3g + báizhǐ 5-2g + huángqín 5-2g + shārén 5-2g + guālóugēn 2-0g + dàhuáng 1-0g.

Xìngsūyǐnyòukē 5g + yínqiàosǎn 5g.

Huángqín 5g + báizhǐ 4g + zhìgāncǎo 3g + shārén 3g + guālóugēn 3g + dàhuáng 0g.

Xìngsūyǐnyòukē 5g + jīnyínhuā 1-0g + liánqiáo 1-0g + báijiāngcán 1-0g + chántuì 1-0g.

Hearing impairment (D034381), Abnormality of the eye (379.90), Conjunctivitis (372.30), Scotoma (D012607), Optic atrophy (377.1), Intellectual disability (D008607), Ataxia (D002524), Lethargy (D053609), Alopecia (704.0), Respiratory distress (D004417), Apnea (D001049), Myelopathy (336.9), Spastic paraparesis (D020336), Hyperventilation (D006985):

Zīshènmíngmùtāng 5g + xǐgānmíngmùtāng 4-0g + juémíngzǐ 1-0g.

Chántuì 5g + zhǐqiào 5-0g + jílí 4-0g.

Júhuā 5g + zhǐqiào 3g + jílí 2g + chántuì 2g.

Xìngrén (cf. Section 1.12), the major herb of Xìngsūyǐnyòukē, was shown to be anti-Parkinson's disease in rats (Saleem et al., 2022). Jīngfángbàidúsǎn "induces perspiration, releases exterior, disperses Wind, eliminates dampness" and is used today for contact dermatitis and other eczema (Wang, 2020). The term bàidú in Jīngfángbàidúsǎn means "to defeat pathogens." A recent molecular docking and network pharmacology study indicated that Jīngfángbàidúsǎn is potentially antiviral through inhibition of virus entry and replication in host cells (Li et al., 2022).

5.14 HARTNUP DISEASE

Hartnup disease, also known as aminoaciduria, Hartnup type, is a disorder where the body cannot absorb nonpolar amino acids such as tryptophan in the intestines and reabsorb them in the kidneys. Hartnup disease is caused by mutations in the *SLC6A19* gene, whose products transport neutral amino acids across the apical membrane of epithelial cells.

TABLE 5.14

GMP Herbal Medicines for a Six-Year-Old Child with Hartnup Disease

Hartnup disease (OrphaCode: 2116)

A disease with a prevalence of ~4 in 100,000

Disease-causing germline mutation(s): collectrin, amino acid transport regulator (*CLTRN* / Entrez: 57393) at Xp22.2

Disease-causing germline mutation(s): solute carrier family 6 member 19 (*SLC6A19* / Entrez: 340024) at 5p15.33

Autosomal recessive

Emotional lability, Hallucinations, Anxiety, Cutaneous photosensitivity, Ataxia, Hypotonia, Hyperreflexia, Migraine, EEG abnormality, Neutral hyperaminoaciduria, Abnormal urinary color

Abnormality of the eye, Strabismus, Abnormality of vision, Photophobia, Nystagmus, Skin rash, Malabsorption

Glossitis, Gingivitis, Hypopigmented skin patches, Intellectual disability, Seizure, Global developmental delay, Encephalitis, Short stature, Irregular hyperpigmentation, Abnormal blistering of the skin

All ages

Hallucinations (D006212), Ataxia (D002524), Hypotonia (D009123), Hyperreflexia (D012021), Migraine (346):

Wúzhūyútāng 5g + máhuángfùzǐxìxīntāng 5g + fùzǐ 3-2g + gānjiāng 3-0g.	Gāncǎo 5g + báizhǐ 5g + shārén 5-4g + huángqín 5-0g + tiānhuā 2-0g + dàhuáng 1-0g.
Gāncǎoxiǎomàidàzǎotāng 5g + guìzhījiālónggǔmǔlìtāng 5g + fúshén 2g + yuǎnzhì 2g.	Mǔlì 5g + gāncǎo 3g + báisháo 3g + shúdìhuáng 3g + biējiǎ 3g + màiméndōng 3g + ējiāo 2g + huǒmárén 2g + fúshén 2g.
Gāncǎoxiǎomàidàzǎotāng 5g + shēnlíngbáizhúsǎn 5g + shíchāngpú 1g + yuǎnzhì 1g.	
Gāncǎoxiǎomàidàzǎotāng 5g + wēndǎntāng 5g + bózǐrén 1g + fúshén 1g + yuǎnzhì 1g.	

Abnormality of the eye (379.90), Strabismus (378.7, 378.6, 378.31), Photophobia (D020795), Nystagmus (379.53, 379.55, 379.50), Skin rash (782.1):

Qǐjúdìhuángwán 5g + dāngguīyǐnzǐ 5g + gǒuqǐzǐ 1g.	Báizhǐ 5g + gāncǎo 5-4g + shārén 5-3g + huángqín 5-3g + tiānhuā 2-0g + dàhuáng 1-0g.
Qǐjúdìhuángwán 5g + zīshènmíngmùtāng 5g + xǐgānmíngmùtāng 5-0g.	

Glossitis (529.0), Gingivitis (523.0, 523.1), Intellectual disability (D008607), Seizure (345.9):

Fángfēngtōngshèngsǎn 5g + liánggésǎn 3-2g + shígāo 2-1g + gānlùyǐn 2-1g + qīngwèisǎn 2-1g + zhīmǔ 1-0g.	Báizhǐ 5g + zhìgāncǎo 4g + shārén 4g + xìxīn 1g + dàhuáng 1-0g.
Gānlùyǐn 5g + qīngwèisǎn 5g + dǎochìsǎn 5g + báijí 2g.	Báizhǐ 5g + gāncǎo 4g + shārén 4g + huángqín 4-0g + xìxīn 2-1g + dàhuáng 1-0g.

Fángfēngtōngshèngsǎn "relaxes exterior, attacks interior, dispels Wind, and clears heat" through the induction of perspiration and purgation in order to eliminate pathogens/heat. It was shown to modulate gut microbiota in mice with diet-induced obesity (Fujisaka et al., 2020) and may, therefore, improve cognitive function through the microbiota-gut-brain axis. Liánggésǎn "cools diaphragm, clears heat, quenches fire, passes stools" and is used today for functional digestive disorders, hemorrhoids, and diseases of the oral soft tissues (Wang, 2019).

5.15 CEREBROTENDINOUS XANTHOMATOSIS

Cerebrotendinous xanthomatosis (CTX), also called sterol 27-hydroxylase deficiency, is a bile acid synthesis disorder, a lipid storage disorder, or a disorder of the white matter of the CNS. CTX is caused by mutations in the *CYP27A1* gene, whose products break down cholesterol in mitochondria

TABLE 5.15

GMP Herbal Medicines for a One-Year-Old Infant with Cerebrotendinous Xanthomatosis

Cerebrotendinous xanthomatosis (OrphaCode: 909)

A disease with a prevalence of ~4 in 100,000

Disease-causing germline mutation(s): cytochrome P450 family 27 subfamily A member 1 (*CYP27A1* / Entrez: 1593) at 2q35

Autosomal recessive

Visual impairment, Juvenile cataract, Abnormal enzyme/coenzyme activity

Optic disc pallor, Nystagmus, Abnormality of visual evoked potentials, Behavioral abnormality, Decreased nerve conduction velocity, Osteoporosis, Optic neuropathy, Abnormality of finger, Intellectual disability, Seizure, Ataxia, Spasticity, Dysarthria, Gait disturbance, Abnormal cerebellum morphology, Specific learning disability, Dystonia, Hyperreflexia, Pes cavus, Chronic diarrhea, Abnormality of extrapyramidal motor function, Orofacial dyskinesia, Paraparesis, Abnormal globus pallidus morphology, Abnormality of tibia morphology, Babinski sign, Distal amyotrophy, Abnormality of the Achilles tendon, Abnormal auditory evoked potentials, Abnormal pyramidal sign, Progressive psychomotor deterioration, Abnormality of somatosensory evoked potentials, Abnormal retinal vascular morphology, Peripheral neuropathy, Tendon xanthomatosis, Abnormality of the cerebellar peduncle, Neurodevelopmental delay, Abnormal motor evoked potentials, Hyperintensity of cerebral white matter on MRI, Cognitive impairment, Abnormality of the plantar skin of foot

Abnormality of the neck, Abnormal eyelid morphology, Proptosis, Optic atrophy, Agitation, Depression, Autism, Aggressive behavior, Short attention span, Hallucinations, Hypothyroidism, Osteopenia, Cholelithiasis, Abnormality of the hand, Cerebellar atrophy, Parkinsonism, Increased serum lactate, Gliosis, Global brain atrophy, Resting tremor, Long-tract signs, Increased susceptibility to fractures, Abnormality of femur morphology, Thoracic kyphosis, Precocious atherosclerosis, Premature coronary artery atherosclerosis, Premature loss of teeth, Prolonged neonatal jaundice, Attention deficit hyperactivity disorder, CNS demyelination, Prematurely aged appearance, Hypermyelinated retinal nerve fibers, Abnormality of the vertebral spinous processes, Abnormality of the elbow, Abnormal atrial septum morphology, Personality disorder, Elevated brain choline level by MRS, Elevated brain lactate level by MRS, Suicidal ideation, Axonal degeneration, Abnormality of the dentate nucleus, Mitochondrial respiratory chain defects

Neonatal, Infancy

Nystagmus (379.53, 379.55, 379.50), Osteoporosis (733.0), Seizure (345.9), Ataxia (D002524), Spasticity (D009128), Dysarthria (D004401), Dystonia (D004421), Hyperreflexia (D012021), Orofacial dyskinesia (333.82), Paraparesis (D020335):

Bǔzhōngyìqìtāng 5g + qǐjúdìhuángwán 4g + tiānmá 1g + shíchāngpú 1-0g + yuǎnzhì 1-0g + acupuncture.

Èrchéntāng 5g + yùpíngfēngsǎn 5g + shíchāngpú 1g + yuǎnzhì 1g.

Yùpíngfēngsǎn 5g + gāncǎo 1g.

Huángqí 5g + báizhú 3-2g + fángfēng 3-2g.

Shānyào 5g + shānzhūyú 2g + wǔwèizǐ 2g + chēqiánzǐ 2g + gǒuqǐzǐ 2g + tùsīzǐ 2g + fùpénzǐ 2g.

Gāncǎo 5g + báizhǐ 5g + jīnyínhuā 5g + shārén 4g + huángqín 4g + dàhuáng 0g.

Zhǐqiào 5g + júhuā 5g + chántuì 5g.

Proptosis (376.30), Optic atrophy (377.1), Autism (299.0), Hallucinations (D006212), Hypothyroidism (244.9), Gliosis (D005911) [Other specified disorders of nervous system (349.89)], Resting tremor (D014202):

Gāncǎoxiǎomàidàzǎotāng 5g + yìqìcōngmíngtāng 5-0g + shíchāngpú 1g + yuǎnzhì 1g + acupuncture.

Liùwèidìhuángwán 5g + shíchāngpú 1g + acupuncture.

Gāncǎo 5g + zhīmǔ 5-3g + huángqín 5-0g + huángbò 4-0g + shénqū 2-0g + dàhuáng 1-0g + huánglián 1-0g.

Báizhú 5g + shíchāngpú 5g + hángjú 5g + gǒuqǐzǐ 5g + shénqū 5g + fúshén 5g + màiyá 5g + huángqí 5g + yuǎnzhì 5g + dǎngshēn 5g + acupuncture.

to form a bile acid that digests fats. CTX is characterized by the development of benign, fatty tumors (xanthomas) in the brain and connective tissue such as the tendon and eye lens.

Fángfēng (cf. Section 2.38) "stops pain, cramps and diarrhea" and was shown to be reviewed and summarized to have anti-inflammatory, analgesic, antioxidant, antiproliferative, antitumor, immunoregulatory, febrifugal analgesic, and anticonvulsive activities (Yang et al., 2020; Wang et al., 1991). Èrchéntāng (cf. Section 1.8) is used today for chronic bronchitis and glaucoma (Wang, 2019). Zhīmǔ was introduced in Section 2.35 to protect the central nervous system; it is used today for neuralgia, neuritis, radiculitis, and headaches (Wang, 2020).

5.16   PORPHYRIA CUTANEA TARDA

Porphyria cutanea tarda (PCT) is an acquired liver disorder characterized by painful blistering of the skin that is exposed to sunlight. PCT is caused by the deficiency of an enzyme called *uroporphyrinogen decarboxylase*, which catalyzes the fifth step in heme production in the liver. The enzyme deficiency can be acquired after conception or inherited from a mutated *UROD* gene in a parent's germ cells.

Dānshēn was introduced in Section 3.15 to remove "blood stasis," the degree of which was found to correlate with the serum index of liver fibrosis in patients with hepatopathy and blood stasis TCM syndrome (Tang et al., 1997). Dānshēn was indeed shown to alleviate hepatic inflammation, fatty

---

TABLE 5.16

GMP Herbal Medicines for a 60-Year-Old Adult with Porphyria Cutanea Tarda

Porphyria cutanea tarda (OrphaCode: 101330)

A disease with a prevalence of ~4 in 100,000

Disease-causing germline mutation(s) (loss of function): uroporphyrinogen decarboxylase (*UROD* / Entrez: 7389) at 1p34.1

Modifying germline mutation: homeostatic iron regulator (*HFE* / Entrez: 3077) at 6p22.2

Autosomal dominant, Multigenic/multifactorial

Exacerbated by tobacco use, Cutaneous photosensitivity, Abnormal blistering of the skin, Fragile skin, Porphyrinuria, Abnormal circulating porphyrin concentration

Abnormal enzyme/coenzyme activity, Abnormal erythrocyte enzyme activity, Increased serum ferritin, Elevated hepatic iron concentration, Alcoholism, Chronic hepatitis, Poor wound healing, Pain, Increased urinary porphobilinogen, Increased serum iron

Decreased hepcidin level, Systemic lupus erythematosus, Stage 5 chronic kidney disease, Diabetes mellitus, Hepatic steatosis, Hematological neoplasm, Scaling skin, Recurrent bacterial skin infections, Cutaneous abscess, Hypertrichosis, Hypopigmentation of the skin, Hyperpigmentation of the skin, Hirsutism, Scarring, Corneal scarring, Ectropion, Elevated hepatic transaminase, Periportal fibrosis, Hepatic lobular inflammation, Portal inflammation, Hepatocellular carcinoma, Increased fecal porphyrin, Viral hepatitis

Adult

Chronic hepatitis (570, 571.4, 571.41), Pain (D010146):

Yīnchénwǔlíngsǎn 5g + lóngdǎnxiègāntāng 5g + jīnyínhuā 2-1g + dàqīngyè 2-0g + púgōngyīng 2-0g + shānzhīzǐ 1-0g + yīnchén 1-0g.

Yīnchénwǔlíngsǎn 5g + jiāwèixiāoyáosǎn 4g + huángliánjiědútāng 4g + jīnyínhuā 1g.

Yīnchénwǔlíngsǎn 5g + huángliánjiědútāng 3-2g + jīnyínhuā 1g + shānzhīzǐ 1-0g + yīnchén 1-0g + púgōngyīng 1-0g.

Dānshēn 5g + báihuāshéshécǎo 5g + yīnchén 5g + wǔjiāpí 3g + huángshuǐqié 3g + huángqín 3g + dīngshùxiǔ 3-0g + huánglián 2-0g.

Shānyào 5g + dānshēn 5g + gāncǎo 5g + chìsháo 5g + hǔzhàng 5g + cháihú 5g + yīnchén 5g + liánqiáo 5g.

Chuānqī 5g + dānshēn 5g + báihuāshéshécǎo 5g + yīnchén 5g + huángshuǐqié 3g + huángqín 3g + huánglián 2g.

Systemic lupus erythematosus (710.0), Diabetes mellitus (250), Hepatic steatosis (571.0), Hirsutism (D006628), Scarring (D002921) [Scar conditions and fibrosis of skin (709.2)], Ectropion (374.1), Elevated hepatic transaminase (573.9):

Jiāwèixiāoyáosǎn 5g + xuèfǔzhúyūtāng 3g + zhǐbódìhuángwán 3g + dānshēn 1g + báixiānpí 1g + dìfūzǐ 1g + mǔdānpí 1g + jīnyínhuā 1g + huángqín 1g.

Jiāwèixiāoyáosǎn 5g + zhǐbódìhuángwán 5g + lóngdǎnxiègāntāng 5g + xiāofēngsǎn 5-0g.

Xiāofēngsǎn 5g + jiědúsìwùtāng 2g + zhēnrénhuómìngyǐnqùchuānshānjiǎ 2g.

Yùnǚjiān 5g + lóngdǎnxiègāntāng 5g + zhǐbódìhuángwán 2g.

Báizhǐ 5-2g + huángqín 5-0g + zhìgāncǎo 4-2g + shārén 4-2g + guālóugēn 2-0g + huángbò 2-0g + xìxīn 1-0g + dàhuáng 0g.

Báisháo 5g + dìhuáng 5g + màiméndōng 4g + wǔwèizǐ 2g + huǒmárén 2g + mǔlì 2g + zhìgāncǎo 2g + ējiāo 2g + guībǎn 2g + biējiǎ 2g.

Báizhú 5g + fùzǐ 5g + cháihú 5g + báisháo 4g + fúlíng 4g + tiānhuā 2g + dǎngshēn 2g + shēngjiāng 2g + wúzhūyú 2g + guìzhī 2g + huángqín 2g + gāncǎo 1g + mǔlì 1g + gānjiāng 1g + huánglián 1g.

degeneration, and haptic fibrogenesis in acute/chronic alcoholic liver disease and non-alcoholic fatty liver disease in mice (Hong et al., 2017). Wǔjiāpí (Cortex Acanthopanacis) "reduces rheumatism, strengthens muscles/bones, promotes urination" and is used today for neuralgia, neuritis, and radiculitis (Wang, 2020). Xuèfǔzhúyūtāng, introduced in Section 2.45 to "disperse blood stasis," was shown to lower the serum liver fibrosis index in patients with hepatopathy and blood stasis TCM syndrome (Tang et al., 1997). Combined therapy of Zhībódìhuángwán or Jiāwèixiāoyáosǎn was found to improve the survival of patients with systemic lupus erythematosus in Taiwan (Ma et al., 2016).

5.17 ACATALASEMIA

Acatalasemia, also called catalase deficiency, is the absence or low levels of an antioxidant enzyme called *catalase* in the cells. Hydrogen peroxide, a harmful metabolic product of cellular respiration, is broken down by catalase into oxygen and water. Acatalasemia is usually asymptomatic but may induce oral ulceration. Acatalasemia is caused by mutations in the *CAT* gene, which encodes catalase.

TABLE 5.17
GMP Herbal Medicines for a 40-Year-Old Adult with Acatalasemia

Acatalasemia (OrphaCode: 926)

A disease with a prevalence of ~3 in 100,000

Disease-causing germline mutation(s): catalase (*CAT* / Entrez: 847) at 11p13

Autosomal recessive

Reduced catalase activity

Oral ulcer

Severe periodontitis, Gingival bleeding, Gingivitis, Microcytic anemia, Type II diabetes mellitus, Old-aged sensorineural hearing impairment, Gangrene

All ages

Gingival bleeding (D005884), Gingivitis (523.0, 523.1), Old-aged sensorineural hearing impairment (D011304), Gangrene (D005734) [Gangrene (785.4)]:

Yùnǔjiān 5g + gānlùyǐn 5g + qīngwèisǎn 5g + xuánshēn 1-0g.	Báizhǐ 5-4g + huángqín 5-0g + zhìgāncǎo 4-2g + shārén 4-2g + tiānhuā 2-0g + xìxīn 1g + dàhuáng 1-0g.
Gānlùyǐn 5g + qīngwèisǎn 5-4g + xuánshēn 1-0g + gǔsuìbǔ 1-0g + shígāo 1-0g + dìhuáng 1-0g.	Dàqīngyè 5g + báihuāshéshécǎo 5g + bàijiàngcǎo 5g + yúxīngcǎo 5g + huángqín 5g + púgōngyīng 5g + gāncǎo 2g + acupuncture.
	Huángbò 5g + shārén 3g + guībǎn 3g + zhìgāncǎo 2g + fùzǐ 2g.

Dàqīngyè (Folium Isatidis) was shown to alleviate liver injury in mice by enhancing the endogenous antioxidant system (Ding & Zhu, 2020). Yùnǔjiān (cf. Section 1.51) "clears the Stomach, nourishes yin" and is used today for the skin, gingival, and periodontal diseases (Wang, 2019). Qīngwèisǎn (cf. Sections 1.69 and 3.24) "clears the Stomach, quenches fire, cools Blood, reduces swelling" and is used today for diseases of the oral soft tissues (Wang, 2019).

5.18 GLYCOGEN STORAGE DISEASE DUE TO ACID MALTASE DEFICIENCY

Glycogen storage disease due to acid maltase deficiency—also known as alpha-1,4-glucosidase acid deficiency; glycogen storage disease type 2; glycogenosis due to acid maltase deficiency; and Pompe disease—is a multisystemic, hereditary condition characterized by skeletal muscle weakness affecting mobility and respiration. Pompe disease is caused by mutations in the *GAA* gene, whose products convert glycogen into glucose. The accumulation of glycogen in skeletal muscle, smooth muscle, and cardiac muscle causes the symptoms of Pompe disease.

TABLE 5.18

GMP Herbal Medicines for a 29-Year-Old Adult with Glycogen Storage Disease Due to Acid Maltase Deficiency

Glycogen storage disease due to acid maltase deficiency (OrphaCode: 365)

A disease with a prevalence of ~3 in 100,000

Disease-causing germline mutation(s): alpha glucosidase (*GAA* / Entrez: 2548) at 17q25.3

Autosomal recessive

Muscle weakness, Progressive proximal muscle weakness, Oligosacchariduria, Abnormal enzyme/coenzyme activity

Hyporeflexia, Motor delay, Areflexia, Failure to thrive, Cardiomegaly, Left ventricular hypertrophy, Respiratory insufficiency, Hepatomegaly, Difficulty walking, Respiratory insufficiency due to muscle weakness, Exertional dyspnea, Elevated circulating creatine kinase concentration, Gowers sign, EMG: myopathic abnormalities, Exercise intolerance, Difficulty climbing stairs, Lower limb muscle weakness, Feeding difficulties in infancy, Respiratory tract infection, Fatigue, Increased lactate dehydrogenase activity, Heart murmur, Glycogen accumulation in muscle fiber lysosomes, Elevated serum alanine aminotransferase

Macroglossia, Difficulty in tongue movements, Facial hypotonia, Hearing impairment, Ptosis, Osteoporosis, Dysarthria, Hypertrophic cardiomyopathy, Dysphagia, Respiratory distress, Transient ischemic attack, Inability to walk, Vasculitis, Scoliosis, Respiratory failure, Hyperlordosis, Generalized muscle weakness, Dilatation of the cerebral artery, Shortened PR interval, Impaired mastication, Cranial nerve paralysis, Infantile muscular hypotonia, Diaphragmatic weakness, Sleep apnea, Chronic pain, Thoracic aortic aneurysm, Orthopnea, Fatigable weakness of swallowing muscles, Fatigable weakness of respiratory muscles, Basilar artery calcification, Left ventricular outflow tract obstruction, Abnormal internal carotid artery morphology

Antenatal, Neonatal, Infancy, Childhood, Adolescent, Adult

Muscle weakness (D018908):

Dúhuójìshēngtāng 5g + shūjīnghuóxuètāng 4g + sháoyàogāncǎotāng 4-0g + acupuncture.

Dúhuójìshēngtāng 5g + jìshēngshènqìwán 5-0g + dùzhòng 1g + niúxī 1-0g + yánhúsuǒ 1-0g + gǒujǐ 1-0g + gǔsuìbǔ 1-0g + xùduàn 1-0g.

Dúhuójìshēngtāng 5g + sháoyàogāncǎotāng 2g + mòyào 1g + rǔxiāng 1g + acupuncture.

Báizhú 5g + fùzǐ 5g + báisháo 5-4g + fúlíng 5-4g + dǎngshēn 5-2g + cháihú 5-0g + tiānhuā 2-0g + shēngjiāng 2-0g + guìzhī 2-0g + huángqín 2-0g + gāncǎo 1-0g + mǔlì 1-0g + gānjiāng 1-0g.

Báizhú 5g + fúlíng 5-4g + zhìgāncǎo 4-3g + gānjiāng 4-0g + niúxī 3-2g + fùzǐ 3-2g + guìzhī 3-0g + ròuguì 3-0g + zhǐshí 3-0g + dàhuáng 1-0g.

Areflexia (D012021), Difficulty walking (D051346), Fatigue (D005221), Heart murmur (D006337):

Qīngshǔyìqìtāng 5g + shēngmàiyǐn 4-0g + huáshí 2-0g + gāncǎo 1-0g.

Bǔzhōngyìqìtāng 5g + huángqí 1-0g + dǎngshēn 1-0g + wǔwèizǐ 1-0g + màiméndōng 1-0g.

Shēngmá 5g + gāncǎo 5g + báizhú 5g + cháihú 5g + huángqí 5g + dāngguī 5g + dǎngshēn 5g + fúlíng 5-0g + chénpí 5-0g.

Shēngmá 5g + xuánshēn 5g + dìhuáng 5g + hòupò 5g + zhǐshí 5g + màiméndōng 5g + dàhuáng 1g.

Dàzǎo 5g + bànxià 5g + shēngjiāng 5g + báisháo 5g + zhǐshí 5g + cháihú 5g + huángqín 5g + dàhuáng 1g.

Shēngmá 5g + chìsháo 5g + qiánhú 5g + sāngbáipí 5g + cháihú 5g + jīngjiè 5g + huángqín 5g + gégēn 5g.

Hearing impairment (D003638), Ptosis (374.3), Osteoporosis (733.0), Dysarthria (D004401), Hypertrophic cardiomyopathy (425.1), Respiratory distress (D004417), Cranial nerve paralysis (352.9), Sleep apnea (780.57), Chronic pain (D059350):

Língguìshùgāntāng 5g + xiōngqióng 2-1g + dāngguī 2-1g + gǎoběn 2-0g + cāngzhú 1-0g.

Língguìshùgāntāng 5g + sǎnzhǒngkuìjiāntāng 5g + shēngjiāng 1g + báisháo 1g.

Fúlíng 5g + mǔlì 4g + hǎigé 4g + hǎipiāoxiāo 4g + jílí 4g + dàfùpí 3g + wǔlíngzhī 3g + gāncǎo 3g + sāngbáipí 3g + zǐsūyè 3g + júhuā 3g + cāngěrzǐ 3g + púgōngyīng 3-0g + xīnyí 2-0g.

Dǎngshēn 5g + gǒuqǐzǐ 2g + júhuā 2g + zhìgāncǎo 1g + fùzǐ 0g + gānjiāng 0g.

Zhìgāncǎo 5g + gǒuqǐzǐ 5g + júhuā 5g + rénshēn 2g + fùzǐ 2g + dàhuáng 0g.

Qīngshǔyìqìtāng "clears summer heat, dispels dampness, benefits Qi, generates saliva" and is used for the effects of heat and light (Wang, 2019). Heavy sweating in summer heat depletes the body's salt and moisture levels, which can cause painful muscle cramps. Shēngmàiyǐn was introduced in Section 3.20 for cardiac dysrhythmias. Xiōngqiōng (Radix Chuanxiong) "activates circulation, moves Qi, dispels wind, stops pain" and is used for the absence of menstruation, peptic ulcers, and headaches (Wang, 2020). Gǎoběn (Rhizoma et Radix Ligustici) "dispels wind, disperses coldness, removes dampness, stops pain" and is used for headaches and migraines (Wang, 2020).

5.19 CITRULLINEMIA TYPE I

Citrullinemia type I (CTLN1), also known as classic citrullinemia or argininosuccinic acid synthetase deficiency, is characterized by an abnormal accumulation of ammonia in the body fluids, including the blood. CTLN1 is caused by mutations in the *ASS1* gene, whose products detoxify ammonia in the body via the urea cycle.

TABLE 5.19

GMP Herbal Medicines for a One-Year-Old Infant with Citrullinemia Type I

Citrullinemia type I (OrphaCode: 247525)

A disease with a prevalence of ~2 in 100,000

Disease-causing germline mutation(s) (loss of function): argininosuccinate synthase 1 (*ASS1* / Entrez: 445) at 9q34.11

Autosomal recessive

Hyperammonemia, Elevated plasma citrulline

Hepatic failure

Abnormality of the nervous system, Seizure, Lethargy, Spasticity, Failure to thrive, Respiratory alkalosis, Vomiting, Intellectual disability, moderate, Hepatic encephalopathy, Intellectual disability, borderline, Feeding difficulties

All ages

Hyperammonemia (D022124) [Disorders of urea cycle metabolism (270.6)]:

Xiǎocháihútāng 5g + wǔlíngsǎn 5g.

Wǔlíngsǎn 5g + píngwèisǎn 5g + shānzhā 1g + shénqū 1g + màiyá 1g.

Shàngzhōngxiàtōngyòngtòngfēngwán 5g.

Xiǎojiànzhōngtāng 5g + yùpíngfēngsǎn 5-0g + bǔzhōngyìqìtāng 5-0g.

Gāncǎo 5g + báizhǐ 5g + shārén 5g + dàhuáng 1-0g.

Báizhǐ 5g + zhìgāncǎo 5g + shārén 5g + dàhuáng 1-0g.

Xuánshēn 5g + dìhuáng 5g + hòupò 5g + zhǐshí 5g + màiméndōng 5g + dàhuáng 2g.

Seizure (345.9), Lethargy (D053609), Spasticity (D009128), Vomiting (D014839), Hepatic encephalopathy (572.2):

Yùpíngfēngsǎn 5g + guìzhītāng 5g.

Yìgānsǎn 5g + yùpíngfēngsǎn 5-0g + bǎohéwán 5-0g + tiānmá 2g + gōuténg 2g.

Cháihújiālónggǔmǔlìtāng 5g.

Bǎohéwán 5g + mázǐrénwán 2g + gāncǎo 1g.

Gāncǎo 5g + báizhǐ 5-0g + shārén 5-0g + huángqín 5-0g + dàhuáng 1-0g.

Huángqín 5g + báizhǐ 2g + gāncǎo 2g + shārén 2g + tiānhuā 1g + dàhuáng 0g.

Liver disease and kidney failure are the two most common causes of acquired hyperammonemia. We therefore see Xiǎocháihútāng and Wǔlíngsǎn in the prescription, where the former is for liver disease and the latter is for kidney disease. Yùpíngfēngsǎn contains Fángfēng as the major herb, which "relieves rheumatism, arrests spasm and stops diarrhea" (cf. Sections 2.38 and 5.15).

5.20 KEARNS-SAYRE SYNDROME

Kearns-Sayre syndrome is a multisystem condition characterized by progressive weakness of the ocular muscles and degeneration of the photoreceptors in the retina, followed by problems with other body systems, including the heart and proximal muscles. Kearns-Sayre syndrome is caused by

TABLE 5.20

GMP Herbal Medicines for a 15-Year-Old Adolescent with Kearns-Sayre Syndrome

Kearns-Sayre syndrome (OrphaCode: 480)

A disease with a prevalence of ~2 in 100,000

Candidate gene tested: mitochondrially encoded ATP synthase membrane subunit 8 (*MT-ATP8* / Entrez: 4509) at mitochondria

Disease-causing germline mutation(s): ribonucleotide reductase regulatory TP53 inducible subunit M2B (*RRM2B* / Entrez: 50484) at 8q22.3

Candidate gene tested: mitochondrially encoded tRNA-Leu (UUA/G) 1 (*MT-TL1* / Entrez: 4567) at mitochondria

Autosomal recessive, Mitochondrial inheritance, Not applicable

Progressive external ophthalmoplegia, Third-degree atrioventricular block, Abnormality of retinal pigmentation

Hearing impairment, Anterior hypopituitarism, Ataxia, Hypotonia, Reduced tendon reflexes, Ragged-red muscle fibers, Skeletal muscle atrophy, EMG abnormality, Progressive intervertebral space narrowing

Delayed skeletal maturation, Hemiplegia/hemiparesis

Infancy, Childhood, Adolescent, Adult

Progressive external ophthalmoplegia (378.72):

Qǐjúdìhuángwán 5g + zīshènmíngmùtāng 5g.

Yìqìcōngmíngtāng 5g + qǐjúdìhuángwán 5-4g + shíchāngpú 1-0g + yuǎnzhì 1-0g + gāncǎo 0g.

Qǐjúdìhuángwán 5g + bǔzhōngyìqìtāng 5g + shíchāngpú 1-0g + yìzhìrén 1-0g + yuǎnzhì 1-0g.

Xiǎojiànzhōngtāng 5g + huángqí 1g + dāngguī 0g.

Zhǐqiào 5-4g + jílí 5-4g + chántuì 5-0g.

Chántuì 5g + zhǐqiào 4g + jílí 4g + sīguāluò 0g.

Báizhǐ 5g + gāncǎo 4g + shārén 4g + huángqín 4g + tiānhuā 2g + dàhuáng 1g.

Hearing impairment (D003638), Ataxia (D002524), Hypotonia (D009123), Skeletal muscle atrophy (D009133):

Wǔlíngsǎn 5g + língguìshùgāntāng 5g.

Língguìshùgāntāng 5g + zhēnwǔtāng 5g + niúxī 1g + chēqiánzǐ 1g.

Língguìshùgāntāng 5g + bànxià 1g + fùzǐ 1g + shārén 1g + dàhuáng 0g.

Rénshēn 5g + bànxià 5-4g + huángqín 5-0g + gānjiāng 5-0g.

deletions in the mtDNA of the mitochondria that use oxygen to convert food into chemical energy for cellular use.

Rénshēn (cf. Sections 1.15, 2.33, and 2.49) was shown to delay age-related hearing loss and progressive vestibular dysfunction in mice (Tian et al., 2014); it was also reviewed to improve hearing thresholds in patients with sensorineural hearing loss and alleviate the symptoms of tinnitus (Castañeda et al., 2019). A compound isolated from Fúlíng (cf. Section 1.21) was shown to inhibit ear inflammation in mice (Yasukawa et al., 1998). Wǔlíngsǎn, Língguìshùgāntāng, and Zhēnwǔtāng all contain Fúlíng.

5.21 LYSOSOMAL ACID LIPASE DEFICIENCY

Lysosomal acid lipase deficiency, or LAL deficiency, is characterized by accumulation of lipids, including low-density lipoproteins in the cells and tissues throughout the body, including the liver and blood vessel walls, leading to liver failure, heart attack, and stroke. LAL deficiency is caused by mutations in the *LIPA* gene, whose products break down cholesteryl esters and triglycerides in the lysosomes within cells.

Zhīzǐ (Fructus Gardeniae) "quenches fire, removes anguish, clears heat, helps draining, cools Blood, detoxifies, reduces swelling, stops pain" and is used today for nonpsychotic mental disorders and sleep disturbances (Wang, 2020). Zhīzǐ, being cold and bitter in TCM nature and taste, extinguishes heat over the body. In TCM, jaundice is said to be caused by "damp evil" (due to external pathogens or internal toxins) affecting the TCM gallbladder and liver. If the patient manifests a fever, Yīnchén (cf. Sections 1.57 and 4.21) is combined with Zhīzǐ to counteract the "damp-heat jaundice."

TABLE 5.21

GMP Herbal Medicines for a Five-Year-Old Child with Lysosomal Acid Lipase Deficiency

Lysosomal acid lipase deficiency (OrphaCode: 275761)

A disease with a prevalence of ~2 in 100,000

Disease-causing germline mutation(s) (loss of function): lipase A, lysosomal acid type (*LIPA* / Entrez: 3988) at 10q23.31

Autosomal recessive

Jaundice, Xanthomatosis, Hepatic fibrosis, Hepatic failure, Decreased liver function, Microvesicular hepatic steatosis, Hepatosplenomegaly, Vacuolated lymphocytes, Nausea and vomiting, Abdominal pain, Hypertriglyceridemia, Steatorrhea, Elevated hepatic transaminase, Hypercholesterolemia, Elevated alkaline phosphatase, Abdominal distention, Fatal liver failure in infancy, Adrenal calcification, Cognitive impairment

Xanthelasma, Stroke, Weight loss, Diarrhea, Esophageal varix, Precocious atherosclerosis, Coronary atherosclerosis

Renal salt wasting, Primary adrenal insufficiency, Pruritus, Global developmental delay, Failure to thrive, Ascites, Anemia, Acidosis, Dehydration, Hypersplenism, Vomiting, Pulmonary arterial hypertension, Hyperkalemia, Psychomotor deterioration, Hypotension, Hyponatremia, Hypernatriuria, Cachexia, Bone-marrow foam cells, Malnutrition, Hypovolemia, Feeding difficulties, Abnormal urine potassium concentration

Neonatal, Infancy, Childhood, Adolescent, Adult

Jaundice (D007565), Decreased liver function (573.9), Abdominal pain (D015746), Elevated hepatic transaminase (573.9):

Xiǎocháihútāng 5g + yīnchénwǔlíngsǎn 5g + wǔwèizǐ 2-0g + hǔzhàng 2-0g.

Gāncǎo 5g + yīnchén 5g + jīnyínhuā 5-0g + huángqín 5-0g.

Xiǎocháihútāng 5g + gānlùxiāodúdān 5g + yīnchén 1g + huángshuǐqié 1g.

Yīnchén 5g + gāncǎo 2g + báizhú 2g + mǔdānpí 2g + fúlíng 2g + màiyá 2g.

Xiǎocháihútāng 5g + sìjūnzǐtāng 5g + yīnchén 1g + yùjīn 1g.

Yīnchén 5g + zhǐzǐ 5g + huángqín 5g + dàhuáng 1g.

Cháihúshūgāntāng 5g + bǎohéwán 2g + gāncǎo 0g.

Gāncǎo 5g + báizhǐ 5g + shārén 5g + dàhuáng 0g.

Weight loss (D015431), Diarrhea (D003967):

Guìzhītāng 5g + xìngrén 1-0g + hòupò 1-0g + gāncǎo 1-0g + dàhuáng 0g.

Zhìgāncǎo 5g + dàhuáng 1-0g.

Gāncǎo 5g + hòupò 5-0g + zhǐshí 5-0g + dàhuáng 1-0g.

Pruritus (D011537), Ascites (789.5), Anemia (285.9), Dehydration (276.51), Hypersplenism (289.4), Vomiting (D014839), Cachexia (D002100):

Shēnlíngbáizhúsǎn 5g.

Gāncǎo 5g + jīnyínhuā 5-0g.

Xiāngshāliùjūnzǐtāng 5g + shénqū 1g + màiyá 1g.

Xuánshēn 5g + dìhuáng 5g + màiméndōng 5g + zhìgāncǎo 2g + dàhuáng 0g.

Sìjūnzǐtāng 5g + xìngsūyǐnyòukē 5-0g.

Bǎohéwán 5g.

Xuánshēn 5g + dìhuáng 5g + màiméndōng 5g + gāncǎo 2-0g + dàhuáng 0g.

5.22 CLASSIC HOMOCYSTINURIA

Classic homocystinuria, also known as homocystinuria due to cystathionine beta-synthase deficiency, is characterized by a buildup of homocysteine and methionine in the blood and excretion of homocysteine in the urine. Classic homocystinuria is caused by mutations in the *CBS* gene, whose products convert the amino acid homocysteine to a molecule called *cystathionine*. Excess homocysteine and related compounds in the body lead to the signs and symptoms of classic homocystinuria in Table 5.22.

TABLE 5.22

GMP Herbal Medicines for a Three-Year-Old Child with Classic Homocystinuria

Classic homocystinuria (OrphaCode: 394)

A disease with a prevalence of ~2 in 100,000

Disease-causing germline mutation(s): cystathionine beta-synthase (*CBS* / Entrez: 875) at 21q22.3

Autosomal recessive

(Continued)

TABLE 5.22 *(Continued)*

GMP Herbal Medicines for a Three-Year-Old Child with Classic Homocystinuria

Dental crowding, Osteoporosis, Ectopia lentis, Arachnodactyly, Intellectual disability, Disproportionate tall stature, Recurrent fractures, Abnormality of amino acid metabolism

Myopia, Amblyopia, Pectus excavatum, Pectus carinatum, Hypertension, Joint stiffness, Pulmonary embolism, Sparse scalp hair, Cerebral ischemia, Scoliosis, Kyphosis, Genu valgum, Arterial thrombosis, Venous thrombosis, Arteriovenous malformation

High palate, Glaucoma, Cataract, Retinal detachment, Optic atrophy, Behavioral abnormality, Psychosis, Urticaria, Seizure, Subcutaneous hemorrhage, Anorexia, Esophageal varix, Intracranial hemorrhage, Gastrointestinal hemorrhage, Hepatomegaly, Elevated hepatic transaminase, Hemiplegia/hemiparesis, Abnormality of retinal pigmentation, Hernia Childhood

Osteoporosis (733.0), Ectopia lentis (743.37), Intellectual disability (D008607):

Liùwèidìhuángwán 5g + shēnlíngbáizhúsǎn 5g + gǔsuìbǔ 2g + bǔgǔzhǐ 2g.

Liùwèidìhuángwán 5g + jiāwèixiāoyáosǎn 5g + gǔsuìbǔ 2g + xùduàn 2g.

Xiāngshāliùjūnzǐtāng 5g + liùwèidìhuángwán 5-0g + gǔsuìbǔ 2-0g + bǔgǔzhǐ 2-0g + shānzhā 1-0g + shénqū 1-0g + màiyá 1-0g.

Báizhú 5g + fùzǐ 5g + cháihú 5g + báisháo 4g + fúlíng 4g + tiānhuā 2g + dǎngshēn 2g + wǔwèizǐ 2g + xìxīn 2g + gāncǎo 1g + mǔlì 1g + gānjiāng 1g.

Báizhú 5g + fùzǐ 5g + cháihú 5g + báisháo 4-3g + fúlíng 4-3g + dǎngshēn 3-2g + tiānhuā 2g + guìzhī 2g + huángqín 2g + gāncǎo 2-1g + mǔlì 2-1g + gānjiāng 2-1g.

Gāncǎo 5g + báizhǐ 5g + jīnyínhuā 5g + huángqín 5g + shārén 4g + dàhuáng 0g.

Màiyá 5g + shānyào 2g + báizhú 2g + huángqí 2g.

Myopia (367.1), Amblyopia (368.01, 368.00), Hypertension (401-405.99):

Sāngjúyǐn 5g + zhǐqiào 5-1g + chántuì 5-0g.

Jiāwèixiāoyáosǎn 5g + zhǐqiào 2g + jílí 2g + chántuì 2g.

Hángjú 5g + gǒuqǐzǐ 5g + shíchāngpú 3-2g + yuǎnzhì 3-2g + gāncǎo 2-0g.

Jílí 5-3g + chántuì 5-0g + zhǐqiào 5-0g + júhóng 5-0g.

Glaucoma (365), Cataract (366.8), Retinal detachment (361.9), Optic atrophy (377.1), Psychosis (295.4, 295.7), Seizure (345.9), Anorexia (D000855), Intracranial hemorrhage (D020300), Gastrointestinal hemorrhage (D006471), Elevated hepatic transaminase (573.9), Hernia (618.6):

Qǐjúdìhuángwán 5g + bǔzhōngyìqìtāng 5g + shíchāngpú 1g + yuǎnzhì 1g + acupuncture.

Qǐjúdìhuángwán 5g + língguìshùgāntāng 5g + tiānmá 1g + shíchāngpú 1g + gōuténg 1g + acupuncture.

Qǐjúdìhuángwán 5g + yìqìcōngmíngtāng 5g + tiānmá 1g + shíchāngpú 1g + yuǎnzhì 1g + acupuncture.

Tiānwángbǔxīndān 5g + bǔzhōngyìqìtāng 5g + shíchāngpú 1g + yuǎnzhì 1g + acupuncture.

Huángbò 5g + shārén 4g + gāncǎo 2g + dìhuáng 2g + bǎihé 2g + zhǐzǐ 2g + dàndòuchǐ 2g + liánqiáo 2g.

Hángjú 5g + shíchāngpú 3g + gǒuqǐzǐ 3g + yuǎnzhì 3g + nǚzhēnzǐ 2g + gāncǎo 2g.

Gǒuqǐzǐ 5g + júhuā 5g + dāngguī 5g + fángfēng 3g + dìhuáng 2g + xìxīn 2g + huánglián 2g.

Xuánshēn 5g + dìhuáng 5g + màiméndōng 5g + shíchāngpú 3g + gǒuqǐzǐ 3g + júhuā 3g + dāngguī 3g + yuǎnzhì 3g + xìxīn 2g.

Liùwèidìhuángwán (cf. Sections 3.19 and 4.5) was shown to treat postmenopausal osteoporosis patients with kidney-yin deficiency (Ge et al., 2018). Báizhú (cf. Section 4.8) was shown to protect against bone loss in mice by inhibiting osteoclast differentiation (Ha et al., 2013). Huángbò (cf. Sections 1.61, 4.19, and 5.2) was demonstrated to be neuroprotective in PC-12 cells (Jung et al., 2013), which are derived from rat pheochromocytoma for the study of neuroscience. Huángbò was also shown to be hemostatic in mice (Liu et al., 2018).

5.23 CYSTINOSIS

Cystinosis, also known as a protein defect of cystine transport, is accumulation of the amino acid cystine within cells, forming crystals in cells that can damage tissues and organs of the body, including the kidneys and eyes. Cystinosis is caused by mutations in the *CTNS* gene, whose products move cystine out of lysosomes where amino acids are digested and recycled.

TABLE 5.23

GMP Herbal Medicines for a One-Year-Old Infant with Cystinosis

Cystinosis (OrphaCode: 213)

A disease with a prevalence of ~2 in 100,000

Disease-causing germline mutation(s): cystinosin, lysosomal cystine transporter (*CTNS* / Entrez: 1497) at 17p13.2
Autosomal recessive

Proteinuria, Nephropathy, Renal tubular dysfunction, Photophobia, Stereotypy, Hypothyroidism, Delayed puberty, Muscle weakness, Failure to thrive, Dehydration, Polydipsia, Vomiting, Hypophosphatemia, Hypokalemia, Myopathy, Aminoaciduria, Short stature, Corneal opacity, Nephrogenic diabetes insipidus, Fatigue, Type I diabetes mellitus
Renal insufficiency, Retinopathy, Rickets

Visual impairment, Intellectual disability, mild, Gait disturbance, Portal hypertension, Fever, Malabsorption, Dysphasia, Cranial nerve paralysis, Abnormal pyramidal sign

Infancy, Childhood, Adolescent, Adult

Proteinuria (791.0), Photophobia (D020795), Stereotypy (307.3), Hypothyroidism (244.9), Muscle weakness (D018908), Polydipsia (D059606), Vomiting (D014839), Myopathy (359.9), Nephrogenic diabetes insipidus (588.1), Fatigue (D005221):

Bìxièfēnqīngyǐn 5g + jìshēngshènqìwán 5-0g + tǔfúlíng 1-0g + yìmǔcǎo 1-0g + bìxiè 1-0g.

Qīngxīnliánzǐyǐn 5g + bìxièfēnqīngyǐn 5g.

Zhūlíngtāng 5g + jìshēngshènqìwán 5g + báimáogēn 1g + chēqiánzǐ 1g.

Shānyào 5g + báizhú 5g + báisháo 5g + ējiāo 5g + gǒuqǐzǐ 5g + huángqí 5g + dāngguī 5g + dǎngshēn 5g + suānzǎorén 5-0g + shúdìhuáng 5-0g + gāncǎo 3g.

Chìxiǎodòu 5g + chēqiánzǐ 5-0g + yìmǔcǎo 5-0 + dāngguī 3-2g + báimáogēn 3-0g + dàhuáng 0g.

Renal insufficiency (586), Retinopathy (362.9):

Qǐjúdìhuángwán 5g + shēnlíngbáizhúsǎn 5-0g.

Qǐjúdìhuángwán 5g + bǔzhōngyìqìtāng 5-0g.

Shēnlíngbáizhúsǎn 5g + qǐjúdìhuángwán 4-0g + guīpítāng 4-0g + gāncǎo 1-0g.

Jílí 5g + zhǐqiào 3-0g + júhóng 2-0g.

Júhuā 5g + júhóng 5-0g.

Gāncǎo 5g + báizhǐ 5g + shārén 5g + dàhuáng 0g.

Visual impairment (D014786), Portal hypertension (572.3), Fever (D005334), Cranial nerve paralysis (352.9):

Xiǎojiànzhōngtāng 5g + yùpíngfēngsǎn 5g.

Shēnlíngbáizhúsǎn 5g + yùpíngfēngsǎn 5-0g + gāncǎo 1-0g.

Shēnlíngbáizhúsǎn 5g + bǎohéwán 1-0g.

Xìngsūyǐnyòukē 5g + xīnyíqīngfèitāng 5g.

Gāncǎo 5g + báizhǐ 5-0g + shārén 5-0g + huángqín 2-0g + dàhuáng 1-0g.

Zhǐqiào 5g + jílí 5g.

Zhìgāncǎo 5g + báizhǐ 2g + shārén 2g + dàhuáng 0g.

Xiǎojiànzhōngtāng is a classic formula for the psychosomatic disorders of the digestive organs, as we will see its frequent use in Chapter 13 on gastroenterologic diseases. The formula was reported to successfully treat children with chronic primary headache (Terasawa et al., 2015). Furthermore, Xiǎojiànzhōngtāng was shown to protect the DNA of human lymphocytes upon oxidative stress, although the component herbs of the formula, being antioxidant individually, were not found to be genoprotective (Szeto et al., 2013).

REFERENCES

Arita, R., Ono, R., Saito, N., Suzuki, S., Kikuchi, A., Ohsawa, M., Tadano, Y., Akaishi, T., Kanno, T., Abe, M., Onodera, K., Takayama, S., & Ishii, T. (2022). Refractory chest pain in mild to moderate Coronavirus disease 2019 successfully treated with Saikanto, a Japanese traditional medicine. *Tohoku Journal of Experimental Medicine, 257*(3), 241–249. https://doi.org/10.1620/tjem.2022.j040

Castañeda, R., Natarajan, S., Jeong, S. Y., Hong, B. N., & Kang, T. H. (2019). Traditional oriental medicine for sensorineural hearing loss: Can ethnopharmacology contribute to potential drug discovery? *Journal of Ethnopharmacology, 231*, 409–428. https://doi.org/10.1016/j.jep.2018.11.016

Chen, W. C., Shih, C. C., Lu, W. A., Li, P. C., Chen, C. J., Hayakawa, S., Shimizu, K., & Chien, C. T. (2006). Combination of Wu Lin San and Shan Zha ameliorates substance P-induced hyperactive bladder via the inhibition of neutrophil NADPH oxidase activity. *Neuroscience Letters, 402*(1–2), 7–11. https://doi. org/10.1016/j.neulet.2006.03.037

Choi, M. J., Choi, B. T., Shin, H. K., Shin, B. C., Han, Y. K., & Baek, J. U. (2015). Establishment of a comprehensive list of candidate antiaging medicinal herb used in Korean medicine by text mining of the classical Korean medical literature, "Dongeuibogam," and preliminary evaluation of the Antiaging effects of these herbs. *Evidence-Based Complementary and Alternative Medicine, 2015*, 1–29. https://doi.org/10.1155/2015/873185

Ding, C., & Zhu, H. (2020). Isatidis Folium alleviates acetaminophen-induced liver injury in mice by enhancing the endogenous antioxidant system. *Environmental Toxicology, 35*(11), 1251–1259. https://doi.org/10.1002/tox.22990

Ding, R., Wang, Y., Zhu, J., Lü, W., Wei, G., Gu, Z., An, Z., & Huo, J. (2020). Danggui Sini decoction protects against oxaliplatin-induced peripheral neuropathy in rats. *Journal of Integrative Neuroscience, 19*(4), 663. https://doi.org/10.31083/j.jin.2020.04.1154

Du, H., Kuang, T., Qiu, S., Xu, T., Huan, C. G., & Fan, G. (2019). Fecal medicines used in traditional medical system of China: A systematic review of their names, original species, traditional uses, and modern investigations. *Chinese Medicine, 14*(1). https://doi.org/10.1186/s13020-019-0253-x

Fong, S. Y. K., Li, C., Ho, Y. C., Li, R., Wang, Q., Wong, Y. C., Xue, H., & Zuo, Z. (2017). Brain uptake of bioactive flavones in Scutellariae Radix and its relationship to anxiolytic effect in mice. *Molecular Pharmaceutics, 14*(9), 2908–2916. https://doi.org/10.1021/acs.molpharmaceut.7b00029

Fujisaka, S., Usui, I., Nawaz, A., Igarashi, Y., Okabe, K., Furusawa, Y., Watanabe, S., Yamamoto, S., Sasahara, M., Watanabe, Y., Nagai, Y., Yagi, K., Nakagawa, T., & Tobe, K. (2020). Bofutsushosan improves gut barrier function with a bloom of *Akkermansia muciniphila* and improves glucose metabolism in mice with diet-induced obesity. *Scientific Reports, 10*(1). https://doi.org/10.1038/s41598-020-62506-w

Ge, J., Xie, L., Chen, J., Li, S., Xu, H., Lai, Y., Qiu, L., & Ni, C. (2018). Liuwei Dihuang Pill (六味地黄丸) treats postmenopausal osteoporosis with Shen (Kidney) Yin deficiency via Janus Kinase/Signal transducer and activator of transcription signal pathway by up-regulating cardiotrophin-like cytokine factor 1 expression. *Chinese Journal of Integrative Medicine, 24*(6), 415–422. https://doi.org/10.1007/s11655-016-2744-2

Guo, J., Wu, W., Sheng, M., Yang, S., & Tan, M. J. (2013). Amygdalin inhibits renal fibrosis in chronic kidney disease. *Molecular Medicine Reports, 7*(5), 1453–1457. https://doi.org/10.3892/mmr.2013.1391

Ha, H., An, H., Shim, K., Kim, T., Lee, K. J., Hwang, Y., & Ma, J. (2013). Ethanol extract of *Atractylodes macrocephala* protects bone loss by inhibiting osteoclast differentiation. *Molecules, 18*(7), 7376–7388. https://doi.org/10.3390/molecules18077376

Hong, M., Li, S., Wang, N., Tan, H., Cheung, F. M., & Feng, Y. (2017). A biomedical investigation of the hepatoprotective effect of *Radix salviae miltiorrhizae* and network pharmacology-based prediction of the active compounds and molecular targets. *International Journal of Molecular Sciences, 18*(3), 620. https://doi.org/10.3390/ijms18030620

Jiang, N., Wei, S., Zhang, Y., He, W., Pei, H., Huang, H., Wang, Q., & Liu, X. (2021). Protective effects and mechanism of Radix Polygalae against neurological diseases as well as effective substance. *Frontiers in Psychiatry, 12*. https://doi.org/10.3389/fpsyt.2021.688703

Jin, M.-Y., & Li, Z.-Y. (2023). Analysis and pharmacovigilance of traditional Chinese medicine prescriptions in cardiovascular department based on data mining. *Yaowu Liuxingbingxue Zazhi, 32*(3), 241–248. [Article in Chinese] https://ywlxbx.whuznhmedj.com/en/journal/35.html

Jung, H. W., Jin, G., Kim, S. Y., Kim, Y. S., & Park, Y. (2013). Neuroprotective effect of methanol extract of Phellodendri Cortex against 1-methyl-4-phenylpyridinium (MPP+)-induced apoptosis in PC-12 cells. *Cell Biology International, 33*(9), 957–963. https://doi.org/10.1016/j.cellbi.2009.06.006

Kurauchi, Y., Ryu, S., Tanaka, R., Haruta, M., Sasagawa, K., Seki, T., Ohta, J., & Katsuki, H. (2024). Goreisan regulates cerebral blood flow according to barometric pressure fluctuations in female C57BL/6J mice. *Journal of Pharmacological Sciences, 154*(2), 47–51. https://doi.org/10.1016/j.jphs.2023.12.001

Li, J., Zhang, K., Bao, J., Yang, J., & Wu, C. (2022). Potential mechanism of action of Jing Fang Bai Du San in the treatment of COVID-19 using docking and network pharmacology. *International Journal of Medical Sciences, 19*(2), 213–224. https://doi.org/10.7150/ijms.67116

Li, Z., Wang, Y., Jiang, Y., Ma, D., Jiang, P., Zhou, G., Yang, J., Dong, F., Zhao, H., Zhang, Y., & Li, X. (2020). Xiao-Qing-Long-Tang maintains cardiac function during heart failure with reduced ejection fraction in salt-sensitive rats by regulating the imbalance of cardiac sympathetic innervation. *Evidence-Based Complementary and Alternative Medicine, 2020*, 1–11. https://doi.org/10.1155/2020/9467271

Liao, W., Jin, Q., Liu, J., Ruan, Y., Li, X., Shen, Y., Zhang, Z., Wang, Y., Wu, S., Zhang, J., Kang, L., & Wu, C. (2021). Mahuang decoction antagonizes acute liver failure via modulating tricarboxylic acid cycle and amino acids metabolism. *Frontiers in Pharmacology, 12*. https://doi.org/10.3389/fphar.2021.599180

Liu, X., Wang, Y., Yan, X., Zhang, M., Zhang, Y., Cheng, J., Lü, F., Qu, H., Wang, Q., & Zhao, Y. (2018). Novel Phellodendri Cortex (Huang Bo)-derived carbon dots and their hemostatic effect. *Nanomedicine*, *13*(4), 391–405. https://doi.org/10.2217/nnm-2017-0297

Liu, Y., Yuan, M., Zhang, C., Li, H., Liu, J., Wei, A., Ye, Q., Zeng, B., Li, M., Guo, Y., & Guo, L. (2021). *Puerariae Lobatae* radix flavonoids and puerarin alleviate alcoholic liver injury in zebrafish by regulating alcohol and lipid metabolism. *Biomedicine & Pharmacotherapy*, *134*, 111121. https://doi.org/10.1016/j.biopha.2020.111121

Ma, Y. C., Lin, C. C., Li, C. I., Chiang, J. H., Li, T., & Lin, J. G. (2016). Traditional Chinese medicine therapy improves the survival of systemic lupus erythematosus patients. *Seminars in Arthritis and Rheumatism*, *45*(5), 596–603. https://doi.org/10.1016/j.semarthrit.2015.09.006

Saleem, U., Hussain, L., Shahid, F., Anwar, F., Chauhdary, Z., & Zafar, A. (2022). Pharmacological potential of the standardized methanolic extract of *Prunus armeniaca* L. in the haloperidol-induced Parkinsonism rat model. *Evidence-Based Complementary and Alternative Medicine*, *2022*, 1–15. https://doi.org/10.1155/2022/3697522

Shimizu, T., Murakami, K., Matsumoto, C., Kido, T., & Isohama, Y. (2023). Goreisan alleviates cerebral edema: Possibility of its involvement in inhibiting aquaporin-4 function. *Traditional & Kampo Medicine*, *10*(2), 168–176. https://doi.org/10.1002/tkm2.1380

Ștefănescu, R., Tero-Vescan, A., Negroiu, A., Aurică, E., & Vari, C. (2020). A comprehensive review of the phytochemical, pharmacological, and toxicological properties of *Tribulus terrestris* L. *Biomolecules*, *10*(5), 752. https://doi.org/10.3390/biom10050752

Szeto, Y. T., Cheng, N., Pak, S., & Kalle, W. (2013). Genoprotective effect of the Chinese herbal decoction Xiao Jian Zhong Tang. *Natural Product Communications*, *8*(3), 389–392. https://doi.org/10.1177/1934578x1300800328

Tang, S., Ren, J., Kong, L., Ge, Y., Liu, C., Han, Y., Sun, H., & Wang, X. (2023). Ephedrae Herba: A review of its phytochemistry, pharmacology, clinical application, and alkaloid toxicity. *Molecules*, *28*(2), 663. https://doi.org/10.3390/molecules28020663

Tang, Z. M., Ru, Q. J., & Zhang, Z. E. (1997). [Clinical study on relationship between liver-blood stasis and liver fibrosis]. *Zhongguo Zhong Xi Yi Jie He Za Zhi*, *17*(2), 81–83. [Article in Chinese] https://pubmed.ncbi.nlm.nih.gov/9812662

Terasawa, K., Sumikoshi, M., Raimura, M., Kobayashi, T., & Chino, A. (2015). Five cases of chronic primary headache in children successfully treated with Shokenchuto. *Nihon Touyou Igaku Zasshi*, *66*(2), 93–98. https://doi.org/10.3937/kampomed.66.93

Tian, C., Kim, Y. J., Lim, H. J., Kim, Y. S., Park, H. Y., & Choung, Y. (2014). Red ginseng delays age-related hearing and vestibular dysfunction in C57BL/6 mice. *Experimental Gerontology*, *57*, 224–232. https://doi.org/10.1016/j.exger.2014.06.013

Wang, F. R., Xu, Q. P., & Li, P. (1991). [Comparative studies on the febrifugal analgesic and anticonvulsive activities of water extracts from cultivated and wild *Saposhnikovia divaricata*]. *Zhong Xi Yi Jie He Za Zhi*, *11*(12), 730–732. [Article in Chinese] https://pubmed.ncbi.nlm.nih.gov/1821340

Wang, S.-C. (2019). Therapeutic classes of CHEG formulas. In S.-C. Wang (Ed.), *Clinical herbal prescriptions: Principles and practices of herbal formulations from deep learning health insurance herbal prescription big data* (pp. 16–89). World Scientific Publishing. https://doi.org/10.1142/11211

Wang, S.-C. (2020). Modern therapeutic uses of CHEG herbs and herb pairs. In S.-C. Wang (Ed.), *Veterinary herbal pharmacopoeia* (pp. 35–233). Nova Science Publishers. https://doi.org/10.52305/GHTR1903

Yang, M., Wang, C., Wang, W., Xu, J., Wang, J., Zhang, C., & Li, M. (2020). *Saposhnikovia divaricata*— An ethnopharmacological, phytochemical and pharmacological review. *Chinese Journal of Integrative Medicine*, *26*(11), 873–880. https://doi.org/10.1007/s11655-020-3091-x

Yasukawa, K., Kaminaga, T., Kitanaka, S., Tai, T., Nunoura, Y., Natori, S., & Takido, M. (1998). 3β-p-hydroxybenzoyldehydrotumulosic acid from *Poria cocos*, and its anti-inflammatory effect. *Phytochemistry*, *48*(8), 1357–1360. https://doi.org/10.1016/s0031-9422(97)01063-7

Zhao, F., Zhang, C., Xiao, D., Zhang, W., Zhou, L., Gu, S., & Qu, R. (2020). Radix Scutellariae ameliorates stress-induced depressive-like behaviors via protecting neurons through the TGFβ3-Smad2/3-Nedd9 signaling pathway. *Neural Plasticity*, *2020*, 1–13. https://doi.org/10.1155/2020/8886715

Zhao, H., Xu, J., Wang, R., Tang, W., Kong, L., Wang, W., Wang, L., Zhang, Y., & Ma, W. (2021). Plantaginis Semen polysaccharides ameliorate renal damage through regulating NLRP3 inflammasome in gouty nephropathy rats. *Food & Function*, *12*(6), 2543–2553. https://doi.org/10.1039/d0fo03143g

6 GMP Herbal Medicine for Rare Ophthalmic Disorders

Mobile digital devices such as smartphones are becoming indispensable in our lives. Prolonged smartphone use is common, as is ocular discomfort such as dry eyes and blurred vision. Ophthalmic symptoms are a price we pay for the convenience and connectivity offered by a modern lifestyle. On the other hand, the early-onset rare ophthalmic disorders of this chapter are mainly autosomal dominantly inherited.

Chrysanthemum Flower (Júhuā), Goji Berry (Chinese Wolfberry; Gǒuqǐzǐ), Bitter Orange (Zhǐqiào), Caltrop Fruit (Puncture-Vine Fruit; Jílí), Cicada Molting (Chántuì), Chinese Wild Ginger (Xìxīn), Golden Thread Root (Huánglián), Chinese Angelica Root (female Ginseng; Dāngguī), Siler Root (Fángfēng), Cassia Seed (Juémíngzǐ), Rehmannia Root (Dìhuáng), Sweetflag Rhizome (Shíchāngpú), Licorice Root (Gāncǎo), Chinese Senega Root (Yuǎnzhì), Lycium, Chrysanthemum and Rehmannia Pill (Qǐjúdìhuángwán), Enrich the Kidneys and Improve Vision Decoction (Zīshènmíngmùtāng), Gardenia and Vitex Combination (Xǐgānmíngmùtāng), Ginseng, Astragalus and Pueraria Combination (Yìqìcōngmíngtāng), Mulberry Leaf and Chrysanthemum Drink (Sāngjúyǐn), Free and Easy Wanderer Plus (Augmented Rambling Powder; Jiāwèixiāoyáosǎn), Lindera Formula (Wūyàoshùnqìsǎn), Six Ingredient Pill with Rehmannia (Liùwèidìhuángwán), Tonify the Middle and Augment the Qi Decoction (Bǔzhōngyìqìtāng), Poria, Cinnamon, Atractylodis and Licorice Decoction (Língguìshùgāntāng), and Clear Summerheat and Augment the Qi Decoction (Qīngshǔyìqìtāng) are the frequently discussed GMP single-herb and multi-herb products for the signs and symptoms of the most common rare ophthalmic disorders. Among them, Júhuā, Gǒuqǐzǐ, and Qǐjúdìhuángwán are best known for their benefits to the eye.

6.1 VERNAL KERATOCONJUNCTIVITIS

Vernal keratoconjunctivitis, also known as spring catarrh, is a chronic allergic inflammation of the bilateral ocular surface, including the cornea and eyelids. Symptoms of vernal keratoconjunctivitis are self-limiting but become worse in warm and dry weather. The condition, which most likely affects adolescent boys, typically resolves as one ages after puberty.

In addition to the eye-benefiting herbs Gǒuqǐzǐ and Júhuā introduced earlier in the book, more ophthalmic herbs, including Mùzéicǎo (cf. Section 4.17), Juémíngzǐ (Semen Cassiae), Xiàkūcǎo (cf. Section 1.6), Mìménghuā (Flos Buddlejae), Qīngxiāngzǐ (Semen Celosiae), and

---

TABLE 6.1

GMP Herbal Medicines for a 12-Year-Old Boy with Vernal Keratoconjunctivitis

Vernal keratoconjunctivitis (OrphaCode: 70476)

A disease with a prevalence of ~3 in 10,000

Not applicable

Abnormal cornea morphology, Abnormal conjunctiva morphology, Abnormal sclera morphology, Photophobia, Lacrimation abnormality, Pruritus, Corneal neovascularization, Punctate keratitis, Allergy

Scarring

Childhood

(Continued)

 DOI: 10.1201/9781032726625-6

TABLE 6.1 *(Continued)*
GMP Herbal Medicines for a 12-Year-Old Boy with Vernal Keratoconjunctivitis

Photophobia (D020795), Pruritus (D011537), Corneal neovascularization (370.6):

Xǐgānmíngmùtāng 5g + zìshènmíngmùtāng 5-0g + mùzéicǎo 1-0g + juémíngzǐ 1-0g + xiàkūcǎo 1-0g + qīngxiāngzǐ 1-0g + chōngwèizǐ 1-0g + mìménghuā 1-0g + gǔjīngcǎo 1-0g.

Xǐgānmíngmùtāng 5g + yínqiàosǎn 5g + juémíngzǐ 2g.

Xǐgānmíngmùtāng 5g + jīngfángbàidúsǎn 5g + juémíngzǐ 1g + xiàkūcǎo 1g + júhuā 1g.

Sāngjúyǐn 5g + zhǐqiào 1g + júhuā 1-0g + chántuì 1-0g + sīguāluò 0g.

Gǒuqǐzǐ 5g + júhuā 5g + dìhuáng 4-3g + dāngguī 4-3g + fángfēng 4-2g + xìxīn 2-1g + huánglián 2-1g.

Báizhǐ 5g + gāncǎo 4g + shārén 4g + dàhuáng 0g.

their pairings (Wang, 2020), are disclosed in Table 6.1. The phrase míngmù in Xǐgānmíngmùtāng and Zìshènmíngmùtāng literally means "eye-clearing." Yínqiàosǎn (cf. Section 1.13), cooler than Sāngjúyǐn in TCM nature, is administered at the onset of a "wind heat" infection; it is also employed for conditions of the skin, such as dermatomycosis (Wang, 2019). Xìxīn (cf. Section 2.43) has been used to treat colds (Liu et al., 2023) and is used today for allergic rhinitis, chronic rhinitis, and acute sinusitis (Wang, 2020).

6.2 RETINOPATHY OF PREMATURITY

Retinopathy of prematurity (ROP) is also known as retrolental fibroplasia. The fetal environment is hypoxic and when the fetus is prematurely born, it is exposed to a relatively hyperoxic environment. ROP is caused by a mismatch of oxygen needs during retinal development in preterm babies.

Qiānlǐguāng (Herba Senecionis Scandentis) and Qīngxiāngzǐ are combined for disorders of the eye (Wang, 2020). Overconsumption of Qiānlǐguāng can damage the liver (Li et al., 2008); therefore, one should be careful about the dosage. Employment of Jílí and/or Chántuì for the eye appeared in previous sections, such as Sections 1.3 and 5.3. The prescription in the table is thought to also strengthen the immunity of ROP babies, as Jīngfángbàidúsǎn was initially formulated for a "wind-cold-damp" epidemic (cf. Section 5.13).

TABLE 6.2
GMP Herbal Medicines for a One-Year-Old Baby with Retinopathy of Prematurity

Retinopathy of prematurity (OrphaCode: 90050)

A disease with a prevalence of ~3 in 10,000

Major susceptibility factor: LDL receptor-related protein 5 (*LRP5* / Entrez: 4041) at 11q13.2

Major susceptibility factor: frizzled class receptor 4 (*FZD4* / Entrez: 8322) at 11q14.2

Major susceptibility factor: norrin cystine knot growth factor NDP (*NDP* / Entrez: 4693) at Xp11.3

Not applicable

Small for gestational age, Premature birth, Abnormal retinal vascular morphology

Blindness, Abnormal macular morphology, Retinal arteriolar tortuosity, Vitreous hemorrhage, Tractional retinal detachment

Neonatal, Infancy

Blindness (D001766), Vitreous hemorrhage (D014823):

Xǐgānmíngmùtāng 5g + jīngfángbàidúsǎn 5-0g + jīnyínhuā 2-0g + liánqiáo 1-0g + mìménghuā 1-0g + gāncǎo 1-0g.

Qiānlǐguāng 5g + qīngxiāngzǐ 5g + huángqín 5g.

Qīngxiāngzǐ 5g + liánqiáo 5g + júhuā 5-0g.

Jílí 5g + chántuì 5g.

Gāncǎo 5g + jīnyínhuā 5-0g + gǒuqǐzǐ 5-0g + júhuā 5-0g + xìxīn 2-0g + huánglián 2-0g.

Júhuā 5g + zhǐqiào 2-1g + jílí 2-0g + júhóng 2-0g + sīguāluò 0g.

Chántuì 5g + zhǐqiào 2g + júhóng 2g.

6.3 RETINITIS PIGMENTOSA

Retinitis pigmentosa, an inherited retinal degeneration with slow progression, is caused by mutations in at least 1 of 84 genes, many of which involve prevention of death of the photoreceptor rod cells and cone cells in the retina of the eye. Clinical presentations of retinitis pigmentosa start with night blindness, followed by peripheral vision loss. Severity of the degeneration partially correlates with the mode of inheritance, which ranges from autosomal, X-linked to mitochondrial.

TABLE 6.3

GMP Herbal Medicines for a 17-Year-Old Adolescent with Retinitis Pigmentosa

Retinitis pigmentosa (OrphaCode: 791)

A disease with a prevalence of ~3 in 10,000

Disease-causing germline mutation(s): S-phase cyclin A associated protein in the ER (*SCAPER* / Entrez: 49855) at 15q24.3

Disease-causing germline mutation(s): intraflagellar transport 88 (*IFT88* / Entrez: 8100) at 13q12.11

Disease-causing germline mutation(s) (loss of function): receptor accessory protein 6 (*REEP6* / Entrez: 92840) at 19p13.3

Disease-causing germline mutation(s): Rho/Rac guanine nucleotide exchange factor 18 (*ARHGEF18* / Entrez: 23370) at 19p13.2

Disease-causing germline mutation(s): Bardet-Biedl syndrome 1 (*BBS1* / Entrez: 582) at 11q13.2

Disease-causing germline mutation(s): KIAA1549 (*KIAA1549* / Entrez: 57670) at 7q34

Disease-causing germline mutation(s): Abelson helper integration site 1 (*AHI1* / Entrez: 54806) at 6q23.3

Disease-causing germline mutation(s): AGBL carboxypeptidase 5 (*AGBL5* / Entrez: 60509) at 2p23.3

Disease-causing germline mutation(s): ATP binding cassette subfamily A member 4 (*ABCA4* / Entrez: 24) at 1p22.1

Disease-causing germline mutation(s): photoreceptor disc component (*PRCD* / Entrez: 768206) at 17q25.1

Disease-causing germline mutation(s): pre-mRNA processing factor 3 (*PRPF3* / Entrez: 9129) at 1q21.2

Disease-causing germline mutation(s): pre-mRNA processing factor 31 (*PRPF31* / Entrez: 26121) at 19q13.42

Disease-causing germline mutation(s): pre-mRNA processing factor 8 (*PRPF8* / Entrez: 10594) at 17p13.3

Disease-causing germline mutation(s): peripherin 2 (*PRPH2* / Entrez: 5961) at 6p21.1

Disease-causing germline mutation(s): retinol dehydrogenase 12 (*RDH12* / Entrez: 145226) at 14q24.1

Disease-causing germline mutation(s): retinal G protein coupled receptor (*RGR* / Entrez: 5995) at 10q23.1

Disease-causing germline mutation(s): rhodopsin (*RHO* / Entrez: 6010) at 3q22.1

Disease-causing germline mutation(s): retinaldehyde binding protein 1 (*RLBP1* / Entrez: 6017) at 15q26.1

Disease-causing germline mutation(s): retinal outer segment membrane protein 1 (*ROM1* / Entrez: 6094) at 11q12.3

Disease-causing germline mutation(s): RP1 axonemal microtubule associated (*RP1* / Entrez: 6101) at 8q11.23-q12.1

Disease-causing germline mutation(s): RP2 activator of ARL3 GTPase (*RP2* / Entrez: 6102) at Xp11.3

Disease-causing germline mutation(s): RP9 pre-mRNA splicing factor (*RP9* / Entrez: 6100) at 7p14.3

Disease-causing germline mutation(s): retinoid isomerohydrolase RPE65 (*RPE65* / Entrez: 6121) at 1p31.3

Disease-causing germline mutation(s): retinitis pigmentosa GTPase regulator (*RPGR* / Entrez: 6103) at Xp11.4

Disease-causing germline mutation(s): S-antigen visual arrestin (*SAG* / Entrez: 6295) at 2q37.1

Disease-causing germline mutation(s): Bardet-Biedl syndrome 2 (*BBS2* / Entrez: 583) at 16q13

Disease-causing germline mutation(s): bestrophin 1 (*BEST1* / Entrez: 7439) at 11q12.3

Disease-causing germline mutation(s): carbonic anhydrase 4 (*CA4* / Entrez: 762) at 17q23.1

Disease-causing germline mutation(s): ceramide kinase like (*CERKL* / Entrez: 375298) at 2q31.3

Disease-causing germline mutation(s): tetratricopeptide repeat domain 8 (*TTC8* / Entrez: 123016) at 14q31.3

Disease-causing germline mutation(s): TUB like protein 1 (*TULP1* / Entrez: 7287) at 6p21.31

Disease-causing germline mutation(s): usherin (*USH2A* / Entrez: 7399) at 1q41

Disease-causing germline mutation(s): clarin 1 (*CLRN1* / Entrez: 7401) at 3q25.1

Disease-causing germline mutation(s): cyclic nucleotide gated channel subunit alpha 1 (*CNGA1* / Entrez: 1259) at 4p12

Disease-causing germline mutation(s): crumbs cell polarity complex component 1 (*CRB1* / Entrez: 23418) at 1q31.3

Disease-causing germline mutation(s): cone-rod homeobox (*CRX* / Entrez: 1406) at 19q13.33

Disease-causing germline mutation(s): ADP ribosylation factor like GTPase 6 (*ARL6* / Entrez: 84100) at 3q11.2

Disease-causing germline mutation(s): fascin actin-bundling protein 2, retinal (*FSCN2* / Entrez: 25794) at 17q25.3

Disease-causing germline mutation(s): heparan-alpha-glucosaminide N-acetyltransferase (*HGSNAT* / Entrez: 138050) at 8p11.21-p11.1

(Continued)

TABLE 6.3 *(Continued)*

GMP Herbal Medicines for a 17-Year-Old Adolescent with Retinitis Pigmentosa

Disease-causing germline mutation(s): inosine monophosphate dehydrogenase 1 (*IMPDH1* / Entrez: 3614) at 7q32.1

Disease-causing germline mutation(s): MER proto-oncogene, tyrosine kinase (*MERTK* / Entrez: 10461) at 2q13

Disease-causing germline mutation(s): nuclear receptor subfamily 2 group E member 3 (*NR2E3* / Entrez: 10002) at 15q23

Disease-causing germline mutation(s): neural retina leucine zipper (*NRL* / Entrez: 4901) at 14q11.2-q12

Disease-causing germline mutation(s): OFD1 centriole and centriolar satellite protein (*OFD1* / Entrez: 8481) at Xp22.2

Disease-causing germline mutation(s): phosphodiesterase 6A (*PDE6A* / Entrez: 5145) at 5q32

Disease-causing germline mutation(s): phosphodiesterase 6B (*PDE6B* / Entrez: 5158) at 4p16.3

Disease-causing germline mutation(s): semaphorin 4A (*SEMA4A* / Entrez: 64218) at 1q22

Disease-causing germline mutation(s): cyclic nucleotide gated channel subunit beta 1 (*CNGB1* / Entrez: 1258) at 16q21

Disease-causing germline mutation(s): TOP1 binding arginine/serine rich protein, E3 ubiquitin ligase (*TOPORS* / Entrez: 10210) at 9p21.1

Disease-causing germline mutation(s): prominin 1 (*PROM1* / Entrez: 8842) at 4p15.32

Disease-causing germline mutation(s): lecithin retinol acyltransferase (*LRAT* / Entrez: 9227) at 4q32.1

Disease-causing germline mutation(s): eyes shut homolog (*EYS* / Entrez: 346007) at 6q12

Disease-causing germline mutation(s): isocitrate dehydrogenase (NAD(+)) 3 non-catalytic subunit beta (*IDH3B* / Entrez: 3420) at 20p13

Disease-causing germline mutation(s): spermatogenesis associated 7 (*SPATA7* / Entrez: 55812) at 14q31.3

Disease-causing germline mutation(s): guanylate cyclase activator 1B (*GUCA1B* / Entrez: 2979) at 6p21.1

Disease-causing germline mutation(s): kelch like family member 7 (*KLHL7* / Entrez: 55975) at 7p15.3

Disease-causing germline mutation(s): small nuclear ribonucleoprotein U5 subunit 200 (*SNRNP200* / Entrez: 23020) at 2q11.2

Disease-causing germline mutation(s): photoreceptor cilium actin regulator (*PCARE* / Entrez: 388939) at 2p23.2

Disease-causing germline mutation(s): phosphodiesterase 6G (*PDE6G* / Entrez: 5148) at 17q25.3

Disease-causing germline mutation(s): interphotoreceptor matrix proteoglycan 2 (*IMPG2* / Entrez: 50939) at 3q12.3

Disease-causing germline mutation(s): FAM161 centrosomal protein A (*FAM161A* / Entrez: 84140) at 2p15

Disease-causing germline mutation(s): zinc finger protein 513 (*ZNF513* / Entrez: 130557) at 2p23.3

Disease-causing germline mutation(s): cadherin-related family member 1 (*CDHR1* / Entrez: 92211) at 10q23.1

Disease-causing germline mutation(s): dehydrodolichyl diphosphate synthase subunit (*DHDDS* / Entrez: 79947) at 1p36.11

Disease-causing germline mutation(s): pre-mRNA processing factor 6 (*PRPF6* / Entrez: 24148) at 20q13.33

Disease-causing germline mutation(s): male germ cell associated kinase (*MAK* / Entrez: 4117) at 6p24.2

Disease-causing germline mutation(s): retinol binding protein 3 (*RBP3* / Entrez: 5949) at 10q11.22

Disease-causing germline mutation(s): cilia and flagella associated protein 418 (*CFAP418* / Entrez: 157657) at 8q22.1

Disease-causing germline mutation(s): intraflagellar transport 140 (*IFT140* / Entrez: 9742) at 16p13.3

Disease-causing germline mutation(s) (loss of function): zinc finger protein 408 (*ZNF408* / Entrez: 79797) at 11p11.2

Disease-causing germline mutation(s): ADP ribosylation factor like GTPase 2 binding protein (*ARL2BP* / Entrez: 23568) at 16q13

Disease-causing germline mutation(s) (loss of function): NIMA-related kinase 2 (*NEK2* / Entrez: 4751) at 1q32.3

Disease-causing germline mutation(s): intraflagellar transport 172 (*IFT172* / Entrez: 26160) at 2p23.3

Disease-causing germline mutation(s) (loss of function): TUB bipartite transcription factor (*TUB* / Entrez: 7275) at 11p15.4

Disease-causing germline mutation(s) (loss of function): kizuna centrosomal protein (*KIZ* / Entrez: 55857) at 20p11.23

Disease-causing germline mutation(s): solute carrier family 7 member 14 (*SLC7A14* / Entrez: 57709) at 3q26.2

Disease-causing germline mutation(s) (loss of function): pre-mRNA processing factor 4 (*PRPF4* / Entrez: 9128) at 9q32

Disease-causing germline mutation(s): RP1 like 1 (*RP1L1* / Entrez: 94137) at 8p23.1

Disease-causing germline mutation(s): aryl hydrocarbon receptor (*AHR* / Entrez: 196) at 7p21.1

Disease-causing germline mutation(s): interphotoreceptor matrix proteoglycan 1 (*IMPG1* / Entrez: 3617) at 6q14.1

Candidate gene tested: isocitrate dehydrogenase (NAD(+)) 3 catalytic subunit alpha (*IDH3A* / Entrez: 3419) at 15q25.1

Disease-causing germline mutation(s): DEAH-box helicase 38 (*DHX38* / Entrez: 9785) at 16q22.2

Disease-causing germline mutation(s): ADP ribosylation factor like GTPase 3 (*ARL3* / Entrez: 403) at 10q24.32

Disease-causing germline mutation(s): protein O-linked mannose N-acetylglucosaminyltransferase 1 (beta 1,2-) (*POMGNT1* / Entrez: 55624) at 1p34.1

Autosomal dominant, Autosomal recessive, Mitochondrial inheritance, X-linked recessive

(Continued)

TABLE 6.3 *(Continued)*

GMP Herbal Medicines for a 17-Year-Old Adolescent with Retinitis Pigmentosa

Abnormal testis morphology, Hypogonadism, Conductive hearing impairment, Sensorineural hearing impairment, Wide nasal bridge, Anteverted nares, Visual impairment, Abnormal electroretinogram, Photophobia, Blindness, Nystagmus, Optic atrophy, Atypical scarring of skin, Intellectual disability, Progressive night blindness, Abnormality of retinal pigmentation, Abnormal retinal vascular morphology, Hypoplasia of penis

Glaucoma, Cataract, Keratoconus, Ophthalmoplegia, Hyperinsulinemia, Obesity

Hyperreflexia, Type II diabetes mellitus

Childhood, Adolescent, Adult

Conductive hearing impairment (D006314), Sensorineural hearing impairment (389.1), Visual impairment (D014786), Photophobia (D020795), Blindness (D001766), Nystagmus (379.53, 379.55, 379.50), Optic atrophy (377.1), Intellectual disability (D008607):

Xīnyíqīngfèitāng 5g + língguìshùgāntāng 5-0g + zīshèntōngěrtāng 4-0g + shíchāngpú 1g + lùlùtōng 1g + cāngěrzǐ 1-0g.

Xīnyíqīngfèitāng 5g + yìqìcōngmíngtāng 5g + shíchāngpú 1g + lùlùtōng 1g + yuǎnzhì 1-0g.

Yìqìcōngmíngtāng 5g + qǐjúdìhuángwán 5-0g + língguìshùgāntāng 5-0g + shíchāngpú 1g + yuǎnzhì 1g.

Jiāwèixiāoyáosǎn 5g + língguìshùgāntāng 5g + shíchāngpú 1g + chēqiánzǐ 1g + héyè 1g + yuǎnzhì 1g.

Shíchāngpú 5g + hángjú 5 + gǒuqǐzǐ 5g + yuǎnzhì 5-4g + huángqí 5-3g + fúlíng 5-0g + dǎngshēn 5-0g + dāngguī 4-0g + shānzhūyú 4-0g + wǔwèizǐ 2-0g.

Gǒuqǐzǐ 5g + tùsīzǐ 5-0g + fúshén 5-0g + shíchāngpú 4-3g + yuǎnzhì 4-3g + júhuā 4-0g + dǎngshēn 3-0g + wǔwèizǐ 2-0g + huángqí 2-0g.

Glaucoma (365), Cataract (366.8), Keratoconus (371.6), Ophthalmoplegia (378.56), Obesity (278.00):

Jiāwèixiāoyáosǎn 5g + qǐjúdìhuángwán 5g + nǚzhēnzǐ 1g + hànliáncǎo 1g + juémíngzǐ 1g + tùsīzǐ 1g.

Jiāwèixiāoyáosǎn 5g + qǐjúdìhuángwán 5g + zīshènmíngmùtāng 5g + xiàkūcǎo 1-0g + cǎojuémíng 1-0g + mìmēnghuā 1-0g + juémíngzǐ 1-0 + mùzéicǎo 1-0g + jílí 1-0g.

Qǐjúdìhuángwán 5g + xǐgānmíngmùtāng 5g + cǎojuémíng 1g + tùsīzǐ 1g.

Qǐjúdìhuángwán 5g + zīshènmíngmùtāng 5g + dānshēn 1g + chēqiánzǐ 1g + xiàkūcǎo 1g + cǎojuémíng 1g.

Jílí 5g + nǚzhēnzǐ 2g + chuānxiōng 2g + tiānméndōng 2g + gǒuqǐzǐ 2g + júhuā 2g + huángqín 2g + dāngguī 2g + shúdìhuáng 2-0g + yuǎnzhì 2-0g + xiàkūcǎo 2-0g + yùzhú 2-0g.

Júhuā 5g + gǒuqǐzǐ 4-2g + dìhuáng 3g + fángfēng 3-2g + dāngguī 3-2g + juémíngzǐ 3-0g + xìxīn 2-1g + huánglián 2-0g.

Jílí 5g + chántuì 5-4g + júhuā 5-0g + zhǐqiào 5-0g + júhóng 4g + sīguāluò 4-0g.

Hyperreflexia (D012021):

Qīngshǔyìqìtāng 5g + shēngmàiyǐn 4-0g + gégēn 1-0g + dānshēn 1-0g + xiāngrú 1-0g + huòxiāng 1-0g + huánglián 0g.

Qīngshǔyìqìtāng 5g + gānlùyǐn 2-0g + huòxiāngzhèngqìsǎn 2-0g.

Qīngshǔyìqìtāng 5g + huòxiāngzhèngqìsǎn 5-0g + xiāngrú 1-0g.

Shēngmá 5g + chìsháo 5g + qiánhú 5g + sāngbáipí 5g + cháihú 5g + huángqín 5g + gégēn 5g + jīngjiè 5-0g + gāncǎo 5-0g.

Shēngmá 5g + zhìgāncǎo 5g + cháihú 5g + huángqín 5g + dāngguī 5g + chuānxiōng 2g + báizhǐ 2g.

Shēngmá 5g + xuánshēn 5g + dìhuáng 5g + hòupò 5g + zhǐshí 5g + màiméndōng 5g + dàhuáng 1-0g.

Shíchāngpú (cf. Sections 1.36 and 1.53) is antiepileptic, sedative, hypnotic, anticonvulsant, anti-tussive, anti-asthmatic, antioxidant, and antitumor and used for neurological disorders, the cardiovascular system, the gastrointestinal system, and respiratory system problems (Wang, 2020; Wen et al., 2023). Xīnyíqīngfèitāng was originally composed for the nose and lungs. It appears in Table 6.3, presumably because conditions of the ear, nose, and throat are closely associated (cf. Sections 1.33 and 1.59). The term tōngěr in Zīshèntōngěrtāng means "ear-opening." Shēngmá (cf. Section 2.13) "opens exterior, exposes exanthems, clears heat, neutralizes pathogens, raises yang Qi" and was reported to have antiosteoporosis, anti–human immunodeficiency virus (HIV), anti-inflammatory, antidiabetic, antimalaria, vasoactive, estrogenic, and antioxidant effects (Li & Yu, 2006; Li et al., 2012). Qīngshǔyìqìtāng, containing Shēngmá, is mainly used for heatstroke, which can cause dehydration and hyperreflexia.

6.4 LIMBAL STEM CELL DEFICIENCY

The cornea is referred to as the window to the eye. The outermost layer of the cornea, called the *corneal epithelium*, prevents foreign materials from entering the eye. The corneal epithelium undergoes constant renewal and regeneration, and limbal stem cells serve as the source of corneal epithelial cell repopulation. Limbal stem cell deficiency can be caused by autoimmunity, trauma, surgeries, and infection.

TABLE 6.4

GMP Herbal Medicines for a 60-Year-Old Adult with Limbal Stem Cell Deficiency

Limbal stem cell deficiency (OrphaCode: 171673)

A disease with a prevalence of ~2 in 10,000

Not applicable

Photophobia, Lacrimation abnormality, Blepharospasm, Reduced visual acuity, Decreased corneal reflex, Epiphora, Conjunctival hyperemia, Ocular pain

Keratitis, Corneal scarring, Opacification of the corneal epithelium, Generalized opacification of the cornea, Corneal neovascularization

Photophobia (D020795), Blepharospasm (333.81), Decreased corneal reflex (D012021), Epiphora (375.2, 375), Ocular pain (D058447):

Wūyàoshùnqìsǎn 5g + báisháo 2-0g.

Wūyàoshùnqìsǎn 5g + zīshènmíngmùtāng 4g + xiōngqióng 1g + gǎoběn 1g.

Wūyàoshùnqìsǎn 5g + xiōngqióng 2-1g + dāngguī 2-0g + báizhǐ 1-0g + gǎoběn 1-0g.

Chuānxiōng 5g + dānshēn 5g + gǒuqǐzǐ 5g + cǎojuémíng 5g + dāngguī 5g + tiānméndōng 5-0g + xuánshēn 5-0g + dìlóng 5-0g + gǒujǐ 5-0g + bózǐrén 5-0g + fúlíng 5-0g + huángqí 5-0g + sāngzhī 5-0g + héshǒuwū 5-0g + guībǎn 5-0g + màiméndōng 5-0g + shúdìhuáng 5-0g.

Shānzhūyú 5g + shānyào 5g + chuānxiōng 5g + ròucōngróng 5g + gǒuqǐzǐ 5g + fúlíng 5g + shúdìhuáng 5g + gāncǎo 3g + xìxīn 2g.

Chuānxiōng 5g + báizhǐ 5g + dìhuáng 5g + fángfēng 5g + zhīzǐ 5g + júhuā 5g + jiāngcán 5g + gāncǎo 3g + bòhé 3g + xìxīn 2g.

Chuānxiōng 5g + dānshēn 5g + báizhú 5g + báisháo 5g + cháihú 5g + fúlíng 5g + liánqiáo 5g + dāngguī 5g + zhìgāncǎo 3g.

Keratitis (370), Corneal neovascularization (370.6):

Qǐjúdìhuángwán 5g + xǐgānmíngmùtāng 5g + zīshènmíngmùtāng 5g.

Xǐgānmíngmùtāng 5g + zīshènmíngmùtāng 5g + mùzéicǎo 1g + juémíngzǐ 1-0g + gǒuqǐzǐ 1-0g + júhuā 1-0g + gǔjīngcǎo 1-0g + chēqiánzǐ 1-0g + mìménghuā 1-0g.

Xǐgānmíngmùtāng 5g + mìménghuā 1-0g + liánqiáo 0g + yúxīngcǎo 0g.

Gǒuqǐzǐ 5g + júhuā 5g + dìhuáng 4-0g + fángfēng 4-0g + dāngguī 4-0g + xìxīn 2-0g + huánglián 2-0g + dàhuáng 1-0g.

A systematic review and meta-analysis of high-quality, randomized controlled trials concluded that formulas containing Chuānxiōng (cf. Sections 1.26 and 2.26) relieve migraine symptoms (Shan et al., 2018). Wūyàoshùnqìsǎn, consisting of Chuānxiōng, was introduced in Sections 2.22 and 2.53 for facial nerve disorders and trigeminal nerve disorders.

6.5 HERPES SIMPLEX VIRUS STROMAL KERATITIS

Herpes simplex virus stromal keratitis is an inflammation of the cornea induced by herpes simplex virus-1 infection. The immune inflammatory responses associated with recurrent herpes simplex virus stromal keratitis can result in long-term visual impairment.

TABLE 6.5
GMP Herbal Medicines for a 47-Year-Old Adult with Herpes Simplex Virus Stromal Keratitis

Herpes simplex virus stromal keratitis (OrphaCode: 137599)

A disease with a prevalence of ~2 in 10,000

Not applicable

Reduced visual acuity, Deep anterior chamber, Corneal stromal edema, Open angle glaucoma

Herpetiform corneal ulceration, Epiphora, Descemet Membrane Folds, Decreased corneal sensation, Corneal perforation

Keratitis, Blindness

All ages

Epiphora (375.2, 375):	
Qǐjúdìhuángwán 5g + zīshènmíngmùtāng 5g + juémíngzǐ 1-0g + tùsīzǐ 1-0g + huángjīng 1-0g + yèjiāoténg 1-0g + mìménghuā 1-0g + mùzéicǎo 1-0g + gǔjīngcǎo 1-0g.	Gǒuqǐzǐ 5g + júhuā 5g + dìhuáng 3g + dāngguī 3g + fángfēng 3-0g + xìxīn 2-1g + huánglián 2-1g.
Keratitis (370), Blindness (D001766):	
Xǐgānmíngmùtāng 5g + mìménghuā 1-0g + juémíngzǐ 1-0g + liánqiáo 0g + yúxīngcǎo 0g + xiàkūcǎo 0g.	Qīngxiāngzǐ 5g + cǎojuémíng 5g + huángqín 5-0g. Gǒuqǐzǐ 5g + júhuā 3g + dìhuáng 2g + fángfēng 2g + dāngguī 2g + xìxīn 1g + huánglián 1g.

The primary functional components in Cǎojuémíng (Semen Cassiae) are pharmacologically antihyperlipidemic, neuroprotective, hepatoprotective, antibacterial, antimutagenic, antidiabetic, antimicrobial, antiestrogenic, antiallergic, and anthelmintic (Dong et al., 2017). It is used alone for constipation and hypercholesterolemia (Wang, 2020); however, when it is paired with Qīngxiāngzǐ, the herb pair treats ill-defined disorders of the eye (Wang, 2020).

6.6   ATOPIC KERATOCONJUNCTIVITIS

Atopic keratoconjunctivitis is inflammation of the cornea and conjunctiva at the same time due to an allergic reaction. Atopic keratoconjunctivitis often occurs in people with a history of atopic dermatitis.

Qǐjúdìhuángwán, Zīshènmíngmùtāng, and Xǐgānmíngmùtāng all contain Júhuā. Qǐjúdìhuángwán "nourishes the Kidney, cultivates the Liver, replenishes Blood and improves eyesight." Zīshènmíngmùtāng "replenishes Qi and Blood, clears heat and improves eyesight." Xǐgānmíngmùtāng "dispels Wind, clears heat, reduces swelling, removes toxins, cultivates Blood and improves eyesight."

TABLE 6.6
GMP Herbal Medicines for a 19-Year-Old Man with Atopic Keratoconjunctivitis

Atopic keratoconjunctivitis (OrphaCode: 163934)

A disease with a prevalence of ~1 in 10,000

Not applicable

Keratitis, Dry skin, Keratoconjunctivitis sicca, Corneal opacity

Abnormal eyelid morphology, Blepharitis, Loss of eyelashes, Corneal neovascularization

Chemosis

All ages

Keratitis (370), Keratoconjunctivitis sicca (375.15):	
Zīshènmíngmùtāng 5g + gégēntāng 4-0g + juémíngzǐ 1g + gǒuqǐzǐ 1-0g + gǔjīngcǎo 1-0g + júhuā 1-0g.	Gǒuqǐzǐ 5g + júhuā 5g + dìhuáng 4-2g + dāngguī 4-2g + fángfēng 4-2g + xìxīn 2-1g + huánglián 2-1g.

(Continued)

TABLE 6.6 *(Continued)*
GMP Herbal Medicines for a 19-Year-Old Man with Atopic Keratoconjunctivitis

Blepharitis (373.0, 373.4), Corneal neovascularization (370.6):

Xīgānmíngmùtāng 5g + zīshènmíngmùtāng 5-0g + qǐjúdìhuángwán 5-0g + xiàkūcǎo 1-0g + mìmēnghuā 1-0g + juémíngzǐ 1-0 + mùzéicǎo 1-0g.

Xīgānmíngmùtāng 5g + lóngdǎnxiègāntāng 5g + mùzéicǎo 1g + juémíngzǐ 1g + xiàkūcǎo 1g + mìmēnghuā 1g + júhuā 1g.

Xiǎocháihútāng 5g + zhúyèshígāotāng 5g + mùzéicǎo 1g + chēqiánzǐ 1g + qīngxiāngzǐ 1g + chōngwèizǐ 1g.

Gǒuqǐzǐ 5g + júhuā 5g + niúbàngzǐ 4g + shègān 4g + xìxīn 1g + huánglián 1g.

Báizhǐ 5g + gāncǎo 4g + shārén 4g + dàhuáng 0g.

Qǐjúdìhuángwán fills TCM kidney and liver yin to support yang, including vision (cf. Section 1.44). If yin remains deficient, Zīshènmíngmùtāng comes to reenforce Qi and blood and also quells excessive fires. On the other hand, Xīgānmíngmùtāng improves vision impaired by infections. Indeed, Xīgānmíngmùtāng was shown to significantly suppress bacterial toxin-induced aqueous flare in rabbits (Nagaki et al., 2001).

6.7 STARGARDT DISEASE

Stargardt disease, also known as fundus flavimaculatus, is a genetic degeneration of a small region in the center of the retina called the *macula,* which is responsible for clear central vision. Stargardt disease is caused by mutations in the genes whose products function in the photoreceptor cells in the retina.

Sīguāluò (cf. Section 1.30) "opens channels, activates collaterals, clears heat, and transforms phlegm." Its pharmacological activities include antimicrobial, anticancer, antioxidant, hypoglycemic, hepatoprotective, gastroprotective, immunomodulatory, antiparasitic, anti-inflammatory, analgesic, and antithyroid (Harfiani et al., 2020); it is used for weight loss, jaundice, blood purification, hypoglycemia, constipation, skin care, strengthening the immune system, wound healing, eye problems, stomach worms, and asthma (Korooni, 2023).

TABLE 6.7
GMP Herbal Medicines for a Three-Year-Old Child with Stargardt Disease

Stargardt disease (OrphaCode: 827)

A disease with a prevalence of ~1 in 10,000

Candidate gene tested: cyclic nucleotide gated channel subunit beta 3 (*CNGB3* / Entrez: 54714) at 8q21.3

Candidate gene tested: peripherin 2 (*PRPH2* / Entrez: 5961) at 6p21.1

Disease-causing germline mutation(s): ATP binding cassette subfamily A member 4 (*ABCA4* / Entrez: 24) at 1p22.1

Disease-causing germline mutation(s): ELOVL fatty acid elongase 4 (*ELOVL4* / Entrez: 6785) at 6q14.1

Disease-causing germline mutation(s): prominin 1 (*PROM1* / Entrez: 8842) at 4p15.32

Autosomal dominant, Autosomal recessive

Reduced visual acuity

Abnormal foveal morphology, Color vision defect, Central scotoma, Macular degeneration, Abnormal choroid morphology, Abnormality of visual evoked potentials, Nyctalopia, Paroxysmal involuntary eye movements, Retinal pigment epithelial atrophy, Retinal pigment epithelial mottling, Abnormality of macular pigmentation, Retinal thinning

Aplasia/Hypoplasia of the macula, Yellow/white lesions of the macula

Childhood, Adolescent, Adult, Elderly

Color vision defect (368.53, 368.5, 368.52, 368.51, 368.54, 368.55), Central scotoma (D012607), Abnormal choroid morphology (363.9), Nyctalopia (368.6):

Sāngjúyǐn 5g + zhǐqiào 2-1g + chántuì 2-0g + jílí 1-0g + júhuā 1-0g.

Qǐjúdìhuángwán 5g + yìqìcōngmíngtāng 5g.

Júhuā 5g + zhǐqiào 3-0g + jílí 3-0g.

Sīguāluò 5g + júhuā 5g.

Jílí 5g + zhǐqiào 5-3g.

6.8 DUANE RETRACTION SYNDROME

Duane retraction syndrome, also known as Stilling-Türk-Duane syndrome, is characterized by a limited inward or outward movement of the affected eye with or without strabismus. Duane retraction syndrome is caused by mutations in the genes whose products are important for the formation

---

TABLE 6.8

GMP Herbal Medicines for a One-Year-Old Infant with Duane Retraction Syndrome

Duane retraction syndrome (OrphaCode: 233)

A malformation syndrome with a prevalence of ~1 in 10,000

Disease-causing germline mutation(s): chimerin 1 (*CHN1* / Entrez: 1123) at 2q31.1

Disease-causing germline mutation(s) (loss of function): MAF bZIP transcription factor B (*MAFB* / Entrez: 9935) at 20q12

Disease-causing germline mutation(s): spalt like transcription factor 4 (*SALL4* / Entrez: 57167) at 20q13.2

Autosomal dominant, Autosomal recessive, Not applicable

Strabismus, Abnormality of eye movement, Oculomotor nerve palsy, Short palpebral fissure

Sensorineural hearing impairment, Anteverted nares, Deeply set eye, Blepharophimosis, Low posterior hairline, Abnormal vertebral segmentation and fusion

Ectopic kidney, Cleft palate, Everted lower lip vermilion, Microcephaly, Facial asymmetry, Micrognathia, Hearing impairment, Preauricular skin tag, Stenosis of the external auditory canal, Wide nasal bridge, Webbed neck, Short neck, Microcornea, Ptosis, Aniridia, Chorioretinal coloboma, Iris coloboma, Abnormal pupil morphology, Nystagmus, Blepharospasm, Amblyopia, Hypopigmented skin patches, Brachydactyly, Preaxial hand polydactyly, Triphalangeal thumb, Seizure, Global developmental delay, Plagiocephaly, Talipes equinovarus, Malformation of the heart and great vessels, Hypoplasia of the radius, Skeletal muscle atrophy, Spina bifida occulta, Abnormal form of the vertebral bodies, Absent radius, Irregular hyperpigmentation, Optic disc hypoplasia, Central heterochromia, Hypoplastic iris stroma, External ear malformation, Aplasia/Hypoplasia of the thumb, Patchy hypopigmentation of hair, Narrow internal auditory canal, Camptodactyly, Anorectal anomaly

Neonatal, Infancy

Strabismus (378.7, 378.6, 378.31), Oculomotor nerve palsy (378.51, 378.52):

Xìngsūyǐnyòukē 5g + xīnyíqīngfèitāng 4-0g + gāncǎo 1-0g.

Xìngsūyǐnyòukē 5g + cāngěrsǎn 5-0g + gāncǎo 1-0g.

Zhúyèshígāotāng 5g + gāncǎo 0g.

Yínqiàosǎn 5g.

Chántuì 5g + jílí 5-0g.

Zhǐqiào 5g.

Júhóng 5g.

Sensorineural hearing impairment (389.1), Deeply set eye (376.5), Blepharophimosis (374.46):

Liùwèidìhuángwán 5g + yìqìcōngmíngtāng 5g + shíchāngpú 1-0g + yuǎnzhì 1-0g + acupuncture.

Liùwèidìhuángwán 5g + língguìshùgāntāng 5-0g + shíchāngpú 1g + yuǎnzhì 1g.

Yìqìcōngmíngtāng 5g + bǔzhōngyìqìtāng 4g + shíchāngpú 1g + yuǎnzhì 1g.

Gāncǎo 5g + shārén 5g + dàhuáng 1g.

Yùzhú 5g + shāshēn 5g + màiméndōng 5g + xuánshēn 2g + dìhuáng 2g + hòupò 2g + zhǐshí 2g + dàhuáng 1g.

Báizhǐ 5-3g + huángqín 5-0g + gāncǎo 4-2g + shārén 4-2g + tiānhuā 2-0g + dàhuáng 0g.

Cleft palate (749.0), Hearing impairment (D003638), Ptosis (374.3), Aniridia (743.45), Nystagmus (379.53, 379.55, 379.50), Blepharospasm (333.81), Amblyopia (368.01, 368.00), Seizure (345.9), Talipes equinovarus (754.51), Skeletal muscle atrophy (D009133):

Liùwèidìhuángwán 5g + jiāwèixiāoyáosǎn 5g + dānshēn 2g + tiānmá 2g + shíchāngpú 2g + xiōngqióng 2g + hángjú 2g + gǒuqǐzǐ 2g + mànjīngzǐ 2g + xiàkūcǎo 2-0g.

Liùwèidìhuángwán 5g + bǔyánghuánwǔtāng 5g + báijiāngcán 1g + hángjú 1g + gǒuqǐzǐ 1g + acupuncture.

Qǐjúdìhuángwán 5g + sìwùtāng 4g + nǚzhēnzǐ 1g + dānshēn 1g + héshǒuwū 1g + hànliáncǎo 1g + chìsháo 1g + hángjú 1g + gǒuqǐzǐ 1g.

Rénshēnyǎngróngtāng 5g + qǐjúdìhuángwán 4g + dānshēn 1g + tiānmá 1g + báijiāngcán 1g + shíchāngpú 1g + xiōngqióng 1g + jílí 1g + chántuì 1g.

Báizhǐ 5g + huángqín 5g + tiānhuā 4g + zhìgāncǎo 4g + shārén 4g + dàhuáng 0g.

Báizhǐ 5g + huángqín 5g + tiānhuā 3g + gāncǎo 3g + shārén 3g + dàhuáng 1-0g + acupuncture.

Gǒuqǐzǐ 5g + júhuā 5g + chìsháo 2g + zhìgāncǎo 2g + jīnyínhuā 2g + dàhuáng 0g.

Huángqín 5g + báizhǐ 3g + jīnyínhuā 2g + gāncǎo 2g + guālóugēn 2g + shārén 2g + dàhuáng 0g.

of the nerves controlling the extraocular muscles that direct eye movement and determine the position of the eye.

Xìngsūyǐnyòukē contains Xìngrén (cf. Section 1.12) and Zǐsūyè (Folium Perillae) as the major herbs. Topical administration of Xìngrén extract was shown to dose-dependently improve all clinical dry eye symptoms in mice with surgical removal of the lacrimal gland (Kim et al., 2016) and to protect against keratoconjunctivitis sicca in rats exposed to urban particulate matter (Hyun et al., 2019). Zǐsūyè extract was reviewed to have an important clinical effect on allergic rhinoconjunctivitis in young populations (Adam et al., 2023). Note that the term yòukē in Xìngsūyǐnyòukē means pediatrics. Chántuì (cf. Sections 1.54, 2.20, and 5.3) "improves vision, relieves convulsions" and was shown to be antiepileptic in epileptic mice (Zhang et al., 2021). Liùwèidìhuángwán was formulated for TCM kidney-yin deficient patients, who manifest "Liver/Kidney deficiency, low back pain, foot soreness, dizziness, thirst, dry tongue, sore throat, and heel pain." It is used today for diabetes, disorders of the lacrimal system, and disorders of the back (Wang, 2019).

6.9 X-LINKED RETINOSCHISIS

X-linked retinoschisis, or X-linked juvenile retinoschisis, is a macular degeneration in boys. X-linked retinoschisis is caused by mutations in a gene that instructs production of extracellular adhesive proteins that help maintain and organize cells in the retina.

TABLE 6.9

GMP Herbal Medicines for a Six-Year-Old Boy with X-Linked Retinoschisis

X-linked retinoschisis (OrphaCode: 792)

A malformation syndrome with a prevalence of ~5 in 100,000

Disease-causing germline mutation(s): retinoschisin 1 (*RS1* / Entrez: 6247) at Xp22.13

X-linked recessive

Abnormality of the eye, Abnormality of eye movement, Glaucoma, Abnormality of vision, Abnormal electroretinogram, Cataract, Retinoschisis

Infancy, Childhood, Adolescent, Adult

Abnormality of the eye (379.90), Glaucoma (365), Cataract (366.8), Retinoschisis (361.10):

Qǐjúdìhuángwán 5g + zǐshènmíngmùtāng 5g + juémíngzǐ 1g + chēqiánzǐ 1g.	Zhǐqiào 5g + jílí 5g + chántuì 5-0g.
Jiāwèixiāoyáosǎn 5g + qǐjúdìhuángwán 5g + juémíngzǐ 1g + qīngxiāngzǐ 1g + chōngwèizǐ 1g + gǔjīngcǎo 1g + mìmēnghuā 1-0g.	Gǒuqǐzǐ 5g + júhuā 5g + dìhuáng 3g + dāngguī 3g + fángfēng 3-2g + xìxīn 1g + huánglián 1g.
Jiāwèixiāoyáosǎn 5g + zhǐqiào 1g + chántuì 1g + jílí 1-0g + júhuā 1-0g.	
Sāngjúyǐn 5g + chántuì 1g.	

The pharmacological activities of Zhǐqiào (cf. Sections 1.31, 1.54, 2.8, 3.3, and 5.1) were reviewed and included gastrointestinal motility regulating, antigastric ulcer, blood pressure regulating, cardioprotective, antiatherosclerotic, antivascular damage, antidepression, anti-obesity, anti-inflammatory, antioxidant, antitumor, immunomodulatory, and enzyme activity affecting (Gao et al., 2021). Juémíngzǐ (cf. Section 6.1) "cleanses the Liver, brightens the eye" and was shown to protect against retinitis pigmentosa in rats (He et al., 2020). The antioxidant-rich extract from Chēqiánzǐ (cf. Sections 3.8 and 5.2) was shown to ameliorate diabetic retinal injury in diabetic rats (Tzeng et al., 2016).

6.10 BEST VITELLIFORM MACULAR DYSTROPHY

Best vitelliform macular dystrophy (BVMD)—also known as Best disease; juvenile-onset vitelliform macular dystrophy; polymorphic vitelline macular degeneration; and vitelliform macular dystrophy type 2—is a genetic macular degeneration characterized by progressive impairment of

TABLE 6.10

GMP Herbal Medicines for a Nine-Year-Old Child with Best Vitelliform Macular Dystrophy

Best vitelliform macular dystrophy (OrphaCode: 1243)

A disease with a prevalence of ~5 in 100,000

Disease-causing germline mutation(s): bestrophin 1 (*BEST1* / Entrez: 7439) at 11q12.3

Autosomal dominant

Visual impairment, Cystoid macular degeneration, Metamorphopsia

Color vision defect

Visual field defect, Choroideremia

Childhood, Adolescent

Visual impairment (D014786), Metamorphopsia (D014786):

Qǐjúdìhuángwán 5g + bǔzhōngyìqìtāng 3-0g.   Zhǐqiào 5g + jílí 5g + chántuì 5-0g.

Qǐjúdìhuángwán 5g + xiāngshāliùjūnzǐtāng
   5-0g + shénqū 1-0g + màiyá 1-0g.

Qǐjúdìhuángwán 5g + zīshènmíngmùtāng
   5-0g + mùzéicǎo 1-0g + juémíngzǐ 1-0g +
   gǔjīngcǎo 1-0g.

Zīshènmíngmùtāng 5g + gǒuqǐzǐ 0g + júhuā 0g.

Color vision defect (368.53, 368.5, 368.52, 368.51, 368.54, 368.55):

Sāngjúyǐn 5g + chántuì 2-1g + zhǐqiào 1g + jílí   Zhǐqiào 5g + júhuā 5g + jílí 5g
   1-0g + júhuā 1-0g.   Zhǐqiào 5g + sāngbáipí 5g

Choroideremia (363.55):

Zīshènmíngmùtāng 5g + bǔzhōngyìqìtāng 5-0g +   Huángqí 5g + tiānmá 1g + mùguā 1g + fúlíng 1g + suǒyáng 1g +
   qǐjúdìhuángwán 4-0g + xǐgānmíngmùtāng   shíchāngpú 1g + dāngguīwěi 1g + táorén 1g + yuǎnzhì 1g + hónghuā 0g.
   4-0g.   Huángqí 5g + chìsháo 1g + fángfēng 1g + xìxīn 1-0g + huánglián 1-0g +

Bǔzhōngyìqìtāng 5g + bāwèidìhuángwán 2g.   dàhuáng 0g.

Yìqìcōngmíngtāng 5g + bǔzhōngyìqìtāng   Báizhǐ 5g + gāncǎo 4g + shārén 4g + huángqín 4g + tiānhuā 1g +
   5-0g + shíchāngpú 0g + yuǎnzhì 0g.   dàhuáng 0g.

---

the central vision. BVMD is caused by mutations in the *BEST1* gene, which expresses as membrane proteins in retinal pigment epithelium that supports and nourishes the retina.

Gǔjīngcǎo (Flos Eriocauli) "dispels wind-heat, improves eyesight, removes shadows" and the mechanisms underlying its treatment for diabetic retinopathy were explored in silico and validated in human retinal endothelial cells (Chen et al., 2022). Yìqìcōngmíngtāng (cf. Sections 1.14 and 1.60), containing Huángqí (cf. Section 1.9), "benefits middle Qi (i.e., Spleen and Stomach energetics), ascends clear yang, smartens up ears, cleans up eyes" and is used for disorders of the ear and migraines (Wang, 2019).

6.11 CENTRAL AREOLAR CHOROIDAL DYSTROPHY

Central areolar choroidal dystrophy (CACD), also called areolar atrophy of the macula, is characterized by a large-area loss of photoreceptors, retinal pigment epithelium and choriocapillaris in the macula. Most CACD cases are caused by mutations in the *PRPH2* gene, which encodes a protein important for the morphogenesis of light-sensing cells.

Niúbàngzǐ (cf. Section 4.17) was shown to ameliorate retinal edema, detachment of the retina, and VEGF expression in the retina of diabetic retinopathy rats (Lu et al., 2012). Shègān (Rhizoma Belamcandae) "clears heat, neutralizes pathogens, eliminates phlegm, and benefits throat." An active compound derived from it was shown to protect against high glucose- and hypoxia-induced

TABLE 6.11

GMP Herbal Medicines for a 30-Year-Old Adult with Central Areolar Choroidal Dystrophy

Central areolar choroidal dystrophy (OrphaCode: 75377)

A disease with a prevalence of ~5 in 100,000

Disease-causing germline mutation(s) (gain of function): guanylate cyclase activator 1A (*GUCA1A* / Entrez: 2978) at 6p21.1

Disease-causing germline mutation(s): peripherin 2 (*PRPH2* / Entrez: 5961) at 6p21.1

Disease-causing germline mutation(s): guanylate cyclase 2D, retinal (*GUCY2D* / Entrez: 3000) at 17p13.1

Autosomal dominant

Hyperautofluorescent macular lesion, Full-thickness macular hole

Visual impairment, Visual loss, Macular atrophy, Reduced visual acuity, Hypopigmentation of the fundus, Slow decrease in visual acuity, Foveal photoreceptor outer segment loss on macular OCT

Chorioretinal atrophy, Retinal pigment epithelial mottling, Absent retinal pigment epithelium, Drusen, Choriocapillaris atrophy, Perifoveal ring of hyperautofluorescence

Adult

Visual impairment (D014786):

Qǐjúdìhuángwán 5g + xǐgānmíngmùtāng 5g + zīshènmíngmùtāng 5g + juémíngzǐ 1g + mùzéicǎo 1-0g + xiàkūcǎo 1-0g + gǔjīngcǎo 1-0g + mìmēnghuā 1-0g. Qǐjúdìhuángwán 5g + bǔzhōngyìqìtāng 5g.	Chántuì 5-4g + jīlí 5-2g + zhǐqiào 5-0g + júhuā 5-0g. Gǒuqǐzǐ 5g + júhuā 5g + niúbàngzǐ 3g + shègān 3g + xìxīn 1g + huánglián 1g. Júhuā 5g + niúbàngzǐ 3g + fángfēng 3g + gǒuqǐzǐ 3g + shègān 3g + xìxīn 2g + huánglián 2g.

injury in rat retinal capillary endothelial cells (Shi et al., 2021). Xiàkūcǎo (cf. Sections 1.6 and 6.1) has been used for red and swollen eyes and its effects on thyroid-associated ophthalmopathy were elucidated (Zhang et al., 2020).

6.12 MACULAR CORNEAL DYSTROPHY

Macular corneal dystrophy (MCD), also known as corneal dystrophy Groenouw type II or Fehr corneal dystrophy, is a corneal stromal dystrophy characterized by development of ill-defined gray-white opacities in the cornea. MCD is caused by mutations in a gene whose products help maintain corneal transparency.

Shígāo (Gypsum Fibrosum) is a component in a modern Chinese herbal formula for the treatment of dry eye disease patients with yin deficiency (Gao et al., 2023). Mìmēnghuā (cf. Section 6.1) granules were shown to alleviate the inflammation of lacrimal gland tissue in rabbits (Jiang et al., 2019). Jīngfángbàidúsǎn has traditionally been used for fever, headache, stiff neck, sore limbs, swollen cheeks, and stuffy nose resulting from a "wind-cold-damp" infection (cf. Sections 5.13 and 6.2).

TABLE 6.12

GMP Herbal Medicines for a Seven-Year-Old Child with Macular Corneal Dystrophy

Macular corneal dystrophy (OrphaCode: 98969)

A disease with a prevalence of ~5 in 100,000

Disease-causing germline mutation(s) (loss of function): carbohydrate sulfotransferase 6 (*CHST6* / Entrez: 4166) at 16q23.1

Autosomal recessive

Corneal crystals, Abnormality of proteoglycan metabolism, Opacification of the corneal stroma, Punctate opacification of the cornea

Recurrent corneal erosions, Severely reduced visual acuity, Decreased corneal thickness

Hyperopic astigmatism, Photophobia, Decreased corneal sensation, Ocular pain

All ages

(Continued)

TABLE 6.12 *(Continued)*
GMP Herbal Medicines for a Seven-Year-Old Child with Macular Corneal Dystrophy

Recurrent corneal erosions (370.0):

Xǐgānmíngmùtāng 5g + mìmēnghuā 1-0g + mùzéicǎo 0g + liánqiáo 0g.

Jīngjièliánqiáotāng 5g + xiàkūcǎo 1g + mìmēnghuā 1g + liánqiáo 1g.

Juémíngzǐ 5g + jīnyínhuā 5g + júhuā 5g + jílí 5g + dàhuáng 2-1g.

Dānshēn 5g + shígāo 5g + juémíngzǐ 5g + mǔdānpí 5g + chìsháo 5g + zhīmǔ 5g + màiméndōng 5g + júhuā 5g + huángqín 5g + mànjīngzǐ 5g + dǎngshēn 5g + dàhuáng 2-0g.

Xuánshēn 5g + yùzhú 5g + dìhuáng 5g + shāshēn 5g + hòupò 5g + zhǐshí 5g + màiméndōng 5g + dàhuáng 1g.

Jīnyínhuā 5g + gāncǎo 2g.

Photophobia (D020795), Ocular pain (D058447):

Xǐgānmíngmùtāng 5g + jīngfángbàidúsǎn 5g.

Xǐgānmíngmùtāng 5g + zīshènmíngmùtāng 5-4g + mùzéicǎo 1-0g + juémíngzǐ 1-0g + xiàkūcǎo 1-0g + mìmēnghuā 1-0g.

Rénshēnbàidúsǎn 5g + xiǎoqīnglóngtāng 5g + chuānxiōngchádiàosǎn 5g + yǎngyīnqīngfèitāng 5g.

Wúzhūyútāng 5g + máhuángfùzǐxìxīntāng 3g + fùzǐ 1g + gānjiāng 1g.

Chántuì 5g + zhǐqiào 5-3g + jílí 5-3g.

Gǒuqǐzǐ 5g + júhuā 5g + niúbàngzǐ 4g + shègān 4g + xìxīn 1g + huánglián 1g.

6.13 CONGENITAL GLAUCOMA

Congenital glaucoma, or buphthalmos (ox eye), is damage of the optic nerve or retina in association with an elevated intraocular pressure due to poor aqueous outflow at birth. The first identified mutated gene associated with congenital glaucoma is the *CYP1B1* gene, whose products are involved in the regulation of fluid secretion inside the eye.

Língguìshùgāntāng extract granules were found to be frequently prescribed to early-stage dementia patients who manifest dizziness and vertigo resulting from balance disorders involving

TABLE 6.13
GMP Herbal Medicines for a One-Year-Old Infant with Congenital Glaucoma

Congenital glaucoma (OrphaCode: 98976)

A disease with a prevalence of ~5 in 100,000

Disease-causing germline mutation(s): cytochrome P450 family 1 subfamily B member 1 (*CYP1B1* / Entrez: 1545) at 2p22.2

Disease-causing germline mutation(s): myocilin (*MYOC* / Entrez: 4653) at 1q24.3

Disease-causing germline mutation(s): latent transforming growth factor beta binding protein 2 (*LTBP2* / Entrez: 4053) at 14q24.3

Disease-causing germline mutation(s) (loss of function): TEK receptor tyrosine kinase (*TEK* / Entrez: 7010) at 9p21.2

Autosomal dominant, Autosomal recessive, Not applicable

Glaucoma, Nevus flammeus

Retinal detachment

Visual loss

Neonatal, Infancy

Glaucoma (365):

Qǐjúdìhuángwán 5g + xǐgānmíngmùtāng 5g + zīshènmíngmùtāng 5g + juémíngzǐ 1-0g.

Língguìshùgāntāng 5g + qǐjúdìhuángwán 4g + mùzéicǎo 1g + niúxī 1g + chēqiánzǐ 1g + chōngwèizǐ 1g.

Wǔlíngsǎn 5g + língguìshùgāntāng 5g + chēqiánzǐ 2g + niúxī 1g.

Sāngjúyǐn 5g + zhǐqiào 1g + chántuì 1g.

Zhǐqiào 5g + jílí 5-4g + chántuì 5-0g + júhuā 5-0g.

Chántuì 5g + jílí 5-0g + júhóng 4-0g.

(Continued)

TABLE 6.13 *(Continued)*
GMP Herbal Medicines for a One-Year-Old Infant with Congenital Glaucoma

Retinal detachment (361.9):

Zīshènmíngmùtāng 5g.	Zhǐqiào 5g + jílí 5g.
Gānlùyǐn 5g + jílí 1g + chántuì 1g.	Júhuā 5g + chántuì 5-0g.
Sāngjúyǐn 5g + zhǐqiào 2-1g + júhuā 2-0g.	Chántuì 5g + júhóng 2g.

the oculomotor, proprioceptive, or vestibular system (Lin et al., 2019). Sāngjúyǐn (or Gānlùyǐn) combined with eye-benefiting herbs such as Jílí is used to treat eye conditions such as conjunctivitis (cf. Section 2.31).

6.14 TRITANOPIA

Tritanopia is blue color blindness. People with tritanopia have difficulty discerning between bluish and greenish colors and also between yellowish and white hues. Tritanopia is caused by mutations in the blue cone pigment gene that produces light-absorbing molecules that mediate vision.

TABLE 6.14
GMP Herbal Medicines for a Two-Year-Old Child with Tritanopia

Tritanopia (OrphaCode: 88629)

A disease with a prevalence of ~5 in 100,000

Disease-causing germline mutation(s): opsin 1, short wave sensitive (*OPN1SW* / Entrez: 611) at 7q32.1

Autosomal dominant

Abnormal retinal morphology, Tritanomaly, Color vision test abnormality

Photophobia, Reduced visual acuity, Pendular nystagmus

Neonatal, Infancy

Abnormal retinal morphology (362.9), Tritanomaly (368.53, 368.5, 368.52, 368.51, 368.54, 368.55):

Qǐjúdìhuángwán 5g + yìqìcōngmíngtāng 5-0g.	Zhǐqiào 5g + jílí 5-0g + chántuì 5-0g.
Qǐjúdìhuángwán 5g + bǔzhōngyìqìtāng 3-0g + gāncǎo 0g.	Jílí 5g + zhǐqiào 3g.
Zīshènmíngmùtāng 5g + yìqìcōngmíngtāng 3g.	

Photophobia (D020795), Pendular nystagmus (379.53, 379.55, 379.50):

Xǐgānmíngmùtāng 5g + zīshènmíngmùtāng 5-0g + gāncǎo 1-0g.	Júhuā 5g + zhǐqiào 5-4g + jílí 4g + chántuì 4-0g.
Zīshènmíngmùtāng 5g + gǒuqǐzǐ 2-0g + júhuā 2-0g.	Chántuì 5g + jílí 5-4g + júhuā 4-0g.

As the eye and kidney share several structural, developmental, and organizational similarities, it has been suggested that retinal microvascular pathology links to and predicts renal injury (Farrah et al., 2020). Qǐjúdìhuángwán and Zīshènmíngmùtāng are TCM formulas that benefit both the kidney and the eye.

6.15 LEBER HEREDITARY OPTIC NEUROPATHY

Leber hereditary optic neuropathy (LHON), also known as Leber optic atrophy, is characterized by progression from initial mild unilateral central vision impairment to severe bilateral vision loss. LHON is caused by point mutations in genes in the mitochondria that convert food to energy for cellular use, and is therefore maternally inherited.

Huángqí, summarized in Section 1.9, treats chronic heart failure (Lu et al., 2011). Shēngmàiyǐn (cf. Sections 2.39, 2.55, 3.20, and 5.18) was shown to reduce myocardial fibrosis and regulate the cardiac

TABLE 6.15

GMP Herbal Medicines for a 20-Year-Old Adult with Leber Hereditary Optic Neuropathy

Leber hereditary optic neuropathy (OrphaCode: 104)

A disease with a prevalence of ~4 in 100,000

Disease-causing germline mutation(s): NADH: ubiquinone oxidoreductase core subunit S2 (*NDUFS2* / Entrez: 4720) at 1q23.3

Disease-causing germline mutation(s) (loss of function): DnaJ heat shock protein family (Hsp40) member C30 (*DNAJC30* / Entrez: 84277) at 7q11.23

Disease-causing germline mutation(s): mitochondrially encoded ATP synthase membrane subunit 6 (*MT-ATP6* / Entrez: 4508) at mitochondria

Candidate gene tested: mitochondrially encoded cytochrome c oxidase I (*MT-CO1* / Entrez: 4512) at mitochondria

Disease-causing germline mutation(s): mitochondrially encoded cytochrome c oxidase III (*MT-CO3* / Entrez: 4514) at mitochondria

Disease-causing germline mutation(s): mitochondrially encoded cytochrome b (*MT-CYB* / Entrez: 4519) at mitochondria

Disease-causing germline mutation(s): mitochondrially encoded NADH: ubiquinone oxidoreductase core subunit 1 (*MT-ND1* / Entrez: 4535) at mitochondria

Disease-causing germline mutation(s): mitochondrially encoded NADH: ubiquinone oxidoreductase core subunit 2 (*MT-ND2* / Entrez: 4536) at mitochondria

Disease-causing germline mutation(s): mitochondrially encoded NADH: ubiquinone oxidoreductase core subunit 4 (*MT-ND4* / Entrez: 4538) at mitochondria

Disease-causing germline mutation(s): mitochondrially encoded NADH: ubiquinone oxidoreductase core subunit 4L (*MT-ND4L* / Entrez: 4539) at mitochondria

Disease-causing germline mutation(s): mitochondrially encoded NADH: ubiquinone oxidoreductase core subunit 5 (*MT-ND5* / Entrez: 4540) at mitochondria

Disease-causing germline mutation(s): mitochondrially encoded NADH: ubiquinone oxidoreductase core subunit 6 (*MT-ND6* / Entrez: 4541) at mitochondria

Mitochondrial inheritance

Slow decrease in visual acuity, Mitochondrial respiratory chain defects

Retinal telangiectasia, Blurred vision, Optic atrophy, Centrocecal scotoma, Central scotoma, Retinal vascular tortuosity

Ataxia, Postural tremor, Myopathy, Ventricular preexcitation, Peripheral neuropathy, Arrhythmia

Adolescent, Adult

Optic atrophy (377.1), Centrocecal scotoma (D012607):

Qǐjúdìhuángwán 5g + yìqìcōngmíngtāng 5-4g + xuèfǔzhúyūtāng 3-0g + shíchāngpú 1-0g + yuǎnzhì 1-0g.	Jílí 5g + chántuì 5g + zhǐqiào 4g. Zhǐqiào 5g + chántuì 5g + jílí 5-4g + júhuā 5-0g.
Qǐjúdìhuángwán 5g + yìqìcōngmíngtāng 5g + bǔyánghuánwǔtāng 5-0g.	
Gānlùyǐn 5g + júhuā 2g + chántuì 1g + zhǐqiào 1g + jílí 1g.	
Jiāwèixiāoyáosǎn 5g + zhǐqiào 2g + júhuā 2g + chántuì 2g.	

Ataxia (D002524), Postural tremor (D014202), Myopathy (359.9), Arrhythmia (D001145) [Cardiac dysrhythmia, unspecified (427.9)]:

Shēngmàiyǐn 5g + zhìgāncǎotāng 5g + dānshēn 1-0g + yùjīn 1-0g.	Huángqí 5g + dǎngshēn 5g + gāncǎo 3g + báizhú 3g + báisháo 3g + fángfēng 3g + qiānghuó 3g + fúlíng 3g + dúhuó 3g + chénpí 3-2g + zéxiè 3-2g + cháihú 3-2g + bànxià 2g + huánglián 2-1g.
Shēngmàiyǐn 5g + bǔzhōngyìqìtāng 5g.	Huángqí 5g + gāncǎo 2g + wǔwèizǐ 1g + dāngguī 1g.
Rénshēnyǎngróngtāng 5g + shēngmàiyǐn 5-0g.	Dǎngshēn 5g + báisháo 4g + fúlíng 4g + fùzǐ 3g + báizhú 2g.
Sìnìtāng 5g + gānlùyǐn 5g + yùzhú 1g.	Zhìgāncǎo 5g + gānjiāng 5g + shēngjiāng 3g + fùzǐ 3g + guìzhī 2g.

immune microenvironment against cardiotoxicity in rats (Ma et al., 2016). Rénshēnyǎngróngtāng "benefits Qi, nourishes nutrition, replenishes the Heart, calms the mind" and was summarized to benefit the heart and brain (Sheng et al., 2019).

6.16   NEUROTROPHIC KERATOPATHY

Neurotrophic keratopathy, also known as neurotrophic keratitis, is a degenerative condition of the cornea due to impaired trigeminal corneal innervation, leading to reduced corneal sensitivity and poor corneal healing. The corneal nerve can be damaged by chemical burns, physical injuries, corneal surgery, contact lens use, and viral herpes infection.

TABLE 6.16

GMP Herbal Medicines for a 68-Year-Old Woman with Neurotrophic Keratopathy

Neurotrophic keratopathy (OrphaCode: 137596)

A disease with a prevalence of ~4 in 100,000

Not applicable

Abnormal fifth cranial nerve morphology, Decreased corneal sensation

Slow decrease in visual acuity

Astigmatism, Recurrent corneal erosions, Corneal scarring, Blurred vision, Lacrimation abnormality, Diabetes mellitus, Corneal stromal edema, Anterior uveitis, Corneal ulceration

Childhood, Adult

Astigmatism (367.2), Recurrent corneal erosions (370.0), Diabetes mellitus (250), Corneal ulceration (370.0):

Qǐjúdìhuángwán 5g + zīshènmíngmùtāng 5g + xǐgānmíngmùtāng 5-0g + juémíngzǐ 1g + nǚzhēnzǐ 1-0g + dānshēn 1-0g + shíhú 1-0g.

Qǐjúdìhuángwán 5g + xǐgānmíngmùtāng 5g + dānshēn 1g + shíhú 1g + juémíngzǐ 1g.

Jiāwèixiāoyáosǎn 5g + qǐjúdìhuángwán 5g + shíhú 1g + juémíngzǐ 1-0g + cǎojuémíng 1-0g + gǔjīngcǎo 1-0g.

Gǒuqǐzǐ 5g + júhuā 5g + dìhuáng 5-2g + fángfēng 5-2g + dāngguī 4-2g + xìxīn 2-1g + huánglián 2-1g + dàhuáng 0g.

Gǒuqǐzǐ (cf. Sections 1.2 and 1.37) "supplements the Liver/Kidney, brightens the eye" and is used to improve digestion, skin, muscle, eye, and respiratory conditions (Wang, 2020). Its beneficial effects on retinal diseases were reviewed (Neelam et al., 2021). In addition, Gǒuqǐzǐ is combined with Dìhuáng (cf. Section 1.10) for the treatment of diabetes (Wang, 2020).

6.17   ACHROMATOPSIA

Achromatopsia, also known as Pingelapese blindness or rod monochromatism, is a condition of the retina characterized by complete or incomplete color blindness. Achromatopsia is caused by mutations in any of the genes whose products make up photoreceptor cells in the retina called *cones*, which are responsible for daylight vision and color vision.

TABLE 6.17

GMP Herbal Medicines for a One-Year-Old Infant with Achromatopsia

Achromatopsia (OrphaCode: 49382)

A disease with a prevalence of ~3 in 100,000

Disease-causing germline mutation(s): phosphodiesterase 6C (*PDE6C* / Entrez: 5146) at 10q23.33

Candidate gene tested: retinitis pigmentosa GTPase regulator (*RPGR* / Entrez: 6103) at Xp11.4

Disease-causing germline mutation(s): cyclic nucleotide gated channel subunit alpha 3 (*CNGA3* / Entrez: 1261) at 2q11.2

(Continued)

TABLE 6.17 *(Continued)*

GMP Herbal Medicines for a One-Year-Old Infant with Achromatopsia

Disease-causing germline mutation(s): cyclic nucleotide gated channel subunit beta 3 (*CNGB3* / Entrez: 54714) at 8q21.3

Disease-causing germline mutation(s): phosphodiesterase 6H (*PDE6H* / Entrez: 5149) at 12p12.3

Disease-causing germline mutation(s): G protein subunit alpha transducin 2 (*GNAT2* / Entrez: 2780) at 1p13.3

Disease-causing germline mutation(s) (loss of function): activating transcription factor 6 (*ATF6* / Entrez: 22926) at 1q23.3

Autosomal recessive

Abnormality of refraction, Color vision defect, Photophobia, Monochromacy, Pendular nystagmus, Undetectable light-adapted electroretinogram, Color vision test abnormality, Inner retinal layer loss on macular OCT

Hypermetropia, Myopia, Central scotoma, Reduced visual acuity, Hypoplasia of the fovea, Absent foveal reflex

Abnormal macular morphology, Abnormal pupillary light reflex, Retinal pigment epithelial mottling, Attenuation of retinal blood vessels, Eccentric visual fixation

Neonatal, Infancy

Color vision defect (368.53, 368.5, 368.52, 368.51, 368.54, 368.55), Photophobia (D020795), Monochromacy (368.53, 368.5, 368.52, 368.51, 368.54, 368.55), Pendular nystagmus (379.53, 379.55, 379.50):

Qǐjúdìhuángwán 5g.	Zhǐqiào 5-4g + jílí 5-0g.
Sāngjúyǐn 5g + zhǐqiào 1g + jílí 1-0g.	Júhuā 5g + jílí 5g.
Gānlùyǐn 5g + zhǐqiào 1g + chántuì 1g.	Chántuì 5g + júhóng 1g.

Hypermetropia (367.0), Myopia (367.1), Central scotoma (D012607):

Sāngjúyǐn 5g + zhǐqiào 2g + jílí 2-0g.	Hángjú 5g + gǒuqǐzǐ 5g + shíchāngpú 4-3g + yuǎnzhì 4-3g + nǚzhēnzǐ 2-0g + huángqí 2-0g + gāncǎo 2-0g.
Jiāwèixiāoyáosǎn 5g + zhǐqiào 2g + jílí 2g + chántuì 2g.	Nǚzhēnzǐ 5g + shíchāngpú 5g + chìsháo 5g + gǒuqǐzǐ 5g + fúshén 5g + mìménghuā 5g + dāngguī 5g + yuǎnzhì 5g + jílí 5g + dǎngshēn 5g + gāncǎo 2g.

Júhuā (cf. Section 1.2) "dispels wind-heat, normalizes the Liver, brightens the eye, clears heat, and neutralizes pathogens." A compound in Júhuā was shown to protect against retinal injury in rats via reduction of DNA damage and oxidative stress (Shen et al., 2016). Júhuā is used today for the eye, skin, headache, digestion, cough, and hypertension (Wang, 2020). In comparison, Hángjú (cf. Section 1.2) is more often used to dispel wind-heat, while Júhuā is used to normalize the TCM liver and improve eyesight.

6.18 CONE ROD DYSTROPHY

Cone rod dystrophy is characterized by the loss of cone cells and rod cells in the retina, which are, respectively, responsible for bright light/central vision and night light/side vision. Cone rod dystrophy is caused by mutations in any of the genes whose activities are important for the structure or function of the cones and rods in the retina. For example, a baby receiving from their parents two copies of the mutated *ABCA4* gene, whose products remove a toxic substance in the photoreceptor cells, will develop cone rod dystrophy.

TABLE 6.18

GMP Herbal Medicines for a Seven-Year-Old Child with Cone Rod Dystrophy

Cone rod dystrophy (OrphaCode: 1872)

A disease with a prevalence of ~2 in 100,000

Disease-causing germline mutation(s): retinitis pigmentosa GTPase regulator (*RPGR* / Entrez: 6103) at Xp11.4

Disease-causing germline mutation(s): peripherin 2 (*PRPH2* / Entrez: 5961) at 6p21.1

Disease-causing germline mutation(s): cilia and flagella associated protein 410 (*CFAP410* / Entrez: 755) at 21q22.3

Disease-causing germline mutation(s): PITPNM family member 3 (*PITPNM3* / Entrez: 83394) at 17p13.2-p13.1

(Continued)

TABLE 6.18 *(Continued)*

GMP Herbal Medicines for a Seven-Year-Old Child with Cone Rod Dystrophy

Disease-causing germline mutation(s): opsin 1, medium wave sensitive (*OPN1MW* / Entrez: 2652) at Xq28

Disease-causing germline mutation(s): cone-rod homeobox (*CRX* / Entrez: 1406) at 19q13.33

Disease-causing germline mutation(s): nicotinamide nucleotide adenylyltransferase 1 (*NMNAT1* / Entrez: 64802) at 1p36.22

Disease-causing germline mutation(s): cilia and flagella associated protein 418 (*CFAP418* / Entrez: 157657) at 8q22.1

Disease-causing germline mutation(s): cadherin-related family member 1 (*CDHR1* / Entrez: 92211) at 10q23.1

Disease-causing germline mutation(s): ATP binding cassette subfamily A member 4 (*ABCA4* / Entrez: 24) at 1p22.1

Disease-causing germline mutation(s): regulating synaptic membrane exocytosis 1 (*RIMS1* / Entrez: 22999) at 6q13

Disease-causing germline mutation(s): RPGR interacting protein 1 (*RPGRIP1* / Entrez: 57096) at 14q11.2

Disease-causing germline mutation(s): calcium voltage-gated channel subunit alpha1 F (*CACNA1F* / Entrez: 778) at Xp11.23

Disease-causing germline mutation(s): cyclic nucleotide gated channel subunit alpha 3 (*CNGA3* / Entrez: 1261) at 2q11.2

Candidate gene tested: aryl hydrocarbon receptor interacting protein like 1 (*AIPL1* / Entrez: 23746) at 17p13.2

Disease-causing germline mutation(s): guanylate cyclase activator 1A (*GUCA1A* / Entrez: 2978) at 6p21.1

Disease-causing germline mutation(s): guanylate cyclase 2D, retinal (*GUCY2D* / Entrez: 3000) at 17p13.1

Disease-causing germline mutation(s): opsin 1, long wave sensitive (*OPN1LW* / Entrez: 5956) at Xq28

Disease-causing germline mutation(s): retina and anterior neural fold homeobox 2 (*RAX2* / Entrez: 84839) at 19p13.3

Disease-causing germline mutation(s): semaphorin 4A (*SEMA4A* / Entrez: 64218) at 1q22

Disease-causing germline mutation(s): prominin 1 (*PROM1* / Entrez: 8842) at 4p15.32

Disease-causing germline mutation(s): calcium voltage-gated channel auxiliary subunit alpha2delta 4 (*CACNA2D4* / Entrez: 93589) at 12p13.33

Disease-causing germline mutation(s): ADAM metallopeptidase domain 9 (*ADAM9* / Entrez: 8754) at 8p11.22

Disease-causing germline mutation(s): unc-119 lipid binding chaperone (*UNC119* / Entrez: 9094) at 17q11.2

Disease-causing germline mutation(s): RAB28, member RAS oncogene family (*RAB28* / Entrez: 9364) at 4p15.33

Disease-causing germline mutation(s) (loss of function): POC1 centriolar protein B (*POC1B* / Entrez: 282809) at 12q21.33

Disease-causing germline mutation(s) (loss of function): DNA damage regulated autophagy modulator 2 (*DRAM2* / Entrez: 128338) at 1p13.3

Disease-causing germline mutation(s) (loss of function): tubulin tyrosine ligase like 5 (*TTLL5* / Entrez: 23093) at 14q24.3

Disease-causing germline mutation(s) (loss of function): TLC domain containing 3B (*TLCD3B* / Entrez: 83723) at 16p11.2

Disease-causing germline mutation(s): activating transcription factor 6 (*ATF6* / Entrez: 22926) at 1q23.3

Autosomal dominant, Autosomal recessive, X-linked recessive

Photophobia, Nyctalopia, Abnormality of retinal pigmentation

Color vision defect

Visual impairment

Childhood, Adolescent, Adult

Photophobia (D020795), Nyctalopia (368.6):

Sāngjúyǐn 5g + zhǐqiào 1-0g + júhuā 1-0g + chántuì 1-0g + jílí 0g.

Zhǐqiào 5g + jílí 5-2g + chántuì 5-0g.
Júhuā 5g + jílí 5g + júhóng 5g + chántuì 5g.

Color vision defect (368.53, 368.5, 368.52, 368.51, 368.54, 368.55):

Qǐjúdìhuángwán 5g + zīshènmíngmùtāng 5-0g + mùzéicǎo 2-0g + chōngwèizǐ 2-0g + mìménghuā 2-0g + gǔjīngcǎo 2-0g + juémíngzǐ 1-0g + chántuì 1-0g.

Qǐjúdìhuángwán 5g + yìqìcōngmíngtāng 5-0g.

Jiāwèixiāoyáosǎn 5g.

Zhǐqiào 5g + jílí 5-3g + júhuā 5-0g + chántuì 4-0g.
Gǒuqǐzǐ 5g + júhuā 5g + dìhuáng 3g + dāngguī 3g + fángfēng 2g + xìxīn 1g + huánglián 1g.
Jílí 5g + júhóng 2g.

Visual impairment (D014786):

Qǐjúdìhuángwán 5g + xǐgānmíngmùtāng 5-4g + juémíngzǐ 2-0g + gǔjīngcǎo 2-0g + mùzéicǎo 1-0g + xiàkūcǎo 1-0g.

Qǐjúdìhuángwán 5g + xiāngshāliùjūnzǐtāng 2g + gāncǎo 0g.

Júhuā 5g + zhǐqiào 4g + jílí 4g.
Gǒuqǐzǐ 5g + júhuā 5g + niúbàngzǐ 4-2g + shègān 4-2g + xìxīn 1g + huánglián 1g.

Chōngwèizǐ (Fructus Leonuri) "enlivens Blood, modulates menstruation, cleanses the Liver, clears the eye" and is used for disorders of the lacrimal system, and disorders of the globe of the eye (Wang, 2020). Chōngwèizǐ is among the component herbs in a modern herbal formula granule for the treatment of dry eye disease (Yang et al., 2020).

6.19 LEBER CONGENITAL AMAUROSIS

Leber congenital amaurosis, also known as amaurosis congenita of Leber, is damage of the retina of both eyes that is present at birth. Leber congenital amaurosis is caused by any of the genes that play roles in the development and function of the retina. For example, mutations in one allele of the *CRX* gene, whose products function as photoreceptor-specific transcription factor for the differentiation of photoreceptors, can cause Leber congenital amaurosis.

TABLE 6.19

GMP Herbal Medicines for a One-Year-Old Infant with Leber Congenital Amaurosis

Leber congenital amaurosis (OrphaCode: 65)

A disease with a prevalence of ~2 in 100,000

Disease-causing germline mutation(s): ubiquitin specific peptidase 45 (*USP45* / Entrez: 85015) at 6q16.2

Disease-causing germline mutation(s): tubulin beta 4B class IVb (*TUBB4B* / Entrez: 10383) at 9q34.3

Disease-causing germline mutation(s): spermatogenesis associated 7 (*SPATA7* / Entrez: 55812) at 14q31.3

Disease-causing germline mutation(s): growth differentiation factor 6 (*GDF6* / Entrez: 392255) at 8q22.1

Disease-causing germline mutation(s): intraflagellar transport 140 (*IFT140* / Entrez: 9742) at 16p13.3

Disease-causing germline mutation(s): nicotinamide nucleotide adenylyltransferase 1 (*NMNAT1* / Entrez: 64802) at 1p36.22

Disease-causing germline mutation(s): RD3 regulator of GUCY2D (*RD3* / Entrez: 343035) at 1q32.3

Disease-causing germline mutation(s) (loss of function): retinol dehydrogenase 12 (*RDH12* / Entrez: 145226) at 14q24.1

Disease-causing germline mutation(s): retinoid isomerohydrolase RPE65 (*RPE65* / Entrez: 6121) at 1p31.3

Disease-causing germline mutation(s) (loss of function): RPGR interacting protein 1 (*RPGRIP1* / Entrez: 57096) at 14q11.2

Disease-causing germline mutation(s): centrosomal protein 290 (*CEP290* / Entrez: 80184) at 12q21.32

Disease-causing germline mutation(s): aryl hydrocarbon receptor interacting protein like 1 (*AIPL1* / Entrez: 23746) at 17p13.2

Disease-causing germline mutation(s): TUB like protein 1 (*TULP1* / Entrez: 7287) at 6p21.31

Disease-causing germline mutation(s): crumbs cell polarity complex component 1 (*CRB1* / Entrez: 23418) at 1q31.3

Disease-causing germline mutation(s): cone-rod homeobox (*CRX* / Entrez: 1406) at 19q13.33

Disease-causing germline mutation(s) (loss of function): guanylate cyclase 2D, retinal (*GUCY2D* / Entrez: 3000) at 17p13.1

Disease-causing germline mutation(s): inosine monophosphate dehydrogenase 1 (*IMPDH1* / Entrez: 3614) at 7q32.1

Disease-causing germline mutation(s) (loss of function): IQ motif containing B1 (*IQCB1* / Entrez: 9657) at 3q13.33

Disease-causing germline mutation(s): lebercilin LCA5 (*LCA5* / Entrez: 167691) at 6q14.1

Disease-causing germline mutation(s): potassium inwardly rectifying channel subfamily J member 13 (*KCNJ13* / Entrez: 3769) at 2q37.1

Disease-causing germline mutation(s): lecithin retinol acyltransferase (*LRAT* / Entrez: 9227) at 4q32.1

Disease-causing germline mutation(s) (loss of function): phosphate cytidylyltransferase 1A, choline (*PCYT1A* / Entrez: 5130) at 3q29

Autosomal dominant, Autosomal recessive

Severely reduced visual acuity, Abnormality of retinal pigmentation, Abnormality of the optic disc

Abnormal electroretinogram, Cataract, Keratoconus, Nystagmus, Seizure, Hypotonia, Encephalocele, Abnormality of neuronal migration, Hemiplegia/hemiparesis, Aplasia/Hypoplasia of the cerebellar vermis

Hearing impairment, Intellectual disability, Global developmental delay

Neonatal, Infancy

(Continued)

TABLE 6.19 *(Continued)*
GMP Herbal Medicines for a One-Year-Old Infant with Leber Congenital Amaurosis

Cataract (366.8), Keratoconus (371.6), Nystagmus (379.53, 379.55, 379.50), Seizure (345.9), Hypotonia (D009123):

Jiāwèixiāoyáosăn 5g + qǐjúdìhuángwán 5g + zīshènmíngmùtāng 5-0g + juémíngzǐ 1g + mùzéicǎo 1-0g + xiàkūcǎo 1-0g + chōngwèizǐ 1-0g + mìmēnghuā 1-0g + gǔjīngcǎo 1-0g + acupuncture.	Hàngjú 5g + gǒuqǐzǐ 5g + shíchāngpú 3g + yuǎnzhì 3g. Hàngjú 5g + gǒuqǐzǐ 5g + fángfēng 2g + xìxīn 2-1g + huánglián 2-1g + dìhuáng 2-0g + dāngguī 1g. Huángqí 5g + chìsháo 1g + fángfēng 1g + xìxīn 0g + huánglián 0g.
Qǐjúdìhuángwán 5g + yìqìcōngmíngtāng 5g + juémíngzǐ 1g + chōngwèizǐ 1-0g + mùzéicǎo 1-0g + xiàkūcǎo 1-0g + acupuncture.	Gǒuqǐzǐ 5g + júhuā 5g + dìhuáng 4g + fángfēng 4g + dāngguī 4g + xìxīn 1g + huánglián 1g.

Hearing impairment (D003638), Intellectual disability (D008607):

Língguìshùgāntāng 5g + gāncǎo 1g + tiáowèichéngqìtāng 0g + dàhuáng 0g.	Rénshēn 5g + bànxià 5g + gāncǎo 5g + shēngjiāng 5g + hòupò 5g.
Língguìshùgāntāng 5g + wǔwèizǐ 1g + gānjiāng 1g + xìxīn 1g + bànxià 1-0g + dàhuáng 0g.	Rénshēn 5g + bànxià 5g + gānjiāng 5g + dàhuáng 0g. Shārén 5g + gāncǎo 5-3g + báizhǐ 5-3g + dàhuáng 0g.

Adjunctive use of Jiāwèixiāoyáosăn was found to be associated with a lower occurrence of retinopathy in female patients with type 2 diabetes and the reduction in retinopathy was shown in human retina cells to be through the antioxidant effect of the herbs (Tsai et al., 2017). Huángqí (cf. Section 1.9) extract was shown to suppress retinal cell apoptosis and repair damaged retinal neovascularization in newborn mice with oxygen-induced retinopathy of prematurity (Liu et al., 2019). Bànxià was introduced in Section 2.3 to be a sedative and hypnotic.

6.20 IDIOPATHIC PANUVEITIS

Idiopathic panuveitis is a generalized inflammation of the uvea, i.e., the iris, ciliary body, and choroid, affecting not only the uvea, but also the retina and vitreous humor. Tuberculosis can cause panuveitis; however, the cause of idiopathic panuveitis is unknown.

TABLE 6.20
GMP Herbal Medicines for a 41-Year-Old Adult with Idiopathic Panuveitis

Idiopathic panuveitis (OrphaCode: 280921)

A disease with a prevalence of ~2 in 100,000

Not applicable

Abnormality of vision, Blurred vision, Reduced visual acuity, Red eye, Vitreous haze, Ocular pain

Cataract, Photophobia, Miosis, Headache, Posterior synechiae of the anterior chamber, Cystoid macular edema, Vitreous snowballs, Conjunctival hyperemia, Vitreous floaters

Childhood, Adolescent, Adult, Elderly

Ocular pain (D058447):

Shūjīnghuóxuètāng 5g + dāngguīniántòngtāng 5g + acupuncture.	Júhuā 5g + júhóng 5g + chántuì 5g + jílí 5-0g. Júhuā 5g + zhǐqiào 4-1g + jílí 4-0g + chántuì 4-0g.
Shūjīnghuóxuètāng 5g + qǐjúdìhuángwán 4g + mùguā 1g + dìlóng 1g + hǎipiāoxiāo 1g + niúxī 1g + sāngjìshēng 1g + nǚzhēnzǐ 1-0g + dìhuáng 0g.	Gǒuqǐzǐ 5g + júhuā 5g + niúbàngzǐ 4-3g + shègān 4-3g + xìxīn 2-1g + huánglián 2-1g.

Cataract (366.8), Photophobia (D020795), Miosis (D015877), Headache (D006261):

Zīshènmíngmùtāng 5g + xǐgānmíngmùtāng 5-0g + juémíngzǐ 1-0g + gǒuqǐzǐ 1-0g + júhuā 1-0g + xiàkūcǎo 1-0g.	Zhǐqiào 5g + jílí 5g + chántuì 5g + júhuā 5-0g. Gǒuqǐzǐ 5g + júhuā 5g + dìhuáng 4g + fángfēng 4g + dāngguī 4g + xìxīn 2-1g + huánglián 2-1g.

Huánglián (cf. Section 1.22) was shown to robustly reduce visceral pain in visceral hyperalgesia rats (Tjong et al., 2011). Mùguā, introduced in Section 2.22 for disorders of the muscle, ligament, and fascia, was shown to alleviate cartilage degradation in rat articular chondrocytes (Yeo et al., 2022). Shūjīnghuóxuètāng is the formula next to Jiāwèixiāoyáosǎn that was associated with a lower chance of retinopathy in diabetic patients of the last section (cf. Section 6.19).

6.21 CHOROIDEREMIA

Choroideremia (CHM), also known as tapetochoroidal dystrophy, is progressive dystrophy of the choroid, retinal pigment epithelium, and retina, characterized by childhood-onset night blindness, followed by peripheral vision loss or tunnel vision, and then complete vision loss. CHM is caused by mutations in the *CHM* gene, whose products play roles in intracellular vesicle trafficking for the transportation of cargo between membrane-enclosed organelles through the cargo containing vesicles.

TABLE 6.21

GMP Herbal Medicines for a Five-Year-Old Boy with Choroideremia

Choroideremia (OrphaCode: 180)

A disease with a prevalence of ~2 in 100,000

Disease-causing germline mutation(s): CHM Rab escort protein (*CHM* / Entrez: 1121) at Xq21.2

X-linked recessive

Abnormality of the eye, Abnormality of vision, Visual impairment, Abnormal electroretinogram, Myopia, Nyctalopia, Abnormality of retinal pigmentation

Progressive visual loss

Childhood, Adolescent, Adult

Abnormality of the eye (379.90), Myopia (367.1), Nyctalopia (368.6):

Qǐjúdìhuángwán 5g + yìqìcōngmíngtāng 5g.	Hángjú 5g + gǒuqǐzǐ 5g + shíchāngpú 3-2g + yuǎnzhì 3-2g + huángqí 1-0g.
Qǐjúdìhuángwán 5g + zīshènmíngmùtāng 5g + shíchāngpú 1-0g + yuǎnzhì 1-0g + mùzéicǎo 1-0g + gǔjīngcǎo 1-0g.	Gǒuqǐzǐ 5g + júhuā 5g + dìhuáng 2g + fángfēng 2g + dāngguī 2g + xìxīn 1g + huánglián 1g + dàhuáng 0g.
Qǐjúdìhuángwán 5g + línguìshùgāntāng 5g + mùzéicǎo 1g + juémíngzǐ 1g + gǔjīngcǎo 1g.	

Water extract of Hángjú, i.e., Júhuā from the Hangzhou area of China, was shown to protect the retina of mice from light damage, which mimics age-related, oxidatively stressed retinal diseases (Gong et al., 2022). Qǐjúdìhuángwán (cf. Sections 1.2, 1.5, and 1.44) was shown to be an effective treatment for dry eye patients using topical eye drops and Qǐjúdìhuángwán, in comparison to dry eye patients using topical eye drops and a placebo (Chang et al., 2005).

6.22 JUVENILE GLAUCOMA

Juvenile glaucoma is glaucoma that develops after the age of 3 years. Most juvenile glaucoma cases are associated with mutations in the *MYOC* gene, whose products function in the structure called the *trabecular meshwork* in the eye that drains the aqueous humor into circulation to regulate the pressure within the eye.

Huángqí (cf. Section 6.19) was concluded to be safe and effective for the treatment of diabetic retinopathy in a systematic review and meta-analysis of randomized controlled trials (Cheng et al., 2013). Dāngguī (cf. Section 2.43) extract was shown to increase tear secretion and repair corneal epithelial cells in rabbits with dry eye syndrome (Chen et al., 2017). Note that Xǐgānmíngmùtāng, Zīshènmíngmùtāng, and Bǔzhōngyìqìtāng all contain Dāngguī, while Bǔzhōngyìqìtāng and Yìqìcōngmíngtāng both contain Huángqí.

TABLE 6.22

GMP Herbal Medicines for a 12-Year-Old Child with Juvenile Glaucoma

Juvenile glaucoma (OrphaCode: 98977)

A disease with a prevalence of ~2 in 100,000

Major susceptibility factor: cytochrome P450 family 1 subfamily B member 1 (*CYP1B1* / Entrez: 1545) at 2p22.2

Disease-causing germline mutation(s): myocilin (*MYOC* / Entrez: 4653) at 1q24.3

Disease-causing germline mutation(s): EGF containing fibulin extracellular matrix protein 1 (*EFEMP1* / Entrez: 2202) at 2p16.1

Autosomal dominant

Visual impairment, Abnormality iris morphology, Abnormality of the optic nerve, Abnormal anterior chamber morphology, Optic neuropathy, Glaucomatous visual field defect, Ocular hypertension, Peripheral visual field loss, Open angle glaucoma

High myopia, Temporal optic disc pallor, Increased cup-to-disc ratio

Childhood, Adolescent

Visual impairment (D014786):

Qǐjúdìhuángwán 5g + xǐgānmíngmùtāng 5g + zīshènmíngmùtāng 5g + mùzéicǎo 1g + juémíngzǐ 1g + mìmēnghuā 1-0g + gǔjīngcǎo 1-0g.

Qǐjúdìhuángwán 5g + xiāngshāliùjūnzǐtāng 3g + shānzhā 1g + shénqū 1g + màiyá 1g.

Qǐjúdìhuángwán 5g + bǔzhōngyìqìtāng 5g + wǔwèizǐ 1g + màiméndōng 1g + dǎngshēn 1g.

Qǐjúdìhuángwán 5g + yìqìcōngmíngtāng 5g + nǚzhēnzǐ 1g + tùsīzǐ 1g.

Gǒuqǐzǐ 5g + júhuā 5g + niúbàngzǐ 4-3g + shègān 4-3g + xìxīn 2-1g + huánglián 2-1g.

Gǒuqǐzǐ 5g + huángqí 5g + dāngguī 5g + jīxuèténg 5g + wǔlíngzhī 4g + tùsīzǐ 4g + púhuáng 4g + fùpénzǐ 4g + bājǐtiān 2g.

Zhǐqiào 5g + jílí 5-4g + chántuì 5-0g.

6.23 AUTOSOMAL DOMINANT OPTIC ATROPHY, CLASSIC FORM

Autosomal dominant optic atrophy, classic form, also known as Kjer optic atrophy, or optic atrophy type 1, is characterized by progressive impairment and loss of bilateral visual acuity and color vision. Autosomal dominant optic atrophy, classic form is associated with mutations in the *OPA1* gene, whose products localize to the mitochondrial membrane and help the biogenesis and stability of the mitochondrial membrane. It is thought that dysfunctional mitochondria resulting from the mutations increase reactive oxygen species to damage the retinal ganglion cells, causing optic atrophy.

Liùwèidìhuángwán combined with acupuncture has been used for patients with tinnitus and TCM liver/kidney-yin deficiency, and the pharmacological mechanisms of Liùwèidìhuángwán

TABLE 6.23

GMP Herbal Medicines for a Five-Year-Old Child with Autosomal Dominant Optic Atrophy, Classic Form

Autosomal dominant optic atrophy, classic form (OrphaCode: 98673)

A disease with a prevalence of ~2 in 100,000

Disease-causing germline mutation(s): OPA1 mitochondrial dynamin like GTPase (*OPA1* / Entrez: 4976) at 3q29

Disease-causing germline mutation(s): dynamin 1 like (*DNM1L* / Entrez: 10059) at 12p11.21

Autosomal dominant

Visual impairment, Optic atrophy

Sensorineural hearing impairment, Color vision defect, Ophthalmoplegia, Sensorimotor neuropathy, Temporal optic disc pallor, Morning glory anomaly, Moderately reduced visual acuity

Ptosis, Central scotoma, Ataxia, Gait disturbance, Myopathy

Childhood, Adolescent, Adult

(Continued)

TABLE 6.23 *(Continued)*
GMP Herbal Medicines for a Five-Year-Old Child with Autosomal Dominant Optic Atrophy, Classic Form

Visual impairment (D014786), Optic atrophy (377.1):

Qǐjúdìhuángwán 5g + zǐshènmíngmùtāng 5g.

Qǐjúdìhuángwán 5g + yìqìcōngmíngtāng 5g + shíchāngpú 1-0g + yuǎnzhì 1-0g.

Qǐjúdìhuángwán 5g + bǔzhōngyìqìtāng 5g + shānzhā 1g + shénqū 1g + màiyá 1g + jīnèijīn 1g.

Qǐjúdìhuángwán 5g + shēnlíngbáizhúsǎn 4g + shānzhā 1g + shénqū 1g + màiyá 1g + jīnèijīn 1g.

Zhǐqiào 5g + jílí 5-2g + chántuì 5-0g + júhuā 5-0g.

Sensorineural hearing impairment (389.1), Color vision defect (368.53, 368.5, 368.52, 368.51, 368.54, 368.55), Ophthalmoplegia (378.56):

Liùwèidìhuángwán 5g + yìqìcōngmíngtāng 5-0g.

Liùwèidìhuángwán 5g + guīpítāng 5-0g + shíchāngpú 1-0g + gǒuqǐzǐ 1-0g + yuǎnzhì 1-0g.

Liùwèidìhuángwán 5g + xiǎocháihútāng 5-0g + shíchāngpú 1-0g + yuǎnzhì 1-0g.

Liùwèidìhuángwán 5g + bǔzhōngyìqìtāng 5-0g + gāncǎo 2-0g.

Shíchāngpú 5g + yuǎnzhì 5g + dǎngshēn 5g + dàzǎo 2g + chuānxiōng 2g + gǒuqǐzǐ 2g + júhuā 2g + dāngguī 2-0g.

Huángqín 5g + gāncǎo 3g + báizhǐ 3g + shārén 3g + dàhuáng 0g.

Huángqín 5g + báizhǐ 4g + zhìgāncǎo 4-2g + shārén 4-2g + guālóugēn 2g + dàhuáng 0g.

Ptosis (374.3), Central scotoma (D012607), Ataxia (D002524), Myopathy (359.9):

Shēnlíngbáizhúsǎn 5g + qǐjúdìhuángwán 5-4g + bǎohéwán 4-0g + màiyá 1-0g + jīnèijīn 1-0g.

Qǐjúdìhuángwán 5g + xiāngshāliùjūnzǐtāng 5g + bǎohéwán 4g + shānzhā 1g + wūméi 1g + shénqū 1g + màiyá 1g.

Qǐjúdìhuángwán 5g + zǐshènmíngmùtāng 4g + mùzéicǎo 1g + cǎojuémíng 1g + mìmēnghuā 1g.

Báizhǐ 5g + gāncǎo 5-4g + shārén 5-4g + dàhuáng 0g.

Huángqí 5g + chìsháo 1g + fángfēng 1g + dàhuáng 0g + xìxīn 0g + huánglián 0g.

Huángqín 5g + báizhǐ 2g + tiānhuā 2g + gāncǎo 2g + shārén 2g + jīnyínhuā 1g + dàhuáng 0g.

for tinnitus were predicted in silico (Wu et al., 2022). Shēnlíngbáizhúsǎn is frequently prescribed to children with functional digestive disorders (Wang, 2019). The formula was shown to regulate the expression of neuropeptides in the hypothalamus of functional diarrheal rats (Li et al., 2018). Shēnlíngbáizhúsǎn may therefore benefit emotion and cognition through the bidirectional communications between the enteric nervous system and the central nervous system.

REFERENCES

Adam, G., Robu, S., Flutur, M., Cioancă, O., Vasilache, I., Adam, A., Mircea, C., Nechita, A., Harabor, V., Harabor, A., & Hăncianu, M. (2023). Applications of *Perilla frutescens* extracts in clinical practice. *Antioxidants*, *12*(3), 727. https://doi.org/10.3390/antiox12030727

Chang, Y., Lin, H., & Li, W. (2005). Clinical evaluation of the traditional Chinese prescription Chi-Ju-Di-Huang-Wan for dry eye. *Phytotherapy Research*, *19*(4), 349–354. https://doi.org/10.1002/ptr.1687

Chen, H., Chen, Z. Y., Wang, T. J., Drew, V. J., Tseng, C. L., Fang, H. W., & Lin, F. H. (2017). Herbal supplement in a buffer for dry eye syndrome treatment. *International Journal of Molecular Sciences*, *18*(8), 1697. https://doi.org/10.3390/ijms18081697

Chen, Y., Sun, J., Zhang, Z., Liu, X., Wang, Q., & Yu, Y. (2022). The potential effects and mechanisms of hispidulin in the treatment of diabetic retinopathy based on network pharmacology. *BMC Complementary Medicine and Therapies*, *22*(1). https://doi.org/10.1186/s12906-022-03593-2

Cheng, L., Gai, Z., Zhou, Y., Lu, X., Zhang, F., Ye, H., & Duan, J. (2013). Systematic review and meta-analysis of 16 randomized clinical trials of *Radix Astragali* and its prescriptions for diabetic retinopathy. *Evidence-Based Complementary and Alternative Medicine*, *2013*, 1–13. https://doi.org/10.1155/2013/762783

Dong, X., Fu, J., Yin, X., Yang, C., Zhang, X., Wang, W., Du, X., Wang, Q., & Ni, J. (2017). *Cassiae* semen: A review of its phytochemistry and pharmacology. *Molecular Medicine Reports*, *16*(3), 2331–2346. https://doi.org/10.3892/mmr.2017.6880

Farrah, T. E., Dhillon, B., Keane, P. A., Webb, D. J., & Dhaun, N. (2020). The eye, the kidney, and cardiovascular disease: Old concepts, better tools, and new horizons. *Kidney International*, *98*(2), 323–342. https://doi.org/10.1016/j.kint.2020.01.039

Gao, T., Jiang, M., Deng, B., Zhang, Z., Fu, Q., & Fu, C. (2021). Aurantii Fructus: A systematic review of ethnopharmacology, phytochemistry and pharmacology. *Phytochemistry Reviews*, *20*(5), 909–944. https://doi.org/10.1007/s11101-020-09725-1

Gao, Y., Lian, H., Deng, S., Duan, Y., Zhang, P., Wang, Z., & Zhang, Y. (2023). Dry eye disease due to meibomian gland dysfunction treated with Pinggan Yuyin Qingre formula: A stratified randomized controlled trial. *Journal of Traditional Chinese Medicine*, *43*(4), 770–779. https://doi.org/10.19852/j.cnki.jtcm.20230526.003

Gong, Y., Wang, X., Wang, Y., Hao, P., Wang, H., Guo, Y., & Zhang, W. (2022). The effect of a chrysanthemum water extract in protecting the retina of mice from light damage. *BMC Complementary Medicine and Therapies*, *22*(1). https://doi.org/10.1186/s12906-022-03701-2

Harfiani, E., Pradana, D. C., & Yusmaini, H. (2020). A review on the phytochemical and pharmacological activitities of *Luffa acutangula* (L.) Roxb. *Jurnal Farmasi Indonesia (Pharmaceutical Journal of Indonesia)*, *17*(2), 396. https://doi.org/10.30595/pharmacy.v17i2.8220

He, S., Ma, X., Meng, Q., Lu, J., Qin, X., Fang, S., & Ma, C. (2020). Effects and mechanisms of water-soluble *Semen* cassiae polysaccharide on retinitis pigmentosa in rats. *Food Science and Technology*, *40*(1), 84–88. https://doi.org/10.1590/fst.32718

Hyun, S., Kim, J., Park, B., Jo, K., Lee, T. G., Kim, J. S., & Kim, C. (2019). Apricot kernel extract and amygdalin inhibit urban particulate matter-induced keratoconjunctivitis sicca. *Molecules*, *24*(3), 650. https://doi.org/10.3390/molecules24030650

Jiang, P., Peng, J., Tan, H., Ouyang, Y., Qin, G., & Peng, Q. (2019). Effects of Buddlejae Flos granules on inflammatory factors TGF-B1, NF-KB, IL-10 and IL-12 in lacrimal gland cells of castrated male rabbits. *Digital Chinese Medicine*, *2*(2), 97–104. https://doi.org/10.1016/j.dcmed.2019.09.004

Kim, C., Jo, K., Lee, I., & Kim, J. (2016). Topical application of apricot kernel extract improves dry eye symptoms in a unilateral exorbital lacrimal gland excision mouse. *Nutrients*, *8*(11), 750. https://doi.org/10.3390/nu8110750

Korooni, Z. (2023). Loofah (*Luffa cylindrica* L.) and its role in medicine, agriculture, and industry: A review. *Safe Future and Agricultural Research Journal (SFARJ)*, *2*(1), 1–5. https://www.sfaresearchjournal.ir/article_172578_2150d6b5471bdbe0f2001a4f7d9504ec.pdf

Li, J.-X., & Yu, Z.-Y. (2006). *Cimicifugae* rhizoma: From origins, bioactive constituents to clinical outcomes. *Current Medicinal Chemistry*, *13*(24), 2927–2951. https://doi.org/10.2174/092986706778521869

Li, S. L., Lin, G., Fu, P. P., Chan, C., Li, M., Jiang, Z. H., & Zhao, Z. (2008). Identification of five hepatotoxic pyrrolizidine alkaloids in a commonly used traditional Chinese medicinal herb, Herba Senecionis scandentis (Qianliguang). *Rapid Communications in Mass Spectrometry*, *22*(4), 591–602. https://doi.org/10.1002/rcm.3398

Li, X., Lin, J., Gao, Y., Han, W., & Chen, D. (2012). Antioxidant activity and mechanism of rhizoma *Cimicifugae*. *Chemistry Central Journal*, *6*(140). https://doi.org/10.1186/1752-153x-6-140

Li, Y., Zhang, W., Ma, J., Chen, M., Lin, B., Yang, X., Li, F., Tang, X., & Wang, F. (2018). Study on the regulation of brain–gut peptide by Shenling Baizhu San in functional diarrhea rats. *Journal of Traditional Chinese Medical Sciences*, *5*(3), 283–290. https://doi.org/10.1016/j.jtcms.2018.07.003

Lin, S., Tzeng, J., & Lai, J. (2019). The core pattern of Chinese herbal formulae and drug–herb concurrent usage in patients with dementia. *Medicine*, *98*(4), e13931. https://doi.org/10.1097/md.0000000000013931

Liu, M., Wang, L., Meng, J., Zheng, B., Qin, S., & Liang, A. (2023). Chemical constituents, pharmacology, and toxicology of Asari Radix et Rhizoma: A review. *Chinese Journal of Experimental Traditional Medical Formulae*, (24), 224–234. https://search.bvsalud.org/gim/resource/fr/wpr-969619

Liu, X., Wang, B., Sun, Y., Jia, Y., & Xu, Z. (2019). Astragalus root extract inhibits retinal cell apoptosis and repairs damaged retinal neovascularization in retinopathy of prematurity. *Cell Cycle*, *18*(22), 3147–3159. https://doi.org/10.1080/15384101.2019.1669998

Lu, L., Zhou, W., Li, Z., Yu, C., Li, C., Luo, M., & Xie, H. (2012). Effects of arctiin on streptozotocin-induced diabetic retinopathy in Sprague-Dawley rats. *Planta Medica*, *78*(12), 1317–1323. https://doi.org/10.1055/s-0032-1314998

Lu, S., Chen, K., Yang, Q., & Sun, H. (2011). Progress in the research of *Radix Astragali* in treating chronic heart failure: Effective ingredients, dose-effect relationship and adverse reaction. *Chinese Journal of Integrative Medicine*, *17*(6), 473–477. https://doi.org/10.1007/s11655-011-0756-5

Ma, S., Li, X., Dong, L., Jin-Li, Z., Zhang, H., & Jia, Y. (2016). Protective effect of Sheng-Mai Yin, a traditional Chinese preparation, against doxorubicin-induced cardiac toxicity in rats. *BMC Complementary and Alternative Medicine*, *16*(1). https://doi.org/10.1186/s12906-016-1037-9

Nagaki, Y., Hayasaka, S., Kadoi, C., Matsumoto, M., Nakamura, N., & Hayasaka, Y. (2001). Effects of Orengedoku-to and Senkanmeimoku-to, traditional herbal medicines, on the experimental herbal medicines, on the experimental elevation of aqueous flare in pigmental rabbits. *American Journal of Chinese Medicine*, *29*(01), 141–147. https://doi.org/10.1142/s0192415x01000150

Neelam, K., Dey, S., Sim, R., Lee, J., & Eong, K. A. (2021). *Fructus lycii*: A natural dietary supplement for amelioration of retinal diseases. *Nutrients*, *13*(1), 246. https://doi.org/10.3390/nu13010246

Shan, C., Xu, Q., Shi, Y., Wang, Y., He, Z., & Zheng, G. (2018). Chuanxiong formulae for migraine: A systematic review and meta-analysis of high-quality randomized controlled trials. *Frontiers in Pharmacology*, *9*, 589. https://doi.org/10.3389/fphar.2018.00589

Shen, Z., Shao, J., Dai, J., Lin, Y., Yang, X., Ma, J., He, Q., Yang, B., Yao, K., & Luo, P. (2016). Diosmetin protects against retinal injury via reduction of DNA damage and oxidative stress. *Toxicology Reports*, *3*, 78–86. https://doi.org/10.1016/j.toxrep.2015.12.004

Sheng, W., Wang, Y., Li, J., & Han, X. (2019). Clinical and basic research on Renshen Yangrong Decoction. *Frontiers in Nutrition*, *6*. https://doi.org/10.3389/fnut.2019.00175

Shi, J., Lv, H., Tang, C., Li, Y., Huang, J., & Zhang, H. (2021). Mangiferin inhibits cell migration and angiogenesis via PI3K/AKT/mTOR signaling in high glucose- and hypoxia-induced RRCECs. *Molecular Medicine Reports*, *23*(6). https://doi.org/10.3892/mmr.2021.12112

Tjong, Y., Ip, S., Lao, L., Fong, H. H. S., Sung, J. J., Berman, B. M., & Che, C. (2011). Analgesic effect of *Coptis chinensis* rhizomes (Coptidis Rhizoma) extract on rat model of irritable bowel syndrome. *Journal of Ethnopharmacology*, *135*(3), 754–761. https://doi.org/10.1016/j.jep.2011.04.007

Tsai, F. J., Li, T. M., Ko, C. H., Cheng, C. F., Ho, T. J., Liu, X., Tsang, H., Lin, T. H., Liao, C., Li, J. P., Huang, S., Lin, J., Lin, C., Liang, W. M., & Lin, Y. (2017). Effects of Chinese herbal medicines on the occurrence of diabetic retinopathy in type 2 diabetes patients and protection of ARPE-19 retina cells by inhibiting oxidative stress. *Oncotarget*, *8*(38), 63528–63550. https://doi.org/10.18632/oncotarget.18846

Tzeng, T., Liu, W. Y., Liou, S., Hong, T., & Liu, I. (2016). Antioxidant-rich extract from Plantaginis Semen ameliorates diabetic retinal injury in a streptozotocin-induced diabetic rat model. *Nutrients*, *8*(9), 572. https://doi.org/10.3390/nu8090572

Wang, S.-C. (2019). Therapeutic classes of CHEG formulas. In S.-C. Wang (Ed.), *Clinical herbal prescriptions: Principles and practices of herbal formulations from deep learning health insurance herbal prescription big data* (pp. 16–89). World Scientific Publishing. https://doi.org/10.1142/11211

Wang, S.-C. (2020). Modern therapeutic uses of CHEG herbs and herb pairs. In S.-C. Wang (Ed.), *Veterinary herbal pharmacopoeia* (pp. 35–233). Nova Science Publishers. https://doi.org/10.52305/GHTR1903

Wen, J., Yang, Y., & Hao, J. (2023). *Acori Tatarinowii* Rhizoma: A comprehensive review of its chemical composition, pharmacology, pharmacokinetics and toxicity. *Frontiers in Pharmacology*, *14*. https://doi.org/10.3389/fphar.2023.1090526

Wu, Z., Zhu, Z., Cao, J., Wu, W., Hu, S., Deng, C., Xie, Q., Huang, X., & You, C. (2022). Prediction of network pharmacology and molecular docking-based strategy to determine potential pharmacological mechanism of Liuwei Dihuang pill against tinnitus. *Medicine*, *101*(46), e31711. https://doi.org/10.1097/md.0000000000031711

Yang, M., Hu, Z., Yue, R., Yang, L., Zhang, B., & Yuan, C. (2020). The efficacy and safety of Qiming granule for dry eye disease: A systematic review and meta-analysis. *Frontiers in Pharmacology*, *11*. https://doi.org/10.3389/fphar.2020.00580

Yeo, C., Ahn, C. R., Kim, J., Kim, Y. W., Park, J., Ahn, K. S., Ha, I., Lee, Y. J., Baek, S. H., & Ha, I. (2022). Chaenomeles Fructus (CF), the fruit of *Chaenomeles sinensis* alleviates IL-1β induced cartilage degradation in rat articular chondrocytes. *International Journal of Molecular Sciences*, *23*(8), 4360. https://doi.org/10.3390/ijms23084360

Zhang, Q., Li, R., Tao, T., Sun, J., Liu, J., Zhang, T., Peng, W., & Wu, C. (2021). Antiepileptic effects of Cicadae Periostracum on mice and its antiapoptotic effects in H_2O_2-stimulated PC12 cells via regulation of PI3K/AKT/NRF2 signaling pathways. *Oxidative Medicine and Cellular Longevity*, *2021*, 1–19. https://doi.org/10.1155/2021/5598818

Zhang, Y., Li, X., Guo, C., Dong, J., & Liao, L. (2020). Mechanisms of Spica Prunellae against thyroid-associated ophthalmopathy based on network pharmacology and molecular docking. *BMC Complementary Medicine and Therapies*, *20*(1). https://doi.org/10.1186/s12906-020-03022-2

7 GMP Herbal Medicine for Rare Skin Diseases

Skin diseases cause such skin changes as inflammation, itchiness, discoloration, blisters, and crusts. Common causes of skin diseases include bacterial/fungal/viral infections, allergy/immunity, malnutrition, and genetics. Half of the rare skin diseases in this chapter have attributable germline or somatic mutations. The rest may involve autoimmunity.

The GMP herbal products that are frequently discussed for rare skin diseases are Rhubarb Root and Rhizome (Dàhuáng), Licorice Root (Gāncǎo), Cardamon Seed (Shārén), Scutellaria Root (Huángqín), Dahurian Angelica Root (Báizhǐ), Trichosanthes Root (Tiānhuā), Bitter Orange (Zhǐqiào), Immature Bitter Orange (Zhǐshí), Figwort Root (Xuánshēn), Five Ingredient Formula with Poria (Wǔlíngsǎn), Enrich the Kidneys and Improve Vision Decoction (Zīshènmíngmùtāng), Lycium, Chrysanthemum and Rehmannia Pill (Qǐjúdìhuángwán), Bamboo and Poria Combination (Warm the Gallbladder Decoction; Wēndǎntāng), Gardenia and Vitex Combination (Xǐgānmíngmùtāng), Jade Windscreen Powder (Yùpíngfēngsǎn), Jade Spring Pill (Yùquánwán), Regulate the Middle Decoction (Lǐzhōngtāng), Aucklandia, Cardamon and the Six Gentlemen Decoction (Xiāngshāliùjūnzǐtāng), Tonify the Middle and Augment the Qi Decoction (Bǔzhōngyìqìtāng), Cinnamon Twig Decoction (Guìzhītāng), Seven Treasure Special Pill for Beautiful Whiskers (Qībǎoměirándān), and Regulate the Stomach and Order the Qi Decoction (Tiáowèichéngqìtāng). Eczema with blisters is considered a form of abnormal fluid distribution in the body, which Wǔlíngsǎn treats.

Acupuncture is frequently prescribed, along with herbal medicines, for the treatment of the skin conditions discussed in this chapter. Acupuncture was reviewed and suggested to be effective for a number of dermatologic conditions (Hwang & Lio, 2021; Van Den Berg-Wolf & Burgoon, 2017).

7.1 APLASIA CUTIS CONGENITA

Aplasia cutis congenita is missing of the skin, at birth, in a section with a size of up to 10 centimeters across the places such as the scalp, face, trunk, and extremities. The outermost layer of the skin is most likely affected, but in rare cases the bone underneath the affected skin can be missing, too. The exact cause of aplasia cutis congenita is unclear, but genetic factors and intrauterine infections and medications are not excluded.

TABLE 7.1

GMP Herbal Medicines for a One-Year-Old Infant with Aplasia Cutis Congenita

Aplasia cutis congenita (OrphaCode: 1114)

A malformation syndrome with a prevalence of ~3 in 10,000

Disease-causing germline mutation(s): plectin (*PLEC* / Entrez: 5339) at 8q24.3

Disease-causing germline mutation(s): integrin subunit beta 4 (*ITGB4* / Entrez: 3691) at 17q25.1

Disease-causing germline mutation(s): BMS1 ribosome biogenesis factor (*BMS1* / Entrez: 9790) at 10q11.21

Disease-causing germline mutation(s) (loss of function): delta like canonical Notch ligand 4 (*DLL4* / Entrez: 54567) at 15q15.1

Disease-causing germline mutation(s): ubiquitin like modifier activating enzyme 2 (*UBA2* / Entrez: 10054) at 19q13.11

Autosomal dominant, Autosomal recessive, Not applicable

(Continued)

DOI: 10.1201/9781032726625-7

TABLE 7.1 *(Continued)*
GMP Herbal Medicines for a One-Year-Old Infant with Aplasia Cutis Congenita

Skull defect, Aplasia cutis congenita over the scalp vertex, Congenital localized absence of skin, Spinal dysraphism

Skin ulcer

Toe syndactyly, Prolonged bleeding time, Abnormality of bone mineral density, Finger syndactyly, Facial palsy

Antenatal, Neonatal

Facial palsy (351.0):

Xiǎocháihútāng 5g + gégēntāng 5-0g + báijiāngcán 2-1g + gōuténg 2-1g + qínjiāo 2-0g + chántuì 2-0g + fángfēng 1-0g + jīngjiè 1-0g + acupuncture.

Wūyàoshùnqìsǎn 5g + xiǎoxùmìngtāng 5-0g + acupuncture.

Yínqiàosǎn 5g + júhuā 2g + jílí 2g + chántuì 2g + zhǐqiào 1g.

Gégēntāng 5g + gāncǎo 0g.

Báizhǐ 5g + zhìgāncǎo 5-3g + shārén 5-3g + huángqín 5-0g + dàhuáng 1-0g + acupuncture.

Báizhǐ 5g + gāncǎo 5-2g + shārén 5-2g + huángqín 5-0g + tiānhuā 3-0g + dàhuáng 1-0g + acupuncture.

Fángfēng 5g + qiānghuó 5g + hòupò 5g + zhǐshí 5g + dàhuáng 1g.

Báizhǐ (cf. Sections 1.7 and 2.40) was demonstrated to produce an antiseizure effect in mice in a dose-dependent manner (Łuszczki et al., 2007); it is used for headaches and rhinitis, among other indications (Wang, 2020). Fángfēng was introduced in Sections 2.38 and 5.15 to relieve pain and cramps. Gégēntāng is annotated in Sections 1.38 and 2.56 for symptoms involving the head and neck, such as rhinitis and migraines (Wang, 2019).

7.2 CHRONIC ACTINIC DERMATITIS

Chronic actinic dermatitis, also known as chronic photosensitivity dermatitis, is itchiness and inflammation of an area of the skin exposed to sunlight and fluorescent light including the face, neck, chest, and backs of the hands. Chronic actinic dermatitis is caused by abnormal reactions of

TABLE 7.2
GMP Herbal Medicines for a 50-Year-Old Man with Chronic Actinic Dermatitis

Chronic actinic dermatitis (OrphaCode: 330064)

A disease with a prevalence of ~3 in 10,000

Not applicable

Eczema, Pruritus, Cutaneous photosensitivity

Epidermal acanthosis, Erythematous papule

Hypopigmented skin patches, Progressive hyperpigmentation, Late-onset atopic dermatitis, Actinic keratosis, Lichenification

Adult

Pruritus (D011537):

Wǔwèixiāodúyǐn 5g + zhēnrénhuómìngyǐn 5-3g + tǔfúlíng 1-0g + báixiānpí 1-0g + dìfūzǐ 1-0g.

Wǔwèixiāodúyǐn 5g + xiāofēngsǎn 5g + huángliánjiědútāng 4-0g + báixiānpí 1g + dìfūzǐ 1g + jīnyínhuā 1-0g + liánqiáo 1-0g + mǔdānpí 1-0g.

Wǔwèixiāodúyǐn 5g + lóngdǎnxiègāntāng 3g + liánqiáo 1g + tǔfúlíng 1-0g + báixiānpí 1-0g + dìfūzǐ 1-0g + jīnyínhuā 1-0g + dàhuáng 0g.

Huángliánjiědútāng 5g + jīnyínhuā 1g + liánqiáo 1g.

Jīnyínhuā 5g + liánqiáo 5g + huángbò 2g.

Tiānhuā 5g + niúbàngzǐ 5g + gāncǎo 5g + dìhuáng 5g + bèimǔ 5g + shègān 5g + liánqiáo 5g.

Tiānhuā 5g + gāncǎo 5g + báizhǐ 5g + shārén 3g + dàhuáng 0g.

Báizhǐ 5g + gāncǎo 4g + shārén 4g + huángqín 4g + tiānhuā 2g + dàhuáng 0g.

Huáshí 5g + yìyǐrén 5g + bànxià 4g + xìngrén 4g + báidòukòu 2g + hòupò 2g + dànzhúyè 2g + tōngcǎo 2g.

Jīnyínhuā 5g + dāngguī 5g + xuánshēn 3-2g + gāncǎo 3-2g + niúxī 2g + chìsháo 2g + dǎodìwúgōng 2g + huángqí 2g.

Jīnyínhuā 5g + dāngguī 5g + niúxī 4-2g + xuánshēn 4-2g + chìsháo 4-2g + zhìgāncǎo 4-2g + dǎodìwúgōng 4-2g + huángqí 4-2g.

the skin to ultraviolet light, and people with chronic actinic dermatitis usually have dermatitis in response to other stimuli, such as cosmetics and sunscreens.

Jīnyínhuā (cf. Sections 3.5 and 3.9) "clears heat, neutralizes pathogens, and disperses wind-heat." It is used today for not only contact dermatitis but also colon cancer (Wang, 2020). Wǔwèixiāodúyǐn, with Jīnyínhuā as the major herb, has traditionally been used to "dissolve boils and carbuncles" and is used today for bullous dermatoses and diffuse connective tissue diseases (Wang, 2019).

7.3 DERMATITIS HERPETIFORMIS

Dermatitis herpetiformis, also known as Duhring-Brocq disease, is characterized by intense itching and burning blisters on the reddened skin of the shoulders, elbows, buttocks, and knees. Dermatitis herpetiformis is due to intolerance of the innate immune system to gluten that can be found in cereals made of wheat, rye, barley, and their derivatives.

TABLE 7.3

GMP Herbal Medicines for a 30-Year-Old Adult with Dermatitis Herpetiformis

Dermatitis herpetiformis (OrphaCode: 1656)

A disease with a prevalence of ~3 in 10,000

Not applicable

Pruritus, Urticaria, Microcytic anemia, Malabsorption, Recurrent fractures, Autoimmunity, Abnormal blistering of the skin, Erythema, Macule, Skin vesicle

Eczema

Edema, Bone pain, Lichenification

All ages

Pruritus (D011537), Erythema (D005483):

Wǔlíngsǎn 5g + fùzǐ 1g + huángqín 1g + tiáowèichéngqìtāng 1-0g + xiǎochéngqìtāng 0g + dǐdāngtāng 0g + dàhuáng 0g.

Wǔlíngsǎn 5g + báisháo 1g + huángqín 1g + tiáowèichéngqìtāng 1-0g + dǐdāngtāng 0g + dàhuáng 0g.

Gāncǎo 5g + báizhǐ 5g + shārén 5-4g + huángqín 5-4g + tiānhuā 3-0g + guālóugēn 2-0g + xìxīn 2-0g + huánglián 1-0g + dàhuáng 1-0g.

Edema (D004487):

Lǐzhōngtāng 5g + bànxià 1g + shārén 1g + fúlíng 1g + dàhuáng 0g.

Lǐzhōngtāng 5g + bǔzhōngyìqìtāng 5g + qīngyānlìgétāng 3g + qínjiāobiējiǎsǎn 3-0g + fángfēng 2g + zhǐqiào 2g + jiégěng 2g + gānjiāng 2g.

Lǐzhōngtāng 5g + bǔzhōngyìqìtāng 5g + qīngyānlìgétāng 3g + chuānxiōngchádiàosǎn 3-0g + liùwèidìhuángwán 3-0g + fángfēng 2g + zhǐqiào 2g + jiégěng 2g + gānjiāng 2g.

Báizhú 5g + báidòukòu 5g + fúlíng 5g + shíchāngpú 4g + shígāo 4g + hòupò 4g + zhǐqiào 4g.

Báizhú 5g + fúlíng 5g + huòxiāng 5-0g + zhǐshí 4g + shénqū 4g + shānzhā 4-0g + xiāngfù 4-0g + cháihú 4-0g + púgōngyīng 4-0g + chénpí 4-0g + shēngmá 2-0g.

Báidòukòu (Fructus Amomi Rotundus) "transforms dampness, moves Qi, warms interior, stops vomiting" and is used today for dyspepsia and gastric ulcer (Wang, 2020). Fúlíng, introduced in Sections 1.21 and 3.3, helps "water draining" and is used today for pruritic disorders, including contact dermatitis and other eczema (Wang, 2020). Lǐzhōngtāng, introduced in Sections 2.28, 2.48, and 3.14 for digestive disorders, is translated to "interior-regulating decoction." The regimens in the table alleviate the connective tissue conditions of the patients.

7.4 BULLOUS PEMPHIGOID

Bullous pemphigoid is a chronic, autoimmune, and blistering disease of the skin, characterized by the formation of large, fluid-filled blisters anywhere on the skin. Bullous pemphigoid is caused by attacks of IgG autoantibodies on hemidesmosomes, which help in the adhesion of basal epithelial cells to the underlying basement membrane of the integumentary system, forming subepidermal blisters.

TABLE 7.4
GMP Herbal Medicines for a 72-Year-Old Adult with Bullous Pemphigoid

Bullous pemphigoid (OrphaCode: 703)

A disease with a prevalence of ~2 in 10,000

Candidate gene tested: major histocompatibility complex, class II, DR beta 1 (*HLA-DRB1* / Entrez: 3123) at 6p21.32

Major susceptibility factor: major histocompatibility complex, class II, DQ beta 1 (*HLA-DQB1* / Entrez: 3119) at 6p21.32

Not applicable

Diabetes mellitus, Eczema, Urticaria, Weight loss, Recurrent infections, Autoimmunity, Abnormal blistering of the skin, Erythema, Macule

Psoriasiform dermatitis

All ages

Diabetes mellitus (250), Weight loss (D015431), Erythema (D005483):

Yùquánwán 5g + báihǔjiārénshēntāng 5-0g + shānyào 2-0g + tiānhuā 2-0g.+ dānshēn 1-0g + chìsháo 1-0g + hónghuā 1-0g.	Gāncǎo 5g + yìzhìrén 5g + gānjiāng 5g + fùpénzǐ 5g + fùzǐ 4-3g + dìfūzǐ 4-0g + guìzhī 4-0g + máhuáng 2-0g + dàhuáng 0g.
	Guālóugēn 5g + shānyào 2g + xuánshēn 2g + shígāo 2g + dìhuáng 2g + màiméndōng 2g + huángqín 2g + huángqí 2g + huánglián 2g + bìxiè 2g + dǎngshēn 2g.
	Tiānhuā 5g + gāncǎo 5g + dìhuáng 5g + mǎchǐxiàn 5g + huángqí 5g + huánglián 5g + huángjīng 5g + dǎngshēn 5g.
	Tiānhuā 5g + fúlíng 5g + jùmài 5g + shānyào 3g + fùzǐ 3g.

Yìzhìrén (Fructus Alpiniae Oxyphyllae) "warms the Kidney, retains semen" and is used today for hyperplasia of prostate and polyuria (Wang, 2020). Gānjiāng (cf. Sections 1.15, 1.46, and 2.16) "warms interior/meridians" to help digestion. Guālóugēn (cf. Section 4.32) "quenches thirst, clears heat" and is used today for polydipsia (Wang, 2020). Shígāo (cf. Section 6.12), being extremely cool in TCM nature, was shown to improve cutaneous pruritus in mice (Ikarashi et al., 2012). Both Yùquánwán, which contains Guālóugēn, and Báihǔjiārénshēntāng, which contains Shígāo, are used today for diabetes mellitus (Wang, 2019).

7.5 PEMPHIGUS VULGARIS

Pemphigus vulgaris is a chronic, autoimmune, blistering disease of the skin and mucous membranes such as the oral mucosa. Pemphigus vulgaris is caused by attacks of IgG autoantibodies on desmosomes that help bind adjacent cells in the epidermis together, forming intraepidermal blisters. Pemphigus vulgaris is potentially life-threatening.

TABLE 7.5
GMP Herbal Medicines for a 55-Year-Old Woman with Pemphigus Vulgaris

Pemphigus vulgaris (OrphaCode: 704)

A disease with a prevalence of ~2 in 10,000

Not applicable

Abnormal oral cavity morphology, Atypical scarring of skin, Urticaria, Weight loss, Recurrent infections, Autoimmunity, Abnormal blistering of the skin, Feeding difficulties in infancy, Acantholysis, Recurrent cutaneous abscess formation

Childhood, Adult, Elderly

Weight loss (D015431), Acantholysis (D000051) [Other specified disorders of skin (709.8)]:

Guìzhītāng 5g + màiyá 2-0g + xiāngfù 2-0g + huángqín 1-0g + xìngrén 1-0g + máhuáng 1-0g + bànxià 1-0g + dàhuáng 0g.	Huángqín 5g + báizhǐ 4g + shārén 3g + zhìgāncǎo 3-0g + tiānhuā 2-1g + xìxīn 1-0g + dàhuáng 1-0g.
Lǐzhōngtāng 5g + bànxià 1g + shārén 1g + fúlíng 1g.	Gāncǎo 5g + shārén 5g + huángbò 5g + gānjiāng 2g + dànzhúyè 2g + liánqiáo 2g.

Huángqín (cf. Sections 1.6 and 5.7) "clears heat, dries dampness, quenches fire, de-toxifies, cools blood, stops bleeding, removes heat, prevents miscarriage" and is used for respiratory, skin, digestive, menstrual conditions, and so on (Wang, 2020). Dànzhúyè (Herba Lophatheri) "clears heat, frees strangury" and is used today for contact dermatitis and other eczema (Wang, 2020). Xiāngfù (Rhizoma Cyperi) "soothes the Liver, regulates Qi, modulates menstruation, stops pain" and is used for disorders of menstruation, chest pain, and benign neoplasm of the skin (Wang, 2020).

7.6 RECESSIVE X-LINKED ICHTHYOSIS

Recessive X-linked ichthyosis, also known as steroid sulfatase deficiency, is characterized by dry and scaly skin. It is caused by mutations in the *STS* gene on the X chromosome. The protein encoded by the *STS* gene breaks down cholesterol sulfate, the accumulation of which on the outer layers of the skin causes excessive skin scaling.

TABLE 7.6

GMP Herbal Medicines for a One-Year-Old Boy with Recessive X-Linked Ichthyosis

Recessive X-linked ichthyosis (OrphaCode: 461)

A disease with a prevalence of ~2 in 10,000

Disease-causing germline mutation(s): filaggrin (*FLG* / Entrez: 2312) at 1q21.3

Disease-causing germline mutation(s): steroid sulfatase (*STS* / Entrez: 412) at Xp22.31

X-linked recessive

Dry skin, Hyperkeratosis, Hypohidrosis, Ichthyosis

Attention deficit hyperactivity disorder, Opacification of the corneal stroma

Cryptorchidism, Autism, Neurological speech impairment

Neonatal

Hypohidrosis (705.0):

Yùpíngfēngsǎn 5g + bǔzhōngyìqìtāng 5g + guìzhītāng 5-0g + fúxiǎomài 2-0g + máhuánggēn 2-0g.

Yùpíngfēngsǎn 5g + guìzhījiālónggǔmǔlìtāng 5-0g + fúxiǎomài 1g + máhuánggēn 1g + huángqí 1-0g.

Huángqí 5g + báizhú 5-2g + fángfēng 5-2g + gāncǎo 5-0g.

Gāncǎo 5g + báizhǐ 5g + shārén 5g + huángqín 5-0g + dàhuáng 0g.

Shígāo 5g + gégēn 5g + dàzǎo 2g + gāncǎo 2g + shēngjiāng 2g + báisháo 2g + jīnyínhuā 2g + huángqín 2g + bòhé 2g + máhuáng 0g.

Cryptorchidism (752.51), Autism (299.0), Neurological speech impairment (D013064):

Gāncǎoxiǎomàidàzǎotāng 5g + wēndǎntāng 5g + shíchāngpú 2-1g + yuǎnzhì 2-1g + dǎngshēn 1-0g + acupuncture.

Xiǎocháihútāng 5g + wēndǎntāng 5g + shíchāngpú 1g + yuǎnzhì 1g + gōuténg 1g.

Cháihújiālónggǔmǔlìtāng 5g + shēnlíngbáizhúsǎn 5g + shānzhī 1g + shénqū 1g + màiyá 1g.

Zhǐqiào 5g + jílí 5-0g + chántuì 5-0g.

Báizhǐ 5g + shārén 5-2g + gāncǎo 5-2g + huángqín 5-0g + tiānhuā 2-0g + dàhuáng 0g.

Yùpíngfēngsǎn, containing Huángqí, Báizhú, and Fángfēng, relieves sweating (cf. Sections 1.29 and 4.7). Guìzhītāng (cf. Sections 1.11, 1.50, 2.30, and 4.1) promotes sweating (Huang et al., 2019). Wēndǎntāng (cf. Section 2.31), containing Zhǐqiào and Gāncǎo, "moves Qi, dissolves phlegm, modulates the Gallbladder and Stomach" and is used today for neurotic disorders and general symptoms such as sleep disturbances (Wang, 2019).

7.7 ALOPECIA TOTALIS

Alopecia totalis is the loss of hair across the entire scalp. The cause of alopecia totalis is believed to be autoimmunity, where the T cells of a person's immune system attack their own hair follicles.

TABLE 7.7
GMP Herbal Medicines for a 31-Year-Old Adult with Alopecia Totalis

Alopecia totalis (OrphaCode: 700)

A disease with a prevalence of ~1 in 10,000

Multigenic/multifactorial

Alopecia, Scalp hair loss

All ages

Alopecia (704.0):

Qībǎoměirándān 5g + nǔzhēnzǐ 1g + héshǒuwū 1g + hànliáncǎo 1-0g + tùsīzǐ 1-0g.

Qībǎoměirándān 5g + jiāwèixiāoyáosǎn 5-0g + rénshēnyǎngróngtāng 4-0g + nǔzhēnzǐ 1g + héshǒuwū 1g + hànliáncǎo 1g.

Biǎnbó 5g + dāngguī 2g.

Héshǒuwū 5g + dāngguī 5g + dùzhòng 2g + fúlíng 2g + tùsīzǐ 2g + huángqí 2g + bǔgǔzhī 2g.

Báizhǐ 5g + huángqín 5-0g + tiānhuā 4-3g + gāncǎo 4-3g + shārén 4-3g + dàhuáng 0g.

Biǎnbó (Cacumen Platycladi) "stops bleeding, cools blood, regenerates hair and darkens hair." The effect and mechanism for its hair growth–promoting capability were verified and identified in shaved mice (Fu et al., 2023). Qībǎoměirándān "replenishes the Liver/Kidney, nourishes Blood, fills essence" and is used today for neurotic disorders, anemias, and disorders of the skin and sub-cutaneous tissue (Wang, 2019). Qībǎoměirándān is made up of Héshǒuwū, Dāngguī, Fúlíng, Tùsīzǐ, Bǔgǔzhī, and two other herbs.

7.8 LOCALIZED SCLERODERMA

Localized scleroderma, or localized fibrosing scleroderma, is thickening and hardening of the skin, and the tissues below the skin, on any area of the body. Localized scleroderma is believed to be caused by an autoimmune inflammation which triggers overproduction of collagen in the affected connective tissue.

Niúxī and Shàngzhōngxiàtōngyòngtòngfēngwán are common herbal products for musculo-skeletal conditions, as we will see their use again for bone diseases in Chapter 10. Huángbò (cf. Section 5.2) treats "damp-heat inundating the lower body," which manifests lower limb flaccid-ity. Its modern uses include skin diseases, leukorrhea, lumbago, and dysmenorrhea (Wang, 2020). Guīlùèrxiānjiāo was shown to increase lower limb muscle strength and decrease articular pain in elderly men with knee osteoarthritis in a case-control study (Tsai et al., 2014).

TABLE 7.8
GMP Herbal Medicines for an Eight-Year-Old Child with Localized Scleroderma

Localized scleroderma (OrphaCode: 90289)

A disease with a prevalence of ~5 in 100,000

Not applicable

Thickened skin

Arthralgia, Localized skin lesion, Stiff skin, Cutaneous sclerotic plaque

Abnormality of the dentition, Abnormality of upper lip, Facial asymmetry, Abnormality of vision, Uveitis, Dental malocclusion, Hyperpigmentation of the skin, Hypopigmented skin patches, Arthritis, Flexion contracture, Gastroesophageal reflux, Migraine, Patchy alopecia, Headache, Autoimmunity, Myopathy, Abnormality of the cheek, Short dental roots, Progressive loss of facial adipose tissue, Erythema, Hemifacial atrophy, Abnormality of facial skeleton, Erythematous plaque, Fasciitis, Upper limb asymmetry, Infra-orbital crease, Sclerosis of finger phalanx

All ages

(Continued)

TABLE 7.8 *(Continued)*
GMP Herbal Medicines for an Eight-Year-Old Child with Localized Scleroderma

Arthralgia (D018771):

Shàngzhōngxiàtōngyòngtòngfēngwán 5g + shūjīnghuóxuètāng 5g + acupuncture.

Shàngzhōngxiàtōngyòngtòngfēngwán 5g + liùwèidìhuángwán 5g + xīnyísǎn 5g + shūgāntāng 5g + shènzhetāng 5g.

Shàngzhōngxiàtōngyòngtòngfēngwán 5g + niúxī 1g + chēqiánzǐ 1-0g + huángbò 1-0g + cāngzhú 1-0g + yìyǐrén 1-0g.

Shàngzhōngxiàtōngyòngtòngfēngwán 5g + dāngguīniāntòngtāng 5g.

Niúxī 5g + huángbò 5g + cāngzhú 5g + yìyǐrén 5-0g.

Niúxī 5g + báisháo 5g + guìzhī 5g + gǔsuìbǔ 5g + xùduàn 5g + mùguā 4g + dāngguī 4g + mòyào 2g + rǔxiāng 2g + acupuncture.

Niúxī 5g + xuánshēn 5g + chìsháo 5g + dǎodìwúgōng 5g + dāngguī 5g + rěndōngténg 2g + zhìgāncǎo 2g + huángqí 2g + dàhuáng 1g.

Dàdīnghuáng 5g + dìwúgōng 5g + gégēn 1g + jiānghuáng 1g + acupuncture.

Gastroesophageal reflux (530.81), Migraine (346), Patchy alopecia (704.01), Headache (D006261), Myopathy (359.9), Erythema (D005483), Fasciitis (729.4):

Guīlüèrxiānjiāo 5g + jiāwèixiāoyáosǎn 2g + zhībódìhuángwán 2g + xiāngshāliùjūnzǐtāng 2g + gāncǎoxiǎomàidàzǎotāng 2-0g.

Guīlüèrxiānjiāo 5g + qíbǎoměirándān 2g + xiǎoqīnglóngtāng 2g + xiāngshāliùjūnzǐtāng 2g + gāncǎo 1g.

Zhībódìhuángwán 5g + cháihújiālónggǔmǔlìtāng 5g + xiāngshāliùjūnzǐtāng 1g + shānzhā 1g + shénqū 1g + màiyá 1g.

Xiǎoqīnglóngtāng 5g + bǔzhōngyìqìtāng 2g + báijí 1g + hǎipiāoxiāo 1g + xiāngshāliùjūnzǐtāng 1g.

Báizhǐ 5g + shārén 5-4g + huángqín 4-0g + gāncǎo 3-0g + tiānhuā 2-0g + xìxīn 2-0g + dàhuáng 1-0g.

Báizhǐ 5g + zhìgāncǎo 5-4g + shārén 5-2g + huángqín 4-2g + guālóugēn 2-0g + dàhuáng 0g.

7.9 DARIER DISEASE

Darier disease is characterized by a flare-up of wart-like blemishes or rough bumps, called *keratosis follicularis*, on the skin. Darier disease is associated with mutations in the *ATP2A2* gene, whose products allow calcium ions to pass into the calcium storage site in cytoplasm in response to cellular signals.

Wǔlíngsǎn (Sections 2.9 and 4.14) treats not only chronic glomerulonephritis (Section 8.4), but also contact dermatitis and other eczema (Wang, 2019). Yuèbìjiāshùtāng (cf. Section 1.51) "disperses

TABLE 7.9
GMP Herbal Medicines for a 22-Year-Old Adult with Darier Disease

Darier disease (OrphaCode: 218)

A disease with a prevalence of ~3 in 100,000

Disease-causing germline mutation(s): ATPase sarcoplasmic/endoplasmic reticulum Ca2+ transporting 2 (*ATP2A2* / Entrez: 488) at 12q24.11

Autosomal dominant

Pruritus, Hypermelanotic macule, Abnormality of the nail, Subungual hyperkeratotic fragments, Acrokeratosis

Palmoplantar keratoderma, Abnormality of skin pigmentation, Thickened skin, Abnormality of the hair, Anal mucosal leukoplakia, Plantar pits

Macule, Skin vesicle

Childhood, Adolescent, Adult

Pruritus (D011537), Abnormality of the nail (703):

Wǔlíngsǎn 5g + zhēnrénhuómìngyǐn 5g + jīngfángbàidúsǎn 5-0g + kǔshēngēn 1-0g.

Wǔlíngsǎn 5g + yuèbìjiāshùtāng 5-0g + báizhǐ 1-0g + dǎngshēn 1-0g + fùzǐ 0g + dàhuáng 0g.

Gāncǎo 5g + báizhǐ 5g + shārén 3g + huángqín 2g + guālóugēn 2g + dàhuáng 0g.

Gāncǎo 5g + báizhǐ 5g + shārén 5-3g + huángqín 5-0g + tiānhuā 2-0g + xìxīn 2-0g + dàhuáng 1-0g.

wind, clears heat, induces sweating, promotes urination" and is used for allergic rhinitis, and contact dermatitis and other eczema (Wang, 2019).

7.10　SOLAR URTICARIA

Solar urticaria is an allergic reaction of the skin in response to exposure to ultraviolet light or visible light. Solar urticaria is caused by IgE-mediated activation and release of histamine by the mast cells in the exposed skin in susceptible individuals.

TABLE 7.10

GMP Herbal Medicines for a 35-Year-Old Adult with Solar Urticaria

Solar urticaria (OrphaCode: 97230)

A disease with a prevalence of ~3 in 100,000

Not applicable

Abnormal lip morphology, Edema, Pruritus, Urticaria, Syncope, Nausea, Headache, Vertigo, Abnormal tongue morphology, Wheezing, Immunologic hypersensitivity, Periorbital edema, Angioedema

Dyspnea

Dermatographic urticaria

All ages

Edema (D004487), Pruritus (D011537), Syncope (D013575), Nausea (D009325), Headache (D006261), Vertigo (386.2), Wheezing (D012135):

Línguìshùgāntāng 5g + fùzǐ 1g + gānjiāng 1g + tiáowèichéngqìtāng 1g + xìxīn 1-0g + dàhuáng 0g.	Rénshēn 5g + bànxià 5g + gānjiāng 5g + huángqín 2-0g + huánglián 2-0g.
Línguìshùgāntāng 5g + báisháo 1g + fùzǐ 1-0g + mázǐrénwán 1-0g + tiáowèichéngqìtāng 1-0g + dàhuáng 0g.	Báizhú 5g + rénshēn 5-3g + huángqín 5-3g + dàhuáng 0g.
	Gāncǎo 5g + báizhú 5g + fúlíng 5g + gānjiāng 5g.
Dyspnea (D004417):	
Máxìnggānshítāng 5g + yínqiàosǎn 5g.	Wǔwèizǐ 5g + zhìgāncǎo 5g + fúlíng 5g + xìxīn 2g + gānjiāng 0g.
Máxìnggānshítāng 5g + cāngěrsǎn 5g + jiégěng 2g + liánqiáo 2g + yúxīngcǎo 2g + yuǎnzhì 2g.	Wǔwèizǐ 5g + bànxià 5g + zhìgāncǎo 5g + cháihú 5g + gānjiāng 5g + huángqín 5g + chénpí 5-0g + dàhuáng 1-0g.
Máxìnggānshítāng 5g + dàzǎo 2g + tínglìzǐ 2g + zhǐshí 1-0g + chénpí 1-0g.	

Línguìshùgāntāng was introduced in Section 1.19 for dampness-removing and vertiginous syndromes. Wǔwèizǐ (Fructus Schisandrae Chinensis) "conserves the Lung, nourishes the Kidney, generates saliva, conserves sweat, astringes semen, stops diarrhea" and is used today for coughs and rhinitis (Wang, 2020). Máxìnggānshítāng (cf. Sections 1.47 and 2.43) was shown to be antitussive in guinea pigs and antipyretic in rats (Lin et al., 2016).

7.11　LARGE CONGENITAL MELANOCYTIC NEVUS

Large congenital melanocytic nevus (LCMN), also known as congenital pigmented nevus, is the formation at birth of a dark mole on the skin of the body, such as the trunk or limbs. As one grows up, the mole will increase in size at the same rate as the body grows and reach a giant size of 40 centimeters across. LCMN is caused by mutations in the *NRAS* gene, whose products transduce extracellular signals to the cellular nucleus to direct cell division and differentiation. The mutation occurs during early development of the fetus and is not inherited.

Huòxiāngzhèngqìsǎn, a formula for "wind-cold" infection and "dampness-retained" ingestion, was shown to alleviate colitis-associated cancer in mice through intestinal microbiota modulation, antioxidation, and antiinflammation (Dong et al., 2022). Yìgānsǎn, introduced in Sections 1.1,

TABLE 7.11

GMP Herbal Medicines for a Two-Year-Old Child with Large Congenital Melanocytic Nevus

Large congenital melanocytic nevus (OrphaCode: 626)

A disease with a prevalence of ~3 in 100,000

Modifying germline mutation: melanocortin 1 receptor (*MC1R* / Entrez: 4157) at 16q24.3

Disease-causing somatic mutation(s): NRAS proto-oncogene, GTPase (*NRAS* / Entrez: 4893) at 1p13.2

Not applicable

Abnormality of skin pigmentation, Nevus, Congenital giant melanocytic nevus

Generalized hirsutism, Neoplasm

Hydrocephalus, Pruritus, Hypopigmented skin patches, Seizure, Subcutaneous nodule, Rhabdomyosarcoma, Neoplasm of the skin, Cutaneous melanoma, Sarcoma

Neonatal, Infancy

Neoplasm (199):

Gānlùyǐn 5g + xiāngshāliùjūnzǐtāng 5g + shānzhā 1g + shénqū 1g + màiyá 1g.	Běishāshēn 5g + yùzhú 5g + hòupò
Gānlùyǐn 5g + qīngwèisǎn 5g.	5g + zhǐshí 5g + xuánshēn 5-4g +
Wǔlíngsǎn 5g + xiāngshāliùjūnzǐtāng 5g + huòxiāngzhèngqìsǎn 5-0g.	dìhuáng 5-4g + màiméndōng 5-4g +
Xiāngshāliùjūnzǐtāng 5g + shēnlíngbáizhúsǎn 5g + huòxiāngzhèngqìsǎn 5-0g + shānzhā 1-0g + báizhú 1-0g + hòupò 1-0g.	dàhuáng 2-0g.

Hydrocephalus (331.4, 331.3), Pruritus (D011537), Seizure (345.9):

Yìgānsǎn 5g + tiānmá 1g + shíchāngpú 1g + yuǎnzhì 1g + gōuténg 1-0g + fúshén 1-0g.	Báizhǐ 5g + gāncǎo 5-3g + shārén 5-3g + huángqín 5-0g + dàhuáng 1-0g.
Xiǎojiànzhōngtāng 5g + tiānmá 1g + shíchāngpú 1g + yuǎnzhì 1g + gōuténg 1g.	Huángqí 5g + chìsháo 1-0g + fángfēng 1-0g.
Bǔyánghuánwǔtāng 5g + tiānmá 1g + shíchāngpú 1g + yuǎnzhì 1g + gōuténg 1-0g.	

1.57, and 2.23 for epilepsy and in Section 1.43 for psychosis, "inhibits Liver Qi, suppresses muscle spasms, calms the mind" and is used today for neurotic disorders (Wang, 2019). Gān means the liver, which in TCM governs emotions. Yìgānsǎn is translated to "Liver-overcoming powder."

7.12 OCULOCUTANEOUS ALBINISM TYPE 2

Oculocutaneous albinism type 2 is characterized by reduced pigmentation of the skin, hair, and eye. Oculocutaneous albinism type 2 is caused by mutations in the *OCA2* gene, which is expressed in melanocytes, a specialized type of cells in the skin, hair, and eye, to produce the color substance, called *melanin*, for pigmentation and thus protection from ultraviolet light.

Zhǐqiào (bitter orange), Jílí (puncture vine caltrop fruit), Chántuì (cicada slough), Júhuā (Chrysanthemum flower), Júhóng (red tangerine peel), Gǒuqǐzǐ (wolfberry) and Gāncǎo (licorice)

TABLE 7.12

GMP Herbal Medicines for a One-Year-Old Infant with Oculocutaneous Albinism Type 2

Oculocutaneous albinism type 2 (OrphaCode: 79432)

A disease with a prevalence of ~3 in 100,000

Disease-causing germline mutation(s): OCA2 melanosomal transmembrane protein (*OCA2* / Entrez: 4948) at 15q12-q13.1

Modifying germline mutation: melanocortin 1 receptor (*MC1R* / Entrez: 4157) at 16q24.3

Autosomal recessive

Abnormality of refraction, Photophobia, Blue irides, Nystagmus, Hypopigmentation of the skin, Heterochromia iridis, Freckling, White eyebrow, Hypopigmentation of hair, Reduced visual acuity, Abnormality of retinal pigmentation, Iris hypopigmentation, Hypoplasia of the fovea, Macular hypopigmentation, White hair, Iris transillumination defect, Optic nerve misrouting

(Continued)

TABLE 7.12 *(Continued)*

GMP Herbal Medicines for a One-Year-Old Infant with Oculocutaneous Albinism Type 2

White eyelashes, Basal cell carcinoma, Squamous cell carcinoma of the skin, Cutaneous melanoma, Posterior staphyloma, Absent skin pigmentation

Neonatal, Infancy

Photophobia (D020795), Nystagmus (379.53, 379.55, 379.50):

Zīshènmíngmùtāng 5g + qǐjúdìhuángwán 2-0g + gǒuqǐzǐ 2-0g + júhuā 2-0g + gāncǎo 0g.	Zhǐqiào 5g + jílí 5-0g + chántuì 5-0g.
Qǐjúdìhuángwán 5g.	Chántuì 5g + zhǐqiào 4g + jílí 4g.
Xǐgānmíngmùtāng 5g + gāncǎo 1-0g + júhuā 1-0g.	Júhuā 5g + júhóng 2g.

are all edible (Xie et al., 2023). Nevertheless, their use by infants should be approved and monitored by licensed herbal medicine practitioners.

7.13 NON-EPIDERMOLYTIC PALMOPLANTAR KERATODERMA, BOTHNIA TYPE

Non-epidermolytic palmoplantar keratoderma (NEPPK), Bothnia type, also known as diffuse palmoplantar keratoderma, Bothnian type, is characterized by diffuse, homogeneous, and excessive thickening of the outermost layer of the skin of the palms and soles. NEPPK, Bothnia type, is caused by mutations in a gene that encodes a water channel protein that is important for fluid secretion.

TABLE 7.13

GMP Herbal Medicines for a Three-Year-Old Child with Non-Epidermolytic Palmoplantar Keratoderma, Bothnia Type

Non-epidermolytic palmoplantar keratoderma, Bothnia type (OrphaCode: 2337)

A disease with a prevalence of ~2 in 100,000

Disease-causing germline mutation(s) (gain of function): aquaporin 5 (*AQP5* / Entrez: 362) at 12q13.12

Autosomal dominant

Diffuse palmoplantar keratoderma

Pruritus, Abnormal blistering of the skin, Erythema, Papule, Skin ulcer

Infancy, Childhood

Pruritus (D011537), Erythema (D005483):

Wǔlíngsǎn 5g + gāncǎo 1-0g + báisháo 1-0g + tiáowèichéngqìtāng 0g + dàhuáng 0g.	Gāncǎo 5g + báizhǐ 5g + shārén 5g + huángqín 2-0g + dàhuáng 1-0g.

Tiáowèichéngqìtāng, translated to "Stomach modulating and Qi lifting decoction," comprises Dàhuáng and Mángxiāo (i.e., Natrii Sulfas; Mirabilite) to "purge heat and unplug obstruction." Elimination of stagnated heat/toxins is believed to alleviate skin conditions.

7.14 PSEUDOXANTHOMA ELASTICUM

Pseudoxanthoma elasticum (PXE), also known as Gronblad-Strandberg-Touraine syndrome, is characterized by mineralization and fragmentation of the elastic fibers in some parts of the body including the skin, eye, and cardiovascular system. PXE is caused by mutations in the *ABCC6* gene, whose products are involved in controlling the deposition of calcium and other minerals in the body.

Huángqín, annotated in detail in Section 5.7, was shown in cells and animal models to be cardioprotective (Chan et al., 2011), skin inflammation protective (Chi et al., 2003), ocular protective (Xiao et al., 2014), CNS neuroprotective (Zhao et al., 2020), and antitumor (Gu et al., 2022).

TABLE 7.14

GMP Herbal Medicines for a 20-Year-Old Adult with Pseudoxanthoma Elasticum

Pseudoxanthoma elasticum (OrphaCode: 758)

A disease with a prevalence of ~2 in 100,000

Disease-causing germline mutation(s) (loss of function): ATP binding cassette subfamily C member 6 (*ABCC6* / Entrez: 368) at 16p13.11

Disease-causing germline mutation(s): ectonucleotide pyrophosphatase/phosphodiesterase 1 (*ENPP1* / Entrez: 5167) at 6q23.2

Autosomal recessive

Thickened nuchal skin fold, Retinopathy, Retinal hemorrhage, Abnormality of the skin, Skin rash, Angioid streaks of the fundus, Malformation of the heart and great vessels, Excessive wrinkled skin, Arterial stenosis, Abnormality of the cerebral vasculature, Lack of skin elasticity

Myopia, Bruising susceptibility, Striae distensae

Nephrocalcinosis, High palate, Visual impairment, Blue sclerae, Abnormality of the thorax, Hypothyroidism, Hypertension, Hyperextensible skin, Pruritus, Multiple lipomas, Acne, Subcutaneous nodule, Mitral valve prolapse, Sudden cardiac death, Angina pectoris, Restrictive cardiomyopathy, Abnormality of thrombocytes, Postural instability, Gastrointestinal hemorrhage, Cerebral calcification, Dilatation, Atherosclerosis, Scoliosis, Abnormality of the endocardium, Hemiplegia/ hemiparesis, Joint hyperflexibility, Metamorphopsia, Telangiectasia of the skin

All ages

Retinopathy (362.9), Abnormality of the skin (702), Skin rash (782.1):

Qǐjúdìhuángwán 5g + dāngguīyǐnzǐ 5g + dānshēn 1g + chēqiánzǐ 1-0g + tùsīzǐ 1-0g + báixiānpí 1-0g + dìfūzǐ 1-0g + chìsháo 1-0g.

Zīshènmíngmùtāng 5g + xiāofēngsǎn 5-4g + báixiānpí 1g + dìfūzǐ 1g + jílí 1-0g + dānshēn 1g + chìsháo 1-0g + tǔfúlíng 1-0g.

Zhēnrénhuómìngyǐn 5g + jiāwèixiāoyáosǎn 4g + qǐjúdìhuángwán 4g + dānshēn 1g + báizhǐ 1g.

Báizhǐ 5g + gāncǎo 5-3g + huángqín 5-2g + shārén 4-3g + guālóugēn 3-2g + júhuā 2-0g + dàhuáng 1-0g.

Báizhǐ 5g + huángqín 5g + zhìgāncǎo 3g + shārén 3g + guālóugēn 2g + huángbò 2-0g + xìxīn 1g + dàhuáng 1-0g.

Myopia (367.1), Bruising susceptibility (D004438), Striae distensae (D057896):

Qǐjúdìhuángwán 5g + zīshènmíngmùtāng 5g.

Qǐjúdìhuángwán 5g + yìqìcōngmíngtāng 5g + shíchāngpú 1-0g + yuǎnzhì 1-0g.

Sāngjúyǐn 5g + zhǐqiào 1g.

Hángjú 5g + gǒuqǐzǐ 5g + shíchāngpú 3g + yuǎnzhì 3g + nǚzhēnzǐ 2-0g + gāncǎo 2-0g.

Zhǐqiào 5-4g + jílí 5-2g + chántuì 5-0g.

Visual impairment (D014786), Hypothyroidism (244.9), Hypertension (401-405.99), Pruritus (D011537), Multiple lipomas (214), Angina pectoris (D000787), Dilatation (442.9), Atherosclerosis (440):

Xǐgānmíngmùtāng 5g + zīshènmíngmùtāng 5g.

Qǐjúdìhuángwán 5g + xǐgānmíngmùtāng 5g + zīshènmíngmùtāng 5-0g + bǔyánghuánwǔtāng 5-0g + juémíngzǐ 1-0g + chōngwèizǐ 1-0g + gǔjīngcǎo 1-0g.

Huángqín 5g + báizhǐ 3-2g + zhìgāncǎo 2g + shārén 2g + tiānhuā 1-0g + guālóugēn 1-0g + dàhuáng 1-0g + huánglián 0g.

Qiānghuó 5g + hòupò 5g + zhǐshí 5g + huángqín 1g + huánglián 1g + dàhuáng 0g.

The multiple bioactive compounds in Huángqín, including flavonoids and glycosides, and the compounds' multiple targets account for the herb's multiple indications.

7.15 OCULOCUTANEOUS ALBINISM TYPE 1

Oculocutaneous albinism (OCA) affects the pigmentation of the skin, hair, iris, and retina. Different types of OCA are caused by different genes undergoing mutation. Oculocutaneous albinism type 1 is caused by mutations in the *TYR* gene, whose enzyme products are responsible for the first step in the production of melanin in melanocytes.

Yínqiàosǎn "clears heat, neutralizes pathogens" and is used for respiratory infections (Kim et al., 2023) with such viruses as adenoviruses, which can also affect the eye through the nasolacrimal system that provides an anatomical bridge between the respiratory and ocular tissues.

TABLE 7.15
GMP Herbal Medicines for a Two-Year-Old Child with Oculocutaneous Albinism Type 1

Oculocutaneous albinism type 1 (OrphaCode: 352731)

A disease with a prevalence of ~2 in 100,000

Disease-causing germline mutation(s) (loss of function): tyrosinase (*TYR* / Entrez: 7299) at 11q14.3

Autosomal recessive

Photophobia, Blue irides, Nystagmus, Abnormality of visual evoked potentials, Cutaneous photosensitivity, Generalized hypopigmentation, Reduced visual acuity, Depigmented fundus, Iris hypopigmentation, Hypoplasia of the fovea, Generalized hypopigmentation of hair, Iris transillumination defect, Optic nerve misrouting, Abnormal morphology of the choroidal vasculature

Strabismus, Amblyopia, White eyebrow, White eyelashes

Thickened skin

Neonatal, Infancy

Photophobia (D020795), Nystagmus (379.53, 379.55, 379.50):	
Xĭgānmíngmùtāng 5g + zīshènmíngmùtāng 5g.	Zhĭqiào 5g + jílí 5g + chántuì 5-0g + júhóng 4-0g.
Zīshènmíngmùtāng 5g + gŏuqĭzĭ 2-0g + júhuā 2-0g + gāncăo 1-0g.	Jílí 5g + chántuì 5g.
Strabismus (378.7, 378.6, 378.31), Amblyopia (368.01, 368.00):	
Sāngjúyĭn 5g + zhĭqiào 1g + jílí 1-0g.	Júhuā 5g + zhĭqiào 4g + jílí 4g.
Yínqiàosăn 5g + jílí 1g + chántuì 1-0g + zhĭqiào 1-0g.	Zhĭqiào 5g + jílí 2g.
Zhĭqiào 5g + chántuì 5g + gānlùyĭn 5g.	

7.16 MUCOUS MEMBRANE PEMPHIGOID

Mucous membrane pemphigoid, also known as cicatricial pemphigoid or mucosynechial pemphigoid, is characterized by the blistering and scarring of the mucous membrane, including the oral mucosa and conjunctiva. Mucous membrane pemphigoid is caused by autoantibodies against the so-called basement membrane zone proteins that glue the epithelium to the underlying tissues. The reason for the immunological attacks is unknown.

TABLE 7.16
GMP Herbal Medicines for a 65-Year-Old Adult with Mucous Membrane Pemphigoid

Mucous membrane pemphigoid (OrphaCode: 46486)

A disease with a prevalence of ~2 in 100,000

Not applicable

Autoimmunity, Oral mucosal blisters

Gingivitis, Atypical scarring of skin

Blindness, Corneal opacity, Abnormal blistering of the skin

Infancy, Childhood, Adolescent, Adult, Elderly

Gingivitis (523.0, 523.1):	
Yùnŭjiān 5g + qīngwèisăn 5g + gānlùyĭn 5-0g.	Báizhĭ 5g + gāncăo 4g + shārén 4g + huángqín 4-3g +
Qīngwèisăn 5g + huángliánjiědútāng 2g + shígāo 1-0g.	guālóugēn 2g + xìxīn 2-1g + dàhuáng 1g.
Qīngwèisăn 5g + gānlùyĭn 4-3g + shígāo 1-0g.	Báizhĭ 5g + zhìgāncăo 4g + shārén 4g + huángqín 4-0g +
	xìxīn 2-1g + dàhuáng 1-0g.
Blindness (D001766):	
Xĭgānmíngmùtāng 5g + mìmēnghuā 1-0g + liánqiáo 0g +	Qiānlĭguāng 5g + qīngxiāngzĭ 5g + căojuémíng 5-0g +
yúxīngcăo 0g.	huángqín 5-0g.
Xĭgānmíngmùtāng 5g + jīngfángbàidúsăn 5g + jīnyínhuā 1g.	Qīngxiāngzĭ 5g + liánqiáo 5g + júhuā 5-0g + căojuémíng
Xĭgānmíngmùtāng 5g + zīshènmíngmùtāng 5g.	5-0g + huángqín 5-0g.

Báizhǐ was summarized in Section 1.7 to be anti-inflammatory and to treat oral soft tissue diseases. Indeed, the topical application of Báizhǐ was demonstrated to ameliorate gingivitis by down-regulating the pro-inflammatory cytokines in the gingival tissue of rats with periodontitis (Lee et al., 2017). Qīngxiāngzǐ (cf. Sections 6.1 and 6.5) "clears Liver heat, improves eyesight, removes shades" and was summarized for its hepatoprotective, antitumor, antidiarrhea, antidiabetic, antioxidant, antihypertensive, and anti-ocular disease activities (Tang et al., 2016).

7.17 MULTIPLE SYMMETRIC LIPOMATOSIS

Multiple symmetric lipomatosis—also known as cephalothoracic lipodystrophy; familial benign cervical lipomatosis; Launois-Bensaude lipomatosis; and Madelung disease—is characterized by the growth of fatty tumors around the head, neck, shoulders, trunk, and hips. Multiple symmetric lipomatosis is caused by mutations in the *MFN2* gene, which encodes a mitochondrial membrane protein and is believed to play a role in obesity pathophysiology.

TABLE 7.17

GMP Herbal Medicines for a 50-Year-Old Man with Multiple Symmetric Lipomatosis

Multiple symmetric lipomatosis (OrphaCode: 2398)

A disease with a prevalence of ~2 in 100,000

Disease-causing germline mutation(s) (loss of function): mitofusin 2 (*MFN2* / Entrez: 9927) at 1p36.22

Autosomal dominant, Autosomal recessive, Mitochondrial inheritance, Not applicable

Multiple lipomas, Joint stiffness, Arthralgia, Abnormal adipose tissue morphology

Insulin resistance, Gait disturbance, Reduced tendon reflexes, Hepatomegaly, Paresthesia, Peripheral neuropathy

Childhood, Adolescent, Adult, Elderly

Multiple lipomas (214), Arthralgia (D018771):

Zhēnrénhuómìngyǐn 5g + sǎnzhǒngkuìjiāntāng 5g + sānléng 1-0g + éshù 1-0g + acupuncture.

Guìzhīfúlíngwán 5g + zhēnrénhuómìngyǐn 3g + xuánshēn 1g + mǔlì 1g + bèimǔ 1g + xiàkūcǎo 1g.

Sǎnzhǒngkuìjiāntāng 5g + xuèfǔzhúyūtāng 4-0g + èrchéntāng 4-0g + xiàkūcǎo 1g + xuánshēn 1-0g + mǔlì 1-0g + bèimǔ 1-0g + hǎizǎo 1-0g + sānléng 1-0g + éshù 1-0g.

Báijièzǐ 5g + kūnbù 5-0g + xiàkūcǎo 5-0g + bèimǔ 3-1g + hǎipiāoxiāo 2-0g + gāncǎo 0g.

Paresthesia (D010292):

Shēntòngzhúyūtāng 5g + dāngguīniàntòngtāng 5-0g + huángbò 1-0g + cāngzhú 1-0g + acupuncture.

Shēntòngzhúyūtāng 5g + shūjīnghuóxuètāng 5-0g + niúxī 1-0g + yánhúsuǒ 1-0g + acupuncture.

Wēilíngxiān 5g + báizhú 3g + qiānghuó 3g + xiāngfù 3g + huángqín 3g + cāngzhú 3g + tiānnánxīng 2g + bànxià 2g + gāncǎo 2g + shēngjiāng 2g + fúlíng 2g + chénpí 2g.

Wēilíngxiān 5g + chuānshānlóng 5g + mùguā 4g + niúxī 4g + hónghuā 4g + huángbò 4g + sānqī 4-0g + wǔjiāpí 4-0g + gǒujǐ 4-0g + dàhuáng 1-0g.

Báijièzǐ was introduced in Section 1.20 for lipoma. Zhēnrénhuómìngyǐn (cf. Sections 1.23 and 1.28) has been considered the holy medicine for swelling and ulcers on the body surface in TCM. Kūnbù (i.e., Kombu, or Kelp) "softens hardening, reduces mass, dissolves phlegm, clears heat, and promotes urination." Xiàkūcǎo (cf. Section 1.6) was shown to suppress the growth of human colon carcinoma cells via activation of a key tumor suppressor (Fang et al., 2017). Guìzhīfúlíngwán (cf. Sections 1.62 and 3.23) was shown to be an effective and safe adjuvant therapy for uterine fibroids in a systematic review and meta-analysis of 28 randomized controlled trials (Lei et al., 2023).

7.18 SYNDROMIC RECESSIVE X-LINKED ICHTHYOSIS

Syndromic recessive X-linked ichthyosis is characterized by skin scaling on the extensor surfaces of the limbs and side of the trunk. Syndromic recessive X-linked ichthyosis is caused by deletion or mutations in the *STS* gene, whose products metabolize cholesterol sulfate, the accumulation of which in skin cells clump skin cells into scales.

TABLE 7.18

GMP Herbal Medicines for a Three-Year-Old Boy with Syndromic Recessive X-Linked Ichthyosis

Syndromic recessive X-linked ichthyosis (OrphaCode: 281090)

A disease with a prevalence of ~1 in 100,000

Role: the phenotype of steroid sulfatase (*STS* / Entrez: 412) at Xp22.31

X-linked recessive

Hyperkeratosis, Hypohidrosis, Ichthyosis

Intellectual disability, Global developmental delay, Dysphasia, Attention deficit hyperactivity disorder, Corneal opacity

Cryptorchidism, Renal insufficiency, Unilateral renal agenesis, Hypogonadism, Autism, Seizure, Lissencephaly, Acute leukemia, Abnormality of the stomach, Abnormality of the abdominal wall, Short stature, Abdominal wall defect, Testicular seminoma

Childhood

Hypohidrosis (705.0):

Yùpíngfēngsǎn 5g + bǔzhōngyìqìtāng 5g + guìzhītāng 5-0g.

Yùpíngfēngsǎn 5-4g + guìzhītāng 5-0g + fúxiǎomài 1g + máhuánggēn 1g + mǔlì 1-0g.

Huángqí 5g + báizhú 4-2g + fángfēng 4-2g.

Máhuánggēn 5g + huángqí 5-4g + fúxiǎomài 5-0g + fángfēng 2-1g + mǔlì 2-0g + gāncǎo 0g.

Intellectual disability (D008607):

Xìngsūyǐnyòukē 5g + xīnyíqīngfèitāng 5g + cāngěrsǎn 5g.

Xiǎojiànzhōngtāng 5g + yùpíngfēngsǎn 5g.

Sìjūnzǐtāng 5g + shānzhā 1g + shénqū 1g + màiyá 1g.

Guìzhītāng 5g + báisháo 1-0g + xìngrén 1-0g + hòupò 1-0g.

Xuánshēn 5g + dìhuáng 5g + màiméndōng 5g + hòupò 5-1g + zhǐshí 5-1g + dàhuáng 1-0g.

Cryptorchidism (752.51), Renal insufficiency (586), Autism (299.0), Seizure (345.9):

Cháihújiālónggǔmǔlìtāng 5g + wēndǎntāng 5g + shíchāngpú 2-1g + yuǎnzhì 2-1g.

Liùwèidìhuángwán 5g + tiānmá 1g + shíchāngpú 1g + bózǐrén 1g + yuǎnzhì 1g + suānzǎorén 1g.

Bāwèidìhuángwán 5g + wēndǎntāng 4g + shíchāngpú 1g + yuǎnzhì 1g + gōuténg 1g.

Huángqín 5g + báizhǐ 4g + gāncǎo 3-2g + shārén 3-2g + dàhuáng 1-0g + acupuncture.

Xuánshēn (cf. Section 1.3) was reviewed and summarized to have anti-amnesic and antidepressant effects in mice (Lee et al., 2021). Xìngsūyǐnyòukē contains Zǐsūyè, which was also shown to be antidepressive in mice (Takeda et al., 2002). Sìjūnzǐtāng and Yùpíngfēngsǎn were shown to improve the immune function of rats with a TCM spleen deficiency by influencing the genetic expression of the JAK-STAT signal pathway in the brain (Xiong & Qian, 2013). Bāwèidìhuángwán was introduced in Section 2.19 for diabetes mellitus, disorders of the back, and chronic glomerulonephritis by "warming/nourishing the lower body and supplementing the Kidney yang." Bāwèidìhuángwán is derived from Liùwèidìhuángwán by adding two warm herbs. Bāwèidìhuángwán is, therefore, more often prescribed to patients with TCM kidney yang deficiency manifesting muscle weakness and back pain.

7.19 NEUROCUTANEOUS MELANOCYTOSIS

Neurocutaneous melanocytosis (NCM), also called neurocutaneous melanosis, is characterized by the presence of large congenital melanocytic nevi on the skin and melanocytic tumors in the CNS. The cause of NCM is not clear; however, post-zygotic mutations in a cell division regulating gene in melanocyte precursor cells may be to blame.

TABLE 7.19

GMP Herbal Medicines for a Three-Year-Old Child with Neurocutaneous Melanocytosis

Neurocutaneous melanocytosis (OrphaCode: 2481)

A disease with a prevalence of ~1 in 100,000

Not applicable

Melanocytic nevus, Thickened skin, Intellectual disability, Seizure, Generalized hirsutism, Numerous congenital melanocytic nevi, Generalized hyperpigmentation

Chorioretinal coloboma, Behavioral abnormality, Hemiparesis, Dandy-Walker malformation, Death in infancy, Ventriculomegaly, Intracranial hemorrhage, Abnormality of neuronal migration, Arnold-Chiari malformation, EEG abnormality, Encephalitis, Meningocele, Neoplasm, Melanoma, Syringomyelia, Venous thrombosis, Cranial nerve paralysis, Aplasia/Hypoplasia of the cerebellum, Abnormality of retinal pigmentation, Renal hypoplasia/aplasia

Childhood

Intellectual disability (D008607), Seizure (345.9):

Cháihújiālónggǔmǔlìtāng 5g + tiānmá 1-0g + shíchāngpú 1-0g + yuǎnzhì 1-0g + chántuì 1-0g + gōuténg 1-0g.	Xuánshēn 5g + dìhuáng 5g + màiméndōng 5g + hòupò 5-1g + zhǐshí 5-1g + dàhuáng 1-0g.
Wēndǎntāng 5g + tiānmá 1g + shíchāngpú 1g + yuǎnzhì 1g + gōuténg 1g.	
Yìgānsǎn 5g + guìzhījiālónggǔmǔlìtāng 5g + shíchāngpú 1g + yuǎnzhì 1g + gōuténg 1g.	

Hemiparesis (D010291), Intracranial hemorrhage (D020300) [Unspecified intracranial hemorrhage (432.9)], Neoplasm (199), Cranial nerve paralysis (352.9):

Xìngsūyǐnyòukē 5g + xīnyíqīngfèitāng 5-0g + shēnlíngbáizhúsǎn 4-0g + bèimǔ 1g + jiégěng 1g + qiánhú 1-0g + acupuncture.	Gāncǎo 5g + báizhǐ 5-0g + shārén 5-0g + dàhuáng 1g.
Xìngsūyǐnyòukē 5g + máxìnggānshítāng 5-0g + bèimǔ 1g + qiánhú 1g + jiégěng 1-0g + sāngbáipí 1-0g + guālóurén 1-0g + acupuncture.	Huángqín 5g + báizhǐ 2g + gāncǎo 2g + jīnyínhuā 2g + shārén 2g + dàhuáng 1g.
Wēndǎntāng 5g + xìngsūyǐnyòukē 5-0g + xiāngshāliùjūnzǐtāng 5-0g + shíchāngpú 2-1g + yuǎnzhì 2-1g + acupuncture.	

Màiméndōng (cf. Section 1.27) was shown to protect against cell injury in PC-12 cells (Liu & Li, 2018) that were originated from a neuroendocrine tumor of the rat adrenal medulla for neuroscience research. Note that heat-, dampness-, and toxin-clearing herbs such as Huángqín, Jīnyínhuā, and Gāncǎo are recommended for hand, foot, and mouth disease due to enteroviruses (Wang et al., 2016), which can cause neurological symptoms such as hemiparesis in children. Xìngsūyǐnyòukē contains Huángqín, Màiméndōng, and Gāncǎo. Furthermore, amygdalin, the main ingredient in Xìngrén (cf. Section 1.12), which is the major herb of Xìngsūyǐnyòukē, was shown to reduce the levels of chronic bee paralysis virus in honeybees (Tauber et al., 2020).

7.20 PEMPHIGUS FOLIACEUS

Pemphigus foliaceus is an autoimmune blistering disease characterized by blistering, erosions, and crusts on the superficial skin without mucosal involvement. Pemphigus foliaceus is caused by the attacks of autoantibodies on the desmogleins in the skin that mediate cell-cell adhesion against mechanical stress.

TABLE 7.20

GMP Herbal Medicines for a 55-Year-Old Adult with Pemphigus Foliaceus

Pemphigus foliaceus (OrphaCode: 79481)

A disease with a prevalence of ~1 in 100,000

Not applicable

Autoimmunity, Acantholysis

Pruritus, Abnormality of the scalp, Crusting erythematous dermatitis, Abnormal blistering of the skin, Erythema,
 Erythematous plaque, Scaling skin, Skin erosion

Oral ulcer, Erythroderma, Abnormal oral mucosa morphology, Skin vesicle

Pruritus (D011537), Erythema (D005483):

Wǔlíngsǎn 5g + lǐzhōngtāng 5-0g + fùzǐ 2-0g + huángqín 1-0g + tiáowèichéngqìtāng 0g.	Gāncǎo 5g + báizhǐ 5g + shārén 5g + huángqín 5-0g + tiānhuā 2-0g + xìxīn 2-0g + dàhuáng 1-0g.

Wǔlíngsǎn was introduced in Sections 1.15 and 7.9 to treat skin conditions. Lǐzhōngtāng was introduced in Sections 2.28 and 3.14 to improve digestion. Tiáowèichéngqìtāng (cf. Section 7.13) was demonstrated to be a laxative in mice (Tseng et al., 2006). Modern Taiwanese complementary medicine using GMP-concentrated herbal extract granules is holistic in the sense that it considers different physiological systems of the body as a whole, where systems interact. So, improving body fluid homeostasis together with nutrient absorption and waste elimination can better help the skin.

REFERENCES

Chan, E., Liu, X. X., Guo, D. J., Kwan, Y. W., Leung, G. P., Lee, S. M., & Chan, S. W. (2011). Extract of *Scutellaria baicalensis* Georgi root exerts protection against myocardial ischemia-reperfusion injury in rats. *American Journal of Chinese Medicine*, 39(04), 693–704. https://doi.org/10.1142/s0192415x 11009135

Chi, Y. S., Lim, H., Park, H., & Kim, H. P. (2003). Effects of wogonin, a plant flavone from *Scutellaria radix*, on skin inflammation: In vivo regulation of inflammation-associated gene expression. *Biochemical Pharmacology*, 66(7), 1271–1278. https://doi.org/10.1016/s0006-2952(03)00463-5

Dong, M., Liu, H., Cao, T., Li, L., Sun, Z., Qiu, Y., & Wang, D. (2022). Huoxiang Zhengqi alleviates azoxymethane/dextran sulfate sodium-induced colitis-associated cancer by regulating Nrf2/NF-κB/NLRP3 signaling. *Frontiers in Pharmacology*, 13. https://doi.org/10.3389/fphar.2022.1002269

Fang, Y., Zhang, L., Feng, J., Lin, W., Cai, Q., & Peng, J. (2017). Spica Prunellae extract suppresses the growth of human colon carcinoma cells by targeting multiple oncogenes via activating miR-34a. *Oncology Reports*, 38(3), 1895–1901. https://doi.org/10.3892/or.2017.5792

Fu, H., Li, W., Weng, Z., Huang, Z., Liu, J., Mao, Q., & Ding, B. (2023). Water extract of cacumen platycladi promotes hair growth through the Akt/GSK3β/β-catenin signaling pathway. *Frontiers in Pharmacology*, 14. https://doi.org/10.3389/fphar.2023.1038039

Gu, Y., Zheng, Q., Fan, G., & Liu, R. (2022). Advances in anti-cancer activities of flavonoids in *Scutellariae radix*: Perspectives on mechanism. *International Journal of Molecular Sciences*, 23(19), 11042. https://doi.org/10.3390/ijms231911042

Huang, X., Ding, C., Liang, H., Xiong, S., & Li, L. (2019). Research on herb pairs of classical formulae of ZHANG Zhong-Jing using big data technology. *Digital Chinese Medicine*, 2(4), 195–206. https://doi.org/10.1016/j.dcmed.2020.01.001

Hwang, J., & Lio, P. A. (2021). Acupuncture in dermatology: An update to a systematic review. *Journal of Alternative and Complementary Medicine*, 27(1), 12–23. https://doi.org/10.1089/acm.2020.0230

Ikarashi, N., Ogiue, N., Toyoda, E., Kon, R., Ishii, M., Toda, T., Aburada, T., Ochiai, W., & Sugiyama, K. (2012). *Gypsum fibrosum* and its major component $CaSO_4$ increase cutaneous aquaporin-3 expression levels. *Journal of Ethnopharmacology*, 139(2), 409–413. https://doi.org/10.1016/j.jep.2011.11.025

Kim, K., Hong, M., Park, Y., Lee, B., Kim, K., Kang, B., & Choi, J. (2023). Effects of herbal medicines (*Eunkyosan/Yin qiao san* and *Samsoeum/Shen su yin*) for treating the common cold: A randomized, placebo-controlled, multicenter clinical trial. *Integrative Medicine Research*, 12(4), 101005. https://doi.org/10.1016/j.imr.2023.101005

Lee, H., Kim, H., Lee, D., Choi, B., & Yang, S. H. (2021). *Scrophulariae radix*: An overview of its biological activities and nutraceutical and pharmaceutical applications. *Molecules, 26*(17), 5250. https://doi.org/10.3390/molecules26175250

Lee, H. J., Lee, H., Kim, M. H., Choi, Y. Y., Ahn, K. S., Um, J., & Lee, S. (2017). *Angelica dahurica* ameliorates the inflammation of gingival tissue via regulation of pro-inflammatory mediators in experimental model for periodontitis. *Journal of Ethnopharmacology, 205*, 16–21. https://doi.org/10.1016/j.jep.2017.04.018

Lei, Y., Yang, L., Yang, H., Li, M., Ou, L., Yang, B., Dong, T., Gao, F., & Wei, P. (2023). The efficacy and safety of Chinese herbal medicine Guizhi Fuling capsule combined with low dose mifepristone in the treatment of uterine fibroids: A systematic review and meta-analysis of 28 randomized controlled trials. *BMC Complementary Medicine and Therapies, 23*(1). https://doi.org/10.1186/s12906-023-03842-y

Lin, Y., Chang, C., & Wu, C. (2016). Antitussive, anti-pyretic and toxicological evaluation of Ma-Xing-Gan-Shi-Tang in rodents. *BMC Complementary and Alternative Medicine, 16*(1). https://doi.org/10.1186/s12906-016-1440-2

Liu, R., & Li, X. (2018). *Radix Ophiopogonis* polysaccharide extracts alleviate MPP+-induced PC-12 cell injury through inhibition of Notch signaling pathway. *International Journal of Clinical and Experimental Pathology, 11*(1), 99–109. https://pubmed.ncbi.nlm.nih.gov/31938091

Łuszczki, J. J., Głowniak, K., & Czuczwar, S. J. (2007). Time–course and dose–response relationships of imperatorin in the mouse maximal electroshock seizure threshold model. *Neuroscience Research, 59*(1), 18–22. https://doi.org/10.1016/j.neures.2007.05.004

Takeda, H., Tsuji, M., Matsumiya, T., & Kubo, M. (2002). Identification of rosmarinic acid as a novel antidepressive substance in the leaves of Perilla frutescens Britton var. acuta Kudo (Perillae Herba). *Nihon Shinkei Seishin Yakurigaku Zasshi, 22*(1), 15–22. https://pubmed.ncbi.nlm.nih.gov/11917505

Tang, Y., Xin, H., & Guo, M. (2016). Review on research of the phytochemistry and pharmacological activities of *Celosia argentea*. *Revista Brasileira De Farmacognosia, 26*(6), 787–796. https://doi.org/10.1016/j.bjp.2016.06.001

Tauber, J. P., Tozkar, C. Ö., Schwarz, R. S., Lopez, D., Irwin, R. E., Adler, L. S., & Evans, J. D. (2020). Colony-level effects of amygdalin on honeybees and their microbes. *Insects, 11*(11), 783. https://doi.org/10.3390/insects11110783

Tsai, C., Chou, Y., Chen, Y., Tang, Y., Ho, H., & Chen, D. (2014). Effect of the herbal drug Guilu Erxian Jiao on muscle strength, articular pain, and disability in elderly men with knee osteoarthritis. *Evidence-Based Complementary and Alternative Medicine, 2014*, 1–9. https://doi.org/10.1155/2014/297458

Tseng, S., Lee, H. H., Chen, L. G., Wu, C. H., & Wang, C. C. (2006). Effects of three purgative decoctions on inflammatory mediators. *Journal of Ethnopharmacology, 105*(1–2), 118–124. https://doi.org/10.1016/j.jep.2005.10.003

Van Den Berg-Wolf, M., & Burgoon, T. (2017). Acupuncture and cutaneous medicine: Is it effective? *Medical Acupuncture, 29*(5), 269–275. https://doi.org/10.1089/acu.2017.1227

Wang, M., Tao, L., & Xu, H. (2016). Chinese herbal medicines as a source of molecules with anti-enterovirus 71 activity. *Chinese Medicine, 11*(1). https://doi.org/10.1186/s13020-016-0074-0

Wang, S.-C. (2019). Therapeutic classes of CHEG formulas. In S.-C. Wang (Ed.), *Clinical herbal prescriptions: Principles and practices of herbal formulations from deep learning health insurance herbal prescription big data* (pp. 16–89). World Scientific Publishing. https://doi.org/10.1142/11211

Wang, S.-C. (2020). Modern therapeutic uses of CHEG herbs and herb pairs. In S.-C. Wang (Ed.), *Veterinary herbal pharmacopoeia* (pp. 35–233). Nova Science Publishers. https://doi.org/10.52305/GHTR1903

Xiao, J. R., Do, C. W., & To, C. H. (2014). Potential therapeutic effects of baicalein, baicalin, and wogonin in ocular disorders. *Journal of Ocular Pharmacology and Therapeutics, 30*(8), 605–614. https://doi.org/10.1089/jop.2014.0074

Xie, X., Guo, H., Liu, J., Wang, J., Li, H., & Deng, Z. (2023). Edible and medicinal progress of *Cryptotympana atrata* (Fabricius) in China. *Nutrients, 15*(19), 4266. https://doi.org/10.3390/nu15194266

Xiong, B., & Qian, H. (2013). Effects of Sijunzi decoction and Yupingfeng powder on expression of janus kinase-signal transducer and activator of transcription signal pathway in the brain of spleen-deficiency model rats. *Journal of Traditional Chinese Medicine, 33*(1), 78–84. https://doi.org/10.1016/s0254-6272(13)60105-3

Zhao, F., Zhang, C., Xiao, D., Zhang, W., Zhou, L., Gu, S., & Qu, R. (2020). Radix Scutellariae ameliorates stress-induced depressive-like behaviors via protecting neurons through the TGFβ3-Smad2/3-Nedd9 signaling pathway. *Neural Plasticity, 2020*, 1–13. https://doi.org/10.1155/2020/8886715

8 GMP Herbal Medicine for Rare Endocrine Diseases

The endocrine system in humans comprises glands, including the hypothalamus, pituitary, pineal, thyroid, parathyroid, thymus, pancreas, adrenal glands, and testicles/ovaries, that secrete signaling molecules, called *hormones*, directly into the bloodstream to target distant organs and glands to regulate our body's growth, development, metabolism, digestion, mood, sleep, and reproduction. Damage of the gland due to infection, medication, gene mutation, or tumor can lead to insufficient or excessive hormone secretion, causing endocrine diseases. Only some of the rare endocrine diseases of this chapter are early-onset genetic.

The single herbs and multi-herb formulas that are most frequently discussed for the signs and symptoms of the rare endocrine diseases are Rhubarb Root and Rhizome (Dàhuáng), Licorice Root (Gāncǎo), Figwort Root (Xuánshēn), Oyster Shell (Mǔlì), Dahurian Angelica Root (Báizhǐ), Prunella Spike (Xiàkūcǎo), Scutellaria Root (Huángqín), Fritillaria Bulb (Bèimǔ), Cardamon Seed (Shārén), Trichosanthes Root (Tiānhuā), Rehmannia Root (Dìhuáng), Immature Bitter Orange (Zhǐshí), Free and Easy Wanderer Plus (Augmented Rambling Powder; Jiāwèixiāoyáosǎn), Disperse the Swelling and Break the Hardness Decoction (Sǎnzhǒngkuìjiāntāng), Five Ingredient Formula with Poria (Wǔlíngsǎn), Lycium, Chrysanthemum and Rehmannia Pill (Qǐjúdìhuángwán), Prepared Licorice Decoction (Zhìgāncǎotāng), Ginseng, Astragalus and Pueraria Combination (Yìqìcōngmíngtāng), Regulate the Stomach and Order the Qi Decoction (Tiáowèichéngqìtāng), Regulate the Middle Decoction (Lǐzhōngtāng), Siler and Platycodon Formula (Fángfēngtōngshèngsǎn), Pogostemon Correct the Qi Powder (Huòxiāngzhèngqìsǎn), Aucklandia, Cardamon and the Six Gentlemen Decoction (Xiāngshāliùjūnzǐtāng), and Drive Out Stasis from the Mansion of Blood Decoction (Xuèfǔzhúyūtāng).

The network of glands secretes hormones to influence one another and the levels of different hormones are maintained in equilibrium through a feedback mechanism; an undersecretion of one hormone can lead to over-secretion of the other, breaking the balance. The hormonal balance is related to the concept of the yin yang balance in traditional Chinese medicine (TCM). Indeed, it was clinically found that individuals with a yin deficiency phenotype are related to disturbances in the hypothalamus-pituitary-adrenal axis, and hypothalamus-pituitary-thyroid axis (Wang et al., 2010). Xuánshēn is renowned for its yin-nourishing effect in TCM.

8.1 PROLACTINOMA

Prolactinoma, also known as pituitary lactotrophic adenoma or prolactin-secreting pituitary adenoma, is a benign tumor of the pituitary gland in the brain, resulting in overproduction of a reproduction hormone called *prolactin,* which stimulates the mammary glands to produce milk. As excessive prolactin reduces levels of sex hormones, prolactinoma can cause infertility in men and women. In addition, as the tumor grows in size, the neighboring regions in the brain are affected, causing headaches, vision problems, and so on.

Mǔdānpí was introduced in Section 4.20 to be anticancer. Zhīmǔ (cf. Sections 2.35, 4.30, and 5.15) was shown to be antiproliferative in human breast cancer cells (Kim et al., 2007). Dúhuójìshēngtāng (cf. Section 2.10) "benefits the Liver/Kidney, replenishes Qi/Blood, dispels wind-dampness, stops numbness/pain" and is used today for disorders of the back and joints (Wang, 2019). Zhúyèshígāotāng (cf. Sections 1.52 and 3.11) is used today for such general symptoms as alteration of consciousness,

DOI: 10.1201/9781032726625-8

TABLE 8.1
GMP Herbal Medicines for a 20-Year-Old Adult with Prolactinoma

Prolactinoma (OrphaCode: 2965)

A disease with a prevalence of ~5 in 10,000

Major susceptibility factor: cadherin-related 23 (*CDH23* / Entrez: 64072) at 10q22.1

Major susceptibility factor: menin 1 (*MEN1* / HGNC:7010) at 11q13

Major susceptibility factor: aryl hydrocarbon receptor interacting protein (*AIP* / Entrez: 9049) at 11q13.2

Autosomal dominant

Male hypogonadism, Hypogonadotrophic hypogonadism, Amenorrhea, Female hypogonadism, Hypogonadism, Abnormality of the menstrual cycle, Impotence, Irregular menstruation, Decreased fertility in females, Low gonadotropins (secondary hypogonadism), Decreased fertility in males, Abnormality of the pituitary gland, Decreased female libido, Erectile dysfunction, Galactorrhea

Progressive visual loss, Gynecomastia, Osteopenia, Osteoporosis, Pallor, Headache, Vomiting, Nausea and vomiting, Hypotension, Decreased circulating ACTH level, Easy fatigability, Secondary growth hormone deficiency, Pituitary hypothyroidism, Abnormality of hair density, Central adrenal insufficiency, Adrenocorticotropin deficient adrenal insufficiency, Adrenocorticotropic hormone deficiency, Fatigue, Dyspareunia

Ptosis, Blindness, Diplopia, Delayed puberty, Anterior hypopituitarism, Growth hormone excess, Sudden loss of visual acuity, Seizure, Cranial nerve paralysis, Vertigo, Cranial nerve VI palsy, Fourth cranial nerve palsy, Internal ophthalmoplegia, Oculomotor nerve palsy, Hemianopia, Heteronymous hemianopia, Bitemporal hemianopia

Childhood, Adolescent, Adult, Elderly

Gynecomastia (778.7), Osteoporosis (733.0), Pallor (D010167), Headache (D006261), Vomiting (D014839), Fatigue (D005221):

Dúhuójìshēngtāng 5g + dùzhòng 1g + jīxuèténg 1-0g + xùduàn 1-0g.

Sānzhǒngkuìjiāntāng 5g + dāngguīsìnìtāng 5-0g + lóngdǎnxiègāntāng 2-0g + jīxuèténg 2-0g + mǔdānpí 1-0g + zhīmǔ 1-0g.

Yòuguīwán 5g + dāngguīsìnìtāng 5g + bājǐtiān 2g + yínyánghuò 2g.

Bāwèidìhuángwán 5g + dúhuójìshēngtāng 5-0g + bājǐtiān 1g + yínyánghuò 1g + ròucōngróng 1-0g + bǔgǔzhī 1-0g.

Bǔzhōngyìqìtāng 5g + guīpítāng 5g + jīxuèténg 1g.

Mǔdānpí 5g + zhīmǔ 5g + gégēn 5-0g + cāngzhú 5-0g + huáihuā 5-0g + shígāo 2-0g.

Huáihuā 5g + cāngzhú 5-2g + jīxuèténg 5-2g + mǔdānpí 2-0g.

Bànzhīlián 5g + cāngzhú 2g + mǔdānpí 2-0g + huáihuā 2-0g.

Ptosis (374.3), Blindness (D001766), Diplopia (D004172), Seizure (345.9), Cranial nerve paralysis (352.9), Vertigo (386.2), Oculomotor nerve palsy (378.51, 378.52), Hemianopia (D006423):

Zhúyèshígāotāng 5g + wēndǎntāng 5g + yìmǔcǎo 2g + xiàkūcǎo 1g + dàhuáng 0g.

Zhúyèshígāotāng 5g + qǐjúdìhuángwán 4g + máxìnggānshítāng 3-0g + yìmǔcǎo 2-0g + zélán 2-0g + xiàkūcǎo 1g + gōuténg 1-0g.

Xiǎocháihútāng 5g + qǐjúdìhuángwán 5g + língguìshùgāntāng 5g + xiàkūcǎo 1g.

Qǐjúdìhuángwán 5g + jiāwèixiāoyáosǎn 4g + xiāngshāliùjūnzǐtāng 4-0g + tiānmá 2-0g + gōuténg 2-0g + xiàkūcǎo 1g + cǎojuémíng 1-0g.

Tiānmágōuténgyǐn 5g + qǐjúdìhuángwán 3g + yìmǔcǎo 1g + zélán 1g + hónghuā 0g.

Huángqín 5g + báizhǐ 5-3g + shārén 4-2g + tiānhuā 2g + gāncǎo 2-0g + dàhuáng 1-0g.

Huángqí 5g + fángfēng 3-1g + gǒuqǐzǐ 3-0g + júhuā 3-0g + dāngguī 3-0g + huánglián 1g + chìsháo 1-0g + xìxīn 1-0g + dàhuáng 0g.

Dìhuáng 5g + fángfēng 5g + gǒuqǐzǐ 5g + júhuā 5g + dāngguī 5g + xìxīn 2g + huánglián 2g.

hallucinations, syncope, convulsions, dizziness/vertigo, sleep disturbance, fever, malaise/fatigue, and excessive sweating (Wang, 2019).

8.2 MODY

MODY (maturity-onset diabetes of the young) is caused by mutations in a single gene, resulting in the disruption of insulin production by, or release from, the pancreatic beta cells and thus high levels of sugar in the patient's blood. The degree of insulin deficiency and age of disease onset depend on the specific mutant gene that causes MODY.

TABLE 8.2
GMP Herbal Medicines for a 25-Year-Old Adult with MODY

MODY (OrphaCode: 552)

A disease with a prevalence of ~3 in 10,000

Disease-causing germline mutation(s): ATP binding cassette subfamily C member 8 (*ABCC8* / Entrez: 6833) at 11p15.1

Disease-causing germline mutation(s): carboxyl ester lipase (*CEL* / Entrez: 1056) at 9q34.13

Disease-causing germline mutation(s): glucokinase (*GCK* / Entrez: 2645) at 7p13

Disease-causing germline mutation(s): hepatocyte nuclear factor 4 alpha (*HNF4A* / Entrez: 3172) at 20q13.12

Disease-causing germline mutation(s): potassium inwardly rectifying channel subfamily J member 11 (*KCNJ11* / Entrez: 3767) at 11p15.1

Disease-causing germline mutation(s): KLF transcription factor 11 (*KLF11* / Entrez: 8462) at 2p25.1

Disease-causing germline mutation(s): neuronal differentiation 1 (*NEUROD1* / Entrez: 4760) at 2q31.3

Disease-causing germline mutation(s): pancreatic and duodenal homeobox 1 (*PDX1* / Entrez: 3651) at 13q12.2

Disease-causing germline mutation(s): HNF1 homeobox A (*HNF1A* / Entrez: 6927) at 12q24.31

Disease-causing germline mutation(s): insulin (*INS* / Entrez: 3630) at 11p15.5

Disease-causing germline mutation(s): paired box 4 (*PAX4* / Entrez: 5078) at 7q32.1

Disease-causing germline mutation(s): BLK proto-oncogene, Src family tyrosine kinase (*BLK* / Entrez: 640) at 8p23.1

Disease-causing germline mutation(s) (loss of function): adaptor protein, phosphotyrosine interacting with PH domain and leucine zipper 1 (*APPL1* / Entrez: 26060) at 3p14.3

Autosomal dominant, Not applicable

Glucose intolerance, Hyperglycemia, Glycosuria, Abnormal oral glucose tolerance, Abnormal C-peptide level, Abnormal insulin level, Hypoinsulinemia, Elevated hemoglobin A1c

Nephropathy, Retinopathy, Hyperinsulinemic hypoglycemia, Insulin-resistant diabetes mellitus, Intrauterine growth retardation, Large for gestational age, Neonatal hypoglycemia, Transient neonatal diabetes mellitus, Overweight

Childhood, Adolescent, Adult

Retinopathy (362.9):

Zīshènmíngmùtāng 5g + yìqìcōngmíngtāng 4-3g + xuèfǔzhúyūtāng 2-0g + tùsīzǐ 1-0g.	Gǒuqǐzǐ 5g + júhuā 5g + dìhuáng 4-0g + dāngguī 4-0g + fángfēng 4-0g + niúbàngzǐ 4-0g + shègān 4-0g + xìxīn 2-1g + huánglián 2-1g.
Qǐjúdìhuángwán 5g + yìqìcōngmíngtāng 5-3g + xuèfǔzhúyūtāng 2g.	Nǚzhēnzǐ 5g + tiānméndōng 2g + mǔdānpí 2g + chuānxiōng 2g + júhuā 2g + huángqín 2g + bǔgǔzhī 2g + fúlíng 2-0g + báizhú 2-0g + fùzǐ 2-0g + bòhé 2-0g + jílí 2-0g.

Nǚzhēnzǐ (cf. Section 1.20) was shown in rats to ameliorate retinal neovascularization (Wu et al., 2016), which can result in vitreous hemorrhage, tractional retinal detachment, and macular edema in patients with diabetic retinopathy. The term cōngmíng in Yìqìcōngmíngtāng means "acuity in auditory-visual perception."

8.3 NON-FUNCTIONING PITUITARY ADENOMA

Non-functioning pituitary adenoma (NFPA) is a benign tumor of the pituitary gland. NFPA presents with no symptoms until the tumor grows too large, pressing against brain regions, including the pituitary gland and optic nerves to cause headaches, vision defects, and hypopituitarism. What causes NFPA is not known.

Màiyá (cf. Section 3.12) was shown in rats to reduce hyperprolactinemia (Wang et al., 2014), which can be caused by a benign tumor in the pituitary gland. Màiyá is used today for problems with digestion and disorder of lactation (Wang, 2020). Báisháo (cf. Section 3.10) was demonstrated to significantly reverse hypertension and also alleviate liver damage in hypertensive rats (Chen et al., 2015); it is used for hypertension (Wang, 2020), which is prevalent in adult patients with hypopituitarism (Deepak et al., 2007). Zhǐshí (cf. Section 3.13) was shown to have anticoagulative and gastrointestinal motility regulative activities in mice (Tan et al., 2017); it is used for constipation and

TABLE 8.3

GMP Herbal Medicines for a 60-Year-Old Adult with Non-Functioning Pituitary Adenoma

Non-functioning pituitary adenoma (OrphaCode: 91349)

A disease with a prevalence of ~3 in 10,000

Not applicable

Male hypogonadism, Hypogonadotrophic hypogonadism, Female hypogonadism, Hypogonadism, Abnormality of the menstrual cycle, Progressive visual loss, Impotence, Growth hormone deficiency, Anterior hypopituitarism, Increased circulating gonadotropin level, Irregular menstruation, Adrenal insufficiency, Decreased fertility in females, Pallor, Vomiting, Nausea and vomiting, Headache, Hypotension, Decreased circulating ACTH level, Low gonadotropins (secondary hypogonadism), Easy fatigability, Secondary growth hormone deficiency, Pituitary hypothyroidism, Increased intraabdominal fat, Anemia of inadequate production, Abnormality of hair density, Central adrenal insufficiency, Adrenocorticotropin deficient adrenal insufficiency, Adrenocorticotropic hormone deficiency, Abnormal muscle physiology, Decreased fertility in males, Fatigue, Abnormality of the pituitary gland, Decreased female libido, Hypopituitarism, Erectile dysfunction

Macroorchidism, Ptosis, Blindness, Diplopia, Panhypopituitarism, Central diabetes insipidus, Diabetes insipidus, Sudden loss of visual acuity, Seizure, Cranial nerve paralysis, Macroorchidism, postpubertal, Vertigo, Cranial nerve VI palsy, Fourth cranial nerve palsy, Internal ophthalmoplegia, Reduced circulating prolactin concentration, Oculomotor nerve palsy, Hemianopia, Increased serum testosterone level, Heteronymous hemianopia, Bitemporal hemianopia

Childhood, Adolescent, Adult

Pallor (D010167), Vomiting (D014839), Headache (D006261), Fatigue (D005221):

Wǔlíngsǎn 5g + píngwèisǎn 5g.

Wǔlíngsǎn 5g + lǐzhōngtāng 5g + bǔzhōngyìqìtāng 5g + fángfēng 2g + zhǐqiào 2g + jiégěng 2g + gānjiāng 2g + ējiāo 2-0g.

Wǔlíngsǎn 5g + lǐzhōngtāng 5g + fùzǐ 2-0g + huángqí 2-0g + báisháo 1-0g.

Xiǎoxùmìngtāng 5g + tiānwángbǔxīndān 5g + gégēnhuángqínhuángliántāng 5g + suānzǎoréntāng 5g.

Màiyá 5g + báizhú 4g + zhǐshí 4g + fúlíng 4-0g + chénpí 4-0g + gāncǎo 3g + báibiǎndòu 3g + qiànshí 2g.

Gāncǎo 5g + báizhú 5g + báisháo 5g + zhīmǔ 5g + liánqiáo 5g + huáshí 5g + dāngguī 5g + dǎngshēn 5g.

Gāncǎo 5g + báizhú 5g + báisháo 5g + báibiǎndòu 5g + fúlíng 5g + huángqí 5g + dàzǎo 2g + shēngjiāng 2g.

Gāncǎo 5g + hòupò 5-2g + zhǐshí 5-2g + dàhuáng 1-0g.

Fùzǐ 5g + xìxīn 5g + dàhuáng 4g + bànxià 4g + fúlíng 4g.

Ptosis (374.3), Blindness (D001766), Diplopia (D004172), Panhypopituitarism (253.2), Diabetes insipidus (253.5), Seizure (345.9), Cranial nerve paralysis (352.9), Vertigo (386.2), Fourth cranial nerve palsy (378.53), Internal ophthalmoplegia (378.56), Oculomotor nerve palsy (378.51, 378.52), Hemianopia (D006423):

Qǐjúdìhuángwán 5g + jiāwèixiāoyáosǎn 4g + bànxiàxièxīntāng 1g + gāncǎoxiǎomàidàzǎotāng 1g + xiāngshāliùjūnzǐtāng 1g.

Qǐjúdìhuángwán 5g + jiāwèixiāoyáosǎn 5-4g + nǚzhēnzǐ 1g + hànliáncǎo 1g + xiàkūcǎo 1g + dānshēn 1-0g + mǔlì 1-0g + bèimǔ 1-0g + cǎojuémíng 1-0g.

Sǎnzhǒngkuìjiāntāng 5g + bànxiàxièxīntāng 1-0g.

Wēndǎntāng 5g + jiāwèixiāoyáosǎn 4g + qǐjúdìhuángwán 4g + xiàkūcǎo 1g.

Báizhú 5g + báisháo 5g + fúlíng 5g + huángqí 5g + dāngguī 5g + yuǎnzhì 5g + suānzǎorén 5g + shúdìhuáng 5g + dǎngshēn 5g + zhìgāncǎo 3-0g.

Báizhǐ 5g + gǒuqǐzǐ 5g + júhuā 5g + huánglián 5g + huángqín 4g + dàhuáng 1g.

Báizhǐ 5g + huángqín 5-2g + tiānhuā 3-2g + gāncǎo 3-2g + shārén 3-2g + jiégěng 3-0g + dàhuáng 0g.

Dānshēn 5g + tiānmá 5g + bèimǔ 5g + dāngguīwěi 5g + chuānxiōng 3g + gǒuqǐzǐ 3g + hǎipiāoxiāo 3g + huángqín 2g + huánglián 2g.

Tiānmá 5g + shíchāngpú 5g + gǒuqǐzǐ 5g + bózǐrén 5g + fúlíng 5g + júhuā 5g + yuǎnzhì 5g + suānzǎorén 5g + zéxiè 5g.

other gastrointestinal diseases (Wang, 2020). Both Wǔlíngsǎn and Lǐzhōngtāng contain Báizhú, which is neuroprotective and antitumor (cf. Sections 2.2 and 3.2).

8.4 THYROID HEMIAGENESIS

Thyroid hemiagenesis is a congenital anomaly characterized by the absence of one, usually the left, thyroid lobe. Since the remaining lobe is able to secrete enough hormones, many people with thyroid hemiagenesis do not have symptoms. Non-Mendelian inheritance, including epigenetic

TABLE 8.4
GMP Herbal Medicines for a One-Year-Old Girl with Thyroid Hemiagenesis

Thyroid hemiagenesis (OrphaCode: 95719)

A morphological anomaly with a prevalence of ~2 in 10,000

Not applicable

Macroglossia, Large fontanelles, Abnormality of the face, Coarse facial features, Jaundice, Hypotonia, Global developmental delay, Growth delay, Umbilical hernia, Constipation, Abdominal distention, Thyroid agenesis, Fatigue, Hypersomnia

Neonatal

Jaundice (D007565), Hypotonia (D009123), Constipation (564.0), Fatigue (D005221), Hypersomnia (327.13):

Wǔlíngsǎn 5g + tiáowèichéngqìtāng 3-1g + báisháo 1-0g + huángqín 1-0g + gāncǎo 1-0g + dàhuáng 0g.	Gāncǎo 5g + báizhǐ 5-3g + shārén 5-3g + dàhuáng 1-0g.
Xiǎocháihútāng 5g + tiáowèichéngqìtāng 2g + guìzhī 1g + dàhuáng 0g.	Báizhǐ 5g + zhìgāncǎo 5g + shārén 5g + dàhuáng 0g.
	Xuánshēn 5g + dìhuáng 5g + màiméndōng 5g + hòupò 5-2g + zhǐshí 5-2g + dàhuáng 1-0g.
	Dàhuáng 5g + gāncǎo 5g + báizhǐ 5-0g + shārén 5-0g.

changes, somatic mutations, and stochastic events in embryogenesis, is suspected to contribute to the development of thyroid hemiagenesis.

Dàhuáng (cf. Section 2.17) "purges, decumulates" and is used today for peptic ulcers and constipation (Wang, 2020). Màiméndōng was introduced in Section 1.27 to be yin-nourishing. Wǔlíngsǎn treats chronic glomerulonephritis (cf. Section 7.9), which can develop and manifest jaundice. Tiáowèichéngqìtāng (cf. Section 7.13) comprises Dàhuáng and is used today for functional digestive disorders (Wang, 2019).

8.5   SECONDARY HYPOPARATHYROIDISM DUE TO IMPAIRED PARATHORMON SECRETION

Secondary hypoparathyroidism due to impaired parathormon secretion is usually caused by damage to the parathyroid glands during a thyroid or neck surgery.

Jiégěng has long been an herb for the throat in TCM (cf. Section 2.57). We will see its frequent use for upper respiratory track conditions in Chapter 12 on rare respiratory diseases. Jiāwèixiāoyáosǎn

TABLE 8.5
GMP Herbal Medicines for a 40-Year-Old Adult with Secondary Hypoparathyroidism Due to Impaired Parathormon Secretion

Secondary hypoparathyroidism due to impaired parathormon secretion (OrphaCode: 140286)

A disease with a prevalence of ~2 in 10,000

Not applicable

Abnormality of the parathyroid gland

Secondary hyperparathyroidism, Abnormal concentration of calcium in blood

Childhood, Adolescent, Adult, Elderly

Abnormality of the parathyroid gland (252.9):

Jiāwèixiāoyáosǎn 5g + zhìgāncǎotāng 5g + zhēnrénhuómìngyǐn 5g + mǔlì 1g + xiàkūcǎo 1g.	Xuánshēn 5g + mǔlì 5g + bèimǔ 5g + jiégěng 5g + liánqiáo 5g + zhìgāncǎo 4g + zhīzǐ 4-2g + dàhuáng 2-0g.
Jiāwèixiāoyáosǎn 5g + sǎnzhǒngkuìjiāntāng 5g + xuánshēn 1g + mǔlì 1g + xiàkūcǎo 1g + bèimǔ 1-0g + hǎizǎo 1-0g.	Jiégěng 5g + zhìgāncǎo 5-3g + xuánshēn 3g + mǔlì 3g + bèimǔ 3g + liánqiáo 3g + shānzhīzǐ 2g + dàhuáng 1-0g.
Xiǎocháihútāng 5g + zhēnrénhuómìngyǐn 5g + sǎnzhǒngkuìjiāntāng 5g + xuánshēn 2g + mǔlì 2g + xiàkūcǎo 2g.	
Zhìgāncǎotāng 5g + sǎnzhǒngkuìjiāntāng 5g + xuánshēn 1g + bèimǔ 1g + xiàkūcǎo 1g + púgōngyīng 1g.	

was found to relieve the symptoms and adverse effects of antithyroid drugs in patients with hyperthyroidism (Ma et al., 2023). Sǎnzhǒngkuìjiāntāng treats goiters as we will see in Chapter 19 on rare otorhinolaryngologic diseases. The physical proximity between the parathyroid and thyroid glands may provide an explanation for the inclusion of Jiāwèixiāoyáosǎn and Sǎnzhǒngkuìjiāntāng in the table for abnormal parathyroid gland.

8.6 CENTRAL PRECOCIOUS PUBERTY

Precocious puberty is the onset of puberty at an age that is earlier than expected. Girls who physically mature before eight years old or boys before nine years old are considered to experience early puberty. If the cause of precocious puberty involves the hypothalamus or pituitary in the brain, such as a brain tumor or infection, it is called central precocious puberty or gonadotropin-dependent precocious puberty. A high-fat diet and obesity in girls are associated with early puberty.

TABLE 8.6

GMP Herbal Medicines for a Seven-Year-Old Child with Central Precocious Puberty

Central precocious puberty (OrphaCode: 759)

A disease with a prevalence of ~2 in 10,000

Autosomal dominant, Not applicable

Isosexual precocious puberty

Increased circulating gonadotropin level, Overgrowth, Accelerated bone age after puberty, Proportionate short stature, Increased body weight, Abnormality of secondary sexual hair, Premature thelarche

Acne, Obesity, Hypothalamic hamartoma, Prenatal maternal abnormality

Infancy, Childhood

Increased body weight (D015430):	
Huòxiāngzhèngqìsǎn 5g + gégēnhuángqínhuángliántāng 4-2g.	Báizhú 5g + fúlíng 5g + huòxiāng 5-0g +
Huòxiāngzhèngqìsǎn 5g + bànxiàxièxīntāng 2g + xiāngshāliùjūnzǐtāng 2g.	shānzhā 4g + zhǐshí 4g + shénqū 4g +
Huòxiāngzhèngqìsǎn 5g + píngwèisǎn 2g.	xiāngfù 4-0g + chénpí 4-0g + púgōngyīng
Huòxiāngzhèngqìsǎn 5g + mùxiāng 1g + huánglián 0g.	4-0g + cháihú 4-0g + báizhǐ 2-0g +
Wǔlíngsǎn 5g + huòxiāngzhèngqìsǎn 5g + mùxiāng 1g.	shēngmá 2-0g.
Obesity (278.00):	
Fángfēngtōngshèngsǎn 5g + shígāo 2g + jīngfángbàidúsǎn 2g + liánggésǎn	Héyè 5g + cǎojuémíng 3g + máhuáng 3-2g +
2g + lóngdǎnxiègāntāng 2g + dàhuáng 1g + zhīmǔ 0g + huángbò 0g.	zéxiè 3-2g + shígāo 2g + chēqiánzǐ 2g +
Fángfēngtōngshèngsǎn 5g + xīnyíqīngfèitāng 4-0g + shānzhā 1-0g +	hǔzhàng 2-0g + dānshēn 2-0g.
gāncǎo 1-0g.	Gāncǎo 5g + zhīmǔ 5g + huángqín 5g +
Èrchéntāng 5g + shānzhā 1g + shénqū 1g + màiyá 1g.	huánglián 1g + dàhuáng 0g.

Huòxiāngzhèngqìsǎn has been used for patients characterized by "dampness and stagnation" in TCM. The formula helps digestion and we will see its use again in Chapter 13 on rare gastroenterologic diseases. Héyè (Folium Nelumbinis) was shown to improve hypertriglyceridemia in a high-fat/high-cholesterol diet induced rat model of hypertriglyceridemia (Kim et al., 2020); it is used today for endocrine disorders and hyperlipidemia (Wang, 2020). Fángfēngtōngshèngsǎn (cf. Sections 1.4 and 5.14) was shown to decrease visceral white adipose tissue volume and adipocyte size in high-fat diet-fed obese mice (Kobayashi et al., 2017).

8.7 THYROID ECTOPIA

Thyroid ectopia is a thyroid in a location other than its normal final position at the front base of the neck. It involves a defective or aberrant embryogenesis of the thyroid gland and is caused by mutations in the genes whose products are transcription factors activating other genes for the development of the thyroid gland during embryogenesis.

TABLE 8.7
GMP Herbal Medicines for a 40-Year-Old Woman with Thyroid Ectopia

Thyroid ectopia (OrphaCode: 95712)

A morphological anomaly with a prevalence of ~1 in 10,000

Disease-causing germline mutation(s): NK2 homeobox 5 (*NKX2-5* / HGNC:2488) at 5q34

Disease-causing germline mutation(s) (loss of function): paired box 8 (*PAX8* / Entrez: 7849) at 2q14.1

Not applicable

Macroglossia, Large fontanelles, Abnormality of the face, Coarse facial features, Abnormality of the thyroid gland, Hypothyroidism, Jaundice, Hypotonia, Muscle weakness, Umbilical hernia, Constipation, Abdominal distention, Ectopic thyroid, Hypersomnia

Global developmental delay, Growth delay, Short stature, Intellectual disability, severe

Neonatal, Infancy

Abnormality of the thyroid gland (246.9), Hypothyroidism (244.9), Jaundice (D007565), Hypotonia (D009123), Muscle weakness (D018908), Constipation (564.0), Hypersomnia (327.13):

Sănzhŏngkuìjiāntāng 5-3g + jiāwèixiāoyáosăn 5-0g + xuánshēn 1g + xiàkūcăo 1g + mŭlì 1-0g + bèimŭ 1-0g + tiānhuā 1-0g.	Xuánshēn 5g + mŭlì 5g + bèimŭ 5g + zhìgāncăo 5g + jiégĕng 5g + liánqiáo 5-4g + shānzhīzĭ 2g + xìngrén 2g.
Sìnìtāng 5g + bànxià 1g + dàhuáng 0g.	Huángqín 5g + báizhĭ 3g + gāncăo 2g + shārén 2g + tiānhuā 1g + dàhuáng 0g.
	Báizhú 5g + fùzĭ 5g + cháihú 5g + báisháo 4g + fúlíng 4g + tiānhuā 2g + shēngjiāng 2g + dăngshēn 2g + guìzhī 2g + huángqín 2g + gāncăo 1g + mŭlì 1g + gānjiāng 1g.

Xuánshēn (cf. Section 1.25) "nourishes yin and quells fires." According to classical Chinese medical texts, the fires that Xuánshēn quenches result from a deficient yin. As hormones belong to yin, hypothyroidism can be considered an example of yin deficiency. Sănzhŏngkuìjiāntāng "quenches fires, de-toxifies, destroys nodules, beats consolidations" and is used for goiters (Wang, 2019). We will see its use for polyps and goiters in Chapters 13 and 19.

8.8 ADDISON DISEASE

Addison disease, also known as autoimmune adrenalitis, is an adrenal insufficiency where the adrenal gland produces too little cortisol and aldosterone hormones. Addison disease is believed to be caused by the immune system's targeting the adrenal gland after an infection or medication.

TABLE 8.8
GMP Herbal Medicines for a 40-Year-Old Woman with Addison Disease

Addison disease (OrphaCode: 85138)

A disease with a prevalence of ~1 in 10,000

Not applicable

Primary adrenal insufficiency, Hypocortisolemia

Hyperpigmentation of the skin, Muscle weakness, Failure to thrive, Weight loss, Diarrhea, Nausea and vomiting, Constipation, Abdominal pain, Anorexia, Hypotension, Autoimmunity, Increased circulating ACTH level, Fatigue

Renal salt wasting, Increased circulating renin level, Normocytic anemia, Hyperuricemia, Hyperkalemia, Hyponatremia, Decreased circulating aldosterone level, Hyperkalemic metabolic acidosis, Androgen insufficiency, Decreased urinary potassium

Delayed puberty, Hypoparathyroidism, Adrenal hypoplasia, Hashimoto thyroiditis, Dry skin, Vitiligo, Seizure, Orthostatic hypotension, Primary ovarian failure, Hypoglycemia, Sparse axillary hair, Vertigo, Celiac disease, Arthralgia, Hypercalcemia, Generalized bone demineralization, Premature ovarian insufficiency, Adrenal calcification, Decreased female libido, Salt craving, Type I diabetes mellitus

All ages

(Continued)

TABLE 8.8 *(Continued)*
GMP Herbal Medicines for a 40-Year-Old Woman with Addison Disease

Muscle weakness (D018908), Weight loss (D015431), Diarrhea (D003967), Constipation (564.0), Abdominal pain (D015746), Anorexia (D000855), Fatigue (D005221):

Wǔlíngsǎn 5g + fùzǐ 1g + huángqín 1g + dǐdāngtāng 0g + dàhuáng 0g.

Wǔlíngsǎn 5g + fùzǐ 1g + huángqín 1g + tiáowèichéngqìtāng 1-0g.

Wǔlíngsǎn 5g + fùzǐ 1g + huángqín 1g + xiǎochéngqìtāng 1g + dàhuáng 0g.

Gāncǎo 5g + hòupò 5-0g + zhǐshí 5-0g + dàhuáng 1-0g.

Hyperuricemia (D033461) [Other abnormal blood chemistry (790.6)]:

Shàngzhōngxiàtōngyòngtòngfēngwán 5g + dāngguīniāntòngtāng 5g + guìzhīsháoyàozhīmǔtāng 5-0g + chēqiánzǐ 1-0g.

Shàngzhōngxiàtōngyòngtòngfēngwán 5g + guìzhīsháoyàozhīmǔtāng 5g + niúxī 1-0g + huángbò 1-0g + cāngzhú 1-0g + yìyǐrén 1-0g + tǔfúlíng 1-0g + bìxiè 1-0g.

Shānzhā 5g + dānshēn 5g + héshǒuwū 5g + juémíngzǐ 5g + gǒuqǐzǐ 5g + zéxiè 5g + fúlíng 5-0g + júhuā 5-0g.

Chìxiǎodòu 5g + chēqiánzǐ 5g + sāngbáipí 5g + liánqiáo 5g + dàzǎo 2g + shēngjiāng 2g + xìngrén 2g + zhìgāncǎo 2g + máhuáng 0g + dàhuáng 0g.

Tǔfúlíng 5g + shānzhā 5g + dānshēn 5g + héshǒuwū 5g + juémíngzǐ 5g + gǒuqǐzǐ 5g + zéxiè 5g.

Hypoparathyroidism (252.1), Vitiligo (709.01), Seizure (345.9), Hypoglycemia (251.2), Vertigo (386.2), Celiac disease (579.0), Arthralgia (D018771), Hypercalcemia (275.42), Premature ovarian insufficiency (256.31):

Sìwùtāng 5g + hànliáncǎo 2-1g + héshǒuwū 2-0g + hónghuā 1g + táorén 1g + nǚzhēnzǐ 1-0g + dānshēn 1-0g + bǔgǔzhǐ 1-0g + jílí 1-0g.

Jiāwèixiāoyáosǎn 5g + bāwèidìhuángwán 5-0g + nǚzhēnzǐ 1g + héshǒuwū 1g + hànliáncǎo 1g + tùsīzǐ 1g + bǔgǔzhǐ 1g + gǒuqǐzǐ 1-0g.

Báizhǐ 5g + zhìgāncǎo 5g + shārén 5-4g + huángqín 5-4g + tiānhuā 2-0g + dàhuáng 0g.

Huángqín 5g + báizhǐ 5-2g + gāncǎo 3-2g + shārén 3-2g + zhīzǐ 2-0g + liánqiáo 2-0g + tiānhuā 2-0g + dàhuáng 0g.

Hòupò was introduced in Section 4.29 for weight loss and muscle repair. A Shānzhā (Fructus Crataegi; hawthorn berry)-containing formula was designed to treat hyperuricemic nephropathy in patients with chronic kidney disease (Lu et al., 2023). Processed Héshǒuwū (Radix Polygoni Multiflori) was reviewed to nourish the TCM liver and kidney, supplement the essence and blood, darken hair, strengthen bones and muscles, eliminate dampness, reduce lipids (Li et al., 2020), and was shown to tonify the liver and kidney by improving the hypothalamic-pituitary-adrenal axis disorder and regulating lipid metabolism in mice (Zhang et al., 2023). Tǔfúlíng (Rhizoma Smilacis Glabrae) was shown to lower serum uric acid and gouty arthritis recurrence rate in patients with gout in a double-blind, randomized, controlled trial (Xie et al., 2017). Bāwèidìhuángwán (cf. Sections 2.19 and 7.18) was formulated to "nourish and benefit Kidney yang," which means the functions and activities of the kidney. Shàngzhōngxiàtōngyòngtòngfēngwán, Dāngguīniāntòngtāng, and Guìzhīsháoyàozhīmǔtāng are the most commonly prescribed TCM formula granules to patients with rheumatoid arthritis in Taiwan (Huang et al., 2015).

8.9 DYSBETALIPOPROTEINEMIA

Dysbetalipoproteinemia, also known as broad-beta disease or familial dyslipidemia type 3, is characterized by high levels of cholesterol and triglycerides in the plasma, predisposing one to atherosclerosis. Dysbetalipoproteinemia is caused by mutations in the *APOE* gene, whose products play roles in catabolism of triglyceride-rich lipoprotein constituents.

An equal-weight combination of Qīngshàngfángfēngtāng (cf. Section 4.3) and Xiāoyáosǎn (cf. Section 1.23) granules was shown to be a safe and effective adjuvant for the treatment of chronic urticaria in a randomized, double-blind, placebo-controlled clinical trial (Yang et al., 2018). Yùquánwán and Báihǔjiārénshēntāng were introduced in Section 7.4 for diabetes; the safety and

TABLE 8.9

GMP Herbal Medicines for a 25-Year-Old Adult with Dysbetalipoproteinemia

Dysbetalipoproteinemia (OrphaCode: 412)

A disease with a prevalence of ~1 in 10,000

Major susceptibility factor: apolipoprotein E (*APOE* / Entrez: 348) at 19q13.32

Autosomal dominant, Multigenic/multifactorial

Abnormality of the skin, Hypertriglyceridemia, Hypercholesterolemia, Increased LDL cholesterol concentration, Decreased HDL cholesterol concentration

Diabetes mellitus, Corneal arcus, Xanthelasma, Hepatomegaly, Hepatic steatosis, Obesity, Atheromatosis, Tendon xanthomatosis

Renal steatosis, Hypothyroidism, Angina pectoris, Acute pancreatitis, Gout, Accelerated atherosclerosis, Peripheral arterial stenosis, Premature coronary artery atherosclerosis, Premature peripheral vascular disease, Aortic atherosclerosis

Childhood, Adolescent, Adult, Elderly

Abnormality of the skin (702):

Qīngshàngfángfēngtāng 5g + huángliánjiědútāng 5g + jīnyínhuā 1g + liánqiáo 1-0g + dàhuáng 0g.

Huángliánjiědútāng 5g + zhúyèshígāotāng 3g + fángjǐhuángqítāng 2g + fángfēngtōngshèngsǎn 2g + xiàkūcǎo 2g + máhuáng 2g + huánglián 2-1g + shānzhā 1g + hónghuā 1g + chénpí 1g + huáshí 1g + héyè 1-0g.

Báizhǐ 5g + gāncǎo 5-4g + tiānhuā 5-0g + shārén 4-3g + huángqín 4-0g + dàhuáng 1-0g.

Huángqín 5g + báizhǐ 4g + zhìgāncǎo 3g + shārén 3g + tiānhuā 2g + xìxīn 1-0g + dàhuáng 0g.

Diabetes mellitus (250), Hepatic steatosis (571.0), Obesity (278.00), Atheromatosis (440):

Yùquánwán 5g + yīnchénwǔlíngsǎn 5g + dānshēn 2g + juémíngzǐ 2g + chìsháo 2g + hónghuā 2g.

Liùwèidìhuángwán 5g + xuèfǔzhúyūtāng 5g + shānzhā 1g.

Báihǔjiārénshēntāng 5g + yùquánwán 5-0g + shānzhā 1-0g + dānshēn 1-0g + juémíngzǐ 1-0g + chìsháo 1-0g + hónghuā 1-0g.

Shānzhā 5g + dānshēn 5g + tiānhuā 5g + dìhuáng 5g + huángqí 5g + huángjīng 5g + huánglián 5-0g + mǎchǐxiàn 5-0g + yùzhú 5-0g + zéxiè 5-0g.

Tiānhuā 5g + dìhuáng 5g + mǎchǐxiàn 5g + huángqí 5g + huánglián 5g + huángjīng 5g + dǎngshēn 5g + dānshēn 5-0g.

Hypothyroidism (244.9), Angina pectoris (D000787), Gout (274, 274.0):

Jiāwèixiāoyáosǎn 5g + xiāngshāliùjūnzǐtāng 5g + bànxiàxièxīntāng 2g + shānzhā 1g + héhuānpí 1g.

Jiāwèixiāoyáosǎn 5g + zhìgāncǎotāng 5g + dānshēn 1g + yùjīn 1g + bǎihé 1-0g + mázǐrénwán 1-0g.

Língguìshùgāntāng 5g + juémíngzǐ 2g + shānzhā 1g + dānshēn 1g + chìsháo 1g + hónghuā 1g + cǎojuémíng 1g.

Sǎnzhǒngkuìjiāntāng 5g + yīnchénwǔlíngsǎn 3g + huàshícǎo 2g + chēqiánzǐ 1g.

Yùzhú 5g + zhǐqiào 5g + sāngzhī 5g + guālóurén 5g + fúlíng 5g + dànzhúyè 5g + sīguāluò 5g + júhuā 5g + gégēn 5g + gǔjīngcǎo 5g + mòyào 4g + rǔxiāng 4g + sānléng 2g + éshù 2g + bǎibù 1-0g.

Báizhú 5g + fùzǐ 5g + cháihú 5-0g + báisháo 4g + fúlíng 4g + dǎngshēn 2g + tiānhuā 2-0g + guìzhī 2-0g + huángqín 2-0g + shēngjiāng 2-0g + wǔwèizǐ 2-0g + xìxīn 2-0g + gāncǎo 1-0g + mǔlì 1-0g + gānjiāng 1-0g + dàhuáng 0g.

efficacy of their adjunctive use for type 2 diabetes mellitus were supported in systematic review and meta-analysis (Peng et al., 2021; Zhou et al., 2022). Mǎchǐxiàn (Herba Portulacae) is popularly used for the treatment of hypotension and diabetes (Uddin et al., 2014; Wang, 2020). Yùzhú was introduced in Section 1.5 for metabolic disorders.

8.10 ACROMEGALY

Acromegaly is overgrowth of parts of the body, such as the nose, ears, hands, and feet. Acromegaly is caused by a tumor of the pituitary gland that releases the growth hormone to the blood or by non-pituitary tumors that produce growth hormone–releasing hormone that signals the pituitary gland to produce the growth hormone.

Shānyào (cf. Section 1.62) was shown to induce the release of the growth hormone in rats (Lee et al., 2007). Tiānméndōng (cf. Section 1.48) "nourishes yin, cleanses the Lung, moisturizes dryness, generates

TABLE 8.10
GMP Herbal Medicines for a 40-Year-Old Adult with Acromegaly

Acromegaly (OrphaCode: 963)

A disease with a prevalence of ~5 in 100,000

Major susceptibility factor: aryl hydrocarbon receptor interacting protein (*AIP* / Entrez: 9049) at 11q13.2

Major susceptibility factor: G protein-coupled receptor 101 (*GPR101* / Entrez: 83550) at Xq26.3

Not applicable

Long penis, Tall stature, Macroglossia, Thick lower lip vermilion, Long face, Coarse facial features, Full cheeks, Mandibular prognathia, Broad forehead, Macrotia, Wide nose, Abnormality of the endocrine system, Anterior hypopituitarism, Growth hormone excess, Hyperhidrosis, Thickened skin, Large hands, Tapered finger, Joint swelling, Broad foot, Deep plantar creases, Osteoarthritis, Arthralgia, Cortical diaphyseal thickening of the upper limbs, Macrodactyly, Deep palmar crease, Pituitary growth hormone cell adenoma, Fatigue

Hypogonadotrophic hypogonadism, Abnormality of the dentition, Synophrys, Widely spaced teeth, Depression, Anxiety, Diabetes mellitus, Hypertension, Abnormal fingernail morphology, Hoarse voice, Frontal bossing, Migraine, Generalized hirsutism, Kyphosis, Paresthesia, Spinal canal stenosis, Abnormal toenail morphology, Sleep apnea, Broad jaw, Cerebral palsy, Palpebral edema, Dysmenorrhea

Impotence, Acanthosis nigricans, Acne, Hypertrophic cardiomyopathy, Mitral regurgitation, Pituitary prolactin cell adenoma, Generalized hyperpigmentation, Wide penis, Dysuria, Hypersomnia, Galactorrhea

Infancy, Childhood, Adolescent, Adult, Elderly

Abnormality of the endocrine system (259.9), Osteoarthritis (715.3), Arthralgia (D018771), Fatigue (D005221):

Liùwèidìhuángwán 5g + jiāwèixiāoyáosǎn 5g + sháoyàogāncǎotāng 5g + shēnlíngbáizhúsǎn 5g + shūjīnghuóxuètāng 5g.

Liùwèidìhuángwán 5g + jiāwèixiāoyáosǎn 5g + shūjīnghuóxuètāng 5g + dāngguīniántòngtāng 5g + dúhuójìshēngtāng 5g + dānshēn 2-0g + niúxī 2-0g.

Zuǒguīwán 5g + shèntòngzhúyūtāng 5g + dāngguīniántòngtāng 5g + dúhuójìshēngtāng 5g + mùguā 2g + niúxī 2g + dùzhòng 2g + xùduàn 2g.

Jiāwèixiāoyáosǎn 5g + yòuguīwán 5g + nǚzhēnzǐ 1g + hànliáncǎo 1g + tùsīzǐ 1g + bǔgǔzhī 1g.

Jiāwèixiāoyáosǎn 5g + zuǒguīwán 5g + shēnlíngbáizhúsǎn 5g + bǔzhōngyìqìtāng 5g + nǚzhēnzǐ 2g + hànliáncǎo 2g + tùsīzǐ 2g.

Shānyào 5g + dānshēn 5g + tiānméndōng 5g + niúxī 5g + báizhú 5g + gǒujǐ 5g + báisháo 5-0g + guìzhī 5-0g + sāngjìshēng 5-0g + xùduàn 5-0g + huángqí 5-0g + dāngguī 5-0g + gāncǎo 3-0g.

Shānyào 5g + chuānxiōng 5g + dānshēn 5g + tiānméndōng 5g + báisháo 5g + gǒujǐ 5g + huángqí 5g + sāngjìshēng 5-0g + niúxī 5-0g + dāngguī 5-0g + guībǎn 5-0g + gāncǎo 3-0g.

Shānzhā 5g + shānyào 5g + dānshēn 5g + tiānméndōng 5g + héshǒuwū 5g + shāshēn 5g + gǒujǐ 5g + sāngjìshēng 5g + huángqí 5g + gāncǎo 3g.

Diabetes mellitus (250), Hypertension (401-405.99), Hoarse voice (D006685), Migraine (346), Paresthesia (D010292), Sleep apnea (780.57), Cerebral palsy (343.0, 343.3, 343.2):

Báihǔjiārénshēntāng 5g + fángfēngtōngshèngsǎn 5-2g + mázǐrénwán 5-0g + xiōngqióng 2-1g + cǎojuémíng 2-1g + yìyǐrén 2-0g + héyè 2-0g + gāncǎo 2-0g + shānzhā 1-0g.

Báihǔjiārénshēntāng 5g + xuèfǔzhúyūtāng 5g + zhībódìhuángwán 5g + dānshēn 1g.

Gōuténgsǎn 5g + fángfēngtōngshèngsǎn 4g + mázǐrénwán 2g + xiōngqióng 1g + cǎojuémíng 1g + gāncǎo 1g.

Jiǔwèiqiānghuótāng 5g + shānyào 2g + cāngzhú 2g + xiōngqióng 1g.

Dìhuáng 5g + xuánshēn 5-3g + tiānhuā 5-2g + cāngzhú 5-2g + huángqí 5-0g + gégēn 5-0g.

Xuánshēn 5g + dìhuáng 5g + màiméndōng 5g + huánglián 5g.

Xuánshēn 5g + tiānhuā 2g + cāngzhú 2g + mǔlì 1g.

Gāncǎo 5g + dàhuáng 1g.

Hypertrophic cardiomyopathy (425.1), Mitral regurgitation (396.3, 746.6), Dysuria (D053159), Hypersomnia (327.13):

Shēngmàiyǐn 5g + zhìgāncǎotāng 5g + dānshēn 2-1g + yùjīn 2-1g + sānqī 1-0g + mùxiāng 1-0g.

Xuèfǔzhúyūtāng 5g + zhìgāncǎotāng 5g + dānshēn 1g + xiāngfù 1g + yùjīn 1g.

Báizhú 5g + fùzǐ 5g + báisháo 3g + fúlíng 3g + dǎngshēn 3g.

Báizhú 5g + fùzǐ 5g + cháihú 5g + báisháo 4g + fúlíng 4g + tiānhuā 2g + dǎngshēn 2g + guìzhī 2g + huángqín 2g + shēngjiāng 2-0g + gāncǎo 1g + mǔlì 1g + gānjiāng 1g.

Báizhú 5g + zhìgāncǎo 5g + zhǐshí 5g + fúlíng 5g + niúxī 2g + ròuguì 2g + fùzǐ 2g.

saliva" and is anti-inflammatory (Lei et al., 2024). Its modern uses include polydipsia and coughs (Wang, 2020). Gǒujǐ (Rhizoma Cibotii) "dispels rheumatism, replenishes the Liver/Kidney, strengthens waist/knee" and is used today for lumbago and pain in joints (Wang, 2020). Gégēn (cf. Section 4.16) has been used extensively in TCM for geriatric diseases, including age-related neurodegenerative, cardio- and cerebrovascular, and endocrine diseases (Zhang et al., 2018). Jiǔwèiqiānghuótāng "promotes sweating, removes dampness, clears internal heat" and is used for allergic rhinitis (Wang, 2019).

8.11 ZOLLINGER-ELLISON SYNDROME

Zollinger-Ellison syndrome, or gastrinoma, is a condition characterized by excessive production of gastric acid by the stomach. Zollinger-Ellison syndrome is caused by a tumor in the pancreas, duodenum, or stomach that secretes a large amount of a hormone called *gastrin*. Too much gastrin in the blood triggers the stomach to produce gastric acid.

TABLE 8.11

GMP Herbal Medicines for a 45-Year-Old Adult with Zollinger-Ellison Syndrome

Zollinger-Ellison syndrome (OrphaCode: 913)

A disease with a prevalence of ~5 in 100,000

Not applicable

Zollinger-Ellison syndrome, Neuroendocrine neoplasm

Diarrhea, Nausea, Episodic abdominal pain, Duodenal ulcer, Peptic ulcer, Esophagitis

Weight loss

Hyperparathyroidism, Growth hormone excess, Thyroid adenoma, Jaundice, Multiple lipomas, Hypercortisolism, Gastrointestinal hemorrhage, Hematochezia, Pituitary adenoma, Hypercalcemia, Elevated circulating parathyroid hormone level, Intestinal obstruction, Pituitary prolactin cell adenoma, Parathyroid hyperplasia, Adrenocortical adenoma, Pituitary corticotropic cell adenoma, Erythema, Pituitary growth hormone cell adenoma, Pituitary null cell adenoma, Increased urinary cortisol level, Lipoma, Extrahepatic cholestasis, Glucagonoma, Increased glucagon level

Adult, Elderly

Neuroendocrine neoplasm (209-209.99):

Shíliùwèiliúqìyǐn 5g + sǎnzhǒngkuìjiāntāng 5-0g + bànzhīlián 2-0g + báihuāshéshécǎo 2-0g + huáihuā 2-0g + cāngzhú 2-0g + sānléng 1-0g + éshù 1-0g.

Xuánshēn 5g + dìhuáng 5g + hòupò 5g + zhǐshí 5g + màiméndōng 5g + yùzhú 5-0g + shāshēn 5-0g + běishāshēn 4-0g + dàhuáng 1-0g.

Lǐzhōngtāng 5g + bǔzhōngyìqìtāng 5g + qīngyānlìgétāng 3g + tiānwángbǔxīndān 3-0g + chuānxiōngchádiàosǎn 3-0g + fángfēng 2g + zhǐqiào 2g + jiégěng 2g + gānjiāng 2-0g.

Tiānméndōng 5g + xìngrén 5g + bèimǔ 5g + zhīmǔ 5g + sāngbáipí 5g + chénpí 5g + màiméndōng 5g + huángqín 3g + gāncǎo 2g.

Huángqín 5g + báizhǐ 4g + tiānhuā 2g + gāncǎo 2g + shārén 2g + dàhuáng 0g.

Diarrhea (D003967), Nausea (D009325), Duodenal ulcer (532), Peptic ulcer (533), Esophagitis (530.1):

Bànxiàxièxīntāng 5g + báitóuwēngtāng 5g + gégēnhuángqínhuángliántāng 5g + huòxiāngzhèngqìsǎn 5g + hǎipiāoxiāo 3-0g + huángliánjiědútāng 2-0g + wūméi 2-0g.

Gāncǎo 5g + huángqín 5g + huánglián 5-0g + gégēn 5-0g + wúzhūyú 1-0g + dàhuáng 0g.

Gégēnhuángqínhuángliántāng 5g + bànxià 1g + fúlíng 1g.

Gāncǎo 5g + báizhú 5g + báisháo 5g + báibiǎndòu 5g + fúlíng 5g + huángqí 5g + dàzǎo 2g + shēngjiāng 2g.

Xiǎobànxiàjiāfúlíngtāng 5g + cāngzhú 2g + yìyǐrén 2g + báijí 1g + hòupò 1g + zhǐshí 1g.

Hyperparathyroidism (252.0), Thyroid adenoma (193), Jaundice (D007565), Multiple lipomas (214), Hypercalcemia (275.42), Intestinal obstruction (560.9):

Sǎnzhǒngkuìjiāntāng 5g + xiǎocháihútāng 5-0g + xuánshēn 1g + bèimǔ 1g + xiàkūcǎo 1g + púgōngyīng 1-0g + mǔlì 1-0g + hǎizǎo 1-0g + biējiǎ 1-0g.

Zhìgāncǎo 5g + jiégěng 5g + báizhǐ 3g + liánqiáo 3g + shēngjiāng 2g + dàhuáng 0g.

Sǎnzhǒngkuìjiāntāng 5g + jiāwèixiāoyáosǎn 5-0g + xuánshēn 1g + bèimǔ 1g + xiàkūcǎo 1g + púgōngyīng 1-0g + mǔlì 1-0g + hǎizǎo 1-0g.

Zhìgāncǎo 5g + jiégěng 5g + xuánshēn 5-3g + mǔlì 5-3g + bèimǔ 5-3g + liánqiáo 5-3g + shānzhīzǐ 2g + dàhuáng 1-0g.

Xuánshēn was introduced in Section 4.11 to be antitumor. Shíliùwèiliúqìyǐn (cf. Section 1.20) was shown to markedly reduce the tumor size in human bladder carcinoma cells-xenografted tumor tissues in nude mice (Ou et al., 2011). Gégēnhuángqínhuángliántāng was concluded to be safe and effective for pediatric diarrhea in a systematic review and meta-analysis of randomized controlled trials (Wang et al., 2022a). Xiǎobànxiàjiāfúlíngtāng, used for nausea and vomiting during pregnancy, is used today for disorders of the stomach function(Wang, 2019). Jiégěng (cf. Sections 2.57 and 8.5) was shown to reduce pulmonary inflammation in mice with pneumonia (Yang et al., 2023).

8.12 CENTRAL DIABETES INSIPIDUS

Central diabetes insipidus (CDI), or neurogenic diabetes insipidus, is characterized by excessive thirst and excessive urination. CDI is caused by impairment in the production, transportation, or storage of the antidiuretic hormone called *arginine vasopressin,* which is produced by the hypothalamus, released by the pituitary gland into the bloodstream, and received by the kidneys to reabsorb water into the body. The impairment can be hereditary or acquired.

TABLE 8.12
GMP Herbal Medicines for a Seven-Year-Old Child with Central Diabetes Insipidus

Central diabetes insipidus (OrphaCode: 178029)

A disease with a prevalence of ~4 in 100,000

Disease-causing germline mutation(s) (loss of function): arginine vasopressin (*AVP* / Entrez: 551) at 20p13

Autosomal dominant, Autosomal recessive, X-linked dominant

Nocturia, Diabetes insipidus, Failure to thrive, Weight loss, Dehydration, Polydipsia, Anorexia

Depression, Anxiety, Lethargy, Excessive daytime somnolence, Fever, Headache

Seizure, Diarrhea, Nausea and vomiting, Hyponatremia

Childhood

Nocturia (D053158), Diabetes insipidus (253.5), Weight loss (D015431), Polydipsia (D059606), Anorexia (D000855):	
Xiāngshāliùjūnzǐtāng 5g + shénqū 1g + màiyá 1g + shānzhā 1-0g + jīnèijīn 1-0g.	Màiyá 5g + shānzhā 3-2g + shénqū 3-2g + jīnèijīn 3-0g.
Xiāngshāliùjūnzǐtāng 5g + bǎohéwán 4-2g.	Gāncǎo 5g + báizhǐ 5-0g + shārén 5-0g + hòupò 5-0g + zhǐshí 5-0g + dàhuáng 1-0g.
Lethargy (D053609), Fever (D005334), Headache (D006261):	
Wǔlíngsǎn 5g + bǔzhōngyìqìtāng 5-0g.	
Wǔlíngsǎn 5g + dǎngshēn 1-0g + báisháo 1-0g + gāncǎo 1-0g.	Gāncǎo 5g + báizhǐ 5g + shārén 5-3g + huángqín 5-0g + tiānhuā 2-0g + xìxīn 2-0g + dàhuáng 1-0g.
Seizure (345.9), Diarrhea (D003967):	
Cháihújiālónggǔmǔlìtāng 5g + wēndǎntāng 5g + tiānmá 2-1g + shíchāngpú 2-1g + yuǎnzhì 2-1g + gōuténg 1-0g.	Huángqí 5g + chìsháo 1-0g + fángfēng 1-0g + xìxīn 0g + huánglián 0g + dàhuáng 0g.
Wēndǎntāng 5g + gāncǎoxiǎomàidàzǎotāng 3g + tiānmá 1g + gōuténg 1g.	Hòupò 5g + zhǐshí 5g + běishāshēn 4g + xuánshēn 4g + yùzhú 4g + dìhuáng 4g + màiméndōng 4g + dàhuáng 0g.
Tiānmágōuténgyǐn 5g + yìgānsǎn 4g + shíchāngpú 1g + yuǎnzhì 1g.	
Gāncǎoxiǎomàidàzǎotāng 5g + cháihújiālónggǔmǔlìtāng 5g + tiānmá 1g + shíchāngpú 1g + yuǎnzhì 1g.	

Màiyá, introduced in Section 3.12 for weight loss, was shown to reduce the risk of diabetic complications through antioxidation in the liver and kidneys of diabetic rats (cf. Section 3.12). Jīnèijīn was shown to be anti-urolithic in rats (cf. Section 4.31) and is used today for digestive conditions and nutritional marasmus (Wang, 2020). Báizhǐ was summarized in Section 1.7 to relieve fatigue, headaches, and fevers. A modified Cháihújiālónggǔmǔlìtāng was shown to reduce the seizure frequency in patients with refractory epilepsy (Wu et al., 2002).

8.13 CUSHING DISEASE

Cushing disease, also known as pituitary corticotroph micro-adenoma, is characterized by high levels of cortisol, a stress hormone, in the body. Cushing disease usually results from long-term, high-dose use of steroid medicine. This disease can also be caused by a benign tumor of the pituitary gland that releases a hormone that stimulates production of cortisol by the adrenal glands above the kidneys.

TABLE 8.13

GMP Herbal Medicines for a 35-Year-Old Woman with Cushing Disease

Cushing disease (OrphaCode: 96253)

A disease with a prevalence of ~4 in 100,000

Major susceptibility factor: cadherin-related 23 (*CDH23* / Entrez: 64072) at 10q22.1

Disease-causing somatic mutation(s): ubiquitin specific peptidase 48 (*USP48* / Entrez: 84196) at 1p36.12

Disease-causing somatic mutation(s): B-Raf proto-oncogene, serine/threonine kinase (*BRAF* / Entrez: 673) at 7q34

Disease-causing somatic mutation(s): ubiquitin specific peptidase 8 (*USP8* / Entrez: 9101) at 15q21.2

Disease-causing somatic mutation(s): nuclear receptor subfamily 3 group C member 1 (*NR3C1* / Entrez: 2908) at 5q31.3

Disease-causing somatic mutation(s): tumor protein p53 (*TP53* / Entrez: 7157) at 17p13.1

Disease-causing somatic mutation(s): ATRX chromatin remodeler (*ATRX* / Entrez: 546) at Xq21.1

Not applicable

Increased circulating cortisol level, Paradoxical increased cortisol secretion on dexamethasone suppression test, Pituitary corticotropic cell adenoma, Increased urinary cortisol level

Amenorrhea, Behavioral abnormality, Emotional lability, Diabetes mellitus, Hypertension, Osteoporosis, Hyperpigmentation of the skin, Thin skin, Bruising susceptibility, Hirsutism, Plethora, Poor wound healing, Acne, Striae distensae, Muscle weakness, Abnormality of the cardiovascular system, Lymphopenia, Truncal obesity, Leukocytosis, Immunodeficiency, Increased circulating ACTH level, Increased body weight, Proximal amyotrophy, Adrenal hyperplasia, Intra-oral hyperpigmentation, Abdominal obesity, Capillary fragility, Dorsocervical fat pad, Fatiguable weakness of proximal limb muscles, Decreased eosinophil count, Impaired glucose tolerance, Moon facies

Depression, Psychotic episodes, Secondary amenorrhea, Oligomenorrhea, Purpura, Stroke, Myocardial infarction, Abnormality of the respiratory system, Sparse scalp hair, Headache, Memory impairment, Large sella turcica, Vertebral compression fractures, Recurrent cutaneous fungal infections, Flushing, Ecchymosis, Suicidal ideation, Abnormal libido, Skin ulcer

Adult

Diabetes mellitus (250), Hypertension (401-405.99), Osteoporosis (733.0), Bruising susceptibility (D004438), Hirsutism (D006628), Striae distensae (D057896), Muscle weakness (D018908), Abnormality of the cardiovascular system (429.2), Lymphopenia (288.51), Truncal obesity (D056128), Immunodeficiency (279.3), Increased body weight (D015430), Abdominal obesity (D056128):

Yùquánwán 5g + yīnchénwǔlíngsǎn 5g + jīnyínhuā 2g + púgōngyīng 2g.	Shānyào 5g + tiānhuā 5g + xuánshēn 5g + dìhuáng 5g + cāngzhú 5g + huángqí 5-0g + dǎngshēn 5-0g + màiméndōng 5-0g + gégēn 5-0g.
Yùquánwán 5g + báihǔjiārénshēntāng 5g + shānyào 2g.	Shígāo 5g + zhīmǔ 5g + màiméndōng 5g + dìhuáng 3g + huánglián 1g.
Yùquánwán 5g + shānyào 3-1g + cāngzhú 2-1g.	Tiānhuā 5g + běishāshēn 5g + xuánshēn 5g + yùzhú 5g + dìhuáng 5g + màiméndōng 5g + gégēn 5g.

Oligomenorrhea (D009839) [Scanty or infrequent menstruation (626.1)], Purpura (D011693), Myocardial infarction (D009203) [Acute myocardial infarction of unspecified site, episode of care unspecified (410.9)], Headache (D006261), Memory impairment (D008569):

Wēnjīngtāng 5g + dāngguīsháoyàosǎn 4-3g + máxìnggānshítāng 3-2g + huángqí 1g + cāngěrzǐ 1g + guìzhī 1-0g + xiāngfù 1-0g.	Báizhú 5g + báisháo 5g + fùzǐ 5g + fúlíng 5g + dǎngshēn 5-0g + táorén 5-0g + gānjiāng 5-0g.
Dāngguīsháoyàosǎn 5g + liùwèidìhuángwán 4g + máxìnggānshítāng 3g + guìzhī 1g + huángqí 1g + mùtōng 1g + fángfēng 1g + xìxīn 0g.	Báizhú 5g + dāngguī 5g + chuānxiōng 4g + báisháo 4g + huángqín 4g + shānzhīzǐ 1g + cháihú 1g.
	Shānyào 5g + gāncǎo 5g + báizhú 5g + báisháo 5g + ējiāo 5g + huángqí 5g + dāngguī 5g + suānzǎorén 5g + dǎngshēn 5g.
	Gāncǎo 5g + fùzǐ 4g + gānjiāng 4g + suānzǎorén 4g.

Cāngzhú (Rhizoma Atractylodis) "dries dampness, strengthens the Spleen, dispels rheumatism" and is used for leukorrhea, diarrhea, rhinitis, eczema, and functional disorder of the stomach (Wang, 2020). Wēnjīngtāng "activates Blood, removes stasis, warms meridians, dispels coldness, benefits Qi, nourishes Blood" and is used today for disorders of menstruation and other abnormal bleeding from the female genital tract (Wang, 2019). Dāngguīsháoyàosǎn was shown to attenuate cognitive impairment via the microbiota-gut-brain axis in amnesic mice through regulation of lipid metabolism (Liu et al., 2022).

8.14 FAMILIAL THYROID DYSHORMONOGENESIS

Familial thyroid dyshormonogenesis is characterized by low levels of thyroid hormones due to impairment in the synthesis of the hormones in the thyroid gland that has occurred since birth. Genetic defects in any step in the enzymatic cascade for normal thyroid hormone synthesis cause familial thyroid dyshormonogenesis.

TABLE 8.14

GMP Herbal Medicines for a One-Year-Old Infant with Familial Thyroid Dyshormonogenesis

Familial thyroid dyshormonogenesis (OrphaCode: 95716)

A disease with a prevalence of ~4 in 100,000

Disease-causing germline mutation(s): solute carrier family 5 member 5 (*SLC5A5* / Entrez: 6528) at 19p13.11

Disease-causing germline mutation(s): thyroid peroxidase (*TPO* / Entrez: 7173) at 2p25.3

Disease-causing germline mutation(s): dual oxidase 2 (*DUOX2* / Entrez: 50506) at 15q21.1

Disease-causing germline mutation(s): dual oxidase maturation factor 2 (*DUOXA2* / Entrez: 405753) at 15q21.1

Disease-causing germline mutation(s): thyroglobulin (*TG* / Entrez: 7038) at 8q24.22

Disease-causing germline mutation(s): iodotyrosine deiodinase (*IYD* / Entrez: 389434) at 6q25.1

Autosomal recessive

Increased thyroid-stimulating hormone level, Decreased circulating thyroxine level

Neurodevelopmental delay, Delayed cranial suture closure, Congenital hypothyroidism, Goiter, Umbilical hernia, Constipation, Large posterior fontanelle, Abnormality of epiphysis morphology, Prolonged neonatal jaundice, Thyroid defect in oxidation and organification of iodide, Delayed proximal femoral epiphyseal ossification, Feeding difficulties in infancy

Macroglossia, Facial edema, Intellectual disability, Hypotonia, Lethargy, Hyporeflexia, Bradycardia, Hypothermia, Neonatal hyperbilirubinemia, Depressed nasal bridge, Positive perchlorate discharge test, Abnormal circulating thyroglobulin level, Reduced radioactive iodine uptake, Increased radioactive iodine uptake

Neonatal, Infancy

Congenital hypothyroidism (243), Goiter (240.9), Constipation (564.0):

Xiǎocháihútāng 5g + xuánshēn 2g + bèimǔ 2g + xiàkūcǎo 2g + mǔlì 2-0g.

Sǎnzhǒngkuìjiāntāng 5g + xuánshēn 1g + mǔlì 1g + bèimǔ 1-0g + xiàkūcǎo 1-0g + dàhuáng 0g.

Jiāwèixiāoyáosǎn 5g + xuánshēn 2g + bèimǔ 2g + xiàkūcǎo 2g.

Xuánshēn 5g + yùzhú 5g + dìhuáng 5g + shāshēn 5g + hòupò 5g + zhǐshí 5g + màiméndōng 5g + dàhuáng 0g.

Xuánshēn 5g + dìhuáng 5g + màiméndōng 5g + hòupò 2-0g + zhǐshí 2-0g + dàhuáng 1-0g.

Intellectual disability (D008607), Hypotonia (D009123), Lethargy (D053609), Bradycardia (D001919) [Other specified cardiac dysrhythmias (427.89)], Hypothermia (D007035):

Guìzhītāng 5g + xìngrén 1g + hòupò 1-0g + dàhuáng 1-0g.

Huángqíwǔwùtāng 5g + gāncǎo 1g + báisháo 1g.

Gāncǎo 5g + shārén 5g + báizhǐ 5-0g + dàhuáng 0g.

The molecular targets and mechanisms of Xiǎocháihútāng for the treatment of thyroid cancer were predicted in silico and verified in cells (Wang et al., 2022b). Xuánshēn was introduced in Section 1.3 for throat pain. Guìzhī (cf. Section 2.30) in Guìzhītāng was shown to inhibit neuroinflammation in murine microglial cells (Ho et al., 2013), inhibit tau aggregation in vitro (George et al., 2013), and protect the neurons in the prefrontal cortex of rats against hyperactivity and oxidative damage induced by Máhuáng (Zheng et al., 2015).

8.15 ATHYREOSIS

Athyreosis is complete absence or lack of function of the thyroid gland. Mutations in the genes whose products control the development and function of the thyroid gland cause athyreosis.

TABLE 8.15

GMP Herbal Medicines for a One-Year-Old Infant with Athyreosis

Athyreosis (OrphaCode: 95713)

A morphological anomaly with a prevalence of ~3 in 100,000

Candidate gene tested: forkhead box E1 (*FOXE1* / Entrez: 2304) at 9q22.33

Candidate gene tested: NK2 homeobox 1 (*NKX2-1* / Entrez: 7080) at 14q13.3

Disease-causing germline mutation(s) (loss of function): solute carrier family 26 member 4 (*SLC26A4* / Entrez: 5172) at 7q22.3

Disease-causing germline mutation(s) (loss of function): thyroid stimulating hormone receptor (*TSHR* / Entrez: 7253) at 14q24-q31

Disease-causing germline mutation(s): NK2 homeobox 5 (*NKX2-5* / HGNC:2488) at 5q34

Disease-causing germline mutation(s) (loss of function): paired box 8 (*PAX8* / Entrez: 7849) at 2q14.1

Autosomal dominant

Macroglossia, Large fontanelles, Abnormality of the face, Coarse facial features, Hypothyroidism, Hypotonia, Muscle weakness, Constipation, Abdominal distention, Thyroid agenesis, Feeding difficulties, Fatigue, Hypersomnia

Global developmental delay, Growth delay, Short stature, Intellectual disability, severe

Hypothyroidism (244.9), Hypotonia (D009123), Muscle weakness (D018908), Constipation (564.0), Fatigue (D005221), Hypersomnia (327.13):

Zhìgāncǎotāng 5g + sǎnzhǒngkuìjiāntāng 5-0g + xuánshēn 2-1g + mǔlì 2-1g + bèimǔ 2-1g + xiàkūcǎo 2-1g + mázǐrénwán 2-0g + dàhuáng 0g.	Gāncǎo 5g + dàhuáng 4-0g.
	Gāncǎo 5g + báizhǐ 5g + shārén 5g + dàhuáng 0g.
Lǐzhōngtāng 5g + mázǐrénwán 5g + gāncǎo 1g + báisháo 1g + dàhuáng 0g.	Gāncǎo 5g + hòupò 5g + zhǐshí 5g + dàhuáng 1g.

Chinese herbal medicine was suggested to be safe and effective for the treatment of chronic fatigue syndrome in a systematic review and meta-analysis of randomized controlled trials (Zhang et al., 2022), in which Gāncǎo (cf. Section 1.1) was identified as the most frequently prescribed herb. A characteristic symptom of hypothyroidism is a slow heart rate and Zhìgāncǎotāng is known to restore the pulse (cf. Section 3.16). Zhìgāncǎotāng was shown to protect against diabetic myocardial infarction (DMI) injury in DMI mice by inhibiting cardiomyocyte apoptosis and reducing inflammatory reactions (Hu et al., 2023).

8.16 THYROID HYPOPLASIA

Thyroid hypoplasia refers to the underdevelopment of the thyroid gland, resulting in permanent thyroid deficiency in the newborn. Mutations in the *SLC26A4, TSHR,* and *PAX8* genes, which are expressed in the thyroid gland for the function and development of the thyroid gland, cause thyroid hypoplasia.

Gāncǎo (cf. Section 1.1) was shown to attenuate thyroiditis in a mouse model of autoimmune thyroiditis (Li et al., 2017). Thyroid deficiency can be considered a form of yin deficiency. The yin-nourishing effect of Xuánshēn (cf. Section 8.7) was demonstrated in vitro with primary splenic lymphocytes and in vivo with mice through the immunoregulatory and antioxidant activities of the compounds in the herb (Gong et al., 2020).

TABLE 8.16
GMP Herbal Medicines for a One-Year-Old Infant with Thyroid Hypoplasia

Thyroid hypoplasia (OrphaCode: 95720)

A morphological anomaly with a prevalence of ~3 in 100,000

Disease-causing germline mutation(s) (loss of function): solute carrier family 26 member 4 (*SLC26A4* / Entrez: 5172) at 7q22.3

Disease-causing germline mutation(s) (loss of function): thyroid stimulating hormone receptor (*TSHR* / Entrez: 7253) at 14q24-q31

Disease-causing germline mutation(s) (loss of function): paired box 8 (*PAX8* / Entrez: 7849) at 2q14.1

Autosomal dominant, Not applicable

Macroglossia, Large fontanelles, Abnormality of the face, Coarse facial features, Hypothyroidism, Jaundice, Hypotonia, Growth delay, Constipation, Abdominal distention, Thyroid hypoplasia, Fatigue

Global developmental delay, Short stature, Intellectual disability, severe

Neonatal, Infancy

Hypothyroidism (244.9), Jaundice (D007565), Hypotonia (D009123), Constipation (564.0), Fatigue (D005221):

Zhìgāncǎotāng 5g + xuánshēn 1g + dìhuáng 1-0g + màiméndōng 1-0g + mǔlì 1-0g + bèimǔ 1-0g + xiàkūcǎo 1-0g + dàhuáng 0g.

Xiǎocháihútāng 5g + gāncǎo 1g + tiáowèichéngqìtāng 1g + dàhuáng 0g.

Xiǎojiànzhōngtāng 5g + gāncǎo 1g + dàhuáng 0g.

Sǎnzhǒngkuìjiāntāng 5g + xuánshēn 1g + mǔlì 1g + bèimǔ 1g + xiàkūcǎo 1g.

Gāncǎo 5g + xuánshēn 2-0g + dìhuáng 2-0g + màiméndōng 2-0g + dàhuáng 2-0g.

Gāncǎo 5g + báizhǐ 5-0g + shārén 5-0g + dàhuáng 2-1g.

Gāncǎo 5g + hòupò 5-0g + zhǐshí 5-0g + dàhuáng 2-1g.

8.17 CRANIOPHARYNGIOMA

Craniopharyngioma is a benign, slow-growing brain tumor derived from the pituitary gland embryonic tissue. Most cases of childhood-onset craniopharyngioma are associated with mutations in the genes, including *BRAF* and *CTNNB1*, whose products play roles in cell signaling.

The life span extension mechanisms of Huángqí (cf. Section 1.9), including its anti-vascular aging, anti-brain aging, and anticancer effects, were reviewed (Liu et al., 2017). Shíchāngpú was introduced in Section 1.36 to open the nine orifices, which include the two eyes, two ears, two nostrils, mouth, tongue, and throat, for our vision, hearing, smell, and taste. A modern study showed

TABLE 8.17
GMP Herbal Medicines for a Nine-Year-Old Child with Craniopharyngioma

Craniopharyngioma (OrphaCode: 54595)

A disease with a prevalence of ~2 in 100,000

Disease-causing somatic mutation(s): B-Raf proto-oncogene, serine/threonine kinase (*BRAF* / Entrez: 673) at 7q34

Disease-causing somatic mutation(s): catenin beta 1 (*CTNNB1* / Entrez: 1499) at 3p22.1

Not applicable

Abnormal hypothalamus morphology

Cerebral calcification, Intracranial cystic lesion, Neoplasm of the anterior pituitary, Enlarged pituitary gland, Hypopituitarism

Hypogonadism, Central diabetes insipidus, Increased circulating prolactin concentration, Papilledema, Excessive daytime somnolence, Obesity, Nausea and vomiting, Headache, Sleep disturbance, Low gonadotropins (secondary hypogonadism), Slow decrease in visual acuity, Progressive visual field defects, Pituitary hypothyroidism, Central adrenal insufficiency, Bitemporal hemianopia, Abnormal visual field test

Hydrocephalus, Hearing impairment, Optic atrophy, Delayed puberty, Growth delay, Increased intracranial pressure, Polyphagia, Cerebral ischemia, Increased susceptibility to fractures, Proportionate short stature, Type II diabetes mellitus, Sleep apnea

All ages

(Continued)

TABLE 8.17 *(Continued)*
GMP Herbal Medicines for a Nine-Year-Old Child with Craniopharyngioma

Papilledema (362.83, 377.0, 377.01), Obesity (278.00), Headache (D006261), Bitemporal hemianopia (D006423):

Liùwèidìhuángwán 5g + jiāwèixiāoyáosăn 5g + acupuncture.	Shíchāngpú 5g + hángjú 5g + gǒuqǐzǐ 5g +
Jiāwèixiāoyáosăn 5g + qǐjúdìhuángwán 5g + acupuncture.	yuǎnzhì 5g + dǎngshēn 5g + gāncǎo 2-0g +
Guìzhītāng 5g + xìngrén 1g + hòupò 1g + dàhuáng 0g + acupuncture.	acupuncture.
Wēndǎntāng 5g + shíchāngpú 1g + yuǎnzhì 1g + acupuncture.	Shíchāngpú 5g + yuǎnzhì 5g + júhóng 3g + júhuā
	3-0g + chántuì 3-0g.
	Zhǐqiào 5g + júhuā 5g + jílí 5g + chántuì 5g.

Hydrocephalus (331.4, 331.3), Hearing impairment (D003638), Optic atrophy (377.1), Polyphagia (D006963), Sleep apnea (780.57):

Yìqìcōngmíngtāng 5g + shíchāngpú 1g + yuǎnzhì 1g + acupuncture.	Huángqí 5g + chìsháo 1g + fángfēng 1g + xìxīn
Liùwèidìhuángwán 5g + yìqìcōngmíngtāng 5-0g + shíchāngpú 1g + yuǎnzhì 1g + acupuncture.	0g + huánglián 0g + dàhuáng 0g + acupuncture.
	Xuánshēn 5g + dìhuáng 5g + màiméndōng 5g +
Liùwèidìhuángwán 5g + tiānwángbǔxīndān 5-0g + shíchāngpú 1g + yuǎnzhì 1g.	hòupò 5-3g + zhǐshí 5-2g + dàhuáng 0g.

that Shíchāngpú improved the learning and memory ability of Alzheimer's disease mice by repairing myelin injury and lowering the tau phosphorylation (Fu et al., 2020).

REFERENCES

Chen, S., Chen, Q., Li, B., Jian-Li, G., Shi, J., & Lv, G. (2015). Antihypertensive effect of Radix paeoniae alba in spontaneously hypertensive rats and excessive alcohol intake and high fat diet induced hypertensive rats. *Evidence-Based Complementary and Alternative Medicine*, *2015*, 1–8. https://doi.org/10.1155/2015/731237

Deepak, D. S., Furlong, N., Wilding, J., & MacFarlane, I. A. (2007). Cardiovascular disease, hypertension, dyslipidaemia and obesity in patients with hypothalamic-pituitary disease. *Postgraduate Medical Journal*, *83*(978), 277–280. https://doi.org/10.1136/pgmj.2006.052241

Fu, Y., Yang, Y., Shi, J., Bishayee, K., Lin, L., Lin, Y., Zhang, S., Ji, L., & Li, C. (2020). Acori tatarinowii rhizoma extract ameliorates Alzheimer's pathological syndromes by repairing myelin injury and lowering Tau phosphorylation in mice. *Die Pharmazie - an International Journal of Pharmaceutical Sciences*, *75*(8), 395–400.

George, R. C., Lew, J. I., & Graves, D. J. (2013). Interaction of cinnamaldehyde and epicatechin with tau: Implications of beneficial effects in modulating Alzheimer's disease pathogenesis. *Journal of Alzheimer's Disease*, *36*(1), 21–40. https://doi.org/10.3233/jad-122113

Gong, P., He, Y., Qi, J., Chai, C., & Yu, B. (2020). Synergistic nourishing 'Yin' effect of iridoid and phenylpropanoid glycosides from Radix Scrophulariae in vivo and in vitro. *Journal of Ethnopharmacology*, *246*, 112209. https://doi.org/10.1016/j.jep.2019.112209

Ho, S., Chang, K., & Chang, P. (2013). Inhibition of neuroinflammation by cinnamon and its main components. *Food Chemistry*, *138*(4), 2275–2282. https://doi.org/10.1016/j.foodchem.2012.12.020

Hu, M., Li, H., Ni, S., & Wang, S. (2023). The protective effects of Zhi-Gan-Cao-Tang against diabetic myocardial infarction injury and identification of its effective constituents. *Journal of Ethnopharmacology*, *309*, 116320. https://doi.org/10.1016/j.jep.2023.116320

Huang, M., Pai, F., Lin, C., Chang, C., Chang, H., Lee, Y., Sun, M., & Yen, H. (2015). Characteristics of traditional Chinese medicine use in patients with rheumatoid arthritis in Taiwan: A nationwide population-based study. *Journal of Ethnopharmacology*, *176*, 9–16. https://doi.org/10.1016/j.jep.2015.10.024

Kim, H.-W., Cho, S.-J., Kim, B.-Y., & Cho, S.-I. (2007). Anti-oxidant effects of *Anemarrhenae Rhizoma* in three different lineages. *The Journal of Internal Korean Medicine*, *28*(3), 608–614. https://www.jikm.or.kr/journal/view.php?number=1254

Kim, H. Y., Hong, M. H., Kim, K. W., Yoon, J. J., Lee, J. E., Kang, D. G., & Lee, H. S. (2020). Improvement of hypertriglyceridemia by roasted *Nelumbinis folium* in high fat/high cholesterol diet rat model. *Nutrients*, *12*(12), 3859. https://doi.org/10.3390/nu12123859

Kobayashi, S., Kawasaki, Y., Takahashi, T., Maeno, H., & Nomura, M. (2017). Mechanisms for the anti-obesity actions of bofutsushosan in high-fat diet-fed obese mice. *Chinese Medicine, 12*(1). https://doi.org/10.1186/s13020-017-0129-x

Lee, H., Jung, D. Y., Ha, H., Son, K., Jeon, S., & Kim, C. (2007). Induction of growth hormone release by dioscin from *Dioscorea batatas* DECNE. *BMB Reports, 40*(6), 1016–1020. https://doi.org/10.5483/bmbrep.2007.40.6.1016

Lei, Y., Wang, B., Zhu, G., Feng, G., Li, W., Han, C., Qi, Q., Yu, X., Song, X., He, Z., Ju, Z., Su, H., & Wang, W. (2024). Isolation and identification of anti-inflammatory active components from Asparagi Radix cochinchinensis based on HPLC-CAD and UPLC-Q/TOF-MS techniques. *Natural Product Communications, 19*(2). https://doi.org/10.1177/1934578x241232269

Li, C., Peng, S., Liu, X., Han, C., Wang, X., Jin, T., Liu, S., Wang, W., Xie, X., He, X., Zhang, H., Shan, L., Fan, C., Shan, Z., & Wang, T. (2017). Glycyrrhizin, a direct HMGB1 antagonist, ameliorates inflammatory infiltration in a model of autoimmune thyroiditis via inhibition of TLR2-HMGB1 signaling. *Thyroid, 27*(5), 722–731. https://doi.org/10.1089/thy.2016.0432

Li, D., Yang, M., & Zuo, Z. (2020). Overview of pharmacokinetics and liver toxicities of Radix polygoni multiflori. *Toxins, 12*(11), 729. https://doi.org/10.3390/toxins12110729

Liu, P., Zhao, H., & Luo, Y. (2017). Anti-aging implications of Astragalus membranaceus (Huangqi): A well-known Chinese tonic. *Aging and Disease, 8*(6), 868. https://doi.org/10.14336/ad.2017.0816

Liu, P., Zhou, X. Y., Zhang, H., Wang, R., Wu, X., Jian, W., Li, W., Yuan, D., Wang, Q., & Zhao, W. (2022). Danggui-Shaoyao-San attenuates cognitive impairment via the Microbiota–Gut–Brain axis with regulation of lipid metabolism in Scopolamine-induced amnesia. *Frontiers in Immunology, 13*. https://doi.org/10.3389/fimmu.2022.796542

Lu, L., Xu, L., He, Y., Shen, J., Xin, J., Zhou, J., Wang, C., Wang, Y., Pan, X., & Gao, J. (2023). Evaluation the effectiveness of the Jiangniaosuan formulation in the treatment of hyperuricemic nephropathy in patients with chronic kidney disease stages 3–4: Study protocol of a randomized controlled trial. *Contemporary Clinical Trials Communications, 32*, 101065. https://doi.org/10.1016/j.conctc.2023.101065

Ma, W., Zhang, X., Zhao, R., Tang, Y., Zhu, X., Liu, L., Xu, M., Wang, G., Peng, P., Liu, J., & Liu, Z. (2023). Effectiveness and potential mechanism of Jiawei-Xiaoyao-San for hyperthyroidism: A systematic review. *Frontiers in Endocrinology, 14*. https://doi.org/10.3389/fendo.2023.1241962

Ou, T., Wang, C., Hung, G., Wu, C., & Lee, H. (2011). Aqueous extract of Shi-Liu-Wei-Liu-Qi-Yin induces G2/M phase arrest and apoptosis in human bladder carcinoma cells via FAS and mitochondrial pathway. *Evidence-Based Complementary and Alternative Medicine, 2011*, 1–10. https://doi.org/10.1093/ecam/nep016

Peng, S., Xie, Z., Zhang, X., Xie, C., Kang, J., Yuan, H., Xu, G., Zhang, X., & Liu, Y. (2021). Efficacy and safety of the Chinese patent medicine Yuquan pill on type 2 diabetes mellitus patients: A systematic review and meta-analysis. *Evidence-Based Complementary and Alternative Medicine, 2021*, 1–14. https://doi.org/10.1155/2021/2562590

Tan, W., Li, Y., Wang, Y., Zhang, Z., Wang, T., Zhou, Q., & Wang, X. (2017). Anti-coagulative and gastrointestinal motility regulative activities of Fructus Aurantii Immaturus and its effective fractions. *Biomedicine & Pharmacotherapy, 90*, 244–252. https://doi.org/10.1016/j.biopha.2017.03.060

Uddin, M. K., Juraimi, A. S., Hossain, S., Nahar, M. a. U., Ali, E., & Rahman, M. (2014). Purslane weed (*Portulaca oleracea*): A prospective plant source of nutrition, Omega-3 fatty acid, and antioxidant attributes. *The Scientific World Journal, 2014*, 1–6. https://doi.org/10.1155/2014/951019

Wang, D., Bi, C., Jiang, H., Li, Y., Zhang, W., Liu, Y., & Liu, Y. (2022a). Efficacy and safety of Gegen Qinlian decoction for pediatric diarrhea: A systematic review and meta-analysis. *Evidence-Based Complementary and Alternative Medicine, 2022*, 1–11. https://doi.org/10.1155/2022/4887259

Wang, K., Qian, R., Li, H., Wang, C., Ding, Y., & Gao, Z. (2022b). Interpreting the pharmacological mechanisms of Sho-saiko-to on thyroid carcinoma through combining network pharmacology and experimental evaluation. *ACS Omega, 7*(13), 11166–11176. https://doi.org/10.1021/acsomega.1c07335

Wang, Q., Ren, X., Shi-Lin, Y., & Wu, H. (2010). Clinical observation on the endocrinal and immune functions in subjects with yin-deficiency constitution. *Chinese Journal of Integrative Medicine, 16*(1), 28–32. https://doi.org/10.1007/s11655-010-0028-9

Wang, S.-C. (2019). Therapeutic classes of CHEG formulas. In S.-C. Wang (Ed.), *Clinical herbal prescriptions: Principles and practices of herbal formulations from deep learning health insurance herbal prescription big data* (pp. 16–89). World Scientific Publishing. https://doi.org/10.1142/11211

Wang, S.-C. (2020). Modern therapeutic uses of CHEG herbs and herb pairs. In S.-C. Wang (Ed.), *Veterinary herbal pharmacopoeia* (pp. 35–233). Nova Science Publishers. https://doi.org/10.52305/GHTR1903

Wang, X., Ma, L., Zhang, E., Zou, J., Guo, H., Peng, S., & Wu, J. (2014). Water extract of *Fructus Hordei Germinatus* shows antihyperprolactinemia activity via dopamine D2 receptor. *Evidence-Based Complementary and Alternative Medicine*, *2014*, 1–7. https://doi.org/10.1155/2014/579054

Wu, H., Liu, C., Tsai, J., Ko, L., & Wei, Y. (2002). Antioxidant and anticonvulsant effect of a modified formula of Chaihu-Longu-Muli-Tang. *American Journal of Chinese Medicine*, *30*(02n03), 339–346. https://doi.org/10.1142/s0192415x02000235

Wu, J., Ke, X., Fu, W., Gao, X., Zhang, H., Wang, W., Ma, N., Zhao, M., Hao, X., & Zhang, Z. (2016). Inhibition of hypoxia-induced retinal angiogenesis by specnuezhenide, an effective constituent of Ligustrum lucidum Ait., through suppression of the HIF-1α/VEGF signaling pathway. *Molecules*, *21*(12), 1756. https://doi.org/10.3390/molecules21121756

Xie, Z., Wu, H., Jing, X., Li, X., Li, Y., Han, Y., Gao, X., Tang, X., Sun, J., Fan, Y., & Wen, C. (2017). Hypouricemic and arthritis relapse-reducing effects of compound tufuling oral-liquid in intercritical and chronic gout. *Medicine*, *96*(11), e6315. https://doi.org/10.1097/md.0000000000006315

Yang, S., Lin, Y., Lin, J., Chen, H., Hu, S., Yang, Y., Yang, Y., Yang, Y., & Fang, Y. (2018). The efficacy and safety of a fixed combination of Chinese herbal medicine in chronic urticaria: A randomized, double-blind, placebo-controlled pilot study. *Frontiers in Pharmacology*, *9*. https://doi.org/10.3389/fphar.2018.01474

Yang, T., Zhao, S., Yuan, Y., Zhao, X., Bu, F., Zhang, Z., Li, Q., Li, Y., Wei, Z., Sun, X., Zhang, Y., & Xie, J. (2023). Platycodonis Radix alleviates LPS-induced lung inflammation through modulation of TRPA1 channels. *Molecules*, *28*(13), 5213. https://doi.org/10.3390/molecules28135213

Zhang, P., Xu, Y.-D., Zhou, P., Zhang, J., Ji, H.-N., Xiao, Y.-Q., & Liu, Y. (2023). Effect and mechanism investigation on improving kidney deficient in mice of Polygoni Multiflori Radix Praeparata based on plasma metabolomics. *Acta Pharmaceutica Sinica*, (12), 1464–1474. https://search.bvsalud.org/gim/resource/es/wpr-978739

Zhang, S., Wang, J., Zhao, H., & Luo, Y. (2018). Effects of three flavonoids from an ancient traditional Chinese medicine *Radix puerariae* on geriatric diseases. *Brain Circulation*, *4*(4), 174–184. https://doi.org/10.4103/bc.bc_13_18

Zhang, Y., Jin, F., Wang, X., Jin, Q., Xie, J., Pan, Y., & Shen, W. (2022). Chinese herbal medicine for the treatment of chronic fatigue syndrome: A systematic review and meta-analysis. *Frontiers in Pharmacology*, *13*. https://doi.org/10.3389/fphar.2022.958005

Zheng, F., Wei, P., Huo, H., Xing, X., Chen, F., Tan, X., & Jia-Bo, L. (2015). Neuroprotective effect of Gui Zhi (Ramulus Cinnamomi) on Ma Huang- (Herb Ephedra-) induced toxicity in rats treated with a Ma Huang-Gui Zhi herb pair. *Evidence-Based Complementary and Alternative Medicine*, *2015*, 1–9. https://doi.org/10.1155/2015/913461

Zhou, M., Yu, R., Liu, X., Lv, X., & Qin, X. (2022). Ginseng-plus-Bai-Hu-Tang combined with Western medicine for the treatment of type 2 diabetes mellitus: A systematic review and meta-analysis. *Evidence-Based Complementary and Alternative Medicine*, *2022*, 1–13. https://doi.org/10.1155/2022/9572384

9 GMP Herbal Medicine for Rare Hematologic Diseases

Blood disorders primarily affect the blood, changing its quantity and functions. Causes of blood disorders include gene mutations, medication side effects, nutritional deficiencies, and other diseases. Many of the rare blood diseases of this chapter are late onset.

The single herbs and multi-herb formulas that are commonly discussed for the signs and symptoms of the rare blood diseases are Rhubarb Root and Rhizome (Dàhuáng), Licorice Root (Gāncǎo), Rehmannia Root (Dìhuáng), Chinese Angelica Root (female Ginseng; Dāngguī), Astragalus Root (Huángqí), Figwort Root (Xuánshēn), Achyranthes Root (Niúxī), Honeysuckle Flower (Jīnyínhuā), Agrimony (Xiānhècǎo), Red Peony Root (Chìsháo), Immature Bitter Orange (Zhǐshí), Magnolia Bark (Hòupò), Scutellaria Root (Huángqín), Tonify the Middle and Augment the Qi Decoction (Bǔzhōngyìqìtāng), Earth Restoring Decoction (Guīpítāng), Relax the Channels and Invigorate the Blood Decoction (Shūjīnghuóxuètāng), Wind Reducing Formula (Xiāofēngsǎn), Generalized Pain Dispel Stasis Decoction (Shēntòngzhúyūtāng), Cinnamon and Angelica Gout Formula (Shàngzhōngxiàtōngyòngtòngfēngwán), Virgate Wormwood and Five Ingredient Powder with Poria (Yīnchénwǔlíngsǎn), Tangkuei and Gelatin Combination (Xiōngguījiāoàitāng), and Bone-Setter's Purple-Gold Special Pill (Zhènggǔzǐjīndān).

Blood in TCM includes not only the blood matter, i.e., blood cells and plasma proteins, but also its movement, driven by Qi, along the channels over the body called *meridians*. In TCM, and also in many other Eastern medical traditions, there exists a universal, vital energy responsible for living things. Blood and Qi are just yin and yang manifestations of the vital energy. The common abnormal patterns related to blood in TCM include blood stasis, blood deficiency, and blood heat (and the associated Qi stagnation, Qi deficiency, and Qi straying) with such clinical manifestations as pain, anemia, and bleeding. We indeed notice Qi/blood-replenishing and pain-relieving herbal products in the GMP herbal regimens for the blood diseases above.

9.1 FETAL AND NEONATAL ALLOIMMUNE THROMBOCYTOPENIA

Fetal and neonatal alloimmune thrombocytopenia (FNAIT) is caused by placental transfer of maternal antibodies against the fetus's platelets, which express antigens inherited from the child's father and differ from the mother's own antigens, leading to destruction and thus low counts of platelets in the fetus or newborn. A shortage of platelets increases the risk of bleeding in the fetus and neonate with FNAIT.

TABLE 9.1

GMP Herbal Medicines for a One-Year-Old Infant with Fetal and Neonatal Alloimmune Thrombocytopenia

Fetal and neonatal alloimmune thrombocytopenia (OrphaCode: 853)

A disease with a prevalence of ~4 in 10,000

Candidate gene tested: glycoprotein Ib platelet subunit alpha (*GP1BA* / Entrez: 2811) at 17p13.2

Candidate gene tested: glycoprotein Ib platelet subunit beta (*GP1BB* / Entrez: 2812) at 22q11.21

Candidate gene tested: integrin subunit alpha 2b (*ITGA2B* / Entrez: 3674) at 17q21.31

Major susceptibility factor: integrin subunit beta 3 (*ITGB3* / Entrez: 3690) at 17q21.32

(Continued)

DOI: 10.1201/9781032726625-9

TABLE 9.1 *(Continued)*

GMP Herbal Medicines for a One-Year-Old Infant with Fetal and Neonatal Alloimmune Thrombocytopenia

Candidate gene tested: integrin subunit alpha 2 (*ITGA2* / Entrez: 3673) at 5q11.2

Candidate gene tested: CD109 molecule (*CD109* / Entrez: 135228) at 6q13

Not applicable

Neonatal alloimmune thrombocytopenia

Petechiae, Purpura, Abnormal bleeding, Spontaneous hematomas, Cephalohematoma

Hematuria, Intracranial hemorrhage, Gastrointestinal hemorrhage, Melena, Ecchymosis

Antenatal, Neonatal

Petechiae (D011693):

Xiāofēngsǎn 5g + jīngfángbàidúsǎn 5-0g + báixiānpí 1-0g + dìfūzǐ 1-0g + jīnyínhuā 1-0g + liánqiáo 1-0g + gāncǎo 0g.

Xiāofēngsǎn 5g + dāngguīyǐnzǐ 5g + báixiānpí 1g + dìfūzǐ 1g.

Xiāofēngsǎn 5g + jiědúsìwùtāng 5g + báixiānpí 1g + dìfūzǐ 1g + zǐcǎo 1g.

Báizhǐ 5g + gāncǎo 4g + shārén 4g + huángqín 4-0g + tiānhuā 2-0g + dàhuáng 1-0g.

Shārén, being antiallergic and anti-inflammatory, is used for allergic rhinitis and psoriasis (cf. Section 3.31). Xiāofēngsǎn treated skin conditions in Sections 1.23, 3.4, and 3.29. Báixiānpí (Cortex Dictamni) "clears heat, dries dampness, dispels Wind, and neutralizes toxins." It was shown to be anti-inflammatory in monocyte/macrophage-like cells derived from mice (Chen et al., 2020) and is used today for contact dermatitis and other eczema (Wang, 2020). The prescriptions in the table are believed to relieve the skin symptoms of the patients.

9.2 HEREDITARY SPHEROCYTOSIS

Hereditary spherocytosis, also known as Minkowski-Chauffard disease, refers to changes in the shape of red blood cells, from the normal biconcave to spherical, caused by mutations in any one of the genes encoding red blood cell membrane proteins. The structurally defective red blood cells are destroyed by the macrophages in the spleen in a process called *hemolysis*. Chronic extravascular hemolysis can lead to anemia and splenomegaly.

TABLE 9.2

GMP Herbal Medicines for a Five-Year-Old Child with Hereditary Spherocytosis

Hereditary spherocytosis (OrphaCode: 822)

A disease with a prevalence of ~3 in 10,000

Disease-causing germline mutation(s): solute carrier family 4 member 1 (Diego blood group) (*SLC4A1* / Entrez: 6521) at 17q21.31

Disease-causing germline mutation(s): spectrin alpha, erythrocytic 1 (*SPTA1* / Entrez: 6708) at 1q23.1

Disease-causing germline mutation(s): spectrin beta, erythrocytic (*SPTB* / Entrez: 6710) at 14q23.3

Disease-causing germline mutation(s): ankyrin 1 (*ANK1* / Entrez: 286) at 8p11.21

Disease-causing germline mutation(s): erythrocyte membrane protein band 4.2 (*EPB42* / Entrez: 2038) at 15q15.2

Autosomal dominant, Autosomal recessive

Increased red cell osmotic fragility

Jaundice, Pallor, Cholelithiasis, Muscle weakness, Splenomegaly, Anemia, Reticulocytosis, Hepatomegaly, Hyperbilirubinemia, Spherocytosis, Spontaneous hemolytic crises, Hypofibrinogenemia, Increased mean corpuscular hemoglobin concentration, Hypercoagulability

Ataxia, Fever, Extramedullary hematopoiesis, Abdominal pain, Myalgia, Restrictive heart failure, Chills, Maculopapular exanthema

All ages

(Continued)

TABLE 9.2 *(Continued)*

GMP Herbal Medicines for a Five-Year-Old Child with Hereditary Spherocytosis

Jaundice (D007565), Pallor (D010167), Muscle weakness (D018908), Anemia (285.9), Reticulocytosis (D045262):

Sìjūnzǐtāng 5g + shēnlíngbáizhúsǎn 5-0g + sìwùtāng 5-0g + bǎohéwán 5-0g.

Zhènggǔzǐjindān 5g + gāncǎo 0g.

Xiǎojiànzhōngtāng 5g + yùpíngfēngsǎn 5g + bǔzhōngyìqìtāng 5g.

Bǔzhōngyìqìtāng 5g + shēnlíngbáizhúsǎn 3g + shānzhā 1g + shénqū 1g + màiyá 1g.

Liùjūnzǐtāng 5g + shānzhā 0g + shénqū 0g + màiyá 0g.

Jīnyínhuā 5g + liánqiáo 5g.

Jīnyínhuā 5g + dāngguī 5-0g + xuánshēn 3-0g + gāncǎo 3-0g + dǎodìwúgōng 3-0g + chìsháo 3-0g + huángqí 3-0g + báizhǐ 2-0g + shārén 2-0g + dàhuáng 0g.

Běishāshēn 5g + xuánshēn 5g + dìhuáng 5g + màiméndōng 5g + hòupò 5-2g + zhǐshí 5-2g + yùzhú 5-0g + dàhuáng 2-0g.

Ataxia (D002524), Fever (D005334), Abdominal pain (D015746), Myalgia (D063806):

Bǔzhōngyìqìtāng 5g + rénshēnyǎngróngtāng 5-0g + xiāngshāliùjūnzǐtāng 5-0g + shénqū 1-0g + màiyá 1-0g + jīnèijīn 1-0g + gāncǎo 0g.

Bāxiāntāng 5g.

Huángqíwǔwùtāng 5-2g + dàzhēnjiāotāng 5-0g.

Yùpíngfēngsǎn 5g + guìzhītāng 5g + xìngrén 1g + hòupò 1g.

Huángqí 5g + dǎngshēn 5g + gāncǎo 3g + báizhú 3g + báisháo 3g + fángfēng 3g + qiānghuó 3g + fúlíng 3g + chénpí 3g + zéxiè 3g + dúhuó 3g + bànxià 2-0g + cháihú 2-0g + huánglián 2-0g.

Huángqí 5g + zhìgāncǎo 4-2g + wǔwèizǐ 1-0g + dāngguī 1-0g.

Huángqí 5g + chìsháo 1g + fángfēng 1g + dāngguī 1-0g + xìxīn 0g + huánglián 0g + dàhuáng 0g.

Dāngguī (cf. Sections 2.43 and 3.9) "nourishes Blood, promotes circulation" and has been used to modulate a variety of hematologic anomalies (Bradley et al., 1999; Wang, 2020). Dǎngshēn (cf. Section 4.20) was reviewed to improve an athlete's recovery from fatigue (Yu et al., 2023). Sìwùtāng, containing Dāngguī, "replenishes Blood, regulates menstruation" and is used nowadays for iron-deficiency anemias and other unspecified anemias (Wang, 2019). Bāxiāntāng also contains Dāngguī and is used today for paralytic syndromes (Wang, 2019).

9.3 HEREDITARY ELLIPTOCYTOSIS

Hereditary elliptocytosis is a change in red blood cell shape from the typical biconcave disc to an oval, due to mutations in the genes coding for the red blood cell membrane and skeletal proteins. As abnormally shaped red blood cells are degraded faster than normal red blood cells in the spleen, severity of hereditary elliptocytosis depends on the extent of red blood cell deformity.

Shúdìhuáng was introduced in Section 3.18 for anemia of the mother. Jīxuèténg was introduced in Section 4.24 to "replenish Blood" and is used today for the absence of menstruation (Wang,

TABLE 9.3

GMP Herbal Medicines for a 17-Year-Old Adolescent with Hereditary Elliptocytosis

Hereditary elliptocytosis (OrphaCode: 288)

A disease with a prevalence of ~3 in 10,000

Disease-causing germline mutation(s): spectrin alpha, erythrocytic 1 (*SPTA1* / Entrez: 6708) at 1q23.1

Disease-causing germline mutation(s): spectrin beta, erythrocytic (*SPTB* / Entrez: 6710) at 14q23.3

Disease-causing germline mutation(s): erythrocyte membrane protein band 4.1 (*EPB41* / Entrez: 2035) at 1p35.3

Disease-causing germline mutation(s): glycophorin C (Gerbich blood group) (*GYPC* / Entrez: 2995) at 2q14.3

Autosomal dominant, Autosomal recessive

Abnormal erythrocyte morphology

Elliptocytosis, Increased red cell osmotic fragility

Jaundice, Splenomegaly, Hemolytic anemia, Reticulocytosis, Hyperbilirubinemia, Neonatal hyperbilirubinemia, Stomatocytosis, Poikilocytosis, Congenital hemolytic anemia, Prolonged neonatal jaundice

All ages

(Continued)

TABLE 9.3 *(Continued)*

GMP Herbal Medicines for a 17-Year-Old Adolescent with Hereditary Elliptocytosis

Elliptocytosis (282.1):

Sìwùtāng 5g + bǔzhōngyìqìtāng 5g + guīpítāng 5-0g.

Rénshēnyǎngróngtāng 5g + bǔzhōngyìqìtāng 5-0g + guīpítāng 5-0g.

Rénshēnyǎngróngtāng 5g + sìwùtāng 5g + dānshēn 1g.

Shíquándàbǔtāng 5g + bǔzhōngyìqìtāng 5g.

Shèngyùtāng 5g + bǔzhōngyìqìtāng 5g + gāncǎo 0g.

Huángqí 5g + zhìgāncǎo 3-2g + wǔwèizǐ 2-1g + dāngguī 1g.

Huángqí 5g + jīxuèténg 5g + gǒuqǐzǐ 4g + dāngguī 4g + wǔlíngzhī 3g + tùsīzǐ 3g + fùpénzǐ 3g + bājǐtiān 2g.

Huángqí 5g + dǎngshēn 5g + shúdìhuáng 5-0g + chuānxiōng 4g + báisháo 4g + dìhuáng 4g + dāngguī 4g + guìzhī 4-0g + héshǒuwū 4-0g.

Shúdìhuáng 5g + báizhú 4g + fùzǐ 4g + báisháo 3g + fúlíng 3g + báijièzǐ 2g + dǎngshēn 2g + gāncǎo 1g + shēngjiāng 1g + guìzhī 1g + máhuáng 1g + huánglián 0g.

Gāncǎo 5g + huángqí 2g + wǔwèizǐ 1g + dāngguī 1g.

Jaundice (D007565), Reticulocytosis (D045262), Congenital hemolytic anemia (282):

Zhènggǔzǐjīndān 5g + sháoyàogāncǎotāng 5-0g + shūjīnghuóxuètāng 5-0g + acupuncture.

Shíquándàbǔtāng 5g + guīpítāng 5-0g.

Lóngdǎnxiègāntāng 5g + jīnyínhuā 1g + liánqiáo 1g + púgōngyīng 1g.

Bāzhēntāng 5g + guīpítāng 5g + xiānhècǎo 1g + ējiāo 1g + jīxuèténg 1g.

Jīnyínhuā 5g + dāngguī 5g + xuánshēn 3-2g + gāncǎo 3-2g + dǎodìwúgōng 3-2g + niúxī 3-2g + chìsháo 3-2g + huángqí 3-2g.

Jīnyínhuā 5g + dāngguī 5g + niúxī 2g + xuánshēn 2g + chìsháo 2g + zhìgāncǎo 2g + dǎodìwúgōng 2g + huángqí 2g.

Běishāshēn 5g + yùzhú 5g + hòupò 5g + zhǐshí 5g + dàhuáng 0g.

2020). Rénshēnyǎngróngtāng, Shíquándàbǔtāng, and Shèngyùtāng all contain Huángqí, Dāngguī, and Shúdìhuáng, and are all used today for iron-deficiency anemias and other unspecified anemias (Wang, 2019). Jīnyínhuā (cf. Section 3.5) was reviewed to be hepatoprotective (Li et al., 2020). Zhènggǔzǐjīndān "nourishes Blood, enlivens Blood, disperses stasis, and stops pain."

9.4 ESSENTIAL THROMBOCYTHEMIA

Essential thrombocythemia, or essential thrombocytosis, is overproduction of platelets in the bone marrow caused by a gene mutation that renders hematopoietic cells to become more sensitive to growth factors. High platelet counts can lead to the formation of clots in blood vessels, increasing the risk of strokes, heart attacks, and pulmonary embolism.

TABLE 9.4

GMP Herbal Medicines for a 60-Year-Old Adult with Essential Thrombocythemia

Essential thrombocythemia (OrphaCode: 3318)

A disease with a prevalence of ~3 in 10,000

Biomarker tested: tet methylcytosine dioxygenase 2 (*TET2* / Entrez: 54790) at 4q24

Disease-causing somatic mutation(s): Janus kinase 2 (*JAK2* / Entrez: 3717) at 9p24.1

Disease-causing somatic mutation(s): MPL proto-oncogene, thrombopoietin receptor (*MPL* / Entrez: 4352) at 1p34.2

Disease-causing somatic mutation(s): calreticulin (*CALR* / Entrez: 811) at 19p13.13

Disease-causing somatic mutation(s): SH2B adaptor protein 3 (*SH2B3* / Entrez: 10019) at 12q24.12

Biomarker tested: tumor protein p53 (*TP53* / Entrez: 7157) at 17p13.1

Multigenic/multifactorial, Not applicable

Myocardial infarction, Abnormality of thrombocytes, Transient ischemic attack, Prolonged bleeding time, Paresthesia, Arterial thrombosis, Increased megakaryocyte count, Abnormality of bone marrow cell morphology, Abnormal platelet morphology, Amaurosis fugax, Abnormality of the cerebral vasculature, Chest pain, Venous thrombosis

Splenomegaly

(Continued)

TABLE 9.4 *(Continued)*
GMP Herbal Medicines for a 60-Year-Old Adult with Essential Thrombocythemia

Acute leukemia, Myelodysplasia, Myelofibrosis
All ages

Paresthesia (D010292), Amaurosis fugax (D020757), Chest pain (D002637):

Shēntòngzhúyūtāng 5g + shūjīnghuóxuètāng 5g + yánhúsuǒ 2-0g + jiānghuáng 1-0g + acupuncture.	Wēilíngxiān 5g + chuānshānlóng 5g + sānqī 4g + mùguā 4g + niúxī 4g + hónghuā 4g + huángbò 4g + gǒujǐ 4-0g + wǔjiāpí 4-0g + dàhuáng 1-0g.
Shēntòngzhúyūtāng 5g + dúhuójìshēngtāng 5g + yánhúsuǒ 1-0g + jīxuèténg 1-0g + acupuncture.	Chuānwū 5g + wǔlíngzhī 2g + tiānnánxīng 2g + mùxiāng 2g + gāncǎo 2g + dìlóng 2g + yánhúsuǒ 2g + táorén 2g + huíxiāng 2g + chénpí 2g + dāngguī 2g.
Shēntòngzhúyūtāng 5g + juānbìtāng 5g + yánhúsuǒ 1g + acupuncture.	Wēilíngxiān 5g + báizhú 3g + qiānghuó 3g + xiāngfù 3g + huángqín 3g + cāngzhú 3g + tiānnánxīng 2g + gāncǎo 2g + shēngjiāng 2g + fúlíng 2g + chénpí 2g + bànxià 2-0g.
Shēntòngzhúyūtāng 5g + sháoyàogāncǎotāng 4g + yánhúsuǒ 1g + guìzhī 1g + acupuncture.	

Wēilíngxiān (cf. Sections 2.1, 2.33, and 2.54) is used today for gouty arthropathy, pain in joints, monoplegia, and so on (Wang, 2020). Chuānshānlóng (cf. Section 2.37) is used for pain in joints, low back pain, chest pain, and backaches (Wang, 2020). Chuānwū was introduced in Sections 2.12 and 2.42 for musculoskeletal pain and chest pain. Shēntòngzhúyūtāng (cf. Sections 2.1, 2.4, and 2.42) is used today for disorders of soft tissues and joints, such as peripheral enthesopathies and allied syndromes (Wang, 2019).

9.5 HEREDITARY THROMBOPHILIA DUE TO CONGENITAL ANTITHROMBIN DEFICIENCY

People with hereditary thrombophilia due to congenital antithrombin deficiency easily form blood clots in the veins of their legs and lungs. Hereditary thrombophilia due to congenital antithrombin deficiency is caused by mutations in the *SERPINC1* gene, whose products regulate blood coagulation cascade.

TABLE 9.5
GMP Herbal Medicines for a 19-Year-Old Adult with Hereditary Thrombophilia Due to Congenital Antithrombin Deficiency

Hereditary thrombophilia due to congenital antithrombin deficiency (OrphaCode: 82)

A disease with a prevalence of ~3 in 10,000

Disease-causing germline mutation(s): serpin family C member 1 (*SERPINC1* / Entrez: 462) at 1q25.1

Autosomal dominant

Reduced antithrombin III activity, Reduced antithrombin antigen

Pulmonary embolism, Deep venous thrombosis, Superficial thrombophlebitis, Recurrent thromboembolism, Pregnancy exposure
Arterial thrombosis, Spontaneous abortion, Retinal vein occlusion, Portal vein thrombosis, Hepatic vein thrombosis,
  Mesenteric venous thrombosis, Recurrent spontaneous abortion

Adolescent, Adult

Retinal vein occlusion (362.35):

Zīshènmíngmùtāng 5g + xǐgānmíngmùtāng 5-4g + qǐjúdìhuángwán 5-0g + juémíngzǐ 2-1g + xiàkūcǎo 1-0g + mànjīngzǐ 1-0g.	Gǒuqǐzǐ 5g + júhuā 5g + niúbàngzǐ 3g + bèimǔ 3g + shègān 3g + xìxīn 1g + huánglián 1g.
Zīshènmíngmùtāng 5g + jiāwèixiāoyáosàn 3g + xuèfǔzhúyūtāng 3g + juémíngzǐ 1g + xiàkūcǎo 1g + júhuā 1g + gōuténg 1g.	Gǒuqǐzǐ 5g + júhuā 5g + dìhuáng 4-3g + fángfēng 4-3g + dāngguī 4-3g + xìxīn 2-1g + huánglián 2-1g.
	Nǚzhēnzǐ 5g + tiānméndōng 2g + báizhú 2g + chuānxiōng 2g + fùzǐ 2g + júhuā 2g + huángqín 2g + bǔgǔzhī 2g.

Nǚzhēnzǐ was introduced in Sections 1.20 and 8.2 to benefit the eye. Bèimǔ (cf. Section 4.27) was shown to decrease the blood viscosity in rats through a decrease of blood lipids and anti-peroxidation of lipids (Jiang et al., 1993). Mànjīngzǐ (Fructus Viticis) was demonstrated to atten-uate trigeminal hyperalgesia in rats with a nitroglycerin-induced migraine (Wen et al., 2020). Both Mànjīngzǐ and Gōuténg (cf. Section 2.43) are used today for headaches and migraines (Wang, 2020).

9.6   POLYCYTHEMIA VERA

Polycythemia vera, also known as acquired primary erythrocytosis or Osler-Vaquez disease, is over-production of red blood cells. It is caused by somatic gene mutations that stimulate erythropoiesis in the bone marrow independent of erythropoietin secretion from the kidneys or liver. A higher frac-tion of red blood cells in the blood thickens the blood and slows blood flow, causing tissue damage.

Sānqī (Radix et Rhizoma Notoginseng) has been used for strokes and the herb pair Sānqī-Dānshēn was shown to synergistically protect human cardiovascular endothelial cells from cel-lular impairments in vitro (Zhou et al., 2019). Huángliánjiědútāng, being bitter in TCM taste and cool in TCM nature, "quells fires in the upper, middle and also the lower body." The term jiědú means detoxification. Huángliánjiědútāng is anti-inflammatory and treats a range of skin condi-tions, including burns, furuncles, and carbuncles.

TABLE 9.6

GMP Herbal Medicines for a 65-Year-Old Man with Polycythemia Vera

Polycythemia vera (OrphaCode: 729)

A disease with a prevalence of ~3 in 10,000

Disease-causing somatic mutation(s): Janus kinase 2 (*JAK2* / Entrez: 3717) at 9p24.1

Disease-causing somatic mutation(s): MPL proto-oncogene, thrombopoietin receptor (*MPL* / Entrez: 4352) at 1p34.2

Disease-causing somatic mutation(s): tet methylcytosine dioxygenase 2 (*TET2* / Entrez: 54790) at 4q24

Not applicable

Gingival bleeding, Tinnitus, Epistaxis, Hypertension, Bruising susceptibility, Angina pectoris, Splenomegaly, Weight loss, Abdominal pain, Hepatomegaly, Headache, Vertigo, Acute leukemia, Myelodysplasia, Myelofibrosis

Respiratory insufficiency, Arthralgia, Fatigue

Pruritus, Stroke, Portal hypertension, Pulmonary embolism, Gastrointestinal hemorrhage, Budd-Chiari syndrome, Intermittent claudication, Arterial thrombosis, Venous thrombosis, Portal vein thrombosis

All ages

Gingival bleeding (D005884), Tinnitus (D014012), Hypertension (401-405.99), Bruising susceptibility (D004438), Angina pectoris (D000787), Weight loss (D015431), Abdominal pain (D015746), Headache (D006261), Vertigo (386.2):

Zhēnwǔtāng 5g + fùzǐ 1g + gānjiāng 1-0g + xìxīn 1-0g + dǐdāngtāng 0g + dàhuáng 0g.	Sānqī 5g + dānshēn 5g + tiānmá 5g + bèimǔ 5g + báijí 3g + qínjiāo 3g + chuānliànzǐ 3-0g + yánhúsuǒ 3-0g + chuānxiōng 3-0g + jiǔcàizǐ 3-0g + huánglián 2-0g + dàhuáng 0g.
Línngguìshùgāntāng 5g + fùzǐ 1g + gānjiāng 1g + tiáowèichéngqìtāng 1g + dàhuáng 0g.	Sānqī 5g + dānshēn 5g + tiānmá 5g + juémíngzǐ 5-3g + jiǔcàizǐ 3g + qínjiāo 3g + chuānxiōng 3-0g + gǒuqǐzǐ 3-0g + niúxī 3-0g.
	Gāncǎo 5g + báizhǐ 5g + shārén 5g + huángqín 5g + dàhuáng 0g.

Arthralgia (D018771), Fatigue (D005221):

Shàngzhōngxiàtōngyòngtòngfēngwán 5g + shūjīnghuóxuètāng 5g + dāngguīniàntòngtāng 5-0g + dúhuójìshēngtāng 5-0g.	Niúxī 5g + báisháo 5g + guìzhī 5g + gǔsuìbǔ 5g + xùduàn 5g + mùguā 4g + dāngguī 4g + mòyào 2g + rǔxiāng 2g.
Shàngzhōngxiàtōngyòngtòngfēngwán 5g + sháoyàogāncǎotāng 2-0g + niúxī 1g + huángbò 1g + cāngzhú 1g + yìyǐrén 1g + mòyào 1-0g + rǔxiāng 1-0g.	Niúxī 5g + huángbò 5g + cāngzhú 5g + dùzhòng 5-0g + yìyǐrén 5-0g + chuānxiōng 4g + fángjǐ 4g + lóngdǎncǎo 4g + shārén 2g.
Guìzhīsháoyàozhīmǔtāng 5g + niúxī 1g + huángbò 1g + cāngzhú 1g + yìyǐrén 1g.	Gāncǎo 5g + chìsháo 5g + huángqí 5g + fùzǐ 3g + máhuáng 3g.

(Continued)

TABLE 9.6 *(Continued)*
GMP Herbal Medicines for a 65-Year-Old Man with Polycythemia Vera

Pruritus (D011537), Portal hypertension (572.3), Intermittent claudication (D007383):

Xiǎocháihútāng 5g + yīnchénwǔlíngsǎn 5g + huángliánjiědútāng 5g + dānshēn 2-0g + chìsháo 2-0g + hónghuā 2-0g + cǎojuémíng 2-0g.

Jiāwèixiāoyáosǎn 5g + xiāngshāliùjūnzǐtāng 5g + bāwèidìhuángwán 3g + shānzhā 1g + héhuānpí 1g.

Lóngdǎnxiègāntāng 5g + yīnchén 2g + dàqīngyè 1g + jīnyínhuā 1g.

Yīnchénwǔlíngsǎn 5g + huángliánjiědútāng 5g + shānzhā 2g + dānshēn 2g + chìsháo 2g + hónghuā 2g + cǎojuémíng 2g.

Yīnchén 5g + fúlíng 5g + zhūlíng 5g + zéxiè 5g + báizhú 3-2g.

Yīnchén 5g + fùzǐ 3g + fúlíng 3g + bànxià 2g + xìxīn 2g + dàhuáng 1g.

Yīnchén 5g + chēqiánzǐ 4g + zhīzǐ 4g + huángqín 4g + huánglián 1g + dàhuáng 0g.

Hǔzhàng 5g + nǚzhēnzǐ 3g + tiānhuā 3g + shíhú 3g + hànliáncǎo 3g + zhìgāncǎo 3g + chuānliànzǐ 2g + héshǒuwū 2g + shāshēn 2g + gǒuqǐzǐ 2g + màiméndōng 2g + júhuā 2g + huángjīng 2g.

9.7 IMMUNE THROMBOCYTOPENIA

Immune thrombocytopenia, or immune thrombocytopenic purpura, is a low count of platelets, which, in the case of an injury, clump to clot blood vessels and seal the wound. Immune thrombocytopenia is an autoimmune condition where antibodies attack one's own platelets.

TABLE 9.7
GMP Herbal Medicines for a 58-Year-Old Woman with Immune Thrombocytopenia

Immune thrombocytopenia (OrphaCode: 3002)

A disease with a prevalence of ~2 in 10,000

Candidate gene tested: Fc gamma receptor IIc (gene/pseudogene) (*FCGR2C* / Entrez: 9103) at 1q23.3

Not applicable

Thrombocytopenia, Thromboembolism

Petechiae, Purpura, Arterial thrombosis

Gingival bleeding, Epistaxis, Bruising susceptibility, Gastrointestinal hemorrhage

All ages

Thrombocytopenia (287.5):

Guīpítāng 5g + bǔzhōngyìqìtāng 5-0g + xiānhècǎo 1g + báimáogēn 1-0g + dìhuáng 1-0g + mǔdānpí 1-0g + ējiāo 1-0g + ǒujiē 1-0g.

Guīpítāng 5g + xiōngguījiāoàitāng 5-0g + xiānhècǎo 1g + báimáogēn 1-0g + dìhuáng 1-0g + mǔdānpí 1-0g + ējiāo 1-0g + jíxuèténg 1-0g + dìyú 1-0g.

Guīpítāng 5g + jiāwèixiāoyáosǎn 5-0g + xiānhècǎo 1g + báimáogēn 1-0g + dìhuáng 1-0g + mǔdānpí 1-0g + ējiāo 1-0g.

Běishāshēn 5g + dìhuáng 5g + mǔdānpí 5g + zhǐqiào 5g + yīnchén 5g + huángqín 5g + báizhú 4-0g + fùzǐ 4-0g.

Shúdìhuáng 5g + báizhú 4g + fùzǐ 4g + báisháo 3g + fúlíng 3g + báijièzǐ 2g + dǎngshēn 2g + gāncǎo 1g + shēngjiāng 1g + máhuáng 1g + huánglián 0g.

Báisháo 5g + dìhuáng 5g + ējiāo 5g + dāngguī 5g + dàzǎo 3g + niúxī 3g + mǔdānpí 3g + xiāngfù 3g + huángbò 3g.

Ējiāo 5g + huángqín 5g + gāncǎo 1g.

Purpura (D011693):

Xiāofēngsǎn 5g + jīngfángbàidúsǎn 5-0g + dìfūzǐ 1-0g + shéchuángzǐ 1-0g + yìyǐrén 1-0g + báixiānpí 1-0g + jílí 1-0g.

Báizhǐ 5g + gāncǎo 4g + shārén 4g + huángqín 4g + tiānhuā 2-0g + dàhuáng 1-0g.

Gingival bleeding (D005884), Epistaxis (D004844) [Epistaxis (784.7)], Bruising susceptibility (D004438), Gastrointestinal hemorrhage (D006471) [Hemorrhage of gastrointestinal tract, unspecified (578.9)]:

Gānlùyǐn 5g + xiānhècǎo 2-1g + báijí 2-1g + huáihuā 2-0g + cāngzhú 2-0g.

Xiānhècǎo 5g + báijí 5g + huáihuā 5g + dìhuáng 5-0g + hànliáncǎo 5-0g + mǔdānpí 5-0g + jíxuèténg 5-0g.

Gāncǎo 5g + jīnyínhuā 5g + huángqín 5g + huánglián 5g + dāngguī 5g + dàhuáng 1g.

Běishāshēn, introduced in Sections 1.6 and 1.63 for coughs and lung cancer, has been used for bloody phlegm and is a component in a decoction for curing cold with blood, bleeding, and nourishing the lungs (Yang et al., 2019). A modified Guīpítāng was shown to promote the suppression of autoantibodies in patients with chronic immune thrombocytopenic purpura (Yamaguchi et al., 1993). Guīpítāng plus an antibiotic was shown to be more effective for treating thrombocytopenia in dogs than the antibiotic alone (Wong & Shiau, 2020). Xiānhècǎo was introduced in Section 4.9 for bleeding, while Báijí was introduced in Section 4.28 for hematemesis and melena.

9.8 VON WILLEBRAND DISEASE

Von Willebrand disease is a hereditary blood-clotting disorder where the affected individuals have insufficient or deficient proteins called the von Willebrand factor, which helps glue platelets to form clots. Von Willebrand disease is caused by mutations in the gene that transcribe and translate to von Willebrand factor proteins. Depending on the specific mutation in the gene, the von Willebrand disease trait can be autosomal dominant or autosomal recessive.

TABLE 9.8

GMP Herbal Medicines for a Nine-Year-Old Child with von Willebrand Disease

Von Willebrand disease (OrphaCode: 903)

A disease with a prevalence of ~1 in 10,000

Disease-causing germline mutation(s): von Willebrand factor (*VWF* / Entrez: 7450) at 12p13.31

Autosomal dominant, Autosomal recessive

Abnormality of thrombocytes, Abnormality of coagulation, Abnormal platelet function

Abnormal mitral valve morphology

Deviation of finger, Venous insufficiency

All ages

Abnormality of coagulation (287.9):

Xiōngguījiāoàitāng 5g + guīpítāng 3g.	Xiānhècǎo 5g + xuánshēn 5g + dìhuáng 5g + mǔdānpí 5g + chìsháo
Xiōngguījiāoàitāng 5g + xiānhècǎo 1g +	5g + huáihuā 5g + jīnyínhuā 5-0g + liánqiáo 5-0g + qiàncǎo 5-0g +
báimáogēn 1-0g + dìhuáng 1-0g + mǔdānpí	zǐcǎo 5-0g + gāncǎo 3-0g.
1-0g + ējiāo 1-0g + ǒujiē 1-0g.	Xuánshēn 5g + dìhuáng 5g + màiméndōng 5g + zhìgāncǎo 2g +
	dàhuáng 0g.
	Xiānhècǎo 5g + báihuāshéshécǎo 5g + mǔdānpí 5g + xuánshēn 2g +
	chìsháo 2g + dàhuáng 0g.
	Xiānhècǎo 5g + mǔdānpí 5g + báisháo 2g + dùzhòng 2g + dǎngshēn 2g.

Venous insufficiency (459.81):

Dāngguīsìnìtāng 5g + niúxī 1g + shēngjiāng	Dìhuáng 5g + mǔdānpí 5g + chìsháo 5g + hónghuā 5g + guìzhī 5g +
1-0g + wúzhūyú 1-0g + fùzǐ 1-0g.	táorén 5g + huángbò 5g + dāngguī 5g + dàhuáng 3-0g.
Sháoyàogāncǎotāng 5g + niúxī 1g + huángbò	
1g + cāngzhú 1g + yìyǐrén 1g.	
Dǐdāngtāng 5g + niúxī 1g + mùguā 1-0g.	

Mǔdānpí was introduced in Section 4.30 for hemorrhagic diseases. Chìsháo (cf. Section 2.36) "clears heat, cools Blood, dissolves stasis and stops pain." It was summarized to improve microcirculation, dilate blood vessels, prevent myocardial ischemia, and prevent thrombosis (Tan et al., 2020). Dāngguīsìnìtāng was introduced in Section 2.12 for diffuse diseases of connective tissue, which can develop lipodermatosclerosis that is in association with venous insufficiency (Gonzalez et al., 2006).

9.9 SICKLE CELL ANEMIA

Sickle cell anemia is characterized by a shortage of red blood cells, which carry oxygen in the lungs and travel to the rest of the body through the bloodstream. Normal red blood cells are round. The red blood cells in people with sickle cell anemia are sickle shaped. The misshapen red blood cells die earlier in the body than normal red blood cells, leading to anemia. Sickle cell anemia is caused by mutations in the *HBB* gene, whose products are a subunit of hemoglobin in red blood cells that binds to oxygen.

TABLE 9.9

GMP Herbal Medicines for a Two-Year-Old Child with Sickle Cell Anemia

Sickle cell anemia (OrphaCode: 232)

A disease with a prevalence of ~1 in 10,000

Disease-causing germline mutation(s): hemoglobin subunit beta (*HBB* / Entrez: 3043) at 11p15.4

Autosomal recessive

Chronic hemolytic anemia

Hemolytic anemia, Recurrent infections, Pain

Osteoporosis, Abnormality of the spleen, Iron deficiency anemia, Thrombocytosis, Reticulocytosis, Leukocytosis, Osteomyelitis, Avascular necrosis, Pigment gallstones, Chest pain

Abnormality of the nervous system, Cholestasis, Abnormality of the vasculature, Elevated serum creatinine, Unconjugated hyperbilirubinemia, Persistence of hemoglobin F, Hypoxemia, Increased lactate dehydrogenase activity

All ages

Pain (D010146):

Xiǎojiànzhōngtāng 5g + shānzhā 1g + shénqū 1g + màiyá 1-0g + jīnèijīn 1-0g.

Guìzhītāng 5g + báisháo 1g + dàhuáng 0g.

Xuánshēn 5g + dìhuáng 5g + màiméndōng 5g + hòupò 5-2g + zhǐshí 5-2g + dàhuáng 1-0g.

Gāncǎo 5g + báizhǐ 5g + shārén 5g + dàhuáng 0g.

Osteoporosis (733.0), Reticulocytosis (D045262), Avascular necrosis (732.3, 733.41, 733.42, 733.43, 733.44), Chest pain (D002637):

Zuǒguīwán 5g + shēntòngzhúyūtāng 5g + gǔsuìbǔ 2g + xùduàn 2g.

Zuǒguīwán 5g + zhènggǔzǐjīndàn 5g + gǔsuìbǔ 2-1g + xùduàn 2-1g + bǔgǔzhī 2-0g.

Shēnlíngbáizhúsǎn 5g + sānqī 2g + gǔsuìbǔ 2g + xùduàn 2g + gāncǎo 1g.

Jīnyínhuā 5g + dāngguī 5g + xuánshēn 2g + gāncǎo 2g + chìsháo 2g + huángqí 2g + niúxī 2-0g + dǎodìwúgōng 2-0g.

Jīnyínhuā 5g + dāngguī 5g + niúxī 2g + xuánshēn 2g + chìsháo 2g + zhìgāncǎo 2g + huángqí 2g.

Báizhú 5g + fùzǐ 5g + cháihú 5g + báisháo 4g + fúlíng 4g + tiānhuā 2g + dǎngshēn 2g + guìzhī 2g + huángqín 2g + gāncǎo 1g + mǔlì 1g + gānjiāng 1g.

Cholestasis (576.2), Hypoxemia (D000860):

Wǔlíngsǎn 5g + píngwèisǎn 5-0g.

Xiǎocháihútāng 5g + báisháo 1-0g + guìzhī 1-0g + gāncǎo 1-0g + dàhuáng 0g.

Guìzhītāng 5g + xiǎocháihútāng 5-0g + gāncǎo 0g.

Gāncǎo 5g + júhuā 5-0g + júhóng 5-0g + chántuì 5-0g + jīlí 5-0g.

Júhuā 5g + zhǐqiào 3g.

Júhóng 5g + jīlí 3g.

Xuánshēn and Gāncǎo are among the top 10 frequently prescribed herbs for patients with cancer pain (cf. Section 3.29). Xiǎojiànzhōngtāng was concluded to be more effective than conventional Western medicine in the treatment of gastric ulcers in a systematic review and meta-analysis of randomized controlled trials (Sun et al., 2017). We see from the table that a strategy of TCM formular prescriptions for children with pain is to improve their digestion and thus growth. An active constituent in Jīnyínhuā (cf. Section 7.2) was shown to promote osteoblastic differentiation in mouse bone marrow stromal cells (Liu et al., 2019). Zuǒguīwán (cf. Section 1.48) "nourishes yin, replenishes the Kidney, fills essence, benefits marrow" and is used for disorders of the bone and cartilage (Wang, 2019).

9.10 HEMOLYTIC ANEMIA DUE TO RED CELL PYRUVATE KINASE DEFICIENCY

Hemolysis is a process when old or faulty red blood cells are destroyed in the spleen. If hemolysis occurs too often, the body has a shortage of red blood cells, leading to hemolytic anemia. Hemolytic anemia due to red cell pyruvate kinase deficiency, also known as pyruvate kinase deficiency of erythrocytes, is caused by deficiency in the pyruvate kinase enzyme, encoded by the *PKLR* gene, in the red blood cells.

TABLE 9.10

GMP Herbal Medicines for a One-Year-Old Infant with Hemolytic Anemia Due to Red Cell Pyruvate Kinase Deficiency

Hemolytic anemia due to red cell pyruvate kinase deficiency (OrphaCode: 766)

A disease with a prevalence of ~5 in 100,000

Disease-causing germline mutation(s): pyruvate kinase L/R (*PKLR* / Entrez: 5313) at 1q22

Autosomal recessive

Splenomegaly, Anemia, Reticulocytosis, Chronic hemolytic anemia, Unconjugated hyperbilirubinemia, Reduced red cell pyruvate kinase activity

Hydrops fetalis, Increased serum ferritin, Increased serum iron, Congenital hemolytic anemia, Prolonged neonatal jaundice

Abnormal erythrocyte morphology, Poikilocytosis, Anisocytosis, Elevated transferrin saturation

Neonatal, Infancy

Anemia (285.9), Reticulocytosis (D045262):

Shēnlíngbáizhúsǎn 5g + gāncǎo 1-0g + màiyá 1-0g.	Dàzǎo 5g + gāncǎo 5g + báizhú 5g + fúlíng 5g + huángqí 5g + dǎngshēn 5-0g.
Sìjūnzǐtāng 5g + shēnlíngbáizhúsǎn 5-0g.	Zhǐqiào 5g + jílí 5-0g.
Bǎohéwán 5g + gāncǎo 0g.	Gāncǎo 5g + báizhǐ 3-0g + shārén 3-0g + dàhuáng 0g.

Hydrops fetalis (D015160), Congenital hemolytic anemia (282):

Xiāngshāliùjūnzǐtāng 5g.	Běishāshēn 5g + yùzhú 5g + hòupò 5-3g + zhǐshí 5-3g + xuánshēn 3-0g + dìhuáng 3-0g + màiméndōng 3-0g + dàhuáng 1-0g.
Liùjūnzǐtāng 5g + shānzhā 1g + shénqū 1g + màiyá 1g + jīnèijīn 1g.	
Xiǎocháihútāngqùrénshēn 5g + bǎihégùjīntāng 2-1g + qínjiāobiējiǎsǎn 2-0g + wūméi 1-0g + qínjiāo 0g + biējiǎ 0g.	Běishāshēn 5g + xuánshēn 5g + yùzhú 5g + dìhuáng 5g + màiméndōng 5g + hòupò 5-4g + zhǐshí 5-4g + dàhuáng 1-0g.
Sìjūnzǐtāng 5g + sìwùtāng 5g.	

The hematopoietic effects of Dàzǎo (cf. Section 2.8), including regulation of erythropoiesis, potential capacity in recycling heme iron during erythrophagocytosis, and bi-directional regulation of immune response, were demonstrated in cell and animal models and summarized in a recent review (Chen & Tsim, 2020). Sìjūnzǐtāng was introduced in Sections 1.17 and 1.56 for digestion. Liùjūnzǐtāng (cf. Section 1.56) is Sìjūnzǐtāng plus Chénpí (cf. Section 2.47) and Bànxià (cf. Section 12.10), both of which "dry dampness." Liùjūnzǐtāng therefore improves the digestion and at the same time alleviates hydrops of the baby.

9.11 ACQUIRED IDIOPATHIC SIDEROBLASTIC ANEMIA

Acquired idiopathic sideroblastic anemia, also known as refractory anemia with ringed sideroblasts, is characterized by more than 15% of ringed sideroblasts among the red blood cell precursors in the bone marrow. Dysfunctional production and processing of heme, which is a component of hemoglobin that contains iron to bind oxygen, cause a ring of iron-laden mitochondria to form around the nucleus of a sideroblast that develops into a red blood cell. Sideroblastic anemia can be acquired through copper deficiency, or lead, arsenic, and zinc poisoning.

TABLE 9.11

GMP Herbal Medicines for a 67-Year-Old Adult with Acquired Idiopathic Sideroblastic Anemia

Acquired idiopathic sideroblastic anemia (OrphaCode: 75564)

A disease with a prevalence of ~5 in 100,000

Disease-causing somatic mutation(s): tet methylcytosine dioxygenase 2 (*TET2* / Entrez: 54790) at 4q24

Disease-causing somatic mutation(s): splicing factor 3b subunit 1 (*SF3B1* / Entrez: 23451) at 2q33.1
Not applicable

Refractory anemia with ringed sideroblasts, Anemia of inadequate production

Pallor, Normochromic anemia, Normocytic anemia, Erythroid hyperplasia, Megaloblastic erythroid hyperplasia

Abnormal fingernail morphology, Splenomegaly, Thrombocytopenia, Hypochromic anemia, Hepatomegaly, Myelodysplasia, Hyposegmentation of neutrophil nuclei, Dysplastic granulopoesis, Abnormal number of granulocyte precursors, Abnormal megakaryocyte morphology, Chronic infection

Adult

Pallor (D010167):

Dàcháihútāng 5g + xuèfǔzhúyūtāng 5g + mázǐrénwán 5g.	Zhǐshí 5g + hòupò 4g + dàhuáng 1g + huǒmárén 1-0g.
Dàcháihútāng 5g + fángfēngtōngshèngsǎn 5g + shānzhā 1-0g + dānshēn 1-0g + héshǒuwū 1-0g + cǎojuémíng 1-0g + juémíngzǐ 1-0g + dàhuáng 1-0g.	Zhǐshí 5g + chénpí 5g + lùlùtōng 5g + jīxuèténg 5g + mùxiāng 4g + láifúzǐ 4g + dāngguīwěi 4g.
Sìnìtāng 5g + zhìgāncǎotāng 5g + dānshēn 2g + xiāngfù 2g + yùjīn 2g.	Zhǐshí 5g + qiānghuó 4g + hòupò 4g + fángfēng 2g + huángqín 1g + huánglián 1g + dàhuáng 0g.
	Qīngpí 5g + gégēn 5g + jīxuèténg 5g + ròudòukòu 3g + wēilíngxiān 3g.

Thrombocytopenia (287.5):

Guīpítāng 5g + xiānhècǎo 1g + báimáogēn 1-0g + ējiāo 1-0g + ǒujié 1-0g + dìhuáng 1-0g + mǔdānpí 1-0g + chìsháo 1-0g.	Xiānhècǎo 5g + dìhuáng 5g + mǔdānpí 5g + chìsháo 5g + jīnyínhuā 5g + liánqiáo 5g + gāncǎo 3g.
Xiōngguījiāoàitāng 5g + guīpítāng 3g + rénshēnyǎngróngtāng 3-0g + xiānhècǎo 1g + huángqí 1g + báimáogēn 1-0g + tùsīzǐ 1-0g + ējiāo 1-0g + dǎngshēn 1-0g.	Dìhuáng 5g + dǎngshēn 5g + dāngguī 5-4g + báizhú 5-0g + guìzhī 5-0g + huángqí 5-0g + huángjīng 5-0g + bǔgǔzhī 5-0g + běishāshēn 5-0g + mǔdānpí 4-2g + fùzǐ 2-0g.
	Báizhú 5g + dìhuáng 5g + mǔdānpí 5g + zhǐqiào 5g + yīnchén 5g + màiyá 5g + huángqín 5g.

Zhǐshí (cf. Sections 3.13 and 8.3) was shown to alleviate inflammation and modulate gut microbiota in mice with colitis (Chen et al., 2022). In TCM, the progression of an affliction is conceptualized into six distinct phases, where Shaoyang and Yangming represent the second and third stages, respectively. In the Shaoyang phase, external pathogenic factors have just infiltrated the body, triggering an immune response from the body. Subsequently, in the Yangming phase, the intruder persists in its growth and advances closer to the internal organs. This continuum unfolds until the body's defenses ultimately falter, allowing the intruder to triumph by destroying the vital organs, an event marking the culmination of intrusion and the demise of the host. Dàcháihútāng was designed to "mediate between the offense and defense" while the disease progression is in the Shaoyang stage and to "purge the stagnated heat" while the disease is in the Yangming stage. Dàcháihútāng was shown to be antihypercholesterolemic in hypercholesterolemic rabbits (Yoshie et al., 2004).

9.12 AUTOIMMUNE HEMOLYTIC ANEMIA, WARM TYPE

Autoimmune hemolytic anemia, warm type (wAIHA), refers to the destruction of healthy red blood cells by autoantibodies that tag the red blood cells of oneself at body temperature. wAIHA is attributed to genetic predispositions and medications.

Dāngguīniántòngtāng was introduced in Section 2.32 for the disorders of joints. Dàqīngyè (cf. Section 5.17) "clears heat, neutralizes pathogens, cools Blood, and removes spots." It was shown

TABLE 9.12

GMP Herbal Medicines for a 54-Year-Old Adult with Autoimmune Hemolytic Anemia, Warm Type

Autoimmune hemolytic anemia, warm type (OrphaCode: 90033)

A disease with a prevalence of ~5 in 100,000

Multigenic/multifactorial

Pallor, Autoimmune hemolytic anemia, Headache, Exertional dyspnea, Autoimmunity, Fatigue

Splenomegaly, Arthralgia, Lymphoproliferative disorder

Jaundice, Congestive heart failure, Tachycardia, Fever, Systemic lupus erythematosus, Chronic lymphatic leukemia, Abnormal urinary color

All ages

Pallor (D010167), Autoimmune hemolytic anemia (283.0), Headache (D006261), Fatigue (D005221):

Bǔzhōngyìqìtāng 5g + guīpítāng 5g.	Bànzhīlián 5g + báihuāshéshécǎo 5g.
Bǔzhōngyìqìtāng 5g + jìshēngshènqìwán 5-0g + dānshēn 2-0g + báijí 1-0g + dùzhòng 1-0g + huángqíjiànzhōngtāng 1-0g + wēilíngxiān 1-0g + guìzhī 1-0g + xùduàn 1-0g.	Huángqí 5g + shúdìhuáng 5g + dǎngshēn 5g + shānyào 3g + shēngmá 2g + zhìgāncǎo 2g + cháihú 2g + chénpí 2g + shēngjiāng 1g + dāngguī 1g + chìsháo 0g + fángfēng 0g + xìxīn 0g + huánglián 0g.
Huángqíwǔwùtāng 5g + dāngguīsìnìtāng 4g + dānshēn 1g + zhúrú 1g + qínjiāo 1g + gōuténg 1g.	Báizhú 5g + fúlíng 5g + dǎngshēn 5g + xiǎohuíxiāng 4g + bànxià 4g + zhìgāncǎo 2g + fùzǐ 1g.
Bǔyánghuánwǔtāng 5g + dúhuójìshēngtāng 5g.	

Arthralgia (D018771):

Shàngzhōngxiàtōngyòngtòngfēngwán 5g + shūjīnghuóxuètāng 5g + dāngguīniántòngtāng 5-0g + niúxī 1-0g + acupuncture.	Niúxī 5g + huángbò 5g + cāngzhú 5g + yìyǐrén 5-0g + dàhuáng 1-0g.
Shàngzhōngxiàtōngyòngtòngfēngwán 5-2g + sháoyàogāncǎotāng 5-0g + shūjīnghuóxuètāng 5-0g + mòyào 1-0g + rǔxiāng 1-0g + acupuncture.	Chuānwū 5g + wǔlíngzhī 2g + tiānnánxīng 2g + mùxiāng 2g + gāncǎo 2g + dìlóng 2g + yánhúsuǒ 2g + táorén 2g + huíxiāng 2g + chénpí 2g + dāngguī 2g.

Jaundice (D007565), Congestive heart failure (428, 428.0), Fever (D005334), Systemic lupus erythematosus (710.0), Chronic lymphatic leukemia (204.1):

Yīnchénwǔlíngsǎn 5g + huángliánjiědútāng 5-0g + dàqīngyè 2-1g + jīnyínhuā 2-1g + púgōngyīng 2-1g + zhǐqiào 2-0g.	Dàqīngyè 5g + bǎnlángēn 5g + jīnyínhuā 5g + bàijiàngcǎo 5g + liánqiáo 5g + zǐhuādìdīng 5g + púgōngyīng 5g + gāncǎo 2-0g.
	Xuánshēn 5g + dìhuáng 5g + màiméndōng 5g + hòupò 5-2g + zhǐshí 5-2g + shāshēn 5-0g + dàhuáng 2-0g.

in mice to be antiviral (Deng et al., 2013), hepatoprotective (Ding & Zhu, 2020), anti-atopic (Min et al., 2023), and is used for coughs, pruritic disorder, and so on (Wang, 2020). Bǎnlángēn (Radix Isatidis) was reviewed to exert antiviral activities by regulating the immune system (Zhou & Zhang, 2013); it is used today for influenza (Wang, 2020).

9.13 HEMOPHILIA A

Hemophilia A, also known as congenital Factor VIII deficiency, is a hereditary bleeding disorder due to insufficient or defective coagulation factor VIII, which helps the formation of blood clots. Mutations in the *F8* gene, which instructs the liver to make coagulation factor VIII proteins, cause hemophilia A.

Chántuì (cf. Section 2.20) was shown to improve hemorheology in rats (Liu et al., 2004). Zhǐsòusǎn "stops coughing, transforms phlegm, relaxes exterior, inflates the Lung" and is used for symptoms involving respiratory system and other chest symptoms including chronic bronchitis (Wang, 2019). Children with respiratory infections often also experience joint pain. Xiāoyáosǎn (cf. Section 3.25) "soothes the Liver, relieves depression, strengthens the Spleen, and nourishes Blood." It, combined

TABLE 9.13

GMP Herbal Medicines for a Four-Year-Old Boy with Hemophilia A

Hemophilia A (OrphaCode: 98878)

A disease with a prevalence of ~5 in 100,000

Disease-causing germline mutation(s): coagulation factor VIII (*F8* / Entrez: 2157) at Xq28

X-linked recessive

Joint swelling, Arthralgia, Reduced factor VIII activity, Bleeding with minor or no trauma

Thromboembolism, Spontaneous hematomas, Oral cavity bleeding

Joint hemorrhage, Gastrointestinal hemorrhage, Abnormality of the elbow, Intramuscular hematoma, Intraventricular hemorrhage

Neonatal, Infancy, Childhood

Arthralgia (D018771), Reduced factor VIII activity (286.0):

Shēnlíngbáizhúsǎn 5g + shānzhā 1g + shénqū 1g + màiyá 1g + jīnèijīn 1g.

Xuèfǔzhúyūtāng 5g + bǔzhōngyìqìtāng 5g + gāncǎo 1g.

Xiǎojiànzhōngtāng 5g + báizhǐ 2g + shígāo 2g.

Xuánshēn 5g + dìhuáng 5g + màiméndōng 5g + hòupò 5-1g + zhǐshí 5-1g + dàhuáng 1-0g.

Joint hemorrhage (719.1), Gastrointestinal hemorrhage (D006471) [Hemorrhage of gastrointestinal tract, unspecified (578.9)]:

Xiāoyáosǎn 5g + cháihújiālónggǔmǔlìtāng 1g + wēndǎntāng 0g.

Xiāoyáosǎn 5g + gégēntāng 2g + táohéchéngqìtāng 1g + píngwèisǎn 1-0g.

Xiāoyáosǎn 5g + dúhuójìshēngtāng 2g + wēndǎntāng 2-1g + yǐzìtāng 2-0g + táohéchéngqìtāng 1-0g.

Zhǐqiào 5-4g + chántuì 5-4g + jílí 5-0g + júhuā 5-0g.

with anxiolytics, was shown to be more effective for the treatment of anxiety than anxiolytics, which might adversely cause sexual dysfunction and gastrointestinal bleeding (Wang et al., 2023).

9.14 HEMOPHILIA B

Hemophilia B, also known as congenital factor IX deficiency or Christmas disease, is a genetic bleeding disorder due to the deficiency of coagulation factor IX. Hemophilia B is caused by mutations in the *F9* gene, whose products, i.e., factor IX, interact with other coagulation factors to set off a cascade of chemical reactions leading to blood clotting.

TABLE 9.14

GMP Herbal Medicines for a Five-Year-Old Boy with Hemophilia B

Hemophilia B (OrphaCode: 98879)

A disease with a prevalence of ~3 in 100,000

Disease-causing germline mutation(s): coagulation factor IX (*F9* / Entrez: 2158) at Xq27.1

X-linked recessive

Hematuria, Poor wound healing, Intracranial hemorrhage, Prolonged bleeding time, Prolonged partial thromboplastin time, Spontaneous, recurrent epistaxis, Prolonged bleeding after surgery, Joint hemorrhage, Prolonged bleeding after dental extraction, Reduced factor IX activity, Intramuscular hematoma, Cephalohematoma, Delayed onset bleeding, Menometrorrhagia

Neonatal, Infancy, Childhood

Hematuria (D006417) [Hematuria, unspecified (599.70)], Intracranial hemorrhage (D020300) [Unspecified intracranial hemorrhage (432.9)], Joint hemorrhage (719.1):

Sāngpiāoxiāosǎn 5g + bǔzhōngyìqìtāng 5-3g + yìzhìrén 2-1g + shānyào 2-0g + wūyào 2-0g + fùpénzǐ 1-0g + shíchāngpú 1-0g + bǔgǔzhǐ 1-0g.

Liùwèidìhuángwán 5g + sāngpiāoxiāosǎn 5g + shānyào 1g + wūyào 1g + yìzhìrén 1g + acupuncture.

Jílí 5g + júhuā 4g + chántuì 4g + zhǐqiào 2g.

Jílí 5g + chántuì 5-0g + zhǐqiào 4-0g.

Huángqín 5g + báizhǐ 3g + zhìgāncǎo 2g + shārén 2g + guālóugēn 1g + dàhuáng 1g.

Báizhǐ 5g + gāncǎo 4g + shārén 4g + dàhuáng 0g + acupuncture.

Jílí (cf. Section 1.35) showed a significant dose-dependent protection against uroliths induced by glass bead implantation in albino rats (Anand et al., 1994). Jílí was also shown to cause a diverse response of regional cerebral blood flow and pial arterial diameter in rats (Gang et al., 1998). An add-on GMP herbal extract granule formula containing Sāngpiāoxiāosǎn (cf. Section 1.26) was shown to improve the lower urinary tract symptoms of patients with benign prostatic hyperplasia (Yeh et al., 2020).

9.15 PAROXYSMAL NOCTURNAL HEMOGLOBINURIA

Paroxysmal nocturnal hemoglobinuria (PNH), also known as Marchiafava-Micheli disease, is an acquired condition of the hematopoietic stem cells and can present with recurrent episodes of hemoglobin in the urine as a result of hemolysis. People with PNH can also develop repeated blood clots. PNH is caused by somatic mutations in the *PIGA* gene in some hematopoietic stem cells. The

---

TABLE 9.15

GMP Herbal Medicines for a 35-Year-Old Adult with Paroxysmal Nocturnal Hemoglobinuria

Paroxysmal nocturnal hemoglobinuria (OrphaCode: 447)

A disease with a prevalence of ~2 in 100,000

Disease-causing somatic mutation(s): phosphatidylinositol glycan anchor biosynthesis class A (*PIGA* / Entrez: 5277) at Xp22.2

Not applicable

Abnormal erythrocyte enzyme activity

Hemolytic anemia, Anemia, Hemoglobinuria, Asthenia

Thromboembolism, Reticulocytosis, Dyspnea, Headache, Episodic abdominal pain, Deep venous thrombosis, Increased blood urea nitrogen, Venous thrombosis, Unconjugated hyperbilirubinemia, Hemosiderinuria, Chronic kidney disease, Reduced haptoglobin level, Increased lactate dehydrogenase activity, Conjunctival icterus, Decreased serum iron, Chest pain

Renal insufficiency, Proteinuria, Impotence, Hypertension, Jaundice, Lethargy, Stroke, Myocardial infarction, Thrombocytopenia, Pancytopenia, Leukopenia, Acute kidney injury, Pulmonary embolism, Budd-Chiari syndrome, Arterial thrombosis, Erythroid hyperplasia, Mesenteric venous thrombosis, Odynophagia

All ages

Anemia (285.9), Hemoglobinuria (791.2):

Jiāwèixiāoyáosǎn 5g + qǐjúdìhuángwán 5g + guīpítāng 5-0g + shēnlíngbáizhúsǎn 5-0g.	Dàzǎo 5g + chuānxiōng 5g + gāncǎo 5g + ējiāo 5g + gǒuqǐzǐ 5g + bózǐrén 5g + huángqí 5g + dāngguī 5g + shúdìhuáng 5g + suǒyáng 5g.
Bǔzhōngyìqìtāng 5g + guīpítāng 5g + jiāwèixiāoyáosǎn 5-0g + liùwèidìhuángwán 5-0g.	Ējiāo 5g + huángqín 5g + xiānhècǎo 2g + gāncǎo 1g + huánglián 1g.
Liùwèidìhuángwán 5g + jiāwèixiāoyáosǎn 5g + sìwùtāng 5g.	Dìhuáng 5g + dùzhòng 5g + ējiāo 5g + huángqí 5g + dǎngshēn 5g.
Bāzhēntāng 5g + jiāwèixiāoyáosǎn 5g.	

Reticulocytosis (D045262) [Other nonspecific findings on examination of blood (790.99)], Dyspnea (D004417), Headache (D006261), Chest pain (D002637):

Wǔlíngsǎn 5g + dāngguīniàntòngtāng 5g + niúxī 1g + chēqiánzǐ 1-0g + huángbò 1-0g + cāngzhú 1-0g + yìyǐrén 1-0g + acupuncture.	Wǔwèizǐ 5g + bànxià 5g + zhìgāncǎo 5g + cháihú 5g + gānjiāng 5g + huángqín 5g.
Xuèfǔzhúyūtāng 5g + sháoyàogāncǎotāng 5g + cháihúshūgāntāng 5g + acupuncture.	Wǔwèizǐ 5g + bājǐtiān 5g + ròucōngróng 5g + chēqiánzǐ 5g + gǒuqǐzǐ 5g + fúshén 5g + yínyánghuò 5g + tùsīzǐ 5g + fùpénzǐ 5g + suǒyáng 5g + xùduàn 5g.
Máxìnggānshítāng 5g + cāngěrsǎn 5g + jiégěng 2g + liánqiáo 2g + yúxīngcǎo 2g.	Dānshēn 5g + dìhuáng 5g + héshǒuwū 5g + fúlíng 5g + dǎngshēn 5g + kuǎndōnghuā 3g + báizhú 3g + mùguā 3g + báisháo 3g + qiàncǎo 3g + dāngguī 3g.
Dāngguīsìnìtāng 5g + báizhú 2g + fùzǐ 2g + báisháo 2g + fúlíng 2g + dǎngshēn 1g + shēngjiāng 1g + wúzhūyú 1g + dàhuáng 1g.	Tǔfúlíng 5g + báixiānpí 4g + dìfūzǐ 4g + shéchuángzǐ 4g + bìxiè 4g + huáshí 4g + tōngcǎo 2g + zéxiè 2g + yìyǐrén 2g.

(Continued)

TABLE 9.15 *(Continued)*

GMP Herbal Medicines for a 35-Year-Old Adult with Paroxysmal Nocturnal Hemoglobinuria

Renal insufficiency (586), Proteinuria (791.0), Hypertension (401-405.99), Jaundice (D007565), Lethargy (D053609), Thrombocytopenia (287.5), Pancytopenia (284.1), Leukopenia (288.50):

Zhēnwǔtāng 5g + zhūlíngtāng 5g + jìshēngshènqìwán 5g + dīngshùxiǔ 2g + shuǐdīngxiāng 2g + báimáogēn 2g + yìmǔcǎo 2-0g + huángqí 2-0g.	Báizhú 5g + zhìgāncǎo 5g + zhǐshí 5g + fúlíng 5g + niúxī 2g + fùzǐ 2g + guìzhī 2-0g + ròuguì 2-0g + dàhuáng 1-0g.
Liùwèidìhuángwán 5g + guīpítāng 5g + sānqī 1g + xiānhècǎo 1g + ējiāo 1g + dàhuáng 0g.	Dìhuáng 5g + zhìgāncǎo 5g + ējiāo 5g + huángqín 5g + huánglián 5g + dàhuáng 1g.
Jìshēngshènqìwán 5g + guīpítāng 5g + dānshēn 1g + huángqí 1g.	Běishāshēn 5g + zhìgāncǎo 5g + xuánshēn 4g + yùzhú 4g + dìhuáng 4g + màiméndōng 4g + dàhuáng 1g.
	Huángqí 5g + chìsháo 1g + fángfēng 1g + dàhuáng 0g.

protein products of *PIGA* form anchors on the surface of hematopoietic stem cells to protect them from attack by the immune system.

Ējiāo was introduced in Section 3.21 to "nourish Blood." Bózǐrén (cf. Section 2.35) "nourishes the Heart, calms the mind, moistens bowels, passes stools" and is used for palpitations, hypertension, and sleep disturbances (Wang, 2020). Dùzhòng (cf. Section 1.4) "nourishes the Liver/Kidney, strengthens muscles/bones, prevents miscarriage." It was reviewed to have been used for lumbar pain, knee pain, osteoporosis, improve learning and memory abilities, hepatoprotection, paralysis, intestinal hemorrhoids, vaginal bleeding, itching in the vaginal or scrotum, dampness and residual draining of urine, abortion, pregnancy bleeding, spermatorrhea, soreness and pain in the feet, foot fungus, and antiaging (Huang et al., 2021) and is used today for lumbago and so on (Wang, 2020). Bāzhēntāng, resulting from a combination of Sìwùtāng (cf. Section 9.2) and Sìjūnzǐtāng (cf. Section 1.17), "coordinates nutrition and defense, nourishes Qi and Blood" and is used today for anemias (Wang, 2019).

REFERENCES

Anand, R., Patnaik, G. K., Kulshreshtha, D. K., & Dhawan, B. N. (1994). Activity of certain fractions of *Tribulus terrestris* fruits against experimentally induced urolithiasis in rats. *Indian J Exp Biol*, *32*(8), 548–552. https://pubmed.ncbi.nlm.nih.gov/7959935

Bradley, R. R., Cunniff, P. J., Pereira, B. J., & Jaber, B. L. (1999). Hematopoietic effect of *Radix angelicae sinensis* in a hemodialysis patient. *American Journal of Kidney Diseases*, *34*(2), 349–354. https://doi.org/10.1016/s0272-6386(99)70367-7

Chen, J., & Tsim, K. W. (2020). A review of edible jujube, the *Ziziphus jujuba* fruit: A heath food supplement for anemia prevalence. *Frontiers in Pharmacology*, *11*. https://doi.org/10.3389/fphar.2020.593655

Chen, S., Zhou, Q. Y., Chen, L., Liao, X., Li, R., & Xie, T. (2022). The *Aurantii Fructus Immaturus* flavonoid extract alleviates inflammation and modulate gut microbiota in DSS-induced colitis mice. *Frontiers in Nutrition*, *9*. https://doi.org/10.3389/fnut.2022.1013899

Chen, Y., Ruan, J., Sun, F., Wang, H., Yang, S., Zhang, Y., Yan, J., Yu, H., Guo, Y., Zhang, Y., & Wang, T. (2020). Anti-inflammatory limonoids from *Cortex Dictamni. Frontiers in Chemistry*, *8*. https://doi.org/10.3389/fchem.2020.00073

Deng, Y., Liu, Y. Y., Zhao, L., Li, J., Lingmin, Z., Xiao, H., Ding, X., & Yang, Z. (2013). Antiviral activity of *Folium Isatidis* derived extracts in vitro and in vivo. *American Journal of Chinese Medicine*, *41*(04), 957–969. https://doi.org/10.1142/s0192415x1350064x

Ding, C., & Zhu, H. (2020). Isatidis folium alleviates acetaminophen-induced liver injury in mice by enhancing the endogenous antioxidant system. *Environmental Toxicology*, *35*(11), 1251–1259. https://doi.org/10.1002/tox.22990

Gang, S.-Y., Han, J.-H., & Kim, K.-Y. (1998). Effect of *Fructus Tribuli* extract on regional cerebral blood flow and pil arterial diameter. *The Korea Journal of Herbology*, *13*(1), 187–187. https://koreascience.kr/article/JAKO199810102466478.page

Gonzalez, F., Magalhães, F. P., Freitas, A. P. V. B., Filho, H. C. L., & Santiago, M. B. (2006). Lipodermatosclerosis in patients with diffuse connective tissue diseases. *European Journal of Internal Medicine*, *17*(4), 288–289. https://doi.org/10.1016/j.ejim.2005.11.030

Huang, L., Lyu, Q., Zheng, W., Qiao, Y., & Cao, G. (2021). Traditional application and modern pharmacological research of *Eucommia ulmoides* Oliv. *Chinese Medicine*, *16*(1). https://doi.org/10.1186/s13020-021-00482-7

Jiang, W., Yang, Y., & Li, Y. (1993). Effects of some drugs for resolving phlegm on blood rheological property in rats. *Journal of Traditional Chinese Medicine*, (12)1993. https://pesquisa.bvsalud.org/portal/resource/pt/wpr-518710

Li, Y., Li, W., Fu, C., Song, Y., & Fu, Q. (2020). *Lonicerae japonicae flos* and *Lonicerae flos*: A systematic review of ethnopharmacology, phytochemistry and pharmacology. *Phytochemistry Reviews*, *19*(1), 1–61. https://doi.org/10.1007/s11101-019-09655-7

Liu, S., Li, J., Wang, L., Wang, Q., Liang, Y., Zhu, F., Li, J., Qi, R. Yu, J., & Lin, L. (2004). The effect of periostracum cicadae on hemorheology in rats. *Acta Chinese Medicine and Pharmacology*, *3*, 56–58. [Article in Chinese] https://qikan.cqvip.com/Qikan/Article/Detail?id=11116309

Liu, Y., Yang, T., Chen, T., Hao, J., Gai, Y., & Zhang, W. (2019). (R)-dehydroxyabscisic alcohol β-D-apiofuranosyl-(1"→6')-β-D-glucopyranoside enhances the osteoblastic differentiation of ST2 cells via the BMP/WNT pathways. *Molecular Medicine Reports*, *19*(1), 461–467. https://doi.org/10.3892/mmr.2018.9690

Min, G., Kim, T., Kim, J. H., Cho, W., Yang, J., & Ma, J. (2023). Anti-atopic effect of isatidis folium water extract in TNF-A/IFN-Γ-induced HACAT cells and DNCB-induced atopic dermatitis mouse model. *Molecules*, *28*(9), 3960. https://doi.org/10.3390/molecules28093960

Sun, Y., Zhang, J., & Chen, Y. (2017). Efficacy and safety of Jianzhong decoction in treating peptic ulcers: A meta-analysis of 58 randomised controlled trials with 5192 patients. *BMC Complementary and Alternative Medicine*, *17*(1). https://doi.org/10.1186/s12906-017-1723-2

Tan, Y., Chen, H., Li, J., & Wu, Q. (2020). Efficacy, chemical constituents, and pharmacological actions of *Radix paeoniae Rubra* and *Radix paeoniae Alba*. *Frontiers in Pharmacology*, *11*. https://doi.org/10.3389/fphar.2020.01054

Wang, S.-C. (2019). Therapeutic classes of CHEG formulas. In S.-C. Wang (Ed.), *Clinical herbal prescriptions: Principles and practices of herbal formulations from deep learning health insurance herbal prescription big data* (pp. 16–89). World Scientific Publishing. https://doi.org/10.1142/11211

Wang, S.-C. (2020). Modern therapeutic uses of CHEG herbs and herb pairs. In S.-C. Wang (Ed.), *Veterinary herbal pharmacopoeia* (pp. 35–233). Nova Science Publishers. https://doi.org/10.52305/GHTR1903

Wang, Y., Chen, X., Wei, W., Ding, Y., Guo, R. S., Xing, J., & Wang, J. (2023). Efficacy and safety of the Chinese herbal medicine Xiao Yao San for treating anxiety: A systematic review with meta-analysis and trial sequential analysis. *Frontiers in Pharmacology*, *14*. https://doi.org/10.3389/fphar.2023.1169292

Wen, W., Chen, H., Fu, K., Wei, J., Qin, L., Pan, T., & Xu, S. (2020). *Fructus Viticis* methanolic extract attenuates trigeminal hyperalgesia in migraine by regulating injury signal transmission. *Experimental and Therapeutic Medicine*, *19*(1), 85–94. https://doi.org/10.3892/etm.2019.8201

Wong, C. M., & Shiau, D.-S. (2020). The effectiveness of integrating Gui Pi Tang with conventional medicine in the treatment of thrombocytopenia in dogs: A retrospective study. *Am J Trad Chin Vet Med*, *15*(2), 39–52.

Yamaguchi, K., Kakemoto, H., Kawakatsu, T., Fukuroi, T., Suzuki, M., Yanabu, M., Nomura, S., Kokawa, T., & Yasunaga, K. (1993). Effects of Kami-kihi-to (Jia- Wei-Gui-Pi-Tang) on autoantibodies in patients with chronic immune thrombocytopenic purpura. *American Journal of Chinese Medicine*, *21*(03n04), 251–255. https://doi.org/10.1142/s0192415x93000297

Yang, M., Li, X., Zhang, L., Wang, C., Ji, M., Xu, J., Zhang, K., Liu, J., Zhang, C., & Li, M. (2019). Ethnopharmacology, phytochemistry, and pharmacology of the genus Glehnia: A systematic review. *Evidence-Based Complementary and Alternative Medicine*, *2019*, 1–33. https://doi.org/10.1155/2019/1253493

Yeh, H., Li, T. F., Tsai, C. H., Wu, P., Huang, Y., Huang, W. J., Chen, F. J., Hwang, S. J., Chen, F. P., & Wu, T. (2020). The effects of a Chinese herbal medicine (VGHBPH0) on patients with benign prostatic hyperplasia: A pilot study. *Journal of the Chinese Medical Association*, *83*(10), 967–971. https://doi.org/10.1097/jcma.0000000000000384

Yoshie, F., Iizuka, A., Komatsu, Y., Matsumoto, A., Itakura, H., & Kondo, K. (2004). Effects of Daisaiko-to (Da-Chai-Hu-Tang) on plasma lipids and atherosclerotic lesions in female heterozygous heritable Kurosawa and Kusanagi-hypercholesterolemic (KHC) rabbits. *Pharmacological Research*, *50*(3), 223–230. https://doi.org/10.1016/j.phrs.2004.02.003

Yu, Z., Wang, W., Yang, K., Gou, J., Jiang, Y., & Yu, Z. (2023). Sports and Chinese herbal medicine. *Pharmacological Research. Modern Chinese Medicine*, *9*, 100290. https://doi.org/10.1016/j.prmcm.2023.100290

Zhou, W., & Zhang, X. (2013). Research progress of Chinese herbal medicine *Radix isatidis* (Banlangen). *American Journal of Chinese Medicine*, *41*(04), 743–764. https://doi.org/10.1142/s0192415x1350050x

Zhou, X., Razmovski-Naumovski, V., Kam, A., Chang, D., Li, C. G., Chan, K., & Bensoussan, A. (2019). Synergistic study of a Danshen (*Salvia Miltiorrhizae Radix et Rhizoma*) and Sanqi (*Notoginseng Radix et Rhizoma*) combination on cell survival in EA.hy926 cells. *BMC Complementary and Alternative Medicine*, *19*(1). https://doi.org/10.1186/s12906-019-2458-z

10 GMP Herbal Medicine for Rare Bone Diseases

Bones are living tissues that constantly rebuild throughout our lives. When we are young, we gain bones faster than we lose them; however, as we age after around 25 years of age, the situation is reversed. Bone diseases can be caused by injury, infection, genetics, and poor nutrition. Many rare bone diseases of this chapter are early-onset, autosomal dominant.

Caltrop Fruit (Puncture-Vine Fruit; Jílí), Cicada Molting (Chántuì), Licorice Root (Gāncǎo), Bitter Orange (Zhǐqiào), Rhubarb Root and Rhizome (Dàhuáng), Achyranthes Root (Niúxī), Chinese Senega Root (Yuǎnzhì), Rehmannia Root (Dìhuáng), Sweetflag Rhizome (Shíchāngpú), Figwort Root (Xuánshēn), Relax the Channels and Invigorate the Blood Decoction (Shūjīnghuóxuètāng), Cinnamon and Angelica Gout Formula (Shàngzhōngxiàtōngyòngtòngfēngwán), Peony and Licorice Decoction (Sháoyàogāncǎotāng), Lycium, Chrysanthemum and Rehmannia Pill (Qǐjúdìhuángwán), Mulberry Leaf and Chrysanthemum Drink (Sāngjúyǐn), Sweet Dew Decoction (Gānlùyǐn), Ginseng, Astragalus and Pueraria Combination (Yìqìcōngmíngtāng), Five Ingredient Formula with Poria (Wǔlíngsǎn), Six Ingredient Pill with Rehmannia (Liùwèidìhuángwán), Enrich the Kidneys and Improve Vision Decoction (Zīshènmíngmùtāng), Ginseng Nutritive Decoction (Rénshēnyǎngróngtāng), and Gardenia and Vitex Combination (Xǐgānmíngmùtāng), besides acupuncture, are the most frequently discussed GMP single herbs and GMP multi-herb formulas for the signs and symptoms of the rare bone diseases of this chapter.

10.1 OSTEOCHONDRITIS DISSECANS

Osteochondritis dissecans, also known as König disease, is cracks of a section of the bone and the covering cartilage due to lack of blood supply. Osteochondritis dissecans usually occurs at a joint, such as the elbow, knee, and ankle, but can affect any bone of the body. It is not clear what causes the interruption of blood to the bone but repetitive overload of the joint during sports is suspected.

Shennong Bencao Jing (*The Divine Farmer's Classic of Materia Medica*) says that Cāngzhú (cf. Section 8.13) treats "wind-cold-dampness arthralgia, rigor mortis, spasticity, and jaundice. Niúxī (cf. Sections 3.6 and 3.27) was shown, using rats, to be a lower guiding component herb to augment the anti-inflammatory effect of the resulting formula (Wu et al., 2018); it is used today for pain in the lower leg joint, polymyalgia rheumatica, and sciatica (Wang, 2020). The term tòngfēng in Shàngzhōngxiàtōngyòngtòngfēngwán means gout. The formula was initially designed for pain/

TABLE 10.1

GMP Herbal Medicines for a 13-Year-Old Adolescent with Osteochondritis Dissecans

Osteochondritis dissecans (OrphaCode: 2764)

A disease with a prevalence of ~3 in 10,000

Not applicable

Limitation of joint mobility, Joint swelling, Joint stiffness, Abnormality of the knee, Arthralgia

Abnormal joint morphology, Limited elbow extension, Decreased hip abduction, Limited elbow flexion, Abnormality of skeletal physiology

Gait disturbance, Abnormality of tibia morphology, Quadriceps muscle atrophy

All ages

(Continued)

 DOI: 10.1201/9781032726625-10

TABLE 10.1 *(Continued)*

GMP Herbal Medicines for a 13-Year-Old Adolescent with Osteochondritis Dissecans

Arthralgia (D018771):

Shàngzhōngxiàtōngyòngtòngfēngwán 5g + shūjīnghuóxuètāng 5g + dāngguīniàntòngtāng 5-0g + acupuncture.

Shàngzhōngxiàtōngyòngtòngfēngwán 5g + liùwèidìhuángwán 5g + xīnyísǎn 5g + shūgāntāng 5g + shènzhetāng 5g.

Shàngzhōngxiàtōngyòngtòngfēngwán 5g + dāngguīniàntòngtāng 5-0g + sháoyàogāncǎotāng 3-0g + mùguā 1-0g + niúxī 1-0g + yánhúsuǒ 1-0g + qiānghuó 1-0g + huángbò 1-0g + cāngzhú 1-0g + acupuncture.

Cāngzhú 5g + niúxī 5-4g + huángbò 5-3g + yìyǐrén 5-0g + bīngláng 5-0g + dàhuáng 0g.

Abnormal joint morphology (711, 719.90):

Liùwèidìhuángwán 5g + niúxī 1g + gǔsuìbǔ 1g + xùduàn 1g.

Sháoyàogāncǎotāng 5g + shūjīnghuóxuètāng 5-0g + niúxī 1-0g + mòyào 1-0g + rǔxiāng 1-0g + huángbò 1-0g + cāngzhú 1-0g + xùduàn 1g + mùguā 1-0g.

Dúhuójìshēngtāng 5g + gǔsuìbǔ 2g + xùduàn 2g.

Zuǒguīwán 5g + shūjīnghuóxuètāng 5g + mùguā 1g + niúxī 1g + gǔsuìbǔ 1g + xùduàn 1g.

Xuánshēn 5g + zhìgāncǎo 5g + jīnyínhuā 5g + dāngguī 5g + niúxī 4g + chìsháo 4g + dǎodìwúgōng 4g + huángqí 4g + dàhuáng 0g.

Niúxī 5g + báisháo 5g + guìzhī 5g + gǔsuìbǔ 5g + xùduàn 5g + mùguā 4g + dāngguī 4g + mòyào 2g + rǔxiāng 2g.

Niúxī 5g + chìsháo 5g + zhìgāncǎo 5g + huángqí 5g + chēqiánzǐ 4g + fùzǐ 4g + máhuáng 4g.

Xuánshēn 5g + gāncǎo 5g + mǔlì 5g + bèimǔ 5g + jiégěng 5g + liánqiáo 4g + zhīzǐ 2g.

Xuánshēn 5g + dìhuáng 5g + màiméndōng 5g + hòupò 5-0g + zhǐshí 5-0g + dàhuáng 1-0g.

heat over the body resulting from gout; it is used today for the disorders of joints (Wang, 2019). Shènzhetāng "warms the Spleen, removes dampness, stops pain" and is used today for disorders of the back (Wang, 2019).

10.2 HYPOCALCEMIC VITAMIN D–DEPENDENT RICKETS

Hypocalcemic vitamin D–dependent rickets is also referred to as pseudovitamin D–deficient rickets, vitamin D–dependent rickets type I, or vitamin D–dependency type I. Vitamin D is an important hormonal regulator of calcium and phosphorus metabolism in the body. Mutations in the genes encoding the enzymes that catalyze the bioactivation of endogenous vitamin D precursors in the kidneys cause hypocalcemic vitamin D–dependent rickets.

TABLE 10.2

GMP Herbal Medicines for a One-Year-Old Infant with Hypocalcemic Vitamin D–Dependent Rickets

Hypocalcemic vitamin D–dependent rickets (OrphaCode: 289157)

A disease with a prevalence of ~3 in 10,000

Disease-causing germline mutation(s): cytochrome P450 family 27 subfamily B member 1 (*CYP27B1* / Entrez: 1594) at 12q14.1

Disease-causing germline mutation(s): cytochrome P450 family 2 subfamily R member 1 (*CYP2R1* / Entrez: 120227) at 11p15.2

Autosomal recessive

(Continued)

TABLE 10.2 *(Continued)*
GMP Herbal Medicines for a One-Year-Old Infant with Hypocalcemic Vitamin D–Dependent Rickets

Rickets, Hypocalcemia, Low serum calcitriol

Secondary hyperparathyroidism, Deformed rib cage, Rachitic rosary, Enlargement of the costochondral junction, Motor delay, Tetany, Muscle weakness, Failure to thrive, Hypophosphatemia, Bone pain, Increased susceptibility to fractures, Delayed epiphyseal ossification, Osteomalacia, Sparse bone trabeculae, Thin and bony cortex, Generalized aminoaciduria, Genu varum, Femoral bowing, Tibial bowing, Enlargement of the wrists, Enlargement of the ankles, Subperiosteal bone resorption, Elevated circulating parathyroid hormone level, Irregular and rachitic-like metaphyses, Flat occiput, Postnatal growth retardation, Wide cranial sutures, Elevated alkaline phosphatase of bone origin

Generalized hypotonia, Frontal bossing, Difficulty walking, Short stature

Delayed eruption of teeth, Irritability, Protuberant abdomen, Hypocalcemic seizures, Hypoplasia of dental enamel

Neonatal, Infancy

Tetany (D013746), Muscle weakness (D018908):

Rénshēnyǎngróngtāng 5g + xiǎojiànzhōngtāng 5-0g + shénqū 1-0g + màiyá 1-0g.

Rénshēnyǎngróngtāng 5g + bǔzhōngyìqìtāng 5-0g.

Rénshēnyǎngróngtāng 5g + xiāngshāliùjūnzǐtāng 5-0g.

Rénshēnyǎngróngtāng 5g + shēnlíngbáizhúsǎn 5-0g.

Guīpítāng 5g + xiāngshāliùjūnzǐtāng 3-0g + bǎohéwán 2-0g + shénqū 1-0g + màiyá 1-0g + jīnèijīn 1-0g.

Shāshēn 5g + yùzhú 3g + gāncǎo 3-0g + xuánshēn 2-0g + dìhuáng 2-0g + màiméndōng 2-0g + dàhuáng 0g.

Shāshēn 5g + fúshén 5g + gōuténg 5g + gégēn 2g + gǎoběn 2g + xùduàn 2g + chìsháo 2g + yánhúsuǒ 2g + shārén 2-0g + jīngjiè 2-0g + yùzhú 2-0g + cháihú 2-0g + chuānxiōng 2-0g.

Suānzǎorén 5g + shāshēn 5-4g + cháihú 4-2g + zhīzǐ 4-2g + yèjiāoténg 3-2g + gégēn 3-2g + xùduàn 2g + dìgǔpí 2-1g + mǔdānpí 2-1g.

Huángqí 5g + chìsháo 1g + fángfēng 1g.

Difficulty walking (D051346):

Shūjīnghuóxuètāng 5g + sháoyàogāncǎotāng 4-0g + niúxī 1-0g + mòyào 1-0g + rǔxiāng 1-0g + yánhúsuǒ 1-0g + fùzǐ 1-0g + guìzhī 1-0g + jīxuèténg 1-0g + mùguā 1-0g + acupuncture.

Fúlíng 5g + báisháo 2g + báibiǎndòu 2g + dìhuáng 2g + kuǎndōnghuā 2g + bòhé 2g + yùjīn 2g + zhúrú 1g + zhīmǔ 1g + júhuā 1g.

Fúlíng 5g + bànxià 3g + fùzǐ 3g + xìxīn 3-2g + dàhuáng 1-0g.

Fúlíng 5g + gāncǎo 2g + dǎngshēn 2g + fùzǐ 2g + gānjiāng 0g.

Fúlíng 5g + báisháo 4-2g + fùzǐ 4-2g + dǎngshēn 4-2g + báizhú 2-1g + dàhuáng 0g.

Shāshēn (Radix Adenophorae) "nourishes yin, clears the Lung" and was shown to be anti-asthmatic in mice (Roh et al., 2008). It is thought to relieve hyperventilation, which lowers carbon dioxide levels to cause tetany. Fúshén (cf. Section 2.24) is used for gastrojejunal ulcer, sleep disturbances, alcohol-induced mental disorders, and palpitations (Wang, 2020). It was shown to ameliorate arrhythmia in zebrafish (Yang et al., 2021). Use of Rénshēnyǎngróngtāng for frailty and sarcopenia to extend a healthy life expectancy was reviewed (Uto et al., 2018). Shūjīnghuóxuètāng is translated word-for-word to "meridian relaxing and Blood activating decoction" and used today for disorders of joints (cf. Sections 2.21 and 3.12).

10.3 OSTEOGENESIS IMPERFECTA

Osteogenesis imperfecta, also known as brittle bone disease or glass bone disease, is a connective tissue disease characterized by extreme fragility of the bones. It is caused by mutations in the genes encoding collagen, which is abundant in the bones, tendons, and ligaments. Osteogenesis imperfecta has more than five clinical subtypes with varying symptoms and severity, depending on the mutated genes.

Both Gānlùyǐn (cf. Sections 1.38, 4.11, and 5.3) and Qīngwèisǎn (cf. Sections 1.69, 3.24, and 5.17) are used for diseases of the oral tissues. Bǎohéwán was introduced in Sections 1.39 and 4.13 to

TABLE 10.3

GMP Herbal Medicines for a Three-Year-Old Child with Osteogenesis Imperfecta

Osteogenesis imperfecta (OrphaCode: 666)

A disease with a prevalence of ~8 in 100,000

Disease-causing germline mutation(s): prolyl 4-hydroxylase subunit beta (*P4HB* / Entrez: 5034) at 17q25.3

Disease-causing germline mutation(s): SEC24 homolog D, COPII coat complex component (*SEC24D* / Entrez: 9871) at 4q26

Disease-causing germline mutation(s): collagen type I alpha 1 chain (*COL1A1* / Entrez: 1277) at 17q21.33

Disease-causing germline mutation(s): collagen type I alpha 2 chain (*COL1A2* / Entrez: 1278) at 7q21.3

Disease-causing germline mutation(s) (loss of function): membrane-bound transcription factor peptidase, site 2 (*MBTPS2* / Entrez: 51360) at Xp22.12

Disease-causing germline mutation(s): prolyl 3-hydroxylase 1 (*P3H1* / Entrez: 64175) at 1p34.2

Disease-causing germline mutation(s): cartilage associated protein (*CRTAP* / Entrez: 10491) at 3p22.3

Disease-causing germline mutation(s): peptidylprolyl isomerase B (*PPIB* / Entrez: 5479) at 15q22.31

Disease-causing germline mutation(s) (loss of function): mesoderm development LRP chaperone (*MESD* / Entrez: 23184) at 15q25.1

Disease-causing germline mutation(s): cAMP responsive element binding protein 3 like 1 (*CREB3L1* / Entrez: 90993) at 11p11.2

Disease-causing germline mutation(s): serpin family H member 1 (*SERPINH1* / Entrez: 871) at 11q13.5

Disease-causing germline mutation(s): FKBP prolyl isomerase 10 (*FKBP10* / Entrez: 60681) at 17q21.2

Disease-causing germline mutation(s): serpin family F member 1 (*SERPINF1* / Entrez: 5176) at 17p13.3

Disease-causing germline mutation(s) (loss of function): Wnt family member 1 (*WNT1* / Entrez: 7471) at 12q13.12

Disease-causing germline mutation(s) (loss of function): terminal nucleotidyltransferase 5A (*TENT5A* / Entrez: 55603) at 6q14.1

Disease-causing germline mutation(s): bone morphogenetic protein 1 (*BMP1* / Entrez: 649) at 8p21.3

Disease-causing germline mutation(s): transmembrane protein 38B (*TMEM38B* / Entrez: 55151) at 9q31.2

Disease-causing germline mutation(s): Sp7 transcription factor (*SP7* / Entrez: 121340) at 12q13.13

Disease-causing germline mutation(s): secreted protein acidic and cysteine rich (*SPARC* / Entrez: 6678) at 5q33.1

Disease-causing germline mutation(s): interferon induced transmembrane protein 5 (*IFITM5* / Entrez: 387733) at 11p15.5

Autosomal dominant, Autosomal recessive, X-linked recessive

Brachycephaly, Macrocephaly, Prominent occiput, Micrognathia, Convex nasal ridge, Carious teeth, Abnormality of dental enamel, Pectus carinatum, Abnormality of the ribs, Thin ribs, Abnormality of the metaphysis, Gait disturbance, Intrauterine growth retardation, Abnormality of tibia morphology, Decreased skull ossification, Diaphyseal thickening, Abnormality of dental color, Mixed hearing impairment

Abnormality of the dentition, Large fontanelles, Glaucoma, Visual impairment, Blue sclerae, Dentinogenesis imperfecta, Narrow chest, Osteopenia, Osteoporosis, Hyperhidrosis, Malformation of the heart and great vessels, Recurrent fractures, Abnormality of femur morphology, Genu valgum, Femoral bowing, Slender long bone, Abnormal cortical bone morphology, Abnormality of the hip bone, Abnormal form of the vertebral bodies, Short stature, Biconcave vertebral bodies, Joint hyperflexibility, Corneal opacity, Abnormality of long bone morphology, Bone pain, Cutis laxa, Dental malocclusion, Enlarged vertebral pedicles, Fractures of the long bones, Hypercalciuria, Increased susceptibility to fractures, Joint hypermobility, Loss of ability to walk, Multiple rib fractures, Progressive hearing impairment, Vertebral compression fractures

Inguinal hernia, Triangular face, Hearing impairment, Pectus excavatum, Umbilical hernia, Thrombocytopenia, Wormian bones, Scoliosis, Kyphosis, Micromelia, Protrusio acetabuli, Abnormality of the endocardium, Bowing of the long bones, Visceral angiomatosis, Arthralgia, Bruising susceptibility, Calcification of the interosseus membrane of the forearm, Constipation, Delayed eruption of teeth, Dislocated radial head, Dysphagia, Flexion contracture, Growth delay, Hyperplastic callus formation, Intestinal obstruction, Morphological abnormality of the central nervous system, Nephrolithiasis, Osteoarthritis, Paresthesia, Relative macrocephaly, Sensory impairment, Small for gestational age, Trigeminal neuralgia, Ventriculomegaly

All ages

(Continued)

TABLE 10.3 *(Continued)*
GMP Herbal Medicines for a Three-Year-Old Child with Osteogenesis Imperfecta

Carious teeth (521.0, 521.07), Mixed hearing impairment (D046089):

Gānlùyǐn 5g + zhúyèshígāotāng 5-0g.

Gānlùyǐn 5g + xiāngshāliùjūnzǐtāng 5-0g.

Gānlùyǐn 5g + qīngwèisǎn 5-0g.

Gānlùyǐn 5g + bǎohéwán 5-0g.

Gānlùyǐn 5g + gāncǎo 2-0g + báizhǐ 2-0g + shārén 2-0g + dàhuáng 0g.

Báizhǐ 5-3g + shārén 5-3g + gāncǎo 5-2g + huángqín 5-0g + tiānhuā 2-0g + xìxīn 2-0g + dàhuáng 1-0g.

Glaucoma (365), Visual impairment (D014786), Osteoporosis (733.0), Hypercalciuria (D053565):

Sāngjúyǐn 5g + zhǐqiào 2-1g + jílí 2-0g + chántuì 2-0g.

Sāngjúyǐn 5g + júhuā 2-1g + jílí 2-1g + chántuì 2-1g.

Júhuā 5g + zhǐqiào 5-2g + jílí 5-2g + chántuì 5-2g.

Jílí 5-4g + zhǐqiào 5-3g + chántuì 5-0g.

Inguinal hernia (550), Hearing impairment (D003638), Thrombocytopenia (287.5), Arthralgia (D018771), Bruising susceptibility (D004438), Constipation (564.0), Intestinal obstruction (560.9), Nephrolithiasis (592), Osteoarthritis (715.3), Paresthesia (D010292), Sensory impairment (D006987), Trigeminal neuralgia (350.1):

Bǔzhōngyìqìtāng 5g + júhéwán 5g.

Júhéwán 5g + zhǐqiào 1g.

Jílí 5g + zhǐqiào 4-1g + júhuā 4-0g + chántuì 4-0g.

Jílí 5g + chántuì 5g + bīngláng 2g.

Júhuā 5g + jílí 5g + zhǐqiào 4g + chántuì 4g.

improve digestion. Jílí was reviewed to protect the central nervous system (cf. Section 5.9). Júhéwán, elucidated in the text of Section 5.3, is used today for inguinal hernia and functional digestive disorders (Wang, 2019). Different prescriptions in the table address different subgroups of the symptoms.

10.4 STICKLER SYNDROME

Stickler syndrome, also known as hereditary progressive arthroophthalmopathy, is a genetic condition affecting the connective tissues that support the body's joints and organs. Stickler syndrome is caused by mutations in the genes encoding collagen, which is the main structural component of the connective tissue.

TABLE 10.4
GMP Herbal Medicines for a Three-Year-Old Child with Stickler Syndrome

Stickler syndrome (OrphaCode: 828)

A disease with a prevalence of ~5 in 100,000

Disease-causing germline mutation(s): collagen type II alpha 1 chain (*COL2A1* / Entrez: 1280) at 12q13.11

Disease-causing germline mutation(s): collagen type XI alpha 1 chain (*COL11A1* / Entrez: 1301) at 1p21.1

Candidate gene tested: collagen type II alpha 1 chain (*COL2A1* / Entrez: 1280) at 12q13.11

Disease-causing germline mutation(s): collagen type XI alpha 2 chain (*COL11A2* / Entrez: 1302) at 6p21.32

Disease-causing germline mutation(s): collagen type IX alpha 1 chain (*COL9A1* / Entrez: 1297) at 6q13

Disease-causing germline mutation(s) (loss of function): collagen type IX alpha 2 chain (*COL9A2* / Entrez: 1298) at 1p34.2

Disease-causing germline mutation(s) (loss of function): collagen type IX alpha 3 chain (*COL9A3* / Entrez: 1299) at 20q13.33

Disease-causing germline mutation(s): lysyl oxidase like 3 (*LOXL3* / Entrez: 84695) at 2p13.1

Autosomal dominant, Autosomal recessive

Malar flattening, Epicanthus, Hypoplasia of the maxilla, Long philtrum, Visual impairment, Telecanthus, Cataract, Retinal detachment, Myopia, Skeletal dysplasia, Arthralgia, Short nose, Abnormal form of the vertebral bodies, Abnormal vitreous humor morphology, Depressed nasal bridge, Abnormality of epiphysis morphology, Midface retrusion

Macroglossia, Glossoptosis, Cleft palate, Cleft upper lip, Micrognathia, Hearing impairment, Chronic otitis media, Sensorineural hearing impairment, Depressed nasal ridge, Anteverted nares, Astigmatism, Proptosis, Pectus carinatum, Platyspondyly, Arachnodactyly, Hypotonia, Joint dislocation, Disproportionate tall stature, Mitral valve prolapse, Gastroesophageal reflux, Recurrent respiratory infections, Scoliosis, Bone pain, Osteoarthritis, Kyphosis, Genu valgum, Joint hyperflexibility, Arrhythmia

(Continued)

TABLE 10.4 *(Continued)*

GMP Herbal Medicines for a Three-Year-Old Child with Stickler Syndrome

Hypertelorism, Strabismus, Glaucoma, Uveitis, Blindness, Abnormality of dental enamel, Abnormal diaphysis morphology, Ectopia lentis, Slender build, Hip dislocation, Protrusio acetabuli, Skeletal muscle atrophy, Spinal canal stenosis, Short stature, Cachexia, Reduced bone mineral density, Hemiplegia/hemiparesis, Advanced eruption of teeth, Feeding difficulties in infancy, Reduced number of teeth, Short hard palate, Open bite
Neonatal, Infancy, Childhood

Visual impairment (D014786), Cataract (366.8), Retinal detachment (361.9), Myopia (367.1), Skeletal dysplasia (756.56, 756.4), Arthralgia (D018771):

Jiāwèixiāoyáosǎn 5g + zhǐqiào 1g + júhuā 1g + jílí 1g + chántuì 1g.	Chántuì 5-4g + jílí 5-3g + zhǐqiào 4-0g.
Jiāwèixiāoyáosǎn 5g + qǐjúdìhuángwán 5g + mùzéicǎo 1g + juémíngzǐ 1g + gǔjīngcǎo 1g + chōngwèizǐ 1g + qīngxiāngzǐ 1-0g + mìménghuā 1-0g.	Jílí 5-3g + zhǐqiào 5-3g + sāngbáipí 4-0g.
Sāngjúyǐn 5g + zhǐqiào 1g + sīguāluò 0g.	
Qǐjúdìhuángwán 5g + yìqìcōngmíngtāng 5g + nǚzhēnzǐ 1g + juémíngzǐ 1g + gǒuqǐzǐ 1g + acupuncture.	
Zīshènmíngmùtāng 5g + yìqìcōngmíngtāng 4-0g + gǒuqǐzǐ 1g + tùsīzǐ 1g + nǚzhēnzǐ 1-0g + cǎojuémíng 1-0g + mìménghuā 1-0g + juémíngzǐ 1-0g.	

Cleft palate (749.0), Hearing impairment (D003638), Sensorineural hearing impairment (389.1), Astigmatism (367.2), Proptosis (376.30), Hypotonia (D009123), Gastroesophageal reflux (530.81), Osteoarthritis (715.3), Arrhythmia (D001145):

Yìqìcōngmíngtāng 5g + qǐjúdìhuángwán 5-0g + shíchāngpú 1g + yuǎnzhì 1g.	Gǒuqǐzǐ 5g + shíchāngpú 4-3g + hángjú 4-3g + yuǎnzhì 4-3g + nǚzhēnzǐ 2-0g + gāncǎo 2-0g + huángqí 1-0g.
Liùwèidìhuángwán 5g + yìqìcōngmíngtāng 5-0g + shíchāngpú 2-1g + yuǎnzhì 2-1g.	
Jiāwèixiāoyáosǎn 5g + xīnyíqīngfèitāng 5g + shíchāngpú 1g + yuǎnzhì 1g.	Hángjú 5g + gǒuqǐzǐ 5g + shíchāngpú 2g + shénqū 2g + yuǎnzhì 2g + báizhú 1g.
Língguìshùgāntāng 5g + yùpíngfēngsǎn 4g + shíchāngpú 1g + yuǎnzhì 1g.	Shíchāngpú 5g + hángjú 5g + gǒuqǐzǐ 5g + yuǎnzhì 5-3g + shénqū 5-2g + màiyá 2-0g + nǚzhēnzǐ 2-0g + báizhú 1-0g.

Strabismus (378.7, 378.6, 378.31), Glaucoma (365), Blindness (D001766), Ectopia lentis (379.32), Skeletal muscle atrophy (D009133), Cachexia (D002100):

Qǐjúdìhuángwán 5g + yìqìcōngmíngtāng 5-0g + zīshènmíngmùtāng 5-0g + juémíngzǐ 1-0g.	Zhǐqiào 5g + chántuì 5g + jílí 5-0g.
Zhúyèshígāotāng 5g + qǐjúdìhuángwán 5-0g + juémíngzǐ 1-0g + qīngxiāngzǐ 1-0g + chōngwèizǐ 1-0g + gǔjīngcǎo 1-0g + mùzéicǎo 1-0g + gǒuqǐzǐ 1-0g + júhuā 1-0g.	Chántuì 5g + júhóng 4g.
	Jílí 5g + chántuì 5-0g + júhuā 5-0g + júhóng 3-0g.
Xiǎojiànzhōngtāng 5g + xǐgānmíngmùtāng 5g + gāncǎo 0g.	
Yìqìcōngmíngtāng 5g + zīshènmíngmùtāng 5g + shíchāngpú 1g + yuǎnzhì 1g.	

Yìqìcōngmíngtāng (cf. Sections 1.60, 6.10, and 8.2), containing Huángqí, "supplements Qi" and is therefore believed to help not only with hearing and vision but also skeletal muscle atrophy and cachexia of the patient. Chōngwèizǐ, introduced in Section 6.18 for dry eye disease, is used today for disorders of the lacrimal system and disorders of the globe (Wang, 2020). Gǔjīngcǎo, introduced in Section 6.10 for the eye, is used for disorders of the globe, retinal detachment, and epiphora (Wang, 2020).

10.5 ENLARGED PARIETAL FORAMINA

Enlarged parietal foramina, also known as fenestrae parietales symmetricae or hereditary cranium bifidum, are incomplete intramembranous ossification of the parietal bones during skull development of the fetus. Enlarged parietal foramina are caused by mutations in the homeobox genes *ALX4* or *MSX2*, which play important roles in craniofacial morphogenesis.

Gāncǎo (cf. Sections 1.1, 2.7, 2.30, and 3.29) was found to be effective for the prevention and treatment of chemotherapy-induced nausea and vomiting based on a review of clinical trials and

TABLE 10.5
GMP Herbal Medicines for a One-Year-Old Infant with Enlarged Parietal Foramina

Enlarged parietal foramina (OrphaCode: 60015)

A malformation syndrome with a prevalence of ~4 in 100,000

Disease-causing germline mutation(s) (loss of function): ALX homeobox 4 (*ALX4* / Entrez: 60529) at 11p11.2

Disease-causing germline mutation(s) (loss of function): msh homeobox 2 (*MSX2* / Entrez: 4488) at 5q35.2

Autosomal dominant

Symmetrical, oval parietal bone defects

Abnormality of the posterior cranial fossa, Vomiting, Headache, Venous malformation, Scalp tenderness

Antenatal, Neonatal

Vomiting (D014839), Headache (D006261):

Wǔlíngsǎn 5g + píngwèisǎn 5-0g + báisháo 1-0g + huángqín 1-0g + gāncǎo 1-0g.	Gāncǎo 5g + báizhǐ 5-0g + shārén 5-0g + dàhuáng 1-0g.

animal experiments (Lv et al., 2018). "Water retention," characterized by thirst, vomiting upon drinking, headache, and fever, is indicated by Wǔlíngsǎn according to the TCM classic *Shanghan Lun* (*Treatise on Cold Damage Diseases*) compiled by Zhang Zhongjing (150–219 AD) at the end of the Han dynasty. Modern applications of Wǔlíngsǎn to patients with nausea, vomiting, and headache symptoms show efficacy (Kang et al., 2020; Lee et al., 2023).

10.6 HYPOCHONDROPLASIA

Hypochondroplasia, a form of dwarfism with short limbs, is caused by mutations in the *FGFR3* gene coding for a receptor that binds to acidic and basic fibroblast growth hormone and is important for bone formation and maintenance.

Liùwèidìhuángwán is used for not only diabetes (cf. Sections 1.66 and 3.19), but also disorders of the back (cf. Sections 5.22 and 6.8). Xīnyí (cf. Section 1.6) is used today for sinusitis and rhinitis (Wang, 2020). Both Xīnyíqīngfèitāng and Xīnyísǎn contain Xīnyí (cf. Section 1.6), which was

TABLE 10.6
GMP Herbal Medicines for a Five-Year-Old Child with Hypochondroplasia

Hypochondroplasia (OrphaCode: 429)

A disease with a prevalence of ~3 in 100,000

Disease-causing germline mutation(s) (gain of function): fibroblast growth factor receptor 3 (*FGFR3* / Entrez: 2261) at 4p16.3

Autosomal dominant

Brachydactyly, Short toe, Skeletal dysplasia, Micromelia, Abnormal form of the vertebral bodies, Childhood onset short-limb short stature

Abnormality of the metaphysis, Abnormality of pelvic girdle bone morphology, Abnormality of femur morphology, Genu varum, Joint hyperflexibility, Abnormality of the elbow

Macrocephaly, Intellectual disability, Scoliosis, Osteoarthritis, Hyperlordosis, Spinal canal stenosis, Bowing of the long bones, Sleep apnea

Antenatal, Neonatal, Infancy, Childhood, Adolescent, Adult

Skeletal dysplasia (756.56, 756.4):

Liùwèidìhuángwán 5g + dúhuójìshēngtāng 5-0g + xiāngshāliùjūnzǐtāng 5-0g + shēnlíngbáizhúsǎn 5-0g + gǔsuìbǔ 2-0g + xùduàn 2-0g.	Xuánshēn 5g + dìhuáng 5g + màiméndōng 5g + hòupò 5-2g + zhǐshí 5-2g + dàhuáng 1-0g.
Shūjīnghuóxuètāng 5g + niúxī 2-0g + gǔsuìbǔ 2-0g + jīxuèténg 2-0g + xùduàn 2-0g + gāncǎo 1-0g.	

(Continued)

TABLE 10.6 *(Continued)*
GMP Herbal Medicines for a Five-Year-Old Child with Hypochondroplasia

Intellectual disability (D008607), Osteoarthritis (715.3), Sleep apnea (780.57):

Xīnyíqīngfèitāng 5g + cāngěrsǎn 5g + gāncǎo 2g + zǐsūyè 2g + jílí 2g + chántuì 2g + mǔlì 2-0g.

Xiǎoqīnglóngtāng 5g + xīnyísǎn 5-0g + gāncǎo 2-0g + chántuì 2-0g + xīnyí 1-0g + shíchāngpú 0g + yuǎnzhì 0g.

Mǔlì 5g + fúlíng 5g + dàfùpí 3g + gāncǎo 3g + sāngbáipí 3g + hǎigé 3g + hǎipiāoxiāo 3g + jílí 3g + xīnyí 2g + cāngěrzǐ 2g + bīngláng 2-0g + yuǎnzhì 2-0g.

Gāncǎo 5g + sāngbáipí 5-0g + hǎigé 5-0g + júhuā 5-0g + jílí 3-2g + mǔlì 3-2g + cāngěrzǐ 3-1g + báizhú 3-0g + yánhúsuǒ 3-0g + fúlíng 3-0g + xīnyí 3-0g + sāngzhī 2-0g + dàfùpí 2-0g + shénqū 2-0g + yuǎnzhì 1-0g + guìzhī 1-0g.

shown to exert a neuroprotective effect against oxidative stress in mouse hippocampal neuronal cells (Jung et al., 2018).

10.7 PSEUDOACHONDROPLASIA

Pseudoachondroplasia, also known as pseudoachondroplastic spondyloepiphyseal dysplasia, is a form of dwarfism. Pseudoachondroplasia is caused by mutations in the *COMP* gene, which is expressed in cartilage-forming cells, many of which turn into bone in early development. The mutations cause early death of the cartilage-forming cells, affecting bone growth.

TABLE 10.7
GMP Herbal Medicines for a Three-Year-Old Child with Pseudoachondroplasia

Pseudoachondroplasia (OrphaCode: 750)

A disease with a prevalence of ~3 in 100,000

Disease-causing germline mutation(s): cartilage oligomeric matrix protein (*COMP* / Entrez: 1311) at 19p13.11

Autosomal dominant

Joint laxity, Disproportionate short-limb short stature

Platyspondyly, Brachydactyly, Waddling gait, Delayed epiphyseal ossification, Osteoarthritis, Generalized joint laxity, Arthralgia, Lumbar hyperlordosis, Metaphyseal widening, Metaphyseal irregularity, Short long bone, Abnormal form of the vertebral bodies, Shortening of all metacarpals, Increased laxity of fingers, Short phalanx of finger, Limb undergrowth, Irregular epiphyses, Distal joint laxity, Knee joint hypermobility, Wind-swept deformity of the knees

Limited elbow extension, Joint stiffness, Scoliosis, Genu valgum, Genu varum, Flared metaphysis, Hypoplasia of the capital femoral epiphysis, Limited hip extension, Flat acetabular roof, Skeletal myopathy, Irregular carpal bones, Breaking of vertebral bodies, Increased laxity of ankles, Abnormality of femoral epiphysis, Acetabular dysplasia, Irregular acetabular roof, Hypoplastic pelvis, Abnormal ossification involving the femoral head and neck, Cone-shaped epiphysis, Small epiphyses, Short femoral neck

Neonatal, Infancy

Waddling gait (D020233), Osteoarthritis (715.3), Arthralgia (D018771):

Sháoyàogāncǎotāng 5g + dàfùpí 2g + wǔlíngzhī 2g + mǔlì 2g + sāngbáipí 2g + hǎigé 2g + fúlíng 2g + zǐsūyè 2g + jílí 2g + chántuì 2-0g + shuānggōuténg 2-0g + bǎibù 1-0g.

Shēnlíngbáizhúsǎn 5g + yùpíngfēngsǎn 5-0g + bǔzhōngyìqìtāng 5-0g + shānzhā 1-0g + shénqū 1-0g + màiyá 1-0g + huángqí 1-0g + gāncǎo 1-0g.

Èrchéntāng 5g + sāngjúyǐn 4g + biǎndòu 1g + xiāoyáosǎn 1g + xuánshēn 0g + dìhuáng 0g + shúdìhuáng 0g + chuānliànzǐ 0g.

Gāncǎo 5g + mǔlì 5g + sāngbáipí 5g + gǔsuìbǔ 5g + gégēn 5g + jílí 5g + sānléng 2g + mòyào 2g + rǔxiāng 2g + éshù 2g + sāngzhī 2-0g + bājǐtiān 2-0g.

Yánhúsuǒ 5g + sāngbáipí 5g + gāncǎo 3g + mǔlì 3g + hǎipiāoxiāo 3g + gǔsuìbǔ 3g + gégēn 3g + jílí 3g + sānléng 1g + éshù 1g.

Mǔlì 5g + gāncǎo 3g + jílí 3g + sāngzhī 3-0g + hǎigé 3-0g + sānléng 2-1g + yánhúsuǒ 2-1g + éshù 2-1g + hónghuā 2-0g + táorén 2-0g + gégēn 2-0g + bājǐtiān 2-0g + zǐsūyè 2-0g + gǔsuìbǔ 1-0g.

Sāngbáipí (cf. Section 2.45) extract was demonstrated to inhibit osteoclast formation and promote osteoblast proliferation in rabbit bone marrow cells (Guo et al., 2020). Gǔsuìbǔ (cf. Section 2.13) extract was shown to have systemic effects on bone histomorphology, formation, and local bone healing in mice (Wong et al., 2007). Yánhúsuǒ (cf. Section 2.15) was reviewed to have effects on the central nervous system, including antinociceptive, sedative, antiepileptic, antidepressive and antianxiety, acetylcholinesterase inhibitory, and drug abstinence effects (Tian et al., 2020). Sháoyàogāncǎotāng (cf. Sections 2.24 and 2.39) is used today for disorders of soft tissues, joints, and the back (Wang, 2019).

10.8   MULTIPLE OSTEOCHONDROMAS

Multiple osteochondromas, also known as Bessel-Hagen disease or multiple cartilaginous exostoses, are multiple benign bone outgrowths covered by cartilage. Multiple osteochondromas are associated with mutations in the *EXT1* or *EXT2* gene that code for proteins found in the protein processing and packaging site called the *Golgi apparatus* in the cytoplasm of a cell.

TABLE 10.8

GMP Herbal Medicines for a Ten-Year-Old Child with Multiple Osteochondromas

Multiple osteochondromas (OrphaCode: 321)

A disease with a prevalence of ~3 in 100,000

Disease-causing germline mutation(s): exostosin glycosyltransferase 1 (*EXT1* / Entrez: 2131) at 8q24.11

Disease-causing germline mutation(s) (loss of function): exostosin glycosyltransferase 2 (*EXT2* / Entrez: 2132) at 11p11.2

Autosomal dominant

Osteochondroma

Limitation of joint mobility, Abnormal cartilage morphology, Abnormality of the knee, Abnormality of femur morphology, Abnormal bone structure, Deformed forearm bones, Functional motor deficit, Short stature, Pain, Abnormal lower limb bone morphology

Arthritis, Coxa valga, Genu valgum, Abnormality of fibula morphology, Abnormality of tibia morphology, Metaphyseal widening, Short long bone, Myalgia, Sensory impairment, Deformed radius, Abnormal hand morphology, Short lower limbs, Bowing of the long bones, Limited hip movement, Forearm undergrowth, Limb undergrowth, Short metacarpal, Limitation of knee mobility, Bursitis, Femoroacetabular impingement, Tendon pain, Abnormal morphology of ulna, Asymmetric growth, Lower limb asymmetry

Childhood

Pain (D010146):

Zhènggǔzǐjīndān 5g + shūjīnghuóxuètāng 5-0g + acupuncture.	Xuánshēn 5g + dìhuáng 5g + màiméndōng 5g + hòupò 5-2g + zhǐshí 5-2g + dàhuáng 1-0g + acupuncture.
Zhènggǔzǐjīndān 5g + sháoyàogāncǎotāng 5-0g + acupuncture.	Gāncǎo 5g + báizhǐ 5g + shārén 5g + dàhuáng 0g.
Shūjīnghuóxuètāng 5g + sháoyàogāncǎotāng 4-2g + yánhúsuǒ 1-0g + mòyào 1-0g + rǔxiāng 1-0g + jiānghuáng 1-0g + acupuncture.	

Myalgia (D063806), Sensory impairment (D006987), Femoroacetabular impingement (D057925) [Femoroacetabular impingement (719.85)]:

Xuèfǔzhúyūtāng 5g + shūjīnghuóxuètāng 5-0g + chuānqí 1-0g + mòyào 1-0g + rǔxiāng 1-0g + acupuncture.	Chuānqí 5g + yánhúsuǒ 5-0g + acupuncture.
Cháixiàntāng 5g + acupuncture.	Jīnyínhuā 5g + xuánshēn 3g + gāncǎo 3g + dāngguī 3g + shārén 2g + acupuncture.
Fùfāngdānshēnpiàn 5g + gāncǎo 2g.	Dānshēn 5g + báisháo 5g + dìhuáng 5g + fúlíng 5g + huángjīng 5g + kuǎndōnghuā 3g + báibiǎndòu 3g + qiàncǎo 3g + dāngguī 3g.
	Dìlóng 5g + guìzhī 5g + táorén 5g + máhuáng 5g + huángbò 5g + dāngguī 5g + sūmù 5g + gāncǎo 2g + hónghuā 2g.

The term zhènggǔ in Zhènggǔzǐjīndān (cf. Sections 3.9 and 9.3) means "bone righting." Zhènggǔzǐjīndān, Shūjīnghuóxuètāng, and Yánhúsuǒ were found to be most commonly prescribed to fracture patients during the inflammatory phase of fracture healing (Tseng et al., 2018) when pain and swelling at the fracture site predominate within two weeks after fracture. Zhènggǔzǐjīndān is used today for disorders of joint and peripheral enthesopathies (Wang, 2019). The term zhúyū in Xuèfǔzhúyūtāng means "stasis dispersing" and blood stasis causes pain in TCM. Xuèfǔzhúyūtāng was indeed found to be commonly combined with other TCM products for the management of pain in the chest and respiratory system, soft tissues, menstruation, and joints and back (Kuo et al., 2023). Chuānqī (Radix NotoGinseng) "dissolves stasis, stops bleeding, invigorates Blood, terminates pain" and is used for chest pain (Wang, 2020). We observe that acupuncture is a component in many of the prescriptions for pain.

10.9 X-LINKED HYPOPHOSPHATEMIA

X-linked hypophosphatemia, also called X-linked hypophosphatemic rickets, is weak and soft bones related to low blood levels of phosphate, which is required for the formation and maintenance of bones and teeth. Mutations in the *PHEX* gene, which reduce reabsorption of phosphate in the urine by the kidneys, cause X-linked hypophosphatemia.

The term niāntòng in Dāngguīniāntòngtāng (cf. Section 2.32) means to "nip the pain." Shàngzhōngxiàtōngyòngtòngfēngwán, Dāngguīniāntòngtāng, Shūjīnghuóxuètāng, Mòyào (Myrrha), and Rǔxiāng (Olibanum) were among the most commonly prescribed TCM granules to patients with rheumatoid arthritis in Taiwan (Huang et al., 2015). Cāngzhú (cf. Sections 8.13 and 10.1) was shown to be antirheumatic in rats with rheumatoid arthritis (Liu et al., 2020). Yìyǐrén (Semen Coicis) "helps draining, eliminates dampness, strengthens the Spleen, removes paralysis, clears heat, and drains pus."

TABLE 10.9

GMP Herbal Medicines for a Four-Year-Old Child with X-Linked Hypophosphatemia

X-linked hypophosphatemia (OrphaCode: 89936)

A disease with a prevalence of ~2 in 100,000

Disease-causing germline mutation(s) (loss of function): phosphate regulating endopeptidase X-linked (*PHEX* / Entrez: 5251) at Xp22.11

X-linked dominant

Renal phosphate wasting, Hypophosphatemia, Rickets, Hypocalciuria, Elevated alkaline phosphatase, Abnormality of lower-limb metaphyses

Shell teeth, Rachitic rosary, Growth delay, Bone pain, Arthralgia, Genu valgum, Genu varum, Bowing of the legs, Disproportionate short stature, Upper limb metaphyseal widening, Reduced bone mineral density, Abnormality of epiphysis morphology, Bowing of the long bones, Shortening of the talar neck, Flattening of the talar dome, Abnormality of dentin, Delayed ability to stand, Tooth abscess, Delayed ability to walk

Enlargement of the costochondral junction, Beaded ribs, Craniosynostosis, Arthritis, Limitation of joint mobility, Frontal bossing, Flared iliac wings, Trapezoidal distal femoral condyles, Vertebral hyperostosis, Sacroiliac joint synovitis, Thick growth plates, Enthesitis

Infancy, Childhood

Arthralgia (D018771):

Shàngzhōngxiàtōngyòngtòngfēngwán 5g + shūjīnghuóxuètāng 5g + acupuncture.	Niúxī 5g + báisháo 5g + guìzhī 5g + gǔsuìbǔ 5g + xùduàn 5g + mùguā 4g + dāngguī 4g + mòyào 2g + rǔxiāng 2g.
Shàngzhōngxiàtōngyòngtòngfēngwán 5g + sháoyàogāncǎotāng 5-2g + dāngguīniāntòngtāng 5-0g + mùguā 1-0g + niúxī 1-0g.	Niúxī 5g + huángbò 5g + cāngzhú 5g + yìyǐrén 5-0g. Gāncǎo 5g + báizhǐ 5g + shārén 5g + dàhuáng 0g. Zhǐqiào 5g + jílí 5g + chántuì 5g.

10.10　ISOLATED OSTEOPOIKILOSIS

Isolated osteopoikilosis is an abnormal bone growth characterized by multiple, small round hardening of bone tissues, called *bone islands*, in the end and neck regions of a long bone. Isolated osteopoikilosis is caused by mutations in the *LEMD3* gene, whose products control a pathway that is involved in the growth of new bone.

TABLE 10.10

GMP Herbal Medicines for a 37-Year-Old Adult with Isolated Osteopoikilosis

Isolated osteopoikilosis (OrphaCode: 166119)

A disease with a prevalence of ~2 in 100,000

Disease-causing germline mutation(s) (loss of function): LEM domain containing 3 (*LEMD3* / Entrez: 23592) at 12q14.3

Autosomal dominant

Increased bone mineral density, Abnormal bone ossification, Abnormality of limb bone

Sclerotic foci in hand bones, Abnormal pelvis bone ossification, Abnormality of long bone morphology, Abnormal pelvis bone morphology, Hyperostosis, Sclerosis of foot bone

Dacryocystitis, Limitation of joint mobility, Joint stiffness, Sclerotic scapulae, Bone pain, Abnormality of femur morphology, Arthralgia, Sclerotic foci within carpal bones, Neurodevelopmental delay, Hip pain, Ankle pain, Alcoholism, Tarsal sclerosis, Episodic pain, Abnormally ossified vertebrae

Childhood, Adolescent, Adult

Dacryocystitis (375.0, 375.30), Arthralgia (D018771):

Qǐjúdìhuángwán 5g + zīshènmíngmùtāng 5-4g + xǐgānmíngmùtāng 5-0g.	Gǒuqǐzǐ 5g + tùsīzǐ 5g + fùpénzǐ 4g + wǔwèizǐ 2g + chēqiánzǐ 2g.
Xǐgānmíngmùtāng 5g + zīshènmíngmùtāng 5-0g + mìmēnghuā 1-0g + nǚzhēnzǐ 1-0g + gǒuqǐzǐ 1-0g + tùsīzǐ 1-0g.	Gǒuqǐzǐ 5-4g + júhuā 5-4g + dāngguī 5-4g + dìhuáng 5-4g + fángfēng 4g + huánglián 4-1g + xìxīn 2-1g + dàhuáng 0g.
	Chēqiánzǐ 5g + chōngwèizǐ 5g + wǔwèizǐ 3g + xuánshēn 3g + dìhuáng 3g + fángfēng 3g + zhīmǔ 3g + jiégěng 3g + huángqín 3g + dǎngshēn 3g + xìxīn 2g.

Tùsīzǐ (Semen Cuscutae) "replenishes the Kidney, holds semen, nourishes the Liver, brightens eyes, stops diarrhea, prevents miscarriage" and has been a popular herb for reproductive health, as we will see its use in Chapter 19 for gynecologic/obstetric diseases. A homemade Chinese herbal fumigation eye patch containing Tùsīzǐ was shown to prevent myopia in children and adolescents (Guan et al., 2023). Its modern uses include lumbago and disorders of the lacrimal system (Wang, 2020); we therefore see its inclusion in the prescription for dacryocystitis and arthralgia in Table 10.10.

10.11　DIASTROPHIC DYSPLASIA

Diastrophic dysplasia, also called diastrophic dwarfism, is abnormal growth of cartilage and bone characterized by a short stature with short arms and legs and joint problems. Diastrophic dysplasia is caused by mutations in the *SLC26A2* gene, whose products transport sulfate ions across membranes of the cells in developing cartilage that is later converted into bone.

TABLE 10.11

GMP Herbal Medicines for a Two-Year-Old Toddler with Diastrophic Dysplasia

Diastrophic dysplasia (OrphaCode: 628)

A disease with a prevalence of ~1 in 100,000

Disease-causing germline mutation(s) (loss of function): solute carrier family 26 member 2 (*SLC26A2* / Entrez: 1836) at 5q32

Autosomal recessive

(Continued)

TABLE 10.11 *(Continued)*

GMP Herbal Medicines for a Two-Year-Old Toddler with Diastrophic Dysplasia

Macrocephaly, Abnormality of the ribs, Abnormality of the clavicle, Abnormality of the metaphysis, Abnormality of the metacarpal bones, Intrauterine growth retardation, Scoliosis, Micromelia, Abnormal form of the vertebral bodies, Depressed nasal bridge, Abnormality of epiphysis morphology, Bowing of the long bones, Hypoplastic cervical vertebrae, Neonatal short-limb short stature, Short finger, Proximal placement of thumb, Large earlobe, Symphalangism affecting the phalanges of the hand, Increased bone mineral density, Midface retrusion

Cleft palate, Full cheeks, Hypertelorism, Low-set, posteriorly rotated ears, Overfolded helix, Blue sclerae, Hypotonia, Joint dislocation, Hip dysplasia, Joint stiffness, Respiratory insufficiency, Recurrent respiratory infections, Kyphosis, Ulnar deviation of finger, Camptodactyly of finger

Cryptorchidism, Micrognathia, Hearing impairment, Hyperextensible skin, Cerebral calcification, Elbow dislocation, Joint hyperflexibility, Visceral angiomatosis

Neonatal

Cleft palate (749.0), Hypotonia (D009123):

Gānlùyǐn 5g + zhǐqiào 2-1g + jílí 1-0g + chántuì 1-0g.

Sāngjúyǐn 5g + zhǐqiào 1g + chántuì 1-0g + sīguāluò 0g.

Gāncǎo 5g + báizhú 5g + fúlíng 5g + chénpí 5g + màiyá 5g + huángqí 5g + dǎngshēn 5g.

Gāncǎo 5g + báizhǐ 5g + shārén 5g + dàhuáng 1g.

Jílí 5-2g + júhóng 5-0g + chántuì 5-0g + júhuā 5-0g.

Cryptorchidism (752.51), Hearing impairment (D003638):

Wǔlíngsǎn 5g + píngwèisǎn 5-0g + báizhǐ 1-0g + gāncǎo 1-0g.

Chántuì 5g + jílí 5-0g + júhuā 5-0g + júhóng 5-0g.

Júhóng 5g + jílí 2-0g.

According to *Bencao Yanyi* (*Augmented Materia Medica*), authored by TCM pharmacist Kou Zongshi in 1119, Chántuì (cf. Sections 1.54, 2.20, 5.3, and 6.8) treats swelling of the scrotum. Píngwèisǎn was introduced in Section 4.13 for functional digestive disorders. From the components in the prescriptions, we learn that a common strategy of GMP herbal extract granule practitioners for pediatric patients is to promote their growth by improving their digestion.

REFERENCES

Guan, W., Zhang, G., Li, Y., Li, Q., & Wang, L. (2023). Homemade Chinese herbal fumigation eye patch prevents myopia in children and adolescents. American Journal of Translational Research, 15(4), 2765–2772. https://pubmed.ncbi.nlm.nih.gov/37193160

Guo, D.-G., Feng, T.-T., Zhang, M., & Wang, H.-J. (2020). Effect of Cortex Mori extract on the activity of osteoclasts and osteoblasts. Science and Technology of Food Industry, 41(8), 316–320. http://www.spgykj.com/article/doi/10.13386/j.issn1002-0306.2020.08.051?pageType=en

Huang, M., Pai, F., Lin, C., Chang, C., Chang, H., Lee, Y., Sun, M., & Yen, H. (2015). Characteristics of traditional Chinese medicine use in patients with rheumatoid arthritis in Taiwan: A nationwide population-based study. Journal of Ethnopharmacology, 176, 9–16. https://doi.org/10.1016/j.jep.2015.10.024

Jung, Y. S., Weon, J. B., Yang, W. S., Ryu, G., & Je, C. (2018). Neuroprotective effects of Magnoliae Flos extract in mouse hippocampal neuronal cells. Scientific Reports, 8(1). https://doi.org/10.1038/s41598-018-28055-z

Kang, J., Bae, J., & Kong, K. (2020). A case of a functional dyspepsia patient diagnosed with water reversal syndrome treated with Oryeong-san. The Journal of Internal Korean Medicine, 41(5), 806–810. https://doi.org/10.22246/jikm.2020.41.5.806

Kuo, C., Hsu, S., Chen, C., Wu, S., Hung, Y., Hsu, C. Y., Tsai, I., & Hu, W. (2023). Prescription characteristics of Xue-Fu-Zhu-Yu-Tang in pain management: A population-based study using the National Health Insurance Research Database in Taiwan. Frontiers in Pharmacology, 14. https://doi.org/10.3389/fphar.2023.1233156

Lee, H., Jin, C., Kwon, S., Jang, B., Jeon, J. P., Lee, Y., Yang, S., Jung, W., Moon, S., & Cho, K. (2023). Treatment of nausea and vomiting associated with cerebellar infarction using the traditional herbal medicines Banhabaekchulcheonma-tang and Oryeong-san: Two case reports (CARE-complaint). Explore, 19(1), 141–146. https://doi.org/10.1016/j.explore.2021.11.011

Liu, Y., Zhang, B., & Cai, Q. (2020). Study on the pharmacodynamics and metabolomics of five medicinal species in Atractylodes DC. on rats with rheumatoid arthritis. Biomedicine & Pharmacotherapy, 131, 110554. https://doi.org/10.1016/j.biopha.2020.110554

Lv, C., Shi, C., Li, L., Wen, X., & Chen, X. (2018). Chinese herbal medicines in the prevention and treatment of chemotherapy-induced nausea and vomiting. Current Opinion in Supportive and Palliative Care, 12(2), 174–180. https://doi.org/10.1097/spc.0000000000000348

Roh, S., Kim, S., Lee, Y., & Seo, Y. (2008). Effects of Radix Adenophorae and cyclosporine A on an OVA-induced murine model of asthma by suppressing to T cells activity, eosinophilia, and bronchial hyper-responsiveness. Mediators of Inflammation, 2008, 1–11. https://doi.org/10.1155/2008/781425

Tian, B., Tian, M., & Huang, S. (2020). Advances in phytochemical and modern pharmacological research of Rhizoma Corydalis. Pharmaceutical Biology, 58(1), 265–275. https://doi.org/10.1080/13880209.2020.1741651

Tseng, C., Huang, C., Hsu, C., & Tseng, W. (2018). Utilization pattern of traditional Chinese medicine among fracture patients: A Taiwan hospital-based cross-sectional study. Evidence-Based Complementary and Alternative Medicine, 2018, 1–9. https://doi.org/10.1155/2018/1706517

Uto, N., Amitani, H., Atobe, Y., Sameshima, Y., Sakaki, M., Rokot, N. T., Ataka, K., Amitani, M., & Inui, A. (2018). Herbal medicine Ninjin'yoeito in the treatment of sarcopenia and frailty. Frontiers in Nutrition, 5. https://doi.org/10.3389/fnut.2018.00126

Wang, S.-C. (2019). Therapeutic classes of CHEG formulas. In S.-C. Wang (Ed.), Clinical herbal prescriptions: Principles and practices of herbal formulations from deep learning health insurance herbal prescription big data (pp. 16–89). World Scientific Publishing. https://doi.org/10.1142/11211

Wang, S.-C. (2020). Modern therapeutic uses of CHEG herbs and herb pairs. In S.-C. Wang (Ed.), Veterinary herbal pharmacopoeia (pp. 35–233). Nova Science Publishers. https://doi.org/10.52305/GHTR1903

Wong, R. W., Rabie, B., Bendeus, M., & Hägg, U. (2007). The effects of Rhizoma Curculiginis and Rhizoma Drynariae extracts on bones. Chinese Medicine, 2(1), 13. https://doi.org/10.1186/1749-8546-2-13

Wu, J., Li, J., Li, W., Sun, B., Xie, J., Cheng, W., & Zhang, Q. (2018). Achyranthis bidentatae radix enhanced articular distribution and anti-inflammatory effect of berberine in Sanmiao Wan using an acute gouty arthritis rat model. Journal of Ethnopharmacology, 221, 100–108. https://doi.org/10.1016/j.jep.2018.04.025

Yang, N., Liu, Y., Tang, Z., Duan, J., Yan, Y., Song, Z., Wang, M., Zhang, Y., Chang, B., Zhao, M., & Zhao, Y. (2021). Poria cum Radix Pini rescues barium chloride-induced arrhythmia by regulating the cGMP-PKG signalling pathway involving ADORA1 in zebrafish. Frontiers in Pharmacology, 12. https://doi.org/10.3389/fphar.2021.688746

11 GMP Herbal Medicine for Rare Infectious Diseases

Infectious diseases are those caused by pathogenic organisms such as viruses, bacteria, fungi, and parasites. Some infectious diseases can be transmitted from person to person. The rare infectious diseases of this chapter affect people of all ages.

The GMP single herbs that are most frequently discussed for the clinical manifestations of the rare infectious diseases are Licorice Root (Gāncǎo), Rhubarb Root and Rhizome (Dàhuáng), Scutellaria Root (Huángqín), Cardamon Seed (Shārén), Dahurian Angelica Root (Báizhǐ), Aconite Accessory Root (Fùzǐ), Dried Ginger Rhizome (Gānjiāng), Golden Thread Root (Huánglián), Chinese Wild Ginger (Xìxīn), White Peony Root (Báisháo), Poria (Fúlíng), and Trichosanthes Root (Tiānhuā), many of which are antimicrobic and anti-inflammatory. The GMP multi-herb formulas that are most frequently used are Five Ingredient Formula with Poria (Wǔlíngsǎn), Tangkuei and Tribulus Decoction (Dāngguīyǐnzǐ), Evodia Decoction (Wúzhūyútāng), Achyranthes and Plantago Formula (Jìshēngshènqìwán), Ephedra, Aconite and Asarum Decoction (Máhuángfùzǐxìxīntāng), Tonify the Middle and Augment the Qi Decoction (Bǔzhōngyìqìtāng), Rhubarb and Leech Combination (Dǐdāngtāng), Regulate the Stomach and Order the Qi Decoction (Tiáowèichéngqìtāng), Wind Reducing Formula (Xiāofēngsǎn), Ginseng, Poria and Atractylodes Powder (Shēnlíngbáizhúsǎn), Schizonepeta and Siler Formula (Jīngfángbàidúsǎn), and True Warrior Decoction (Zhēnwǔtāng), which are known to relieve diverse symptoms including diarrhea, skin rash, headache, cough, and so on.

11.1 HEMORRHAGIC FEVER-RENAL SYNDROME

Hemorrhagic fever-renal syndrome, also known as hantavirus fever, is a group of illnesses caused by hantavirus infections. Rodents are natural hosts and carriers of hantaviruses; people working with live rodents may get infected through inhalation of aerosolized excreta such as urine, droppings, and saliva from the infected rodents.

Bìxièfēnqīngyǐn (cf. Section 3.16), containing Yìzhìrén, which was introduced in Section 7.4 for prostate enlargement, "warms the Kidney, helps draining, clarifies cleanness, and reduces turbidity."

TABLE 11.1

GMP Herbal Medicines for a 20-Year-Old Adult with Hemorrhagic Fever-Renal Syndrome

Hemorrhagic fever-renal syndrome (OrphaCode: 340)

A disease with a prevalence of ~4 in 10,000

Not applicable

Acute kidney injury, Fever, Elevated serum creatinine, Decreased urine output, Decreased glomerular filtration rate, Capillary leak, Severe infection, Oliguria

Proteinuria, Glomerulonephritis, Blurred vision, Petechiae, Excessive daytime somnolence, Muscle weakness, Tachycardia, Thrombocytopenia, Palpitations, Tubulointerstitial nephritis, Leukocytosis, Vomiting, Nausea, Abdominal pain, Headache, Hypotension, Myalgia, Back pain, Decreased body weight, Acute tubulointerstitial nephritis, Fatigue, Chills, Increased serum interleukin-6

Agitation, Hematuria, Hyperhidrosis, Confusion, Anemia, Diarrhea, Pneumonia, Dyspnea, Respiratory distress, Hyperkalemia, Pleural effusion, Hematemesis, Hyperphosphatemia, Elevated hepatic transaminase, Subconjunctival hemorrhage, Cough, Shock, Ecchymosis, Anuria, Pulmonary edema, Insomnia

All ages

(Continued)

DOI: 10.1201/9781032726625-11

TABLE 11.1 *(Continued)*
GMP Herbal Medicines for a 20-Year-Old Adult with Hemorrhagic Fever-Renal Syndrome

Fever (D005334), Oliguria (D009846):

Wǔlíngsǎn 5g + xìxīn 1-0g + huángqín
1-0g + fùzǐ 1-0g + báisháo 1-0g + báizhǐ
1-0g + dǎngshēn 1-0g + tiáowèichéngqìtāng
0g + dǐdāngtāng 0g + gāncǎo 0g.

Gāncǎo 5g + báizhǐ 5g + shārén 5-0g + huángqín 5-0g + tiānhuā
3-0g + guālóugēn 2-0g + xìxīn 2-0g + dàhuáng 2-0g + huánglián 1-0g.

Proteinuria (791.0), Petechiae (D011693), Muscle weakness (D018908), Thrombocytopenia (287.5), Vomiting (D014839), Nausea (D009325), Abdominal pain (D015746), Headache (D006261), Myalgia (D063806), Back pain (D001416), Decreased body weight (D013851), Fatigue (D005221):

Bìxièfēnqīngyǐn 5g + qīngxīnliánzǐyǐn 5-0g +
shēnlíngbáizhúsǎn 5-0g.
Wǔlíngsǎn 5g + bìxièfēnqīngyǐn 5g +
jìshēngshènqìwán 5-0g.
Wǔlíngsǎn 5g + shēnlíngbáizhúsǎn 5g +
huángqí 1g.
Wǔlíngsǎn 5g + zhūlíngtāng 5g.

Báizhú 5g + fùzǐ 5-3g + báisháo 5-3g + fúlíng 5-3g + dǎngshēn 5-2g +
cháihú 5-0g + tiānhuā 2-0g + guìzhī 2-0g + huángqín 2-0g + mǔlì
1-0g + gānjiāng 1-0g + gāncǎo 1-0g.
Báizhú 5g + dìhuáng 5g + dùzhòng 5g + guìzhī 5g + huángqín 5g +
dǎngshēn 5g + dāngguī 4g.
Báizhú 5g + fúlíng 4-3g + zhìgāncǎo 4-0g + gānjiāng 4-0g + zhūlíng
3-0g + zéxiè 3-0g + ròuguì 2-1g + niúxī 2-0g + fùzǐ 2-0g.
Shúdìhuáng 5g + báizhú 3g + qiànshí 3g + yìyǐrén 3g + shānzhūyú
2g + wǔwèizǐ 2g + báijièzǐ 2g + dùzhòng 2g + dǎngshēn 2g + guìzhī
2g + fúlíng 2g + yìzhìrén 1g + shārén 0g.

Confusion (D003221), Anemia (285.9), Diarrhea (D003967), Dyspnea (D004417), Respiratory distress (D004417), Hematemesis (D006396), Elevated hepatic transaminase (573.9), Cough (D003371):

Wǔlíngsǎn 5g + bǔzhōngyìqìtāng 5g +
guīpítāng 5-0g + jìshēngshènqìwán 5-0g +
huòxiāngzhèngqìsǎn 5-0g.
Lǐzhōngtāng 5g + bǔzhōngyìqìtāng 5-0g +
qínjiāobiējiǎsǎn 3-0g + jìshēngshènqìwán
3-0g + fángfēng 2-0g + ējiāo 2-0g + zhǐqiào
2-0g + gānjiāng 2-0g.
Bǔzhōngyìqìtāng 5g + rénshēnyǎngróngtāng
4-0g + xiāngshāliùjūnzǐtāng 2-0g + huángqí
1-0g + dǎngshēn 1-0g.

Gānjiāng 5g + dǎngshēn 5g + huángqín 3g + huánglián 3g + dàhuáng 0g.
Gānjiāng 5g + rénshēn 4-2g + bànxià 4-2g.
Báizhú 5g + fùzǐ 5g + cháihú 5g + báisháo 4g + fúlíng 4g + tiānhuā
2g + dǎngshēn 2g + wúzhūyú 2g + guìzhī 2g + huángqín 2g + gāncǎo
1g + mǔlì 1g + gānjiāng 1g + huánglián 1g.
Gāncǎo 5g + báizhú 5g + báisháo 5g + báibiǎndòu 5g + chēqiánzǐ 5g +
fúlíng 5g + huángqí 5g + dàzǎo 2g + shēngjiāng 2g.
Wǔwèizǐ 5g + bànxià 5g + zhìgāncǎo 5g + cháihú 5g + gānjiāng 5g +
huángqín 5g.

Qīngxīnliánzǐyǐn contains Huángqín and is used today for nephritis and nephropathy (cf. Section 3.11). Gānjiāng (cf. Section 2.16) extract was shown to significantly improve the ability of mice to recognize novel objects through its synaptogenic effect (Lim et al., 2014). Báibiǎndòu (Semen Lablab Album) was shown to be hypoglycemic in diabetic mice (Han et al., 2021) and play an important role in treating irritable bowel syndrome in a network pharmacology-based study (Meng et al., 2021). It is used today for disorders of functions of the stomach (Wang, 2020). The prescriptions in the table aim to improve the renal, cognitive, and digestive symptoms of the infected individuals.

11.2 BOUTONNEUSE FEVER

Boutonneuse fever, also known as Mediterranean spotted fever, is a bacterial infection by the tick-borne bacterium *Rickettsia conorii*. A bite by a dog tick transmits the bacteria into human blood circulation, leaving a black spot at the site of the tick bite. Symptoms begin in about a week following the bite, including fever, rash, joint pain, and headache.

Dāngguīyǐnzǐ, introduced in Section 3.28, is used today for eczema and urticaria (Wang, 2019). Jìshēngshènqìwán, introduced in Sections 1.61, 3.20, and 4.6, "helps the Kidney yang." Huánglián (cf. Sections 1.22 and 6.20) "clears heat, dries dampness, extinguishes fires and neutralizes pathogens." It was reviewed and summarized to be antibacterial, antiviral, antifungal, antidiabetic,

TABLE 11.2

GMP Herbal Medicines for a 65-Year-Old Adult with Boutonneuse Fever

Boutonneuse fever (OrphaCode: 83313)

A disease with a prevalence of ~3 in 10,000

Not applicable

Skin rash, Fever, Abnormality of the skin of the palm, Abnormality of the plantar skin of foot

Renal insufficiency, Thrombocytopenia, Headache, Lymphadenopathy, Arthralgia, Elevated hepatic transaminase, Myalgia, Increased circulating IgM level, Macule, Cervical lymphadenopathy, Skin detachment, Maculopapular exanthema, Skin nodule

Petechiae, Leukopenia, Diarrhea, Nausea, Abdominal pain, Increased circulating IgG level

All ages

Skin rash (782.1), Fever (D005334):

Jīngfángbàidúsăn 5g + dìfūzĭ 1g + shéchuángzĭ 1g + jílí 1g + jīnchán 1-0g + huánglián 1-0g.

Xiāofēngsăn 5g + dāngguīyĭnzĭ 5-0g + jiĕdúsìwùtāng 5-0g + tŭfúlíng 2-0g + báixiānpí 1g + dìfūzĭ 1g + jílí 1g + yìyĭrén 1-0g + chántuì 1-0g.

Báizhĭ 5g + gāncăo 5-4g + shārén 4-3g + huángqín 4-2g + guālóugēn 3-2g + huánglián 1-0g + dàhuáng 1-0g.

Renal insufficiency (586), Thrombocytopenia (287.5), Headache (D006261), Arthralgia (D018771), Elevated hepatic transaminase (573.9), Myalgia (D063806):

Zhūlíngtāng 5g + zhēnwŭtāng 3g + huángqí 1g.

Zhūlíngtāng 5g + jìshēngshènqìwán 5g + dānshēn 1g + báimáogēn 1g + yìmŭcăo 1-0g + zélán 1-0g + huángqí 1-0g + jīxuèténg 1-0g + xiānhècăo 1-0g.

Rénshēnyăngróngtāng 5g + guīpítāng 5g + jìshēngshènqìwán 4g + dānshēn 1g.

Guīpítāng 5g + liùwèidìhuángwán 4g + huángqí 1g + dăngshēn 1g + dàhuáng 0g.

Guīpítāng 5g + zhēnwŭtāng 4-2g + jìshēngshènqìwán 3-0g + dānshēn 1g + dīngshùxiŭ 1-0g + huángqí 1-0g + jīxuèténg 1-0g + dàhuáng 1-0g.

Báizhú 5g + fùzĭ 5g + cháihú 5g + báisháo 4g + fúlíng 4g + tiānhuā 2g + dăngshēn 2g + guìzhī 2g + huángqín 2g + shēngjiāng 2-0g + wŭwèizĭ 2-0g + xìxīn 2-0g + gāncăo 1g + mŭlì 1g + gānjiāng 1g + dàhuáng 1-0g.

Shānyào 5g + báizhú 5g + dìhuáng 5g + fùzĭ 5g + yīnchén 5g + dăngshēn 5g + mŭdānpí 4g.

Báizhú 5g + báisháo 5-4g + fúlíng 5-4g + fùzĭ 5-3g + dăngshēn 5-2g + gānjiāng 5-0g + zĭwăn 3-0g + gāncăo 2-1g.

Petechiae (D011693), Leukopenia (288.50), Diarrhea (D003967), Nausea (D009325), Abdominal pain (D015746):

Wŭlíngsăn 5g + fùzĭ 1-0g + huángqín 1-0g + báisháo 1-0g + xiăochéngqìtāng 1-0g + tiáowèichéngqìtāng 1-0g + gāncăo 1-0g + dĭdāngtāng 0g.

Gāncăo 5g + báizhĭ 5g + shārén 5-3g + huángqín 5-0g + tiānhuā 2-0g + xìxīn 2-0g + dàhuáng 1-0g.

anticancer, and cardioprotective (Wang et al., 2019) and is used today for a wide spectrum of skin and digestive conditions (Wang, 2020).

11.3 TUBERCULOSIS

Tuberculosis is caused by the bacterium *Mycobacterium tuberculosis*. People are infected through inhalation of the bacteria. Some infected people do not become sick because their immune system keeps the bacteria from multiplying in the body. The latency can last a lifetime. However, when the immune system becomes weak for other reasons, the bacteria begin to grow and the latent tuberculosis becomes active. Active tuberculosis patients show pulmonary symptoms and can spread the bacteria when they cough, sneeze, spit, sing, and speak.

Gāncăo, one of the most commonly used herbs in TCM, "benefits Qi and nourishes the Heart." A Kawasaki disease pediatric patient presenting with persistent fever, poor appetite, vomiting diarrhea, slight cough, runny nose, and throat congestion successfully treated with TCM formulas including Wŭlíngsăn was reported (Zhu et al., 2019). Tiáowèichéngqìtāng, introduced in the text of Sections 7.13

TABLE 11.3

GMP Herbal Medicines for a 22-Year-Old Adult with Tuberculosis

Tuberculosis (OrphaCode: 3389)

A disease with a prevalence of ~2 in 10,000

Major susceptibility factor: solute carrier family 11 member 1 (*SLC11A1* / Entrez: 6556) at 2q35

Not applicable

Weight loss, Fever, Abnormal lung morphology, Fatigue, Cough

All ages

Weight loss (D015431), Fever (D005334), Fatigue (D005221), Cough (D003371):

Wǔlíngsǎn 5g + báisháo 1-0g + huángqín 1-0g + fùzǐ 1-0g + gāncǎo 1-0g + tiáowèichéngqìtāng 1-0g + dǐdāngtāng 0g + dàhuáng 0g.

Guìzhītāng 5g + hòupò 1g + zhǐshí 1g + dàhuáng 0g.

Gāncǎo 5g + hòupò 5-2g + zhǐshí 5-2g + dàhuáng 1-0g.

and 8.4, "harmonizes the Stomach, rectifies Qi, clears heat and removes blockage." The prescriptions in the table improve the symptoms of the patient who manifests signs of frailness and dampness.

11.4 PULMONARY NON-TUBERCULOUS MYCOBACTERIAL INFECTION

Pulmonary non-tuberculous mycobacterial infection is a pulmonary infection caused by non-tuberculous mycobacteria, which are found in the water and soil in the environment and can infect the lungs, skin, soft tissues, and lymph nodes. Immunocompromised individuals are at risk for this infection.

Bǎibù (Radix Stemonae) was shown to inhibit the release of inflammatory mediators to help airways rebuild in COPD rats (Wang et al., 2016) and is used today for bronchitis and coughs (Wang, 2020). Máhuáng, associated with the lung and urinary bladder meridians, has long been used in TCM for the treatment of asthma, liver disease, and skin disease (cf. Section 5.5). It is used today for rhinitis and dermatomycosis (Wang, 2020). The effects of Guālóurén (cf. Section 5.11) on the cardiovascular system, including protection against myocardial ischemia, calcium antagonist, endothelial cell protection, anti-hypoxic, antiplatelet aggregation, expectorant, anti-inflammatory, cytotoxic, and antioxidant activities, were reviewed (Yu et al., 2018).

TABLE 11.4

GMP Herbal Medicines for a 70-Year-Old Adult with Pulmonary Non-Tuberculous Mycobacterial Infection

Pulmonary non-tuberculous mycobacterial infection (OrphaCode: 411703)

A disease with a prevalence of ~6 in 100,000

Not applicable

Elevated erythrocyte sedimentation rate

Bronchiectasis, Cough, Asthenia, Pulmonary opacity, Abnormal sputum

Pericardial effusion, Weight loss, Fever, Diarrhea, Dyspnea, Respiratory distress, Hemoptysis, Pleural effusion, Lymphadenopathy, Chronic obstructive pulmonary disease, Crackles, Mycobacterium abscessus infection, Disseminated non-tuberculous mycobacterial infection, Chest pain

All ages

Bronchiectasis (494), Cough (D003371):

Máxìnggānshítāng 5g + wēndǎntāng 5g + báijièzǐ 1g + láifúzǐ 1g + tínglìzǐ 1g + sūzǐ 1g.

Máxìnggānshítāng 5g + tínglìzǐ 2-1g + dàzǎo 1g + yúxīngcǎo 1-0g + dàhuáng 0g.

Sūzǐjiàngqìtāng 5g + báisháo 1g + shēngjiāng 1-0g.

Qīngfèitāng 5g + máxìnggānshítāng 5g + yínqiàosǎn 5g.

Bǎibù 5g + máhuáng 5-2g + dàqīngyè 3-2g + yúxīngcǎo 3-2g + huángqín 3-2g + gāncǎo 2-1g + wǔwèizǐ 2-1g + xìngrén 2-1g + jiégěng 2-1g + xìxīn 2-1g + tínglìzǐ 1-0g.

Wǔwèizǐ 5g + bànxià 5g + zhìgāncǎo 5g + cháihú 5g + gānjiāng 5g + huángqín 5g + dàhuáng 0g.

(Continued)

TABLE 11.4 *(Continued)*

GMP Herbal Medicines for a 70-Year-Old Adult with Pulmonary Non-Tuberculous Mycobacterial Infection

Pericardial effusion (423.0), Weight loss (D015431), Fever (D005334), Diarrhea (D003967), Dyspnea (D004417), Respiratory distress (D004417), Hemoptysis (D006469), Crackles (D012135), Chest pain (D002637):

Wǔlíngsǎn 5g + fùzǐ 1-0g + huángqín 1-0g + báisháo 1-0g + guālóurén 1-0g + gāncǎo 1-0g + dǐdāngtāng 0g + dàhuáng 0g.

Guālóurén 5g + xièbái 5g + tiānwángbǔxīndān 5g + xuèfǔzhúyūtāng 5g.

Língguìshùgāntāng 5g + báisháo 1g + fùzǐ 1g + suānzǎorén 1g.

Cháihújiālónggǔmǔlìtāng 5g + guālóurén 1g + xièbái 1g.

Gāncǎo 5g + yúxīngcǎo 5g + púgōngyīng 5-0g + báijiāngcán 4g + fángfēng 4g + jiégěng 4g + jīngjiè 4g + bòhé 4g + niúbàngzǐ 4-0g + tǔfúlíng 4-0g + dìlóng 4-0g + xìngrén 4-0g.

Gāncǎo 5g + gānjiāng 5-0g + fùzǐ 5-0g + suānzǎorén 5-0g + mázǐrénwán 5-0g + fúlíng 5-0g + dǎngshēn 3-0g + báizhú 2-0g + dàhuáng 0g.

Gāncǎo 5g + guìzhī 5g + táorén 5g + zhǐqiào 3g + hónghuā 0g + dàhuáng 0g.

11.5 AMOEBIASIS DUE TO FREE-LIVING AMOEBAE

Amoebae, ubiquitous in water and soil worldwide, enter into the human body through the eyes, nose, and broken skin, causing amoebiasis due to free-living amoebae in immunocompromised or immunocompetent individuals, depending on the amoeba genera.

TABLE 11.5

GMP Herbal Medicines for a 55-Year-Old Adult with Amoebiasis Due to Free-Living Amoebae

Amoebiasis due to free-living amoebae (OrphaCode: 68)

A disease with a prevalence of ~5 in 100,000

Not applicable

Photophobia, Behavioral abnormality, Personality changes, Seizure, Fever, Vomiting, Nausea, Headache, Encephalitis, Abnormality of the cerebrospinal fluid, Increased CSF protein, CSF lymphocytic pleiocytosis, Brain imaging abnormality Facial asymmetry, Visual loss, Diplopia, Restlessness, Irritability, Lethargy, Hemiparesis, Confusion, Abnormal cerebellum morphology, Abnormality of the basal ganglia, Abnormality of the spinal cord, Cerebral edema, Aphasia, Abnormality of midbrain morphology, Abnormal cerebral white matter morphology, Increased intracranial pressure, Abnormality of the cerebral cortex, Immunodeficiency, Cranial nerve VI palsy, Fourth cranial nerve palsy, Loss of consciousness, Abnormality of the pons, Facial palsy, Abnormality of the medulla oblongata, Oculomotor nerve palsy, Abnormal hypothalamus morphology, Abnormal brainstem MRI signal intensity, Increased red blood cell count, Stiff neck, Nuchal rigidity, Abnormal cranial nerve physiology, Granuloma

All ages

Photophobia (D020795), Seizure (345.9), Fever (D005334), Vomiting (D014839), Nausea (D009325), Headache (D006261):

Wúzhūyútāng 5g + máhuángfùzǐxìxīntāng 5-2g + fùzǐ 2-0g + gānjiāng 2-0g.

Chántuì 5g + zhǐqiào 5-4g + jílí 5-0g.

Huángqí 5g + chìsháo 1g + fángfēng 1g + xìxīn 0g + huánglián 0g + dàhuáng 0g + acupuncture.

Diplopia (D004172), Lethargy (D053609), Hemiparesis (D010291), Confusion (D003221), Abnormality of the spinal cord (336.9), Aphasia (D001037), Immunodeficiency (279.3), Fourth cranial nerve palsy (378.53), Loss of consciousness (D014474), Facial palsy (351.0):

Wǔlíngsǎn 5g + lǐzhōngtāng 5g + fùzǐ 2-0g.

Máhuángtāng 5g + bànxià 1g + shēngjiāng 1g + xìxīn 1g.

Pǔjìxiāodúyǐn 5g + gégēntāng 2-0g + hónggǔshé 1-0g + hónghuā 0g + gāncǎo 0g + acupuncture.

Gāncǎo 5g + báizhǐ 5g + shārén 5g + huángqín 5g + tiānhuā 2-0g + xìxīn 2-0g + dàhuáng 1-0g.

Wúzhūyútāng was introduced in Section 2.9 for migraines. Pǔjìxiāodúyǐn is translated to "a drink for general relief and detoxification." It, containing Huángqín and Gāncǎo, was specifically formulated for swelling and redness of the head, face, and neck resulting from "wind-heat epidemic," of which COVID-19 is an example. Pǔjìxiāodúyǐn is used today for chronic sinusitis (Wang, 2019).

11.6 MENINGOCOCCAL MENINGITIS

Meningococcal meningitis is an infection and inflammation of the meninges, which envelop the brain and spinal cord, by the bacteria called *Neisseria meningitidis* (meningococcus). Meningococcus is transmitted through saliva during kissing or water sharing and through respiratory secretions during coughing and sneezing. Meningococcal meningitis is a medical emergency and can cause death if left untreated.

Báizhǐ was introduced in Section 1.7 to be anti-inflammatory. Máhuángfùzǐxìxīntāng "warms meridians, releases exterior" and is used today for allergic rhinitis and migraines in the winter (Wang, 2019). We note that Wúzhūyútāng, Máhuángfùzǐxìxīntāng, Fùzǐ, and Gānjiāng

---

TABLE 11.6

GMP Herbal Medicines for an 18-Year-Old Adolescent with Meningococcal Meningitis

Meningococcal meningitis (OrphaCode: 33475)

A disease with a prevalence of ~5 in 100,000

Not applicable

Fever, Increased CSF protein, Hypoglycorrhachia, CSF pleocytosis, Stiff neck, Nuchal rigidity

Photophobia, Petechiae, Skin rash, Anorexia, Headache, Projectile vomiting, Reduced consciousness/confusion, Elevated C-reactive protein level, Sepsis

Renal insufficiency, Abnormality of the anterior fontanelle, Hearing impairment, Irritability, Purpura, Papilledema, Seizure, Lethargy, Drowsiness, Increased intracranial pressure, Hypotension, Paresthesia

All ages

Fever (D005334):

Xīnyíqīngfèitāng 5g + língguìshùgāntāng 5g + bǔzhōngyìqìtāng 5g + cāngěrsǎn 5g + zhǐqiào 1g + wūméi 1g + guālóurén 1g + màiméndōng 1g + zǐsūyè 1g + huángqín 1g + lùlùtōng 1g + cāngěrzǐ 1g.	Báizhǐ 5g + zhìgāncǎo 4g + shārén 4g + dàhuáng 0g.
	Báizhǐ 5g + shārén 3g + gāncǎo 2g + dàhuáng 0g.
	Báizhǐ 5g + huángqín 5g + zhìgāncǎo 3g + shārén 3g + tiānhuā 2g + xìxīn 2-1g + dàhuáng 0g.
Xīnyíqīngfèitāng 5g + jīngfángbàidúsǎn 5g + níngsòuwán 5g + xiǎngshēngpòdíwán 5g + jiégěng 1g + huángqín 1g.	Báizhǐ 5g + huángqín 5g + tiānhuā 4-3g + gāncǎo 4-3g + shārén 4-3g + dàhuáng 1g.
Xīnyíqīngfèitāng 5g + máxìnggānshítāng 5g + cāngěrsǎn 5g + jiégěng 2g + liánqiáo 2g + niúbàngzǐ 2-0g + yúxīngcǎo 2-0g + dōngguāzǐ 2-0g.	
Máhuángtāng 5g + bànxià 1g + xìxīn 1g + shēngjiāng 0g + dàhuáng 0g.	

Photophobia (D020795), Petechiae (D011693), Skin rash (782.1), Anorexia (D000855), Headache (D006261):

Wúzhūyútāng 5g + máhuángfùzǐxìxīntāng 5g + fùzǐ 3-0g + gānjiāng 3-0g + guìzhī 1-0g.	Báizhǐ 5g + gāncǎo 5-4g + shārén 4-3g + huángqín 4-2g + guālóugēn 3-2g + dàhuáng 1-0g.

Renal insufficiency (586), Hearing impairment (D003638), Purpura (D011693), Papilledema (362.83, 377.0, 377.01), Seizure (345.9), Lethargy (D053609), Paresthesia (D010292):

Zhēnwǔtāng 5g + jìshēngshènqìwán 5g + dānshēn 2-1g + huángqí 2-0g + tiānmá 2-0g + dàhuáng 1g + jīnyínhuā 1-0g + sāngbáipí 1-0g + liánqiáo 1-0g.	Huángqí 5g + chìsháo 1g + fángfēng 1g + xìxīn 0g + huánglián 0g + dàhuáng 0g + acupuncture.
Wǔlíngsǎn 5g + jìshēngshènqìwán 5-4g + zhēnwǔtāng 5-0g + guīpítāng 5-0g + dàhuáng 1-0g.	Báizhú 5g + fùzǐ 5g + cháihú 5g + báisháo 4g + fúlíng 4g + tiānhuā 2g + shēngjiāng 2g + dǎngshēn 2g + guìzhī 2g + huángqín 2g + gāncǎo 1g + mǔlì 1g + gānjiāng 1g.

are all warm in TCM nature. The prescription is therefore suitable for patients presenting with yang deficiency.

11.7 DENGUE FEVER

Dengue fever is caused by infection with dengue viruses, which are spread to people through bites by infected *Aedes* mosquitos. An infected person cannot directly transmit dengue to other people. However, an infected person can infect, through blood sucking, an uninfected mosquito, which then spreads the virus to other people. Since mosquitoes prevail in tropical and subtropical climates, global warming can worsen the dengue fever burden.

TABLE 11.7

GMP Herbal Medicines for a Five-Year-Old Child with Dengue Fever

Dengue fever (OrphaCode: 99828)

A disease with a prevalence of ~5 in 100,000

Not applicable

Fever, Headache

Skin rash, Pruritus, Abdominal pain, Arthralgia

Gingival bleeding, Epistaxis, Petechiae, Bruising susceptibility, Lethargy, Cerebral hemorrhage, Ascites, Thrombocytopenia, Leukopenia, Diarrhea, Nausea and vomiting, Gastrointestinal hemorrhage, Hepatomegaly, Hypotension, Hypoproteinemia, Cardiorespiratory arrest

All ages

Fever (D005334), Headache (D006261):

Wǔlíngsǎn 5g + báizhǐ 1-0g + gāncǎo 1-0g + báisháo 1-0g + tiáowèichéngqìtāng 1-0g + dàhuáng 0g.

Gāncǎo 5g + báizhǐ 5g + shārén 5-3g + huángqín 5-0g + tiānhuā 2-0g + dàhuáng 1-0g.

Skin rash (782.1), Pruritus (D011537), Abdominal pain (D015746), Arthralgia (D018771):

Jīngfángbàidúsǎn 5g + dìfūzǐ 1-0g + shéchuángzǐ 1-0g + huánglián 1-0g + jílí 1-0g + chántuì 0g.

Báizhǐ 5g + gāncǎo 5-4g + shārén 4-3g + huángqín 4-2g + guālóugēn 2g + huánglián 1-0g + dàhuáng 1-0g.

Xiāofēngsǎn 5g + dāngguīyǐnzǐ 5g + báixiānpí 1g + dìfūzǐ 1g + jílí 1-0g + tǔfúlíng 1-0g.

Gingival bleeding (D005884), Petechiae (D011693), Bruising susceptibility (D004438), Lethargy (D053609), Cerebral hemorrhage (D002543) [Intracerebral hemorrhage (431)], Ascites (D001201) [Ascites (789.5)], Thrombocytopenia (287.5), Leukopenia (288.50), Diarrhea (D003967), Gastrointestinal hemorrhage (D006471) [Gastrointestinal hemorrhage, unspecified (578.9)], Cardiorespiratory arrest (427.5):

Guīlùèrxiānjiāo 5g + bǔyánghuánwǔtāng 2-0g.

Guīlùèrxiānjiāo 5g + guīpítāng 5-0g.

Sìjūnzǐtāng 5g + sìwùtāng 5g + huángqí 1g.

Sānqī 5g + dàhuáng 5g + dàfùpí 5g + hòupò 5g + huánglián 5g + mùxiāngbīnglángwán 5g + xiāngshāliùjūnzǐtāng 5g.

Sānqī 5g + dānshēn 5g + xiānhècǎo 5g + báimáogēn 5g + ǒujié 5g + sìwùtāng 5g + guīpítāng 5g.

Huángbò 5g + shārén 4-3g + shānzhīzǐ 2g + dìhuáng 2g + bǎihé 2g + dàndòuchǐ 2g + gāncǎo 2g + chìsháo 2g + ējiāo 2g + huángqín 2g + jiānghuáng 2g + jiāngcán 2g + chántuì 2-0g + dàhuáng 0g + huánglián 0g.

Huángbò 5g + shārén 3g + guībǎn 3g + zhìgāncǎo 2g + fùzǐ 2g.

Huángbò was introduced in Section 5.22 to stop bleeding and to protect neurons. Guīlùèrxiānjiāo, introduced in Section 4.20 to "replenish marrow," has been used for patients who are depleted in the TCM kidney, yin and yang. It was shown to enhance the skeletal muscle mass and motor function in mice through upregulation of protein synthesis, myogenic differentiation, glucose homeostasis, and mitochondrial biogenesis (Fang et al., 2023). Sānqī (cf. Section 9.6) was shown to ameliorate the neurological deficit and activities of daily living in patients with ischemic stroke in anterior cerebral circulation within 30 days of onset in a randomized controlled study (He et al., 2011).

11.8 SCRUB TYPHUS

Scrub typhus, also known as Tsutsugamushi fever, is a rickettsial infection transmitted from infected rodents to humans through the bites of microscopic mites called *chiggers*, which can be found in areas of vegetation dominated by scrubs. Scrub typhus is differentiated from other bites by the presence of an eschar, or a black wound, at the site of the bite.

TABLE 11.8
GMP Herbal Medicines for a 31-Year-Old Woman with Scrub Typhus

Scrub typhus (OrphaCode: 83317)

A disease with a prevalence of ~4 in 100,000

Not applicable

Hyperhidrosis, Skin rash, Lethargy, Fever, Myalgia, Reduced consciousness/confusion, Cough

Photophobia, Nausea and vomiting, Abdominal pain, Headache, Hypotension, Lymphadenopathy, Anterior uveitis, Macule, Gangrene

Renal insufficiency, Behavioral abnormality, Seizure, Meningitis, Tremor, Splenomegaly, Abnormal bleeding, Restrictive ventilatory defect, Dyspnea, Encephalitis, Myocarditis

All ages

Skin rash (782.1), Lethargy (D053609), Fever (D005334), Myalgia (D063806), Cough (D003371):

Xiāofēngsǎn 5g + dāngguīyǐnzǐ 5-0g + lóngdǎnxiègāntāng 5-0g + tǔfúlíng 1g + báixiānpí 1g + dìfūzǐ 1g + mǔdānpí 1-0g + chìsháo 1-0g + jílí 1-0g.

Wǔlíngsǎn 5g + fùzǐ 1g + gānjiāng 1g + tiáowèichéngqìtāng 1g.

Guìzhītāng 5g + bànxià 1g + shēngjiāng 1g + guìzhī 1g.

Báizhǐ 5g + gāncǎo 5-4g + shārén 5-4g + huángqín 4-3g + guālóugēn 3-2g + huánglián 1-0g + dàhuáng 1-0g.

Gāncǎo 5g + báizhǐ 5g + shārén 5g + huángqín 5g + tiānhuā 2g + xìxīn 2g + dàhuáng 0g.

Photophobia (D020795), Abdominal pain (D015746), Headache (D006261), Gangrene (D005734) [Gangrene (785.4)]:

Wúzhūyútāng 5-3g + guìzhītāng 5-0g + máhuángfùzǐxìxīntāng 5-0g + fùzǐ 3-1g + gānjiāng 3-0g.

Wúzhūyútāng 5g + zhēnwǔtāng 5g + fùzǐ 1g.

Wǔlíngsǎn 5g + fùzǐ 1g + huángqín 1g.

Zhǐqiào 5g + jílí 5-2g + chántuì 5-0g + júhuā 5-0g.

Renal insufficiency (586), Seizure (345.9), Meningitis (322.9), Tremor (D014202), Dyspnea (D004417), Myocarditis (429.0):

Dàhuáng 5g + chuānliànzǐ 5g + hòupò 5g + wūyào 5g + guālóurén 5g + huánglián 5g + dàchéngqìtāng 5g + tiānwángbǔxīndān 5g + xuèfǔzhúyūtāng 5g.

Dàhuáng 5g + chuānliànzǐ 5g + hòupò 5g + wūyào 5g + huánglián 5g + xiāngshāliùjūnzǐtāng 5g + mázǐrénwán 5-0g + ānzhōngsǎn 5-0g + mùxiāngbīnglángwán 5-0g.

Tiānwángbǔxīndān 5g + cháihújiālónggǔmǔlìtāng 3g + dānshēn 1g + dàhuáng 0g.

Dàhuáng 5g + bèimǔ 5g + guālóu 5g + xìngsūyǐn 5g + sāngjúyǐn 5g + liánggésǎn 5g + cāngěrsǎn 5g.

Báizhú 5g + fúlíng 5-4g + fùzǐ 5-3g + cháihú 5-0g + báisháo 4-0g + gānjiāng 3-1g + tiānhuā 2-0g + shēngjiāng 2-0g + dǎngshēn 2-0g + guìzhī 2-0g + huángqín 2-0g + gāncǎo 1-0g + mǔlì 1-0g + dàhuáng 0g.

Huángqí 5g + chìsháo 2g + fángfēng 2g + xìxīn 1g + huánglián 1g.

Huángqín 5g + báizhǐ 4g + gāncǎo 3g + shārén 2g + dàhuáng 1g + tiānhuā 1g + xìxīn 1g.

Dàhuáng (cf. Section 8.4) is widely used to treat diabetic kidney disease and the compounds and their mechanisms of action were identified and elucidated (Luo et al., 2022). Moreover, Dàhuáng was indicated to prevent and treat cardiovascular diseases by the so-called two-way adjustment mechanism: activating both blood circulation and blood coagulation (Pei et al., 2020). Ānzhōngsǎn "conducts Qi, calms interior, dispels coldness, stops pain" and is used for gastritis and duodenitis (Wang, 2019).

11.9 MALARIA

Malaria is an infection of *Plasmodium* parasites, unicellular organisms, mediated by the bites of *Anopheles* mosquitos that inhabit tropical and subtropical areas of the world. Malaria is transmitted through mosquito saliva, not human saliva. Therefore, malaria is seen in travelers or immigrants

TABLE 11.9

GMP Herbal Medicines for a Three-Year-Old Child with Malaria

Malaria (OrphaCode: 673)

A disease with a prevalence of ~3 in 100,000

Not applicable

Anemia, Acute kidney injury, Fever, Morphological abnormality of the central nervous system, Nausea and vomiting, Headache, Elevated C-reactive protein level

Abnormality of blood and blood-forming tissues, Thrombocytopenia, Respiratory distress, Gait imbalance, Hyperbilirubinemia, Myalgia, Reduced consciousness/confusion, Cognitive impairment

Retinopathy

All ages

Anemia (285.9), Fever (D005334), Headache (D006261):

Sìjūnzǐtāng 5g + sìwùtāng 5-0g + huángqí 1-0g.

Shēnlíngbáizhúsǎn 5g + shānzhā 1-0g + gāncǎo 1-0g + shénqū 1-0g + màiyá 1-0g.

Bǔzhōngyìqìtāng 5g + ypíngfēngsǎn 5-0g + xiāngshāliùjūnzǐtāng 5-0g.

Gāncǎo 5g + shénqū 5g + màiyá 5g.

Gāncǎo 5g + báizhǐ 5g + shārén 5g + xìxīn 5g + dàhuáng 0g.

Huángqí 5g + dǎngshēn 5-0g + gāncǎo 5-0g + báizhú 5-0g.

Abnormality of blood and blood-forming tissues (289.9), Thrombocytopenia (287.5), Respiratory distress (D004417), Myalgia (D063806):

Shēnlíngbáizhúsǎn 5g + bǎohéwán 2-0g + shānzhā 2-0g + shénqū 2-0g + màiyá 2-0g.

Sìjūnzǐtāng 5g + shēnlíngbáizhúsǎn 5-0g + shānzhā 1-0g + shénqū 1-0g + màiyá 1-0g.

Gāncǎo 5g + dìhuáng 5g + mǔdānpí 5g + chìsháo 5g + jīnyínhuā 5g + liánqiáo 5g + huángqín 5g + dànzhúyè 5-0g + bòhé 5-0g.

Gāncǎo 5g + shārén 5g + dàhuáng 0g.

Gāncǎo 5g + báizhú 5g + dǎngshēn 5g.

Xuánshēn 5g + dìhuáng 5g + màiméndōng 5g + gāncǎo 3g + dàhuáng 0g.

Retinopathy (362.9):

Qǐjúdìhuángwán 5g + yìqìcōngmíngtāng 5-0g.

Qǐjúdìhuángwán 5g + xǐgānmíngmùtāng 5-0g.

Qǐjúdìhuángwán 5g + shēnlíngbáizhúsǎn 4-0g + xuèfǔzhúyūtāng 2-0g.

Qǐjúdìhuángwán 5g + zīshènmíngmùtāng 3-0g + chēqiánzǐ 1-0g + tùsīzǐ 1-0g.

Jílí 5g + chántuì 5g + júhóng 5-0g + zhǐqiào 2-0g.

Hángjú 5g + gǒuqǐzǐ 5g + shíchāngpú 2g + yuǎnzhì 2g.

Gāncǎo 5g + báizhǐ 4g + shārén 4g + dàhuáng 0g.

who traveled to countries with *Anopheles* mosquitoes and were bitten by an *Anopheles* mosquito infected with the parasite.

Sìjūnzǐtāng (cf. Sections 1.17 and 1.56) was shown to reduce the decrease of leukocytes, thrombocytes, erythrocytes, and hematocrit in irradiated mice (Hsu et al., 1996). Sìwùtāng (cf. Section 9.2) was shown to promote hematopoiesis and immunity in irradiated mice (Liang et al., 2006). Liánqiáo (cf. Section 1.28) was shown in mice to protect against acute lung injury through its anti-inflammatory effects (Wang et al., 2022).

11.10 BACTERIAL TOXIC-SHOCK SYNDROME

Bacterial toxic-shock syndrome is an acute-onset condition caused by bacterial toxins released from staphylococcus or streptococcus bacteria found in the bloodstream or organs in the body. Risk factors for bacterial toxic-shock syndrome include open wounds on the skin, burns, or staphylococcal or streptococcal infection.

Suānzǎorén (cf. Section 2.44) "nourishes the Heart, benefits the Liver, calms the mind, and conserves sweat." Its pharmacological effects were reviewed and updated, including sedative-hypnotic, antianxiety, antidepressant, anticancer, anti-inflammatory, and anti-Alzheimer's disease (Wang et al., 2022); it is used today for sleep disturbances (Wang, 2020). Sìnìtāng (cf. Sections 1.15, 1.46,

TABLE 11.10
GMP Herbal Medicines for a 65-Year-Old Adult with Bacterial Toxic-Shock Syndrome

Bacterial toxic-shock syndrome (OrphaCode: 36234)

A disease with a prevalence of ~3 in 100,000

Not applicable

Hypotension, Shock, Severe infection

Confusion, Recurrent skin infections, Tachycardia, Metabolic acidosis, Fever, Abdominal pain, Respiratory distress, Increased serum lactate, Myalgia, Abnormality of facial soft tissue, Pain, Fasciitis

Renal insufficiency, Glomerulonephritis, Sinusitis, Skin rash, Meningitis, Arthritis, Thrombocytopenia, Vomiting, Diarrhea, Nausea, Pneumonia, Encephalitis, Peritonitis, Osteomyelitis, Tachypnea, Abnormality of the lower limb, Abnormality of the upper limb, Hypocalcemia, Hypoalbuminemia, Septic arthritis, Elevated circulating creatine kinase concentration, Elevated serum creatinine, Disseminated intravascular coagulation, Abnormal blistering of the skin, Localized skin lesion, Respiratory tract infection, Hepatitis, Myocarditis, Chills, Pharyngitis, Abscess, Capillary leak, Ecchymosis, Severe viral infection, Bacteremia, Severe varicella zoster infection, Increased circulating myelocyte count, Increased circulating metamyelocyte count, Acute cutaneous wound, Scaling skin, Myositis, Cellulitis, Sepsis

All ages

Confusion (D003221), Tachycardia (D013610) [Tachycardia, unspecified (785.0)], Fever (D005334), Abdominal pain (D015746), Respiratory distress (D004417), Myalgia (D063806), Pain (D010146), Fasciitis (729.4):

Wǔlíngsǎn 5g + sìnìtāng 5-0g + zhēnwǔtāng 5-0g + bǔzhōngyìqìtāng 5-0g + fùzǐ 1-0g + xìxīn 1-0g.	Gāncǎo 5g + fùzǐ 5-4g + gānjiāng 5-3g + fúlíng 5-0g + báizhú 5-0g + suānzǎorén 5-0g + dǎngshēn 5-0g.

Renal insufficiency (586), Skin rash (782.1), Meningitis (322.9), Thrombocytopenia (287.5), Vomiting (D014839), Diarrhea (D003967), Nausea (D009325), Tachypnea (D059246), Septic arthritis (711.90, 711.91, 711.92, 711.93, 711.94, 711.95, 711.96, 711.97), Disseminated intravascular coagulation (286.6), Myocarditis (429.0), Cellulitis (D002481) [Cellulitis and abscess of unspecified sites (682.9)]:

Shēnlíngbáizhúsǎn 5g. Zhūlíngtāng 5g. Jīngfángbàidúsǎn 5g.	Báimáogēn 5g + dìhuáng 5g + mǔdānpí 5g + chìsháo 5g + jīnyínhuā 5g + liánqiáo 5g + huángqín 5g + huánglián 5g + huángbò 5-0g + dànzhúyè 5-0g. Gégēn 5g + gāncǎo 2g + huánglián 2g + huángqín 2g. Gégēn 5g + zhìgāncǎo 3g + huángqín 2g + huánglián 2g. Dìhuáng 5g + mǔdānpí 5g + chìsháo 5g + ējiāo 5g + zǐcǎo 5g + huángbò 5g + dāngguī 5g.

1.70, and 2.47) "warms meridians, dispels coldness, restores yang, reverses adversity" and is used for gastritis/duodenitis and general symptoms (Wang, 2019).

11.11 TULAREMIA

Tularemia, also known as rabbit fever, is a bacterial infection caused by the bacteria *Francisella tularensis*, which can infect humans and animals, including rabbits, hares, and rodents. Humans are infected through bites by infected ticks and deer flies, inhalation of contaminated dust, or drinking contaminated water.

TABLE 11.11
GMP Herbal Medicines for a Seven-Year-Old Child with Tularemia

Tularemia (OrphaCode: 3392)

A disease with a prevalence of ~2 in 100,000

Not applicable

Tachycardia, Fever, Leukocytosis, Pneumonia, Headache, Arthralgia, Myalgia, Increased antibody level in blood, Chills, Asthenia

(Continued)

TABLE 11.11 *(Continued)*

GMP Herbal Medicines for a Seven-Year-Old Child with Tularemia

Oral ulcer, Skin rash, Thrombocytopenia, Anemia, Respiratory distress, Pulmonary infiltrates, Pleural effusion, Lymphadenopathy, Localized skin lesion, Cough, Cervical lymphadenopathy, Pharyngitis, Neck pain, Abnormal pulmonary thoracic imaging finding
All ages

Tachycardia (D013610) [Tachycardia, unspecified (785.0)], Fever (D005334), Headache (D006261), Arthralgia (D018771), Myalgia (D063806), Increased antibody level in blood (D006942):

Zhìgāncǎotāng 5g + gāncǎoxiǎomàidàzǎotāng 5-0g.	Gāncǎo 5g + báizhǐ 5g + shārén 5g + huángqín 5-0g + dàhuáng 1-0g.
Zhìgāncǎotāng 5g + yǎngxīntāng 5-0g.	
Zhìgāncǎotāng 5g + bǔzhōngyìqìtāng 5-0g.	Gāncǎo 5g + fùzǐ 5g + gānjiāng 5g + fúlíng 5-0g + suānzǎorén 5-0g + dàhuáng 0g.

Skin rash (782.1), Thrombocytopenia (287.5), Anemia (285.9), Respiratory distress (D004417), Cough (D003371), Neck pain (D019547):

Dāngguīyǐnzǐ 5g + jīngfángbàidúsǎn 5-0g + xiāofēngsǎn 5-0g + báixiānpí 1g + dìfūzǐ 1g.	Huángqí 5g + dāngguī 5g + shúdìhuáng 5g + jīxuèténg 5g + dǎngshēn 5-0g.
Dāngguīyǐnzǐ 5g + guīpítāng 5-0g + ējiāo 1-0g + jīxuèténg 1-0g + báixiānpí 1-0g + dìfūzǐ 1-0g + mǔdānpí 1-0g + chìsháo 1-0g.	Báizhǐ 5g + huángqín 5-0g + gāncǎo 4-2g + shārén 4-2g + guālóugēn 2-0g + huánglián 1-0g + dàhuáng 0g.

Fùzǐ was shown in animal models to be cardioprotective, especially when paired with Gāncǎo (cf. Section 1.16). Modern uses of Fùzǐ include chest pain, palpitations, neuralgia, headache, cardiac dysrhythmia, and pain in joints (Wang, 2020). Yǎngxīntāng "nourishes the Heart, replenishes Blood, settles the mind, anchors the will" and is used for cardiac dysrhythmias and other forms of chronic ischemic heart disease (Wang, 2019).

REFERENCES

Fang, W., Chang, W., Tsai, Y., Hsu, H., Chang, F., Lin, C., & Lo, Y. (2023). Guilu Erxian Jiao enhances protein synthesis, glucose homeostasis, mitochondrial biogenesis and slow-twitch fibers in the skeletal muscle. Journal of Food and Drug Analysis, 31(1), 116–136. https://doi.org/10.38212/2224-6614.3435

Han, J., Zheng, Q., Fang, L., & Huang, X. (2021). Screening and functional evaluation of the glucose-lowering active compounds of total saponins of Baibiandou (Lablab Semen Album). Digital Chinese Medicine, 4(3), 229–240. https://doi.org/10.1016/j.dcmed.2021.09.007

He, L., Chen, X., Zhou, M., Zhang, D., Yang, J., Yang, M., & Zhou, D. (2011). Radix/Rhizoma Notoginseng extract (Sanchitongtshu) for ischemic stroke: A randomized controlled study. Phytomedicine, 18(6), 437–442. https://doi.org/10.1016/j.phymed.2010.10.004

Hsu, H., Yang, J., Lian, S., Ho, Y., & Lin, C. (1996). Recovery of the hematopoietic system by Si-Jun-Zi-Tang in whole body irradiated mice. Journal of Ethnopharmacology, 54(2–3), 69–75. https://doi.org/10.1016/s0378-8741(96)01450-x

Liang, Q., Gao, Y., H, T., Guo, P., Li, Y., Zhou, Z., Wang, T., Ma, Z., B, M., & Wang, S. (2006). Effects of four Si-Wu-Tang's constituents and their combination on irradiated mice. Biological & Pharmaceutical Bulletin, 29(7), 1378–1382. https://doi.org/10.1248/bpb.29.1378

Lim, S., Moon, M., Oh, H. S., Kim, H. G., Kim, S. Y., & Oh, M. S. (2014). Ginger improves cognitive function via NGF-induced ERK/CREB activation in the hippocampus of the mouse. Journal of Nutritional Biochemistry, 25(10), 1058–1065. https://doi.org/10.1016/j.jnutbio.2014.05.009

Luo, J., Piao, C., Jin, D., Wang, L., Zhao, X., Lian, F., & Tong, X. (2022). Mechanism of rhubarb for diabetic kidney disease through the AMPK/NF-κB signaling pathway based on network pharmacology. ChemistrySelect, 7(4). https://doi.org/10.1002/slct.202103534

Meng, M., Bai, C., Wan, B., Zhao, L., Li, Z., Li, D., & Zhang, S. (2021). A network pharmacology-based study on irritable bowel syndrome prevention and treatment utilizing Shenling Baizhu powder. BioMed Research International, 2021, 1–14. https://doi.org/10.1155/2021/4579850

Pei, L., Shen, X., Qu, K., Tan, C., Zou, J., Wang, Y., & Ping, F. (2020). Exploration of the two-way adjustment mechanism of Rhei Radix et Rhizoma for cardiovascular diseases. Combinatorial Chemistry & High Throughput Screening, 23(10), 1100–1112. https://doi.org/10.2174/1386207323666200521120308

Wang, D., Ho, C., & Bai, N. (2022). Ziziphi Spinosae Semen: An updated review on pharmacological activity, quality control, and application. Journal of Food Biochemistry, 46(7). https://doi.org/10.1111/jfbc.14153

Wang, J., Luo, L., Zhao, X., Xue, X., Liao, L., Deng, Y., Zhou, M., Peng, C., & Li, Y. (2022). Forsythiae Fructuse extracts alleviates LPS-induced acute lung injury in mice by regulating PPAR-γ/RXR-α in lungs and colons. Journal of Ethnopharmacology, 293, 115322. https://doi.org/10.1016/j.jep.2022.115322

Wang, J., Wang, L., Lou, G., Zeng, H., Ju, H., Peng, W., & Yang, X. (2019). Coptidis Rhizoma: A comprehensive review of its traditional uses, botany, phytochemistry, pharmacology and toxicology. Pharmaceutical Biology, 57(1), 193–225. https://doi.org/10.1080/13880209.2019.1577466

Wang, S.-C. (2019). Therapeutic classes of CHEG formulas. In S.-C. Wang (Ed.), Clinical herbal prescriptions: Principles and practices of herbal formulations from deep learning health insurance herbal prescription big data (pp. 16–89). World Scientific Publishing. https://doi.org/10.1142/11211

Wang, S.-C. (2020). Modern therapeutic uses of CHEG herbs and herb pairs. In S.-C. Wang (Ed.), Veterinary herbal pharmacopoeia (pp. 35–233). Nova Science Publishers. https://doi.org/10.52305/GHTR1903

Wang, Z., Yang, W., Yang, P., Gao, B., & Luo, L. (2016). Effect of Radix Stemonae concentrated decoction on the lung tissue pathology and inflammatory mediators in COPD rats. BMC Complementary and Alternative Medicine, 16(1). https://doi.org/10.1186/s12906-016-1444-y

Yu, X., Tang, L., Wu, H., Zhang, X., Luo, H., Guo, R., Xu, M., Yang, H., Fan, J., Wang, Z., & Su, R. (2018). Trichosanthis Fructus: Botany, traditional uses, phytochemistry and pharmacology. Journal of Ethnopharmacology, 224, 177–194. https://doi.org/10.1016/j.jep.2018.05.034

Zhu, L., Lao, L., Huang, Y. J., Lin, X., & Liu, J. (2019). A child with Kawasaki disease successfully treated with Chinese herbal medicine: A case report with 12-month follow up. European Journal of Integrative Medicine, 28, 33–38. https://doi.org/10.1016/j.eujim.2019.02.006

12 GMP Herbal Medicine for Rare Respiratory Diseases

Respiratory diseases affect the organs and tissues that enable exchange of oxygen and carbon dioxide between the air in the alveoli and blood in the capillaries in the walls of the alveoli in the lungs. Lung diseases can arise from air pollution, tobacco smoking, genetic factors, and infections. The various rare respiratory diseases of this chapter affect people of different ages by different causes.

The single herbs and multi-herb formulas that are commonly discussed for the signs and symptoms of the rare respiratory diseases are Rhubarb Root and Rhizome (Dàhuáng), Licorice Root (Gāncǎo), Pinellia Tuber (Bànxià), Dried Ginger Rhizome (Gānjiāng), Platycodon Root (Jiégěng), Scutellaria Root (Huángqín), Schisandra Berry (Wǔwèizǐ), Processed Licorice Root (Zhìgāncǎo), Fritillaria Bulb (Bèimǔ), Magnolia Bark (Hòupò), Black Jujube (Dàzǎo), Descurainia Seed (Tínglìzǐ), Bitter Apricot Kernel (Xìngrén), Ephedra, Apricot Kernel, Gypsum, and Licorice Decoction (Máxìnggānshítāng), Five Ingredient Formula with Poria (Wǔlíngsǎn), Frigid Extremities Decoction (Sìnìtāng), Magnolia Flower and Gypsum Combination (Xīnyíqīngfèitāng), Minor Blue Dragon Decoction (Xiǎoqīnglóngtāng), Apricot and Perilla Formula (Pediatrics) (Xìngsūyǐnyòukē), Honeysuckle and Forsythia Powder (Yínqiàosǎn), and Xanthium Powder (Cāngěrsǎn), many of which are known to benefit the throat and lungs. The lung in TCM governs not only respiration but also the exterior, i.e., the skin and hair, for the defense against external pathogens.

12.1 PRIMARY CILIARY DYSKINESIA

Cilia are tiny, hairlike projections that stick out from the surface of the epithelium cells of the airways. They move in a coordinated wavelike motion to move the mucus toward the throat, helping clearance of the mucus. Primary ciliary dyskinesia is a condition of dysfunctional cilia. Accumulation of the bacteria in the mucus causes recurrent lung infections in patients with primary ciliary dyskinesia, which is caused by mutations in any of the genes encoding ciliary proteins.

TABLE 12.1

GMP Herbal Medicines for a One-Year-Old Infant with Primary Ciliary Dyskinesia

Primary ciliary dyskinesia (OrphaCode: 244)

A disease with a prevalence of ~4 in 10,000

Disease-causing germline mutation(s): dynein axonemal heavy chain 1 (*DNAH1* / Entrez: 25981) at 3p21.1

Disease-causing germline mutation(s) (loss of function): tetratricopeptide repeat domain 12 (*TTC12* / Entrez: 54970) at 11q23.2

Disease-causing germline mutation(s): NIMA-related kinase 10 (*NEK10* / Entrez: 152110) at 3p24.1

Disease-causing germline mutation(s) (loss of function): dynein axonemal assembly factor 6 (*DNAAF6* / Entrez: 139212) at Xq22.3

Disease-causing germline mutation(s): cilia and flagella associated protein 221 (*CFAP221* / Entrez: 200373) at 2q14.2

Disease-causing germline mutation(s): sperm flagellar 2 (*SPEF2* / Entrez: 79925) at 5p13.2

Disease-causing germline mutation(s) (loss of function): DnaJ heat shock protein family (Hsp40) member B13 (*DNAJB13* / Entrez: 374407) at 11q13.4

Disease-causing germline mutation(s) (loss of function): outer dynein arm docking complex subunit 4 (*ODAD4* / Entrez: 83538) at 17q21.2

Disease-causing germline mutation(s) (loss of function): multiciliate differentiation and DNA synthesis associated cell cycle protein (*MCIDAS* / Entrez: 345643) at 5q11.2

(Continued)

DOI: 10.1201/9781032726625-12

TABLE 12.1 *(Continued)*

GMP Herbal Medicines for a One-Year-Old Infant with Primary Ciliary Dyskinesia

Disease-causing germline mutation(s): growth arrest specific 2 like 2 (*GAS2L2* / Entrez: 246176) at 17q12

Disease-causing germline mutation(s): OFD1 centriole and centriolar satellite protein (*OFD1* / Entrez: 8481) at Xp22.2

Disease-causing germline mutation(s): dynein axonemal heavy chain 11 (*DNAH11* / Entrez: 8701) at 7p15.3

Disease-causing germline mutation(s): dynein axonemal heavy chain 5 (*DNAH5* / Entrez: 1767) at 5p15.2

Disease-causing germline mutation(s): dynein axonemal intermediate chain 1 (*DNAI1* / Entrez: 27019) at 9p13.3

Disease-causing germline mutation(s): NME/NM23 family member 8 (*NME8* / Entrez: 51314) at 7p14.1

Disease-causing germline mutation(s): dynein axonemal intermediate chain 2 (*DNAI2* / Entrez: 64446) at 17q25.1

Disease-causing germline mutation(s): dynein axonemal assembly factor 2 (*DNAAF2* / HGNC:20188) at 14q21.3

Disease-causing germline mutation(s): radial spoke head component 9 (*RSPH9* / Entrez: 221421) at 6p21.1

Disease-causing germline mutation(s): radial spoke head component 4A (*RSPH4A* / Entrez: 345895) at 6q22.1

Disease-causing germline mutation(s): dynein axonemal assembly factor 1 (*DNAAF1* / Entrez: 123872) at 16q24.1

Disease-causing germline mutation(s): coiled-coil domain containing 39 (*CCDC39* / Entrez: 339829) at 3q26.33

Disease-causing germline mutation(s): coiled-coil domain containing 40 (*CCDC40* / Entrez: 55036) at 17q25.3

Disease-causing germline mutation(s): dynein axonemal light chain 1 (*DNAL1* / Entrez: 83544) at 14q24.3

Disease-causing germline mutation(s): dynein axonemal assembly factor 3 (*DNAAF3* / Entrez: 352909) at 19q13.42

Disease-causing germline mutation(s): coiled-coil domain containing 103 (*CCDC103* / Entrez: 388389) at 17q21.31

Disease-causing germline mutation(s): dynein axonemal assembly factor 5 (*DNAAF5* / Entrez: 54919) at 7p22.3

Disease-causing germline mutation(s) (loss of function): HYDIN axonemal central pair apparatus protein (*HYDIN* / Entrez: 54768) at 16q22.2

Disease-causing germline mutation(s) (loss of function): dynein axonemal assembly factor 11 (*DNAAF11* / Entrez: 23639) at 8q24.22

Disease-causing germline mutation(s) (loss of function): outer dynein arm docking complex subunit 1 (*ODAD1* / Entrez: 93233) at 19q13.33

Disease-causing germline mutation(s) (loss of function): dynein regulatory complex subunit 1 (*DRC1* / Entrez: 92749) at 2p23.3

Disease-causing germline mutation(s) (loss of function): outer dynein arm docking complex subunit 2 (*ODAD2* / Entrez: 55130) at 10p12.1

Disease-causing germline mutation(s) (loss of function): dynein axonemal assembly factor 4 (*DNAAF4* / Entrez: 161582) at 15q21.3

Disease-causing germline mutation(s) (loss of function): radial spoke head component 1 (*RSPH1* / Entrez: 89765) at 21q22.3

Disease-causing germline mutation(s) (loss of function): zinc finger MYND-type containing 10 (*ZMYND10* / Entrez: 51364) at 3p21.31

Disease-causing germline mutation(s): cilia and flagella associated protein 298 (*CFAP298* / Entrez: 56683) at 21q22.11

Disease-causing germline mutation(s): coiled-coil domain containing 65 (*CCDC65* / Entrez: 85478) at 12q13.12

Disease-causing germline mutation(s): sperm associated antigen 1 (*SPAG1* / Entrez: 6674) at 8q22.2

Disease-causing germline mutation(s) (loss of function): cyclin O (*CCNO* / Entrez: 10309) at 5q11.2

Disease-causing germline mutation(s) (loss of function): outer dynein arm docking complex subunit 3 (*ODAD3* / Entrez: 115948) at 19p13.2

Disease-causing germline mutation(s): radial spoke head 3 (*RSPH3* / Entrez: 83861) at 6q25.3

Disease-causing germline mutation(s) (loss of function): growth arrest specific 8 (*GAS8* / Entrez: 2622) at 16q24.3

Disease-causing germline mutation(s): retinitis pigmentosa GTPase regulator (*RPGR* / Entrez: 6103) at Xp11.4

Disease-causing germline mutation(s) (loss of function): serine/threonine kinase 36 (*STK36* / Entrez: 27148) at 2q35

Disease-causing germline mutation(s) (loss of function): forkhead box J1 (*FOXJ1* / Entrez: 2302) at 17q25.1

Disease-causing germline mutation(s) (loss of function): dynein axonemal heavy chain 9 (*DNAH9* / Entrez: 1770) at 17p12

Disease-causing germline mutation(s): leucine rich repeat containing 56 (*LRRC56* / Entrez: 115399) at 11p15.5

Disease-causing germline mutation(s) (loss of function): cilia and flagella associated protein 300 (*CFAP300* / Entrez: 85016) at 11q22.1

Autosomal dominant, Autosomal recessive, X-linked recessive

Chronic otitis media, Recurrent otitis media, Nasal obstruction, Chronic rhinitis, Neonatal respiratory distress, Male infertility, Recurrent sinopulmonary infections, Chronic sinusitis, Respiratory tract infection, Abnormal sperm motility, Productive cough, Abnormal sputum, Nasal polyposis

(Continued)

TABLE 12.1 *(Continued)*

GMP Herbal Medicines for a One-Year-Old Infant with Primary Ciliary Dyskinesia

Abnormality of the genitourinary system, Hearing impairment, Conductive hearing impairment, Delayed speech and
language development, Abnormality of the skeletal system, Clubbing, Abnormal heart morphology, Situs inversus totalis,
Morphological abnormality of the central nervous system, Bronchiectasis, Airway obstruction, Female infertility,
Recurrent mycobacterial infections, Pulmonary situs ambiguus, Peribronchovascular interstitial thickening, Abnormality
of cardiovascular system morphology, Wheezing, Ectopic pregnancy, Lithoptysis, Atelectasis

Neonatal

Male infertility (606):

Yòuguīwán 5g + huánshǎodān 5g + ròucōngróng 1g + yínyánghuò 1g +
tùsīzǐ 1g.

Yòuguīwán 5g + zuǒguīwán 5g + bājǐtiān 2-0g + ròucōngróng 2-0g +
yínyánghuò 2-0g + tùsīzǐ 1-0g + bǔgǔzhǐ 1-0g.

Zuǒguīwán 5g + shēnlíngbáizhúsǎn 5g.

Shēnlíngbáizhúsǎn 5g + bǔzhōngyìqìtāng 5g + guīpítāng 5g.

Xiǎohuíxiāng 5g + mùxiāng 5g + shārén 5g +
ròudòukòu 3g + hòupò 3g + zhǐqiào 3g +
chénpí 3g + láifúzǐ 3g + gǔyá 3g.

Xiǎohuíxiāng 5g + mùxiāng 5g + qiānghuó 5g +
fùzǐ 5g + gānjiāng 5g + dúhuó 5-0g.

Tùsīzǐ 5g + bājǐtiān 4g + gǒuqǐzǐ 4g + fùpénzǐ
4g + chēqiánzǐ 2g + wǔwèizǐ 1g.

Gāncǎo 5g + báizhǐ 5g + shārén 5g + dàhuáng 0g.

Zhǐqiào 5g + jílí 4g + chántuì 4g + sīguāluò 1g.

Hearing impairment (D003638), Conductive hearing impairment (D006314), Delayed speech and language development
(D007805), Abnormal heart morphology (746.9), Situs inversus totalis (759.3), Bronchiectasis (494), Wheezing
(D012135):

Xīnyíqīngfèitāng 5g + máxìnggānshítāng 5g + bèimǔ 2g + guālóurén
2g + yúxīngcǎo 2g.

Máxìnggānshítāng 5g + cāngěrsǎn 4-0g + yínqiàosǎn 4-0g + gāncǎo
2-1g + bèimǔ 2-1g + qiánhú 2-0g + sāngbáipí 2-0g + liánqiáo 2-0g +
yúxīngcǎo 2-0g + guālóurén 1-0g.

Máxìnggānshítāng 5g + wēndǎntāng 3g + bèimǔ 1g + guālóurén 1g +
huángqín 1g + tínglìzǐ 1g.

Xìngsūyǐnyòukě 5g + xīnyíqīngfèitāng 5g + yínqiàosǎn 5g + gāncǎo 1g.

Xiǎoqīnglóngtāng 5g + xiāngshāliùjūnzǐtāng 5g + xīnyíqīngfèitāng 5-0g.

Gāncǎo 5g + shārén 5g + huángqín 5-0g +
huángbò 5-0g + dàhuáng 2-0g.

Ròudòukòu (Semen Myristicae) extract was shown to stimulate mounting behavior of male mice
and also to significantly increase their mating performance without any conspicuous acute toxicity
(Tajuddin et al., 2003). Yòuguīwán (cf. Section 2.19) "benefits Kidney yang" while Zuǒguīwán (cf.
Section 1.48) "benefits Kidney yin." The kidney in TCM is responsible for not only renal functions
but also postnatal growth and development including reproduction. Today, both are used for disorders of bone and cartilage; however, Yòuguīwán is prescribed to both sexes, while Zuǒguīwán is
more often to females (Wang, 2019). Xiǎohuíxiāng, introduced in Section 1.8 for hernia, is also used
for chronic inflammation of the glomeruli in the kidney today (Wang, 2020).

12.2 ADULT ACUTE RESPIRATORY DISTRESS SYNDROME

Adult acute respiratory distress syndrome, or adult ARDS, is due to accumulation of fluid in the
lungs resulting from an acute injury to the lungs, such as pneumonia, burning, and sepsis. ARDS
is life-threatening and its treatment includes mechanical ventilation and medication for the underlying causes.

Wǔwèizǐ, introduced in Section 7.10 for coughs, was shown to inhibit bleomycin-induced idiopathic
pulmonary fibrosis in rats (Guo et al., 2020). Jiégěng (cf. Sections 2.57 and 8.11) has been widely used
for respiratory diseases (Wang, 2020). The bioactive compounds in it were identified and summarized
to have such pharmacological effects as apophlegmatic, antitussive, anti-inflammatory, anticancer,

TABLE 12.2
GMP Herbal Medicines for a 20-Year-Old Adult with Adult Acute Respiratory Distress Syndrome

Adult acute respiratory distress syndrome (OrphaCode: 70578)

A disease with a prevalence of ~3 in 10,000

Not applicable

Dyspnea, Pulmonary infiltrates, Abnormal blood gas level, Hypoxemia, Abnormal serum interleukin level

Metabolic acidosis, Hypotension, Respiratory failure, Abnormality of tumor necrosis factor secretion, Increased serum interleukin-6, Shock, Pulmonary edema, Sepsis

Pneumonia

Adult

Dyspnea (D004417), Hypoxemia (D000860):

Máxìnggānshítāng 5g + cāngěrsǎn 4g + niúbàngzǐ 2g + jiégěng 2g + liánqiáo 2g + yúxīngcǎo 2g + dōngguāzǐ 2-0g + qiánhú 1-0g.	Wǔwèizǐ 5g + yùzhú 5g + dìhuáng 5g + shāshēn 5g + jiégěng 5g + sāngbáipí 5g + fúlíng 5g + chénpí 5g + màiméndōng 5g + zǐwǎn 5g.
Máxìnggānshítāng 5g + dàzǎo 1-0g + tínglìzǐ 1-0g + dàhuáng 0g.	Wǔwèizǐ 5g + bànxià 5g + zhìgāncǎo 5g + cháihú 5g + gānjiāng 5g + huángqín 5g + chénpí 5-0g + dàhuáng 2-0g.

anti-obese, antidiabetic, immunomodulatory, cardiovascular protective, and hepatoprotective (Zhang et al., 2020). Cāngěrsǎn was introduced in Section 1.59 for upper respiratory tract infections.

12.3 ALPHA-1-ANTITRYPSIN DEFICIENCY

Alpha-1-antitrypsin is a protein made by the liver to protect the lungs from being attacked by the neutrophils of our innate immune system. Mutations in the gene encoding alpha-1-antitrypsin causes alpha-1-antitrypsin deficiency, which is also called alpha-1-proteinase inhibitor deficiency. Apart from lung impairment, the liver can also be damaged by accumulation of abnormal alpha-1-antitrypsin in the liver of the patient with alpha-1-antitrypsin deficiency.

Tínglìzǐ (Semen Lepidii; Semen Descurainiae) was shown to alleviate eosinophilic inflammation in the lungs of asthmatic mice (Kim et al., 2019); it is used today for coughs and allergic rhinitis (Wang, 2020). Yīnchénwǔlíngsǎn was introduced in Sections 4.21 and 5.12 for liver diseases.

TABLE 12.3
GMP Herbal Medicines for a 35-Year-Old Adult with Alpha-1-Antitrypsin Deficiency

Alpha-1-antitrypsin deficiency (OrphaCode: 60)

A disease with a prevalence of ~2 in 10,000

Disease-causing germline mutation(s): serpin family A member 1 (*SERPINA1* / Entrez: 5265) at 14q32.13

Autosomal recessive

Hepatic failure, Emphysema

Jaundice, Hepatomegaly, Hepatitis

Nephrotic syndrome

All ages

Emphysema (492.8):

Xiǎoqīnglóngtāng 5g + màiméndōngtāng 5-0g + xìngrén 1-0g + hòupò 1-0g + fúlíng 1-0g + shígāo 1-0g + gāncǎo 0g.	Wǔwèizǐ 5-4g + bànxià 5-4g + cháihú 5-4g + gānjiāng 5-4g + huángqín 5-4g + gāncǎo 5-0g + zhìgāncǎo 5-0g.
Máxìnggānshítāng 5g + tínglìzǐ 2-1g + dàzǎo 1g.	Wǔwèizǐ 5g + yùzhú 5g + dìhuáng 5g + shāshēn 5g + jiégěng 5g + sāngbáipí 5g + fúlíng 5g + chénpí 5g + màiméndōng 5g + zǐwǎn 5g.
	Wǔwèizǐ 5g + bànxià 5g + báizhú 5g + báisháo 5g + fùzǐ 5g + fúlíng 5g + gānjiāng 5g + xìxīn 5g + dàhuáng 1g.
	Tínglìzǐ 5g + dàzǎo 5-2g + jīnyínhuā 5-2g + dàhuáng 1-0g.

(Continued)

TABLE 12.3 *(Continued)*

GMP Herbal Medicines for a 35-Year-Old Adult with Alpha-1-Antitrypsin Deficiency

Jaundice (D007565):

Yīnchénwǔlíngsǎn 5g + huòxiāngzhèngqìsǎn 5g + yèjiāoténg 3g + hǎipiāoxiāo 3g + bózǐrén 2g + chuānxiōng 2-0g + cāngzhú 2-0g + chántuì 2-0g + yúxīngcǎo 2-0g + dàhuáng 1-0g.

Yīnchénwǔlíngsǎn 5g + jiāwèixiāoyáosǎn 4g + qǐjúdìhuángwán 4g + dìlóng 1g + huángqí 1g + mùtōng 1g + fángfēng 1g + xìxīn 0g.

Yīnchénwǔlíngsǎn 5g + lóngdǎnxiègāntāng 5g + huángliánjiědútāng 5-0g.

Yīnchén 5g + bànxià 2g + fùzǐ 2g + xìxīn 1g + dàhuáng 1g.

Yīnchén 5g + zhīzǐ 4g + huángqín 4g + dàhuáng 1g.

Yīnchén 5g + shānzhīzǐ 4-0g + liánqiáo 1-0g + zǐhuādìdīng 1-0g + dàhuáng 1-0g + huǒmárén 1-0g + tōngcǎo 1-0g.

Nephrotic syndrome (581):

Zhūlíngtāng 5g + jìshēngshènqìwán 5g + báimáogēn 1-0g + chēqiánzǐ 1-0g + jīnqiáncǎo 1-0g + niúxī 0g.

Wǔlíngsǎn 5g + liùwèidìhuángwán 5g + jiāwèixiāoyáosǎn 5g + dùzhòng 1g.

Wǔlíngsǎn 5g + jìshēngshènqìwán 5g + dānshēn 1-0g.

Chìxiǎodòu 5g + dānggui 5-2g + chēqiánzǐ 5-0g + yìmǔcǎo 5-0g + báimáogēn 3-0g + dàhuáng 1-0g.

Báimáogēn 5g + chēqiánzǐ 3g + báizhú 2g + fúlíng 2g + dàzǎo 1g + shēngjiāng 1g + shígāo 1g + zhìgāncǎo 1g + máhuáng 1g.

Chēqiánzǐ 5g + jùmài 5g + shānyào 3g + tiānhuā 3g + fúlíng 3g + fùzǐ 2g + dàhuáng 0g.

Dìhuáng 5g + mǔdānpí 4g + shíwěi 2g + zhǐqiào 2g + táorén 2g + zélán 2g + dàhuáng 0g + hónghuā 0g.

Chìxiǎodòu, introduced in Sections 1.66 and 4.12, "eliminates dampness." Báimáogēn benefits the kidney (cf. Sections 1.66 and 3.11) and pairs with Báihuāshéshécǎo to alleviate nephrotic syndrome through anti-inflammatory and hypolipidemic effects in rats (Zou et al., 2021).

12.4 INFANT ACUTE RESPIRATORY DISTRESS SYNDROME

Infant acute respiratory distress syndrome (infant ARDS), or neonatal respiratory distress syndrome, is previously called hyaline membrane disease. Infant ARDS occurs in premature newborns whose lungs lack of production of a substance called *pulmonary surfactant* that helps prevent the lungs from collapsing. Infant ARDS can also occur in full-term babies with a low birth weight.

Sìnìtāng, made up of Gānjiāng, Gāncǎo, and Fùzǐ, is supposed to help energize the body (cf. Sections 1.15, 1.46, and 11.10). Chántuì (cf. Sections 1.54 and 6.8) is a component medicinal in a

---

TABLE 12.4

GMP Herbal Medicines for a One-Year-Old Infant with Infant Acute Respiratory Distress Syndrome

Infant acute respiratory distress syndrome (OrphaCode: 70587)

A disease with a prevalence of ~2 in 10,000

Major susceptibility factor: surfactant protein B (*SFTPB* / Entrez: 6439) at 2p11.2

Major susceptibility factor: surfactant protein C (*SFTPC* / Entrez: 6440) at 8p21.3

Candidate gene tested: ATP binding cassette subfamily A member 3 (*ABCA3* / Entrez: 21) at 16p13.3

Not applicable

Hypoxemia

Abnormality of the thorax, Cyanosis, Premature birth, Tachypnea, Respiratory failure, Nasal flaring, Pulmonary edema, Atelectasis

Tachycardia, Bradycardia, Cardiac arrest, Pneumonia, Hypotension, Respiratory tract infection

Neonatal, Infancy

(Continued)

TABLE 12.4 *(Continued)*

GMP Herbal Medicines for a One-Year-Old Infant with Infant Acute Respiratory Distress Syndrome

Hypoxemia (D000860):

Sìnìtāng 5g + huòxiāngzhèngqìsăn 5g + yèjiāoténg 3g + hăipiāoxiāo 3g + bózĭrén 2g + cāngzhú 2g + chántuì 2g.	Gānjiāng 5g + rénshēn 4-2g + bànxià 4-2g + dàhuáng 1-0g.
Sìnìtāng 5g + fúlíng 2-0g + bànxià 1-0g + rénshēn 1-0g + shēngjiāng 1-0g + guìzhī 1-0g + hòupò 1-0g + zhǐshí 1-0g + dàhuáng 0g.	Gāncăo 5g + gégēn 5g + dàhuáng 1g. Zhìgāncăo 5g + dàhuáng 1g.

Cyanosis (D003490), Tachypnea (D059246):

Wŭlíngsăn 5g + píngwèisăn 5-0g + gāncăo 1-0g + báisháo 1-0g + guìzhī 1-0g + tiáowèichéngqìtāng 1-0g + dàhuáng 0g. Zhēnwŭtāng 5g + gāncăo 1g + báisháo 1g.	Gānjiāng 5g + cōngbái 5-0g + rénshēn 3g + huángqín 3-0g + huánglián 3-0g + fùzĭ 3-0g + ròuguì 2-0g + wúzhūyú 1-0g + xìxīn 1-0g. Gāncăo 5g + hòupò 5-0g + zhǐshí 5-0g + shārén 5-0g + báizhǐ 3-0g + dàhuáng 1-0g.

Cardiac arrest (427.5):

Zhìgāncăotāng 5g + línggúìshùgāntāng 5-0g. Zhìgāncăotāng 5g + yăngxīntāng 5-0g. Zhìgāncăotāng 5g + xiāngshāliùjūnzĭtāng 5-0g. Zhìgāncăotāng 5g + gāncăoxiǎomàidàzăotāng 5-0g. Tiānwángbŭxīndān 5g. Sìjūnzĭtāng 5g + yăngxīntāng 5g.	Chántuì 5g + jílí 3-0g. Zhǐqiào 5g + jílí 5-4g + chántuì 5-4g. Jílí 5g + chántuì 5-0g.

modern Chinese medicine patent formula to treat chronic heart failure (Chen et al., 2023). Zhǐqiào, introduced in Sections 1.31, 5.1, and 6.9 for digestion, is also used for chest pain (Wang, 2020) and its cardioprotective effect was demonstrated in myocardial ischemic rats (Yang et al., 2020). Jílí (cf. Section 5.9) was shown to protect against hypertensive endothelial injury in spontaneously hypertensive rats (Jiang et al., 2017).

12.5 BRONCHOPULMONARY DYSPLASIA

Bronchopulmonary dysplasia (BPD) is abnormal growth and development of the lungs and airways of a premature baby who, as a complication of respiratory distress syndrome or infection, has received breathing assistance such as supplemental oxygen and mechanical ventilation for a prolonged period of time.

Jīngjiè (cf. Section 2.43) "releases exterior, disperses Wind, promotes eruption, resolves ulcer" and is used today for skin and respiratory conditions (Wang, 2020). Moreover, it pairs with Jiāngcán (Bombyx Batryticatus) for the treatment of pneumonia due to respiratory syncytial virus (Wang,

TABLE 12.5

GMP Herbal Medicines for a One-Year-Old Infant with Bronchopulmonary Dysplasia

Bronchopulmonary dysplasia (OrphaCode: 70589)

A malformation syndrome with a prevalence of ~1 in 10,000

Not applicable

Small for gestational age, Premature birth, Abnormal lung morphology, Dyspnea, Emphysema, Respiratory distress, Respiratory failure requiring assisted ventilation, Chronic lung disease, Hyperoxemia, Cough

Right ventricular hypertrophy, Right ventricular failure, Sleep disturbance, Functional respiratory abnormality, Central apnea, Exercise intolerance, Diaphragmatic paralysis, Abnormal respiratory system morphology, Wheezing

Tracheobronchomalacia, Pulmonary sequestration, Atelectasis

Neonatal, Infancy

(Continued)

TABLE 12.5 *(Continued)*
GMP Herbal Medicines for a One-Year-Old Infant with Bronchopulmonary Dysplasia

Dyspnea (D004417), Emphysema (492.8), Respiratory distress (D004417), Cough (D003371):

Máxìnggānshítāng 5g + dàzǎo 2-1g + tínglìzǐ 2-1g + dàhuáng 0g.

Máxìnggānshítāng 5g + gāncǎo 2-1g + mázǐrénwán 1-0g + dàhuáng 0g.

Gāncǎo 5g + xìngrén 5g + fángfēng 5g + jiégěng 5g + jīngjiè 5g + yúxīngcǎo 5g + bòhé 5g + jiāngcán 5g.

Gāncǎo 5g + xìngrén 5g + bèimǔ 5g + qiánhú 5g + jiégěng 5g + sāngbáipí 5g + guālóurén 5g + fúlíng 5g + chénpí 5g + zǐsūyè 5-0g.

Gāncǎo 5g + wǔwèizǐ 3g + fúlíng 3g + xìxīn 1g + gānjiāng 0g.

Right ventricular failure (428, 428.0), Diaphragmatic paralysis (D012133), Wheezing (D012135):

Shēngmàiyǐn 5g + bǔzhōngyìqìtāng 5-0g.

Shēngmàiyǐn 5g + xuèfǔzhúyūtāng 5-0g + sānqī 1-0g + dānshēn 1-0g + yùjīn 1-0g.

Shēngmàiyǐn 5g + língguìshùgāntāng 5-0g + dānshēn 1-0g.

Zhēnwǔtāng 5g + shēngmàiyǐn 4-0g + gāncǎo 0g.

Gāncǎo 5g + fúlíng 5g + báizhú 5-0g + dǎngshēn 5-0g + xìngrén 5-0g + chénpí 5-0g + máhuáng 2-0g.

Dǎngshēn 5g + báizhú 2g + zhìgāncǎo 2g + gānjiāng 2g.

Zhìgāncǎo 5g + rénshēn 3g + dàhuáng 0g.

2020). Sāngbáipí (cf. Sections 2.45, 3.34, and 10.7) was shown to inhibit growth and induce apoptosis of human lung carcinoma cells (Park et al., 2012).

12.6 IDIOPATHIC PULMONARY FIBROSIS

Idiopathic pulmonary fibrosis (IPF) is thickening, stiffening, and eventual scarring of the tissues surrounding the air sacs in the lungs, leading to a progressive and irreversible decline in lung function. The cause of IPF is unknown; however, cigarette smoking, gastroesophageal reflux disease, viral infection, and genetic changes are among the risk factors.

TABLE 12.6
GMP Herbal Medicines for a 60-Year-Old Adult with Idiopathic Pulmonary Fibrosis

Idiopathic pulmonary fibrosis (OrphaCode: 2032)

A disease with a prevalence of ~1 in 10,000

Major susceptibility factor: surfactant protein A1 (*SFTPA1* / Entrez: 653509) at 10q22.3

Major susceptibility factor: desmoplakin (*DSP* / Entrez: 1832) at 6p24.3

Major susceptibility factor: telomerase reverse transcriptase (*TERT* / HGNC:11730) at 5p15.33

Major susceptibility factor: telomerase RNA component (*TERC* / Entrez: 7012) at 3q26.2

Major susceptibility factor: mucin 5B, oligomeric mucus/gel-forming (*MUC5B* / Entrez: 727897) at 11p15.5

Major susceptibility factor: surfactant protein A2 (*SFTPA2* / Entrez: 729238) at 10q22.3

Major susceptibility factor: regulator of telomere elongation helicase 1 (*RTEL1* / Entrez: 51750) at 20q13.33

Major susceptibility factor: family with sequence similarity 13 member A (*FAM13A* / Entrez: 10144) at 4q22.1

Major susceptibility factor: STN1 subunit of CST complex (*STN1* / Entrez: 79991) at 10q24.33

Major susceptibility factor: ATPase phospholipid transporting 11A (*ATP11A* / Entrez: 23250) at 13q34

Major susceptibility factor: dipeptidyl peptidase 9 (*DPP9* / Entrez: 91039) at 19p13.3

Major susceptibility factor: poly(A)-specific ribonuclease (*PARN* / Entrez: 5073) at 16p13.12

Major susceptibility factor: surfactant protein C (*SFTPC* / Entrez: 6440) at 8p21.3

Candidate gene tested: ATP binding cassette subfamily A member 3 (*ABCA3* / Entrez: 21) at 16p13.3

Multigenic/multifactorial

Interstitial pulmonary abnormality

Gastroesophageal reflux, Bronchiectasis, Pulmonary fibrosis, Exertional dyspnea, Cough, Honeycomb lung, Ground-glass opacification on pulmonary HRCT, Reticular pattern on pulmonary HRCT, Crackles, Clubbing of fingers

Pulmonary insufficiency

Adult

(Continued)

TABLE 12.6 *(Continued)*
GMP Herbal Medicines for a 60-Year-Old Adult with Idiopathic Pulmonary Fibrosis

Gastroesophageal reflux (530.81), Bronchiectasis (494), Cough (D003371), Crackles (D012135), Clubbing of fingers (731.2):

Xuánfùdàizhěshítāng 5g + báijí 2g + hǎipiāoxiāo 2g + xiāngshāliùjūnzǐtāng 2g + bànxiàxièxīntāng 2-0g.	Wǔwèizǐ 5g + bànxià 5g + zhìgāncǎo 5g + cháihú 5g + gānjiāng 5g + huángqín 5g + dàhuáng 2-0g.
Qīngfèitāng 5g + xīnyíqīngfèitāng 5-0g + báijí 1g + hǎipiāoxiāo 1g.	
Qīngfèitāng 5g + xiāngshāliùjūnzǐtāng 2-0g + báijí 1g + hǎipiāoxiāo 1g.	Zhìgāncǎo 5g + wǔwèizǐ 4g + bànxià 4g + jiégěng 4g + gānjiāng 4g + xìxīn 4g.
Qīngfèitāng 5g + dìngchuǎntāng 4-0g + báijí 1g + hǎipiāoxiāo 1g.	

Xuánfùdàizhěshítāng "lowers ascending, reduces phlegm" and is used today for bronchitis and gastritis (Wang, 2019). Qīngfèitāng literally means "lung cleansing decoction." It consists of Huángqín, Jiégěng, Wǔwèizǐ, and other herbs and is used for bronchitis and rhinitis (Wang, 2019). The prescriptions in the table are seen to address the respiratory and digestive symptoms of the patient.

12.7 CYSTIC FIBROSIS

Cystic fibrosis, or mucoviscidosis, is characterized by buildup of thick and sticky mucus in the linings of the lungs and gastrointestinal tract, leading to repeated lung infections and impaired nutrient absorption. Cystic fibrosis is caused by mutations in the *CFTR* gene, whose products transport chloride ions into and out of the cells that produce mucus, sweat, and saliva, which is important for the production of thin and freely flowing mucus.

TABLE 12.7
GMP Herbal Medicines for a Three-Year-Old Child with Cystic Fibrosis

Cystic fibrosis (OrphaCode: 586)

A disease with a prevalence of ~1 in 10,000

Modifying germline mutation: serpin family A member 1 (*SERPINA1* / Entrez: 5265) at 14q32.13

Modifying germline mutation: solute carrier family 26 member 9 (*SLC26A9* / Entrez: 115019) at 1q32.1

Modifying germline mutation: solute carrier family 6 member 14 (*SLC6A14* / Entrez: 11254) at Xq23

Modifying germline mutation: solute carrier family 9 member A3 (*SLC9A3* / Entrez: 6550) at 5p15.33

Modifying germline mutation: CEA cell adhesion molecule 3 (*CEACAM3* / Entrez: 1084) at 19q13.2

Modifying germline mutation: CEA cell adhesion molecule 6 (*CEACAM6* / Entrez: 4680) at 19q13.2

Modifying germline mutation: endothelin receptor type A (*EDNRA* / Entrez: 1909) at 4q31.22-q31.23

Modifying germline mutation: glutathione S-transferase mu 3 (*GSTM3* / Entrez: 2947) at 1p13.3

Modifying germline mutation: heme oxygenase 1 (*HMOX1* / Entrez: 3162) at 22q12.3

Modifying germline mutation: glutamate-cysteine ligase catalytic subunit (*GCLC* / Entrez: 2729) at 6p12.1

Modifying germline mutation: homeostatic iron regulator (*HFE* / Entrez: 3077) at 6p22.2

Disease-causing germline mutation(s) (loss of function): CF transmembrane conductance regulator (*CFTR* / Entrez: 1080) at 7q31.2

Modifying germline mutation: transforming growth factor beta 1 (*TGFB1* / Entrez: 7040) at 19q13.2

Modifying germline mutation: dynactin subunit 4 (*DCTN4* / Entrez: 51164) at 5q33.1

Modifying germline mutation: chloride channel accessory 4 (*CLCA4* / Entrez: 22802) at 1p22.3

Modifying germline mutation: syntaxin 1A (*STX1A* / Entrez: 6804) at 7q11.23

Modifying germline mutation: potassium calcium-activated channel subfamily N member 4 (*KCNN4* / Entrez: 3783) at 19q13.31

Modifying germline mutation: macrophage migration inhibitory factor (*MIF* / Entrez: 4282) at 22q11.23

Modifying germline mutation: solute carrier family 11 member 1 (*SLC11A1* / Entrez: 6556) at 2q35

Autosomal recessive

(Continued)

TABLE 12.7 *(Continued)*

GMP Herbal Medicines for a Three-Year-Old Child with Cystic Fibrosis

Exocrine pancreatic insufficiency, Malabsorption, Bronchiectasis, Recurrent respiratory infections, Airway obstruction, Elevated sweat chloride, Absent vas deferens

Failure to thrive

Sinusitis, Depression, Anxiety, Osteopenia, Abnormality of the liver, Gastroesophageal reflux, Rectal prolapse, Asthma, Steatorrhea, Recurrent *Aspergillus* infections, Recurrent *Staphylococcus aureus* infections, Elevated hepatic transaminase, Meconium ileus, Recurrent *Hemophilus influenzae* infections, Reduced forced expiratory volume in one second, Decreased body mass index

All ages

Bronchiectasis (494):

Xìngsūyǐnyòukē 5g + xīnyíqīngfèitāng 5g + dìngchuǎntāng 5g.	Báiqián 5g + bǎibù 5g + xìngrén 5g + qiánhú 5g + jiégěng 5g + jīngjiè 5g + zǐwǎn 5g + máhuáng 5-0g + kuǎndōnghuā 5-0g + chénpí 5-0g + gāncǎo 3-2g.
Xìngsūyǐnyòukē 5g + xīnyíqīngfèitāng 5g + máxìnggānshítāng 5g + yúxīngcǎo 2-0g.	Xìngrén 5g + máhuáng 5g + bànxià 4-3g + chénpí 4-3g + tínglìzǐ 3-0g + gāncǎo 2g + shēngjiāng 2-0g + dàhuáng 1-0g.
Máxìnggānshítāng 5-4g + dìngchuǎntāng 5-0g + yúxīngcǎo 1-0g + dàzǎo 1-0g + tínglìzǐ 1-0g + dàhuáng 0g.	Bǎibù 5g + zǐwǎn 5g + xìngrén 4g + dǎodìwúgōng 4g + jiégěng 4g + jīngjiè 4g + máhuáng 4g + kuǎndōnghuā 4g + gāncǎo 2g + liánqiáo 2g.

Abnormality of the liver (573.9), Gastroesophageal reflux (530.81), Rectal prolapse (569.1), Asthma (493):

Xiǎocháihútāngqùrénshēn 5g + bǎihégùjīntāng 5-2g + qínjiāobiējiǎsǎn 5-2g + wūméi 1g.	Huáihuā 5g.
Èrchéntāng 5g + màiméndōngtāng 5g + dānshēn 5g + běishāshēn 5g + bǎnlángēn 5g + jiégěng 5g + xiānhècǎo 5-0g + huáihuā 5-0g + kuǎndōnghuā 5-0g + jīnyínhuā 5-0g + ǒujié 5-0g.	Gāncǎo 5g + huángqín 5g + huánglián 1-0g + dàhuáng 0g.
	Bànxià 5g + xìngrén 5g + hòupò 5g + fúlíng 5g + chénpí 5g + màiyá 5g.
	Bèimǔ 5g + zhīmǔ 4g + gāncǎo 3g + dàhuáng 0g + huánglián 0g.

Báiqián (Rhizoma et Radix Cynanchi Stauntonii) "dispels phlegm, lowers Qi, stops cough" and is used today for coughs, rhinitis, and bronchitis (Wang, 2020). Xìngrén (cf. Section 1.12) is used for chest pain and coughs. Qiánhú (Radix Peucedani) "disperses wind-heat, lowers Qi, eliminates phlegm" and is used also for coughs, rhinitis, and bronchitis (Wang, 2020). Huáihuā (Flos Sophorae) "cools Blood, stops bleeding" and is used today for digestive conditions including hemorrhoids (Wang, 2020). Bǎihégùjīntāng "nourishes yin, clears heat, moistens the Lung, dissolves phlegm" and is used today for chronical bronchitis (Wang, 2019). Qínjiāobiējiǎsǎn, containing Cháihú (cf. Section 3.2), has been used for patients with "yin deficiency" manifesting "osteopyrexia and tidal fever." The formula is used today for menopause, diffuse connective tissue diseases, and chronic bronchitis (Wang, 2019).

12.8 RECURRENT RESPIRATORY PAPILLOMATOSIS

Recurrent respiratory papillomatosis is benign epithelial tumors called *papillomas* in the combined respiratory tract and upper digestive tract including the nose, mouth, throat, larynx, esophagus, trachea, and lungs. Recurrent respiratory papillomatosis is caused by human papillomavirus (HPV) infection during vaginal childbirth in juvenile patients or oral sex in adult patients.

Xuánshēn was introduced in Section 1.3 for throat pain. Qīngyānlìgétāng "dispels Wind, clears heat, reduces swelling, benefits throat" and is used today for chronic pharyngitis and nasopharyngitis (Wang, 2019). Máxìnggānshítāng was introduced in Sections 1.47, 2.43, 7.10, and 11.4 for symptoms involving the respiratory system and other chest symptoms. Jiégěngtāng, containing Jiégěng (cf. Sections 2.57 and 8.11), has been used for pulmonary abscess (cf. Section 2.57).

TABLE 12.8
GMP Herbal Medicines for a Four-Year-Old Child with Recurrent Respiratory Papillomatosis

Recurrent respiratory papillomatosis (OrphaCode: 60032)

A disease with a prevalence of ~5 in 100,000

Not applicable

Hoarse voice

Dysphonia, Respiratory distress, Abnormal trachea morphology

Failure to thrive, Dysphagia, Respiratory insufficiency, Dyspnea, Hemoptysis, Upper airway obstruction, Recurrent upper respiratory tract infections, Tachypnea, Recurrent pneumonia, Stridor, Wheezing, Nonproductive cough

Childhood, Adolescent, Adult

Hoarse voice (D006685):

Qīngyānlìgétāng 5g + yínqiàosǎn 5g + shāndòugēn 1-0g + gāncǎo 1-0g + shègān 1-0g.	Xuánshēn 5g + yùzhú 5g + dìhuáng 5g + hòupò 5g + zhǐshí 5g + màiméndōng 5g + shāshēn 5-0g + dàhuáng 1-0g.
Xuánshēn 5g + dìhuáng 5g + shāshēn 5g + màiméndōng 5g + xiǎochéngqìtāng 1g.	

Dysphonia (D055154), Respiratory distress (D004417):

Máxìnggānshítāng 5g + dàzǎo 1-0g + tínglìzǐ 1-0g + dàhuáng 0g.	Gāncǎo 5g + dìlóng 5g + fángfēng 5g + jiégěng 5g + jīngjiè 5g + yúxīngcǎo 5g + bòhé 5g + jiāngcán 5g.
Jiégěngtāng 5g + xuánshēn 2g + mǔlì 2g + bèimǔ 2g + dàzǎo 2g + shēngjiāng 2g + liánqiáo 2g + zhīzǐ 1g.	Gāncǎo 5g + jiégěng 5g + xuánshēn 4-3g + mǔlì 4-3g + bèimǔ 4-3g + liánqiáo 4-2g + zhīzǐ 2g.
	Xuánshēn 5g + dìhuáng 5g + hòupò 5g + zhǐshí 5g + màiméndōng 5g + dàhuáng 0g.

Dyspnea (D004417), Hemoptysis (D006469), Tachypnea (D059246), Stridor (D012135), Wheezing (D012135):

Máxìnggānshítāng 5g + tínglìzǐ 1-0g + dàzǎo 1-0g + dàhuáng 0g.	Wǔwèizǐ 5g + bànxià 5g + zhìgāncǎo 5g + cháihú 5g + gānjiāng 5g + huángqín 5g + dàhuáng 1-0g.
	Wǔwèizǐ 5g + yùzhú 5g + dìhuáng 5g + shāshēn 5g + jiégěng 5g + sāngbáipí 5g + fúlíng 5g + chénpí 5g + màiméndōng 5g + zǐwǎn 5g.

12.9   ACUTE INTERSTITIAL PNEUMONIA

Acute interstitial pneumonia, also known as Hamman-Rich syndrome, is a fulminant, idiopathic, and diffuse lung injury, characterized by rapid progression from the initial symptoms to respiratory failure. The cause of acute interstitial pneumonia is unknown.

TABLE 12.9
GMP Herbal Medicines for a 52-Year-Old Adult with Acute Interstitial Pneumonia

Acute interstitial pneumonia (OrphaCode: 79126)

A disease with a prevalence of ~4 in 100,000

Unknown

Dyspnea, Bronchiectasis, Pulmonary infiltrates, Respiratory failure, Hypoxemia, Peribronchovascular interstitial thickening, Ground-glass opacification on pulmonary HRCT, Nodular pattern on pulmonary HRCT, Reticulonodular pattern on pulmonary HRCT, Interlobular septal thickening on pulmonary HRCT

Hypertension, Cyanosis, Fever, Pleural effusion, Tachypnea, Fatigue, Crackles, Nonproductive cough, Decreased DLCO

Pericardial effusion, Pulmonary fibrosis, Lymphadenopathy, Arthralgia, Elevated serum creatinine, Myalgia, Elevated erythrocyte sedimentation rate, Elevated C-reactive protein level, Peripheral edema, Subpleural honeycombing, Reduced hematocrit, Chest pain, Atelectasis

Adult

(Continued)

TABLE 12.9 *(Continued)*
GMP Herbal Medicines for a 52-Year-Old Adult with Acute Interstitial Pneumonia

Dyspnea (D004417), Bronchiectasis (494), Hypoxemia (D000860):

Máxìnggānshítāng 5g + cāngěrsǎn 5-4g + jiégěng 2g + liánqiáo 2g + yúxīngcǎo 2g + niúbàngzǐ 2-0g + dōngguāzǐ 2-0g + qiánhú 1-0g.

Wǔwèizǐ 5g + yùzhú 5g + dìhuáng 5g + shāshēn 5g + jiégěng 5g + sāngbáipí 5g + fúlíng 5g + chénpí 5g + màiméndōng 5g + zǐwǎn 5g.

Máxìnggānshítāng 5g + yínqiàosǎn 5g.

Wǔwèizǐ 5g + bànxià 5g + zhìgāncǎo 5g + cháihú 5g + gānjiāng 5g + huángqín 5g + chénpí 5-0g.

Máxìnggānshítāng 5g + zhǐsòusǎn 4g + bèimǔ 1g + qiánhú 1g.

Hypertension (401-405.99), Cyanosis (D003490), Fever (D005334), Tachypnea (D059246), Fatigue (D005221), Crackles (D012135):

Wǔlíngsǎn 5g + gōuténgsǎn 5g + niúxī 1g + chēqiánzǐ 1g.

Qiānghuó 5g + hòupò 5-3g + zhǐshí 5-3g + huángqín 1-0g + huánglián 1-0g + dàhuáng 1-0g.

Wǔlíngsǎn 5g + tiānmágōuténgyǐn 5g + xuèfǔzhúyūtāng 5-0g.

Zhēnwǔtāng 5g + wǔlíngsǎn 5-0g + fùzǐ 1g + gānjiāng 1-0g + dǐdāngtāng 0g.

Pericardial effusion (423.0), Pulmonary fibrosis (D011658) [Idiopathic pulmonary fibrosis (516.31)], Arthralgia (D018771), Myalgia (D063806), Chest pain (D002637):

Guālóurén 5g + xièbái 5g + tiānwángbǔxīndān 5g + xuèfǔzhúyūtāng 5g + acupuncture.

Guālóurén 5g + xièbái 5g + bànxià 3-0g + guìzhī 3-0g + hòupò 2-0g + zhǐshí 2-0g.

Cháixiàntāng 5g + xuèfǔzhúyūtāng 5-0g + zhìgāncǎotāng 4-0g + dānshēn 1g + yùjīn 1g + sānqī 1-0g + mùxiāng 1-0g.

Fùzǐ 5g + gāncǎo 4g + gānjiāng 4g + suānzǎorén 4g.

Fùzǐ 5g + gāncǎo 4g + shārén 4g + guìbǎn 4g + qiánhú 2g + yuánzhì 2g.

Qiānghuó was introduced in Sections 2.14 and 4.10 for hypertension and fever. Guālóurén (cf. Section 5.11) was found to be among the top five commonly prescribed single herbs for patients with tuberculosis (Yang et al., 2018). Xièbái (Bulbus Allii Macrostemonis) was summarized to be antiplatelet, lipid-lowering, antiatherosclerosis, antitumor, antispasmodic, antibacterial, antioxidant, and insecticidal (Yao et al., 2016), and is used for palpitations and chest pain (Wang, 2020). The term bǔxīn in Tiānwángbǔxīndān means "to nourish the heart." We will see its use for cardiac diseases in Chapter 14.

12.10 AUTOIMMUNE PULMONARY ALVEOLAR PROTEINOSIS

Pulmonary alveolar proteinosis (PAP) is a syndrome where clearance of a fatty substance called *pulmonary surfactant*, which helps the lung inflate, is impaired, leading to pileup of pulmonary surfactant in the air sacs of the lung. Autoimmune PAP is caused by IgG antibodies that block a messenger molecule that regulates digestion of excessive pulmonary surfactant by alveolar macrophages.

TABLE 12.10
GMP Herbal Medicines for a 35-Year-Old Adult with Autoimmune Pulmonary Alveolar Proteinosis

Autoimmune pulmonary alveolar proteinosis (OrphaCode: 747)

A disease with a prevalence of ~3 in 100,000

Major susceptibility factor: major histocompatibility complex, class II, DR beta 1 (*HLA-DRB1* / Entrez: 3123) at 6p21.32

Multigenic/multifactorial, Not applicable

Alveolar proteinosis

Cyanosis, Clubbing, Abnormality of the upper respiratory tract, Dyspnea, Restrictive deficit on pulmonary function testing, Foam cells, Abnormal circulating protein level, Hypoxemia, Increased lactate dehydrogenase activity, Autoimmune antibody positivity, Decreased DLCO

(Continued)

TABLE 12.10 *(Continued)*

GMP Herbal Medicines for a 35-Year-Old Adult with Autoimmune Pulmonary Alveolar Proteinosis

Cough, Crazy paving pattern on pulmonary HRCT, Crackles
Childhood, Adolescent, Adult

Alveolar proteinosis (516.0):

Máxìnggānshítāng 5g + zhǐsòusǎn 4g + bèimǔ 1g + guālóurén 1g + qiánhú 1-0g + sāngbáipí 1-0g + hǎigé 1-0g + huángqín 1-0g + lúgēn 1-0g. Máxìnggānshítāng 5g + yínqiàosǎn 5g. Máxìnggānshítāng 5g + dàzǎo 1g + tínglìzǐ 1g.	Wǔwèizǐ 5g + bànxià 5g + zhìgāncǎo 5g + cháihú 5g + gānjiāng 5g + huángqín 5g + dàhuáng 1-0g. Gāncǎo 5g + yúxīngcǎo 5g + dìlóng 4g + fángfēng 4g + jiégěng 4g + jīngjiè 4g + bòhé 4g + jiāngcán 4g. Zǐwǎn 5g + bǎibù 4g + xìngrén 4g + dǎodìwúgōng 4g + jiégěng 4g + jīngjiè 4g + máhuáng 4g + kuǎndōnghuā 4g + gāncǎo 2g + liánqiáo 2g.

Cyanosis (D003490), Dyspnea (D004417), Hypoxemia (D000860):

Wǔlíngsǎn 5g + fùzǐ 1g + huángqín 1g + tiáowèichéngqìtāng 1g + dǐdāngtāng 0g. Máxìnggānshítāng 5g + dàzǎo 1g + tínglìzǐ 1g + dàhuáng 0g. Sìnìtāng 5g + bànxià 2-1g + dàhuáng 0g.	Gānjiāng 5g + rénshēn 4-2g + bànxià 4-2g + dàhuáng 0g.

Cough (D003371), Crackles (D012135):

Máhuángtāng 5g + bànxià 1g + shēngjiāng 1g + xìxīn 1g + dàhuáng 0g. Dàqīnglóngtāng 5g + jīngfángbàidúsǎn 3-2g + pǔjìxiāodúyǐn 3-2g + mǔlì 1g + lónggǔ 1g.	Gāncǎo 5g + dìlóng 5-4g + fángfēng 5-4g + jiégěng 5-4g + jīngjiè 5-4g + yúxīngcǎo 5-4g + jiāngcán 5-4g + bòhé 5-0g + tǔfúlíng 4-0g.

Bànxià (cf. Section 2.3) "dries dampness, dissolves phlegm, calms adverse rising, stops vomiting, reduces lumps, resolves masses" and is used for both digestive and respiratory conditions such as gastritis and cough (Wang, 2020). Chinese herbal medicine, including Wǔwèizǐ and Gāncǎo, combined with conventional medicine, was concluded to be a more effective strategy for the treatment of connective tissue disease-associated interstitial lung disease in the clinic in a meta-analysis of randomized controlled trials (Yin et al., 2023). Dìlóng (cf. Sections 1.22 and 1.69) protein was shown to ameliorate pulmonary fibrosis in mice (Li et al., 2022). Zǐwǎn (Radix et Rhizoma Asteris) "moistens the Lung, transforms phlegm, stops coughing" and is used today for bronchitis and coughs (Wang, 2020). Zhǐsòusǎn (cf. Section 9.13), which consists of Jiégěng, Jīngjiè, Zǐwǎn, Bǎibù, Gāncǎo, and so on, is translated to "cough stopping powder." Dàqīnglóngtāng was introduced in Section 4.22 for asthma.

12.11 MECONIUM ASPIRATION SYNDROME

Meconium is the first stool of a newborn. Meconium aspiration syndrome refers to a neonatal respiratory distress condition where meconium gets into the newborn's lungs. Meconium aspiration syndrome can happen when the fetus passes the stool while still in the uterus due to, e.g., a prolonged pregnancy. The fetus is further stressed during labor and gasps to suck in meconium-stained amniotic fluid.

Bèimǔ (cf. Section 4.27) "clears heat, removes phlegm, moistens the Lung, stops coughing, dissolves masses, and reduces swelling." It was reviewed and summarized to be antitussive, expectorant, and anti-asthmatic (Chen et al., 2020), and is used for cough (Wang, 2020). Note that GMP herbal extract granule prescriptions to infants are small in size and weight compared with those to adults.

TABLE 12.11

GMP Herbal Medicines for a One-Year-Old Infant with Meconium Aspiration Syndrome

Meconium aspiration syndrome (OrphaCode: 70588)

A disease with a prevalence of ~2 in 100,000

Not applicable

Respiratory distress, Transient pulmonary infiltrates, Caesarian section, Fetal distress, Post-term pregnancy, Abnormal heart rate variability, Abnormal pulmonary thoracic imaging finding

Intrauterine growth retardation, Premature rupture of membranes, Pulmonary arterial hypertension, Pneumothorax, Maternal hypertension, Maternal diabetes, Aspiration pneumonia, Hypoxemia, Meconium stained amniotic fluid, Neonatal asphyxia, Pneumomediastinum, Wheezing, Atelectasis

Neonatal, Infancy

Respiratory distress (D004417):

Xìngsūyǐnyòukē 5g + cāngěrsǎn 5g + xīnyíqīngfèitāng 5-0g.	Bèimǔ 5g + zhìgāncǎo 5g + jiégěng 5g + xuánshēn 4-3g + mǔlì 4-3g + liánqiáo 3-2g + xìngrén 3-0g + zhīzǐ 2-0g + dàhuáng 1-0g.
Xìngsūyǐnyòukē 5g + máxìnggānshítāng 5-3g + xīnyíqīngfèitāng 5-0g + bèimǔ 0g.	Báiqián 5g + xìngrén 5g + bèimǔ 5g + qiánhú 5g + sāngbáipí 5g + guālóurén 5g + huángqín 5g + júhóng 5g + bòhé 5g + gāncǎo 2g.
Xìngsūyǐnyòukē 5g + xīnyíqīngfèitāng 5g + yínqiàosǎn 5-0g + bèimǔ 1-0g.	Báiqián 5g + bǎibù 5g + jiégěng 5g + jīngjiè 5g + chénpí 5g + gāncǎo 3g + zǐwǎn 3g.

Hypoxemia (D000860), Neonatal asphyxia (768.9), Wheezing (D012135):

Wǔlíngsǎn 5g + gāncǎo 1-0g.	Gāncǎo 5g + xìngrén 5-0g + bèimǔ 5-0g + jiégěng 5-0g + fúlíng 5-0g + júhóng 5-0g.
Sìnìtāng 5g.	
Guìzhītāng 5g + xìngrén 1g + hòupò 1g.	Gāncǎo 5g + báizhǐ 5-0g + shārén 3-0g + tiānhuā 2-0g + dàhuáng 0g.
	Gāncǎo 5g + gégēn 5-0g.

REFERENCES

Chen, J., Wei, X., Zhang, Q., Wu, Y., Xia, G., Xia, H., Wang, L., Shang, H., & Lin, S. S. (2023). The traditional Chinese medicines treat chronic heart failure and their main bioactive constituents and mechanisms. *Acta Pharmaceutica Sinica B, 13*(5), 1919–1955. https://doi.org/10.1016/j.apsb.2023.02.005

Chen, T., Zhong, F., Yao, C., Chen, J., Xiang, Y., Dong, J., Yan, Z., & Ma, Y. (2020). A systematic review on traditional uses, sources, phytochemistry, pharmacology, pharmacokinetics, and toxicity of *Fritillariae cirrhosae bulbus. Evidence-Based Complementary and Alternative Medicine, 2020*, 1–26. https://doi.org/10.1155/2020/1536534

Guo, Z., Li, S., Zhang, N., Kang, Q., & Zhai, H. (2020). Schisandra inhibit bleomycin-induced idiopathic pulmonary fibrosis in rats via suppressing M2 macrophage polarization. *BioMed Research International, 2020*, 1–11. https://doi.org/10.1155/2020/5137349

Jiang, Y., Guo, J., Wu, S., & Yang, C. (2017). Vascular protective effects of aqueous extracts of *Tribulus terrestris* on hypertensive endothelial injury. *Chinese Journal of Natural Medicines, 15*(8), 606–614. https://doi.org/10.1016/s1875-5364(17)30088-2

Kim, S., Seo, Y., Kim, H. S., Lee, A. Y., Chun, J. M., Moon, B. C., & Kwon, B. (2019). Anti-asthmatic effects of lepidii seu Descurainiae Semen plant species in ovalbumin-induced asthmatic mice. *Journal of Ethnopharmacology, 244*, 112083. https://doi.org/10.1016/j.jep.2019.112083

Li, S., Yang, Q., Chen, F., Tian, L., Huo, J., Meng, Y., Tang, Q., & Wang, W. (2022). The antifibrotic effect of pheretima protein is mediated by the TGF-β1/Smad2/3 pathway and attenuates inflammation in bleomycin-induced idiopathic pulmonary fibrosis. *Journal of Ethnopharmacology, 286*, 114901. https://doi.org/10.1016/j.jep.2021.114901

Park, S., Yong, G., Eom, H. S., Kim, G., Hyun, J. W., Kim, W., Lee, S., Yoo, Y. H., & Choi, Y. H. (2012). Role of autophagy in apoptosis induction by methylene chloride extracts of Mori cortex in NCI-H460 human lung carcinoma cells. *International Journal of Oncology, 40*(6), 1929–1940. https://doi.org/10.3892/ijo.2012.1386

Tajuddin, T., Ahmad, S., Latif, A., & Qasmi, I. A. (2003). Aphrodisiac activity of 50% ethanolic extracts of *Myristica fragrans* Houtt. (nutmeg) and *Syzygium aromaticum* (L) Merr. & Perry. (clove) in male mice: A comparative study. *BMC Complementary and Alternative Medicine*, *3*(1), 6. https://doi.org/10.1186/1472-6882-3-6

Wang, S.-C. (2019). Therapeutic classes of CHEG formulas. In S.-C. Wang (Ed.), *Clinical herbal prescriptions: Principles and practices of herbal formulations from deep learning health insurance herbal prescription big data* (pp. 16–89). World Scientific Publishing. https://doi.org/10.1142/11211

Wang, S.-C. (2020). Modern therapeutic uses of CHEG herbs and herb pairs. In S.-C. Wang (Ed.), *Veterinary herbal pharmacopoeia* (pp. 35–233). Nova Science Publishers. https://doi.org/10.52305/GHTR1903

Yang, S., Lin, Y., Wu, M., Chiang, J. H., Yang, P., Hsia, T., & Yen, H. (2018). Utilization of Chinese medicine for respiratory discomforts by patients with a medical history of tuberculosis in Taiwan. *BMC Complementary and Alternative Medicine*, *18*(1), 313. https://doi.org/10.1186/s12906-018-2377-4

Yang, Y., Ding, Z., Zhong, R., Xia, T., Wang, W., Zhao, H., Wang, Y., & Shu, Z. (2020). Cardioprotective effects of a *Fructus Aurantii* polysaccharide in isoproterenol-induced myocardial ischemic rats. *International Journal of Biological Macromolecules*, *155*, 995–1002. https://doi.org/10.1016/j.ijbiomac.2019.11.063

Yao, Z., Qin, Z. H., Dai, Y., & Yao, X. (2016). Phytochemistry and pharmacology of Allii Macrostemonis Bulbus, a traditional Chinese medicine. *Chinese Journal of Natural Medicines*, *14*(7), 481–498. https://doi.org/10.1016/s1875-5364(16)30058-9

Yin, X., Zhao, S., Xiang, N., Chen, J., Xu, J., & Zhang, Y. (2023). Efficacy and safety of Chinese herbal medicines combined with cyclophosphamide for connective tissue disease-associated interstitial lung disease: A meta-analysis of randomized controlled trials. *Frontiers in Pharmacology*, *14*. https://doi.org/10.3389/fphar.2023.1064578

Zhang, L., Huang, M., Yang, Y., Huang, M., Shi, J., Zou, L., & Lu, J. (2020). Bioactive platycodins from *Platycodonis Radix*: Phytochemistry, pharmacological activities, toxicology and pharmacokinetics. *Food Chemistry*, *327*, 127029. https://doi.org/10.1016/j.foodchem.2020.127029

Zou, W., Dong, Y., Yang, S., Gong, L., Zhang, Y., Shi, B., La, L., Tang, L., & Liu, M. (2021). Imperatae rhizoma-*Hedyotis diffusa* Willd. herbal pair alleviates nephrotic syndrome by integrating anti-inflammatory and hypolipidaemic effects. *Phytomedicine*, *90*, 153644. https://doi.org/10.1016/j.phymed.2021.153644

13 GMP Herbal Medicine for Rare Gastroenterologic Diseases

Gastroenterologic diseases affect the digestive tract that leads from the mouth, where food enters, to the anus, where feces exit. The common causes of gastroenterologic diseases include viruses, bacteria, parasites, toxins, and medications. Many of the rare gastroenterologic diseases of this chapter are adult onset.

The GMP single herbs and multi-herb formulas that are frequently discussed for the signs and symptoms of the rare gastroenterologic diseases are Rhubarb Root and Rhizome (Dàhuáng), Magnolia Bark (Hòupò), Licorice Root (Gāncǎo), Immature Bitter Orange (Zhǐshí), Scutellaria Root (Huángqín), Figwort Root (Xuánshēn), Rehmannia Root (Dìhuáng), Ophiopogon Tuber (Màiméndōng), Pinellia Tuber (Bànxià), Cardamon Seed (Shārén), Barbated Skullcap Herb (Bànzhīlián), Poria (Fúlíng), Medicated Leaven (Shénqū), Preserve Harmony Pill (Bǎohéwán), Pueraria, Scute and Coptis Decoction (Gégēnhuángqínhuángliántáng), Minor Construct the Middle Decoction (Xiǎojiànzhōngtáng), Ginseng, Poria and Atractylodes Powder (Shēnlíngbáizhúsǎn), Calm the Stomach Powder (Píngwèisǎn), Aucklandia, Cardamon and the Six Gentlemen Decoction (Xiāngshāliùjūnzǐtāng), Five Ingredient Formula with Poria (Wǔlíngsǎn), Disperse the Swelling and Break the Hardness Decoction (Sǎnzhǒngkuìjiāntáng), Gardenia and Hoelen Formula (Wǔlínsǎn), Cinnamon Twig Decoction (Guìzhītāng), Rhubarb and Leech Combination (Dǐdāngtāng), Pogostemon Correct the Qi Powder (Huòxiāngzhèngqìsǎn), and Frigid Extremities Decoction (Sìnìtāng).

In TCM, the stomach, small intestine, large intestine, and spleen cooperate to descend the food and ascend the extracted essences and fluids, accomplishing the digestive job of the body. We discuss digestion-improving herbs and formulas such as Dàhuáng, Hòupò, and Bǎohéwán in the chapter.

13.1 NECROTIZING ENTEROCOLITIS

Necrotizing enterocolitis is severe inflammation and death of the small or large intestine. The inflamed intestine wall can perforate, leaking wastes and bacteria into the bloodstream and abdomen. Necrotizing enterocolitis most likely occurs in premature babies in which an underdeveloped intestine plays a role in causing necrotizing enterocolitis.

TABLE 13.1

GMP Herbal Medicines for a One-Year-Old Baby with Necrotizing Enterocolitis

Necrotizing enterocolitis (OrphaCode: 391673)

A disease with a prevalence of ~4 in 10,000

Not applicable

Premature birth

Small for gestational age, Neutropenia, Leukocytosis, Diarrhea, Hyponatremia, Abdominal distention, Food intolerance, Bloody diarrhea

Edema, Lethargy, Ascites, Gastroschisis, Abnormal heart morphology, Bradycardia, Thrombocytopenia, Acidosis, Metabolic acidosis, Vomiting, Apnea, Increased serum lactate, Peritonitis, Hypotension, Hyperglycemia, Disseminated intravascular coagulation, Temperature instability, Abnormal glucose homeostasis, Shock, Neonatal sepsis

Neonatal

(Continued)

DOI: 10.1201/9781032726625-13

TABLE 13.1 *(Continued)*

GMP Herbal Medicines for a One-Year-Old Baby with Necrotizing Enterocolitis

Diarrhea (D003967):

Gégēnhuángqínhuángliántāng 5g + huòxiāngzhèngqìsǎn 5-0g + bànxià 1-0g + fúlíng 1-0g + dàhuáng 0g.

Huángqíntāng 5g.

Báitóuwēngtāng 5g + gāncǎo 1g.

Bǎohéwán 5g + gāncǎo 0g.

Xiǎojiànzhōngtāng 5g + shānzhā 1g + shénqū 1g + màiyá 1g.

Hòupò 5g + zhǐshí 5g + xuánshēn 4g + dìhuáng 4g + màiméndōng 4g + bèimǔ 3-0g + huánglián 1-0g + dàhuáng 1-0g.

Gāncǎo 5g + hòupò 3g + zhǐshí 3g + dàhuáng 0g.

Gégēn 5g + huánglián 2g.

Báizhǐ 5g + shārén 5g + gāncǎo 5-4g + huángqín 3-0g + dàhuáng 0g.

Edema (D004487), Lethargy (D053609), Gastroschisis (756.73), Abnormal heart morphology (746.9), Thrombocytopenia (287.5), Vomiting (D014839), Apnea (D001049), Disseminated intravascular coagulation (286.6):

Bǎohéwán 5g + shēnlíngbáizhúsǎn 5g.

Bǎohéwán 5g + xiāngshāliùjūnzǐtāng 5g + bǔzhōngyìqìtāng 5-0g.

Xiāngshāliùjūnzǐtāng 5g + shēnlíngbáizhúsǎn 5-0g + bǔzhōngyìqìtāng 5-0g.

Bǔzhōngyìqìtāng 5g.

Sìjūnzǐtāng 5g + xiǎojiànzhōngtāng 5-0g.

Guìzhītāng 5g.

Gāncǎo 5g + shārén 5g + dàhuáng 2-0g.

Zhìgāncǎo 5g + shārén 5-0g + dàhuáng 1-0g.

Xuánshēn 5g + yùzhú 5g + dìhuáng 5g + shāshēn 5g + hòupò 5g + zhǐshí 5g + màiméndōng 5g + dàhuáng 1g.

Gégēn (cf. Sections 4.16, 5.13, and 8.10) has been used for digestive problems, including diarrhea, peptic ulcers, and cardiovascular diseases including essential hypertension and headaches (Wang, 2020; Zhang et al., 2013). Gégēnhuángqínhuángliántāng comprises Gégēn and is used for gastritis and duodenitis (cf. Sections 4.16 and 8.11). Guìzhītāng "dispels Wind from muscles, modulates nutrition and defense" and is believed to improve both the digestion and immunity of an "exterior deficient" patient suffering from a cold (cf. Sections 1.11, 2.30, and 4.1). Huángqíntāng (cf. Section 2.29) "clears heat, arrests diarrhea, harmonizes interior, and stops pain." Báitóuwēngtāng "clears heat, neutralized pathogens, cools Blood, and stops diarrhea." Both formulas are used today for gastritis and duodenitis (Wang, 2019).

13.2 RADIATION PROCTITIS

Radiation proctitis is inflammation and damage of the rectal mucosa as a complication of radiation therapy for malignancies in the pelvis such as cervical, prostate, and rectal cancers. Radiation proctitis can be acute or chronic, with chronic radiation proctitis showing symptoms six months or longer after the initial radiation.

Píngwèisǎn, containing Gāncǎo and Hòupò, is literally translated to "Stomach normalizing powder" and used nowadays for gastritis, esophageal reflux, gastric or duodenal ulcers, and acute or chronic enteritis (Riedlinger et al., 2001). Huòxiāngzhèngqìsǎn (cf. Sections 2.46 and 7.11), also

TABLE 13.2

GMP Herbal Medicines for a 65-Year-Old Adult with Radiation Proctitis

Radiation proctitis (OrphaCode: 70475)

A disease with a prevalence of ~3 in 10,000

Not applicable

Abnormality of the rectum, Hematochezia, Abnormality of the vasculature, Abnormality of connective tissue, Abnormality of gastrointestinal vasculature, Rectal abscess, Abnormal vascular morphology, Rectal fistula

Diarrhea, Intestinal obstruction, Arteritis, Tenesmus, Sepsis

Adult

(Continued)

TABLE 13.2 *(Continued)*

GMP Herbal Medicines for a 65-Year-Old Adult with Radiation Proctitis

Diarrhea (D003967), Intestinal obstruction (560.9):

Wǔlíngsǎn 5g + píngwèisǎn 5g + huòxiāngzhèngqìsǎn 5-0g + mùxiāng 1-0g + shārén 1-0g.	Gāncǎo 5g + hòupò 5-3g + zhǐshí 5-3g + dàhuáng 1-0g,
Wǔlíngsǎn 5g + huángqín 1g + dǐdāngtāng 0g + dàhuáng 0g.	Gāncǎo 5g + huángqín 5g + huánglián 5-1g + huángbò 5-0g + gégēn 5-0g + dàhuáng 0g.
Wǔlíngsǎn 5g + báisháo 1g + huángqín 1g + tiáowèichéngqìtāng 1-0g + dǐdāngtāng 0g + dàhuáng 0g.	

containing Gāncǎo and Hòupò, "resolves exterior, transforms dampness, regulates Qi, and harmonizes interior." It was shown to improve gut microbiome homeostasis in healthy adults and antibiotic-induced gut microbiota dysbiosis mice (Gao et al., 2022) and is used today for gastritis and duodenitis (Wang, 2019).

13.3 SERRATED POLYPOSIS SYNDROME

Serrated polyposis syndrome (SPS), previously called hyperplastic polyposis syndrome, is appearance of saw-edged polyps in the colon or rectum. People with SPS have no symptoms. However, some serrated polyp subtypes can turn into cancer. SPS is caused by gene mutations or CpG island hypermethylation. Table 13.3 shows herbal prescriptions for benign neoplasm of colon.

Bànxià (cf. Section 12.10) is used for flatulence, eructation, and gas pain (Wang, 2020), in addition to other conditions (cf. Section 2.3). Báijí (cf. Sections 4.28 and 9.7) has been serving as a hemostatic agent in TCM. The hemostatic compound and mechanism were elucidated by compound concentration dependent platelet aggregation in rat platelet-rich plasma (Dong et al., 2020). It is used today for peptic ulcers (Wang, 2020). Bànxiàxièxīntāng (cf. Sections 1.12 and 4.28), containing Bànxià, was shown to inhibit human colorectal adenocarcinoma transplanted tumor in nude mice (Yan et al., 2019) and is used for gastritis and duodenitis (Wang, 2019).

TABLE 13.3

GMP Herbal Medicines for a 55-Year-Old Adult with Benign Neoplasm of Colon

Serrated polyposis syndrome (OrphaCode: 157798)

A disease with a prevalence of ~3 in 10,000

Disease-causing germline mutation(s): ring finger protein 43 (*RNF43* / Entrez: 54894) at 17q22

Autosomal dominant, Multigenic/multifactorial, Unknown

Colorectal polyposis

Adenomatous colonic polyposis, Gastric diverticulum

Neoplasm of the large intestine

Adult, Elderly

Benign neoplasm of colon (211.3):

Bànxiàxièxīntāng 5g + sìnìtāng 4g + chuānliànzǐ 1g + dānshēn 1g + yánhúsuǒ 1g + yùjīn 1g.	Bànxià 5g + báizhú 5g + zhǐqiào 5g + huángqín 5g + hòupò 5-4g + báijí 5-0g + màiyá 5-0g + yīnchén 5-0g + chuānliànzǐ 2-0g.
Píngwèisǎn 5g + bǎohéwán 5g + xiāngshāliùjūnzǐtāng 5-0g + shēnlíngbáizhúsǎn 5-0g + huòxiāngzhèngqìsǎn 5-0g.	Běishāshēn 5g + yùzhú 5g + báizhú 5g + zhǐqiào 5g + huángqín 5g + fùzǐ 4g + bànxià 4-0g + yuǎnzhì 4-0g + màiyá 2-0g + hòupò 2-0g.
	Yùzhú 5g + báizhú 5g + huángqí 5g + dǎngshēn 5g + bànxià 4g + hòupò 4g + yuǎnzhì 4g.
Píngwèisǎn 5g + xiāngshāliùjūnzǐtāng 5g + xuánfùdàizhěshítāng 5-0g + bànxiàxièxīntāng 5-0g.	Báizhú 5g + hòupò 5g + zhǐqiào 5g + dǎngshēn 5g + bànxià 4g + guìzhī 4g + huángqín 4g + gānjiāng 1g.

13.4 CONGENITAL SUCRASE-ISOMALTASE DEFICIENCY

Congenital sucrase-isomaltase deficiency, also known as disaccharide intolerance, is a genetic condition affecting individuals to break down sucrose, found in fruits, and maltose, found in grains, into simple sugars. Congenital sucrase-isomaltase deficiency is caused by mutations in the gene, which instructs production of the enzyme responsible for the breaking down in the small intestine.

TABLE 13.4

GMP Herbal Medicines for a Two-Year-Old Child with Congenital Sucrase-Isomaltase Deficiency

Congenital sucrase-isomaltase deficiency (OrphaCode: 35122)

A disease with a prevalence of ~2 in 10,000

Disease-causing germline mutation(s): sucrase-isomaltase (*SI* / Entrez: 6476) at 3q26.1

Autosomal recessive

Diarrhea

Vomiting

Abdominal distention, Abdominal colic

Infancy, Childhood, Adolescent, Adult

Diarrhea (D003967):

Gégēnhuángqínhuángliántāng 5g + mùxiāng 1-0g + bànxià 1-0g + fúlíng 1-0g + dàhuáng 0g.

Báitóuwēngtāng 5g + huòxiāngzhèngqìsǎn 5g + mùxiāng 1g + shārén 1g.

Hòupò 5g + zhǐshí 5g + xuánshēn 4g + dìhuáng 4g + màiméndōng 4g + huánglián 1-0g + dàhuáng 1-0g.

Gégēn 5g + huánglián 3g + huángqín 2g + dàhuáng 0g.

Báizhǐ 5g + zhìgāncǎo 4g + shārén 4g + dàhuáng 0g.

Gāncǎo 5g + báizhǐ 5g + shārén 5g + dàhuáng 1-0g.

Vomiting (D014839):

Xiǎojiànzhōngtāng 5g + yùpíngfēngsǎn 5g.

Bǎohéwán 5g + xiāngshāliùjūnzǐtāng 5-0g + gāncǎo 1-0g + shānzhā 0g + shénqū 0g + màiyá 0g.

Xiǎojiànzhōngtāng 5g + shēnlíngbáizhúsǎn 5-0g + shānzhā 1-0g + shénqū 1-0g + màiyá 1-0g + jīnèijīn 1-0g.

Xuánshēn 5g + dìhuáng 5g + màiméndōng 5g + hòupò 5-1g + zhǐshí 5-1g + dàhuáng 1-0g.

Abdominal colic (D003085):

Bāzhèngsǎn 5g + wǔlínsǎn 5-0g + dǐdāngtāng 5-0g.

Wǔlínsǎn 5g + huàshícǎo 2-1g + jīnyínhuā 1-0g + huángqín 1-0g.

Zhǐshí 5g + chénpí 5g + lùlùtōng 5g + mùxiāng 4g + láifúzǐ 4g + dāngguīwěi 4g + shānzhā 2-0g.

Zhǐshí 5g + hòupò 5g + běishāshēn 4-0g + xuánshēn 4-0g + yùzhú 4-0g + dìhuáng 4-0g + màiméndōng 4-0g + dàhuáng 1-0g + huǒmárén 1-0g.

Zhǐshí 5g + hòupò 4g + fángfēng 2g + qiānghuó 2g + huángqín 2g + huánglián 2g + dàhuáng 1g.

Bāzhèngsǎn plus acupuncture (cf. Section 2.23) was reported to relieve pain in a man with chronic prostatitis with chronic pelvic pain syndrome (Ohlsen, 2013). Dǐdāngtāng was introduced in Section 2.14 to "remove heat and stasis in the lower body." Chénpí (cf. Sections 2.47 and 9.10) "regulates Qi, strengthens the Spleen, dries dampness, dissolves phlegm" and was reviewed and summarized to be antitumor, antioxidant, and anti-inflammatory; have a beneficial effect on the cardiovascular, digestive, and respiratory systems; and have a protective effect on the liver and nerves (Yu et al., 2018). It is used today for coughs, dyspepsia, and so on (Wang, 2020). Lùlùtōng (Fructus Liquidambaris) "dispels Wind, opens collaterals, promotes urination, and removes dampness."

13.5 HIRSCHSPRUNG DISEASE

Hirschsprung disease, also called congenital intestinal aganglionosis, is a birth defect where affected newborns miss nerves in a section of the intestine, usually the colon. As a result, the affected intestine does not move stools through the intestine, causing constipation. Hirschsprung disease is due to mutations in multiple genes that are involved in nerve cell signaling during embryonic development.

Rùnchángwán (cf. Section 4.25), translated to "intestines-soothing pill," was concluded to be efficient and safe for the treatment of functional constipation in a meta-analysis of randomized controlled

---

TABLE 13.5

GMP Herbal Medicines for a Three-Year-Old Boy with Hirschsprung Disease

Hirschsprung disease (OrphaCode: 388)

A disease with a prevalence of ~1 in 10,000

Disease-causing germline mutation(s): ATPase copper transporting alpha (*ATP7A* / Entrez: 538) at Xq21.1

Disease-causing germline mutation(s): ATP binding cassette subfamily D member 1 (*ABCD1* / Entrez: 215) at Xq28

Disease-causing germline mutation(s): erb-b2 receptor tyrosine kinase 2 (*ERBB2* / Entrez: 2064) at 17q12

Disease-causing germline mutation(s): erb-b2 receptor tyrosine kinase 3 (*ERBB3* / Entrez: 2065) at 12q13.2

Disease-causing germline mutation(s): smoothened, frizzled class receptor (*SMO* / Entrez: 6608) at 7q32.1

Disease-causing germline mutation(s): ret proto-oncogene (*RET* / Entrez: 5979) at 10q11.21

Major susceptibility factor: endothelin converting enzyme 1 (*ECE1* / Entrez: 1889) at 1p36.12

Major susceptibility factor: endothelin 3 (*EDN3* / Entrez: 1908) at 20q13.32

Major susceptibility factor: endothelin receptor type B (*EDNRB* / Entrez: 1910) at 13q22.3

Major susceptibility factor: glial cell derived neurotrophic factor (*GDNF* / Entrez: 2668) at 5p13.2

Major susceptibility factor: neurturin (*NRTN* / Entrez: 4902) at 19p13.3

Major susceptibility factor: semaphorin 3C (*SEMA3C* / Entrez: 10512) at 7q21.11

Major susceptibility factor: semaphorin 3D (*SEMA3D* / Entrez: 223117) at 7q21.11

Disease-causing germline mutation(s): sterol regulatory element binding transcription factor 1 (*SREBF1* / Entrez: 6720) at 17p11.2

Autosomal dominant, Autosomal recessive, Multigenic/multifactorial, Not applicable

Nausea and vomiting, Constipation, Abdominal pain, Aganglionic megacolon, Intestinal obstruction, Functional abnormality of the gastrointestinal tract

Weight loss

Sensorineural hearing impairment, Adducted thumb, Intellectual disability, Failure to thrive in infancy, Diarrhea, Short stature, Neoplasm of the thyroid gland, Sepsis, Intestinal polyposis

Neonatal, Infancy, Childhood

Constipation (564.0), Abdominal pain (D015746), Intestinal obstruction (560.9):

Bǎohéwán 5g + rùnchángwán 5g + xuánshēn 2-1g + dìhuáng 2-1g + màiméndōng 2-1g + huángqí 1-0g.

Gāncǎo 5g + dàhuáng 5-0g + huánglián 0g.

Xuánshēn 5g + dìhuáng 5g + hòupò 5g + zhǐshí 5g + màiméndōng 5g + dàhuáng 1g.

Xiǎochéngqìtāng 5g + xuánshēn 2-1g + dìhuáng 2-1g + màiméndōng 2-1g + yùzhú 2-0g + shāshēn 2-0g.

Dàchéngqìtāng 5g + xuánshēn 1g + dìhuáng 1g + màiméndōng 1g.

Weight loss (D015431):

Xiǎojiànzhōngtāng 5g + yùpíngfēngsǎn 5-0g + shēnlíngbáizhúsǎn 5-0g + gāncǎo 1-0g.

Zhìgāncǎo 5g + dàhuáng 0g.

Gāncǎo 5g + báizhǐ 5g + shārén 5g + dàhuáng 0g.

Guìzhītāng 5g + xìngrén 1g + hòupò 1g.

Hòupò 5g + zhǐshí 5g + xuánshēn 4-3g + dìhuáng 4-3g + màiméndōng 4-3g + dàhuáng 1-0g.

Sensorineural hearing impairment (389.1), Intellectual disability (D008607), Diarrhea (D003967), Neoplasm of the thyroid gland (193):

Xìngsūyǐnyòukē 5g + xīnyíqīngfèitāng 5g.

Shēnlíngbáizhúsǎn 5g + bǎohéwán 4-0g + shānzhā 1-0g + shénqū 1-0g + màiyá 1-0g + wūméi 1-0g + jīnèijīn 1-0g.

Gāncǎo 5g + shārén 5g + báizhǐ 5-0g + huángqín 5-0g + dàhuáng 0g.

trials (Zhao et al., 2021). Xiǎojiànzhōngtāng (cf. Sections 5.23 and 9.9) "warms interior, replenishes deficiency, harmonizes the Spleen/Stomach, and relieves acute abdominal pain." It was shown to increase body weight and improve the histopathological manifestations of rats with gastric precancerous lesions (J. Zhang et al., 2023); it is used for disorders of functions of the stomach (Wang, 2019).

13.6   IDIOPATHIC ACHALASIA

Idiopathic achalasia, or achalasia cardia, is a motor disorder of the esophagus characterized by impairment of the involuntary contraction and relaxation movement of the muscles in the esophagus. The precise etiology of idiopathic achalasia is not known, but autoimmunity, viral infection, and neurodegeneration are of suspicion.

TABLE 13.6
GMP Herbal Medicines for a 43-Year-Old Adult with Idiopathic Achalasia

Idiopathic achalasia (OrphaCode: 930)

A disease with a prevalence of ~8 in 100,000

Disease-causing germline mutation(s): cytokine receptor like factor 1 (*CRLF1* / Entrez: 9244) at 19p12

Major susceptibility factor: major histocompatibility complex, class II, DQ alpha 1 (*HLA-DQA1* / Entrez: 3117) at 6p21.32

Major susceptibility factor: major histocompatibility complex, class II, DQ beta 1 (*HLA-DQB1* / Entrez: 3119) at 6p21.32

Disease-causing germline mutation(s): nitric oxide synthase 1 (*NOS1* / Entrez: 4842) at 12q24.22

Autosomal recessive, Not applicable

Dysphagia

Weight loss, Gastroesophageal reflux, Bronchitis, Cough, Chest pain

Recurrent aspiration pneumonia, Malnutrition, Wheezing, Decreased prealbumin level

All ages

Weight loss (D015431), Gastroesophageal reflux (530.81), Bronchitis (466.0, 490, 491), Cough (D003371), Chest pain (D002637):

Guìzhītāng 5g + xìngrén 1g + hòupò 1g + bànxià 1-0g + fúlíng 1-0g + dàhuáng 0g. Xiǎoqīnglóngtāng 5g + xuánfùdàizhěshítāng 4g + báijí 1g + hǎipiāoxiāo 1g.	Zhìgāncǎo 5g + wǔwèizǐ 5-3g + bànxià 5-3g + cháihú 5-3g + gānjiāng 5-3g + huángqín 5-3g + dàhuáng 1-0g.
Wheezing (D012135): Bànxiàhòupòtāng 5g + màiméndōngtāng 5g. Màiméndōngtāng 5g + gégēntāng 5g + niúbàngzǐ 2g + xuánshēn 2g + jiégěng 2g + sāngbáipí 2g + jīngjiè 2g + chántuì 2g. Màiméndōngtāng 5g + xiǎoqīnglóngtāng 4g + xìngrén 1g + hòupò 1g. Màiméndōngtāng 5g + xīnyíqīngfèitāng 3g + gāncǎo 1g + jiégěng 1g.	Jiégěng 5g + gāncǎo 4g + xuánshēn 3g + mǔlì 3g + bèimǔ 3g + liánqiáo 3-2g + zhīzǐ 2g. Jiégěng 5g + gāncǎo 4-3g + wǔwèizǐ 3-2g + fúlíng 2-0g + xìxīn 1g + gānjiāng 0g.

Guìzhītāng (cf. Sections 1.11, 1.50, 2.30, 4.1, and 7.6) is believed to improve both the immune and digestive functions of the patient. Bànxiàhòupòtāng, containing Bànxià and Hòupò, "moves Qi, disperses depression, lowers ascending, and dissipates phlegm." It was shown to improve hoarse voice, foreign body sensation in the throat and esophagus, and swallowing reflex disorder in healthy individuals by stimulation of neuropeptidergic nerves locally (Naito et al., 2003); it is used today for chronic bronchitis and diseases of the esophagus (Wang, 2019). Màiméndōngtāng was introduced in Section 1.61 for symptoms involving the respiratory system and other chest symptoms.

13.7   FAMILIAL ADENOMATOUS POLYPOSIS

Familial adenomatous polyposis, also known as colorectal adenomatous polyposis, is characterized by multiple precancerous polyps in the epithelium of the colon and rectum. The number of polyps increases with age and can reach thousands. Familial adenomatous polyposis is caused

TABLE 13.7

GMP Herbal Medicines for a 39-Year-Old Adult with Familial Adenomatous Polyposis

Familial adenomatous polyposis (OrphaCode: 733)

A disease with a prevalence of ~5 in 100,000

Role: the phenotype of APC regulator of WNT signaling pathway (*APC* / Entrez: 324) at 5q22.2

Autosomal dominant, Autosomal recessive

Colon cancer, Adenomatous colonic polyposis, Neoplasm of the gastrointestinal tract, Congenital hypertrophy of retinal pigment epithelium, Desmoid tumors, Colorectal polyposis

Abnormality of the dentition, Multiple gastric polyps, Duodenal polyposis, Osteoma

Unerupted tooth, Abnormality of the thyroid gland, Papillary thyroid carcinoma, Duodenal adenocarcinoma, Angiofibromas, Odontoma, Increased number of teeth, Neoplasm of the adrenal gland, Abnormality of the cementum

Adult

Colon cancer (153), Neoplasm of the gastrointestinal tract (239.0):

Sānzhǒngkuìjiāntāng 5g + huáihuā 2-1g + cāngzhú 2-1g.

Sānzhǒngkuìjiāntāng 5g + bànzhǐlián 2g + huáihuā 2g + báihuāshéshécǎo 2-0g.

Bànzhǐlián 5g + báihuāshéshécǎo 5-0g.
Bànzhǐlián 5g + huáihuā 5-0g.
Bànzhǐlián 5g + shāndòugēn 4-0g.

Abnormality of the thyroid gland (246.9), Duodenal adenocarcinoma (152.0), Neoplasm of the adrenal gland (194.0):

Sānzhǒngkuìjiāntāng 5g + bànzhǐlián 2g + báihuāshéshécǎo 2-0g.

Jiāwèixiāoyáosǎn 5g + xiāngshāliùjūnzǐtāng 5g.

Jiāwèixiāoyáosǎn 5g + xuèfǔzhúyūtāng 5g + dānshēn 1g + mǔlì 1g + bèimǔ 1g + xiāngfù 1g + xiàkūcǎo 1g.

Jiāwèixiāoyáosǎn 5g + shēnlíngbáizhúsǎn 5g + huòxiāngzhèngqìsǎn 5g + báihuāshéshécǎo 1g + xiàkūcǎo 1g + éshù 1g.

Jiāwèixiāoyáosǎn 5g + guìzhīfúlíngwán 4g + dānshēn 1g + bànzhǐlián 1g + báihuāshéshécǎo 1g + bèimǔ 1g + xiāngfù 1g + hǎipiāoxiāo 1g.

Báizhú 5g + fùzǐ 5g + cháihú 5g + báisháo 4g + fúlíng 4g + tiānhuā 2g + dǎngshēn 2g + guìzhī 2g + huángqín 2g + wǔwèizǐ 2-0g + xìxīn 2-0g + gāncǎo 1g + mǔlì 1g + gānjiāng 1g.

Xuánshēn 5g + yùzhú 5g + dìhuáng 5g + hòupò 5g + zhǐshí 5g + màiméndōng 5g + dàhuáng 0g.

by microdeletion in the *APC* gene, which is a tumor suppressor gene controlling how often a cell divides.

Bànzhǐlián "defeats toxins, resists cancer, reduces swelling, dissolves congelation, dispels stasis, stops pain" and was shown to inhibit colon tumor growth and metastasis in tumor-bearing mice (Yue et al., 2021). Báihuāshéshécǎo "clears heat, neutralizes pathogens, promotes urination, relieves stranguria" and was shown to suppress colorectal cancer growth in mice (Feng et al., 2017). They were introduced in Section 4.4 for cancers. Huáihuā (cf. Section 12.7) was shown to decrease cell viability and increase apoptosis in human colorectal cancer cells in a dose-dependent manner (Lee et al., 2015). Guìzhīfúlíngwán, introduced in Section 1.62 for ovarian cancer, was shown to induce apoptosis in uterine myoma cells collected from patients with uterine leiomyoma (Lee et al., 2019).

REFERENCES

Dong, L., Liu, X., Wu, S., Yao, M., Liu, M., Dong, Y., Huang, J., Li, Y., Huang, Y., Wang, Y., & Liao, S. (2020). Rhizoma Bletillae polysaccharide elicits hemostatic effects in platelet-rich plasma by activating adenosine diphosphate receptor signaling pathway. *Biomedicine & Pharmacotherapy, 130*, 110537. https://doi.org/10.1016/j.biopha.2020.110537

Feng, J., Jin, Y., Peng, J., Wei, L., Cai, Q., Yan, Z., Lai, Z., & Lin, J. (2017). *Hedyotis diffusa willd* extract suppresses colorectal cancer growth through multiple cellular pathways. *Oncology Letters, 14*(6), 8197–8205. https://doi.org/10.3892/ol.2017.7244

Gao, M., Duan, X., Liu, X., Luo, S., Tang, S., Nie, H., Yan, J., Zou, Z., Chen, C., Qi, Y., & Qiu, J. (2022). Modulatory effects of Huoxiang Zhengqi oral Liquid on gut microbiome homeostasis based on healthy adults and antibiotic-induced gut microbial dysbiosis mice model. *Frontiers in Pharmacology, 13*, 841990. https://doi.org/10.3389/fphar.2022.841990

Lee, J. W., Park, G. H., Park, G. H., Song, H. M., Kim, M. K., Kwon, M. J., Koo, J. S., Lee, J. R., Lee, M. H., & Jeong, J. B. (2015). Anti-cancer activity of the flower bud of *Sophora japonica* L. through upregulating activating transcription factor 3 in human colorectal cancer cells. *Korean Journal of Plant Resources*, *28*(3), 297–304. https://doi.org/10.7732/kjpr.2015.28.3.297

Lee, S. M., Choi, E. S., Ha, E., Ji, K. Y., Shin, S. J., & Jung, J. (2019). Gyejibongnyeong-Hwan (Gui Zhi Fu Ling Wan) ameliorates human uterine myomas via apoptosis. *Frontiers in Pharmacology*, *10*, 1105. https://doi.org/10.3389/fphar.2019.01105

Naito, T., Itoh, H., & Takeyama, M. (2003). Effects of Hange-koboku-to (Banxia-houpo-tang) on neuropeptide levels in human plasma and saliva. *Biological & Pharmaceutical Bulletin*, *26*(11), 1609–1613. https://doi.org/10.1248/bpb.26.1609

Ohlsen, B. A. (2013). Acupuncture and traditional Chinese medicine for the management of a 35-year-old man with chronic prostatitis with chronic pelvic pain syndrome. *Journal of Chiropractic Medicine*, *12*(3), 182–190. https://doi.org/10.1016/j.jcm.2013.10.004

Riedlinger, J., Tan, P. W., & Lu, W. (2001). Ping Wei San, a Chinese medicine for gastrointestinal disorders. *Annals of Pharmacotherapy*, *35*(2), 228–235. https://doi.org/10.1345/aph.10122

Wang, S.-C. (2019). Therapeutic classes of CHEG formulas. In S.-C. Wang (Ed.), *Clinical herbal prescriptions: Principles and practices of herbal formulations from deep learning health insurance herbal prescription big data* (pp. 16–89). World Scientific Publishing. https://doi.org/10.1142/11211

Wang, S.-C. (2020). Modern therapeutic uses of CHEG herbs and herb pairs. In S.-C. Wang (Ed.), *Veterinary herbal pharmacopoeia* (pp. 35–233). Nova Science Publishers. https://doi.org/10.52305/GHTR1903

Yan, S., Yue, Y., Wang, J., Li, W., Sun, M., Zeng, L., & Wang, X. (2019). Banxia Xiexin decoction, a traditional Chinese medicine, alleviates colon cancer in nude mice. *Annals of Translational Medicine*, *7*(16), 375. https://doi.org/10.21037/atm.2019.07.26

Yue, G. G., Chan, Y., Liu, W., Gao, S., Wong, C., Lee, J. K., Lau, K., & Lau, C. B. (2021). Effectiveness of *Scutellaria barbata* water extract on inhibiting colon tumor growth and metastasis in tumor-bearing mice. *Phytotherapy Research*, *35*(1), 361–373. https://doi.org/10.1002/ptr.6808

Yu, X., Sun, S., Guo, Y., Liu, Y., Yang, D., Li, G., & Lü, S. (2018). Citri Reticulatae Pericarpium (Chenpi): Botany, ethnopharmacology, phytochemistry, and pharmacology of a frequently used traditional Chinese medicine. *Journal of Ethnopharmacology*, *220*, 265–282. https://doi.org/10.1016/j.jep.2018.03.031

Zhang, J., Bao, S., Chen, J., Chen, T., Wei, H., Zhou, X., Li, J., & Su, Y. (2023). Xiaojianzhong decoction prevents gastric precancerous lesions in rats by inhibiting autophagy and glycolysis in gastric mucosal cells. *World Journal of Gastrointestinal Oncology*, *15*(3), 464–489. https://doi.org/10.4251/wjgo.v15.i3.464

Zhang, Z., Lam, T., & Zuo, Z. (2013). Radix *Puerariae*: An overview of its chemistry, pharmacology, pharmacokinetics, and clinical use. *Journal of Clinical Pharmacology*, *53*(8), 787–811. https://doi.org/10.1002/jcph.96

Zhao, X., Fang, Y., Ye, J., Qin, F., Lu, W., & Gong, H. (2021). A meta-analysis of randomized controlled trials of a traditional Chinese medicine prescription, modified RunChang-Tang, in treating functional constipation. *Medicine*, *100*(20), e25760. https://doi.org/10.1097/md.0000000000025760

14 GMP Herbal Medicine for Rare Cardiac Diseases

Cardiac diseases refer to problems with the heart. The causes of heart diseases include hypercholesterolemia, hypertension, inactivity, obesity, diabetes, and genetics. Many of the rare cardiac diseases of this chapter are inherited but adult onset.

Dried Ginger Rhizome (Gānjiāng), Processed Licorice Root (Zhìgāncǎo), Aconite Accessory Root (Fùzǐ), Codonopsis Root (Dǎngshēn), Salvia Root (Dānshēn), Rhubarb Root and Rhizome (Dàhuáng), Licorice Root (Gāncǎo), Pinellia Tuber (Bànxià), Poria (Fúlíng), Chinese Senega Root (Yuǎnzhì), and White Atractylodis (Báizhú) are the most frequently used single herb products for the rare heart diseases, while Prepared Licorice Decoction (Zhìgāncǎotāng), Pulse Generating Decoction (Shēngmàiyǐn), Emperor of Heaven's Pill to Tonify the Heart (Tiānwángbǔxīndān), Bupleurum plus Dragon Bone and Oyster Shell Decoction (Cháihújiālónggǔmǔlìtāng), Free and Easy Wanderer Plus (Augmented Rambling Powder; Jiāwèixiāoyáosǎn), Tonify the Middle and Augment the Qi Decoction (Bǔzhōngyìqìtāng), Poria, Cinnamon, Atractylodis and Licorice Decoction (Língguìshùgāntāng), Licorice, Wheat and Jujube Decoction (Gāncǎoxiǎomàidàzǎotāng), Frigid Extremities Decoction (Sìnìtāng), Drive Out Stasis from the Mansion of Blood Decoction (Xuèfǔzhúyūtāng), Minor Bupleurum Decoction (Xiǎocháihútāng), and Anemarrhena, Phellodendron and Rehmannia Pill (Zhībódìhuángwán) are the most frequently discussed multi-herb formulas for the conditions in this chapter.

The heart in TCM governs not only heartbeat and blood circulation but also the mind. Therefore, insomnia is treated in TCM by herbs and formulas that enter into the heart meridian.

14.1 ROMANO-WARD SYNDROME

Romano-Ward syndrome is caused by mutations in genes whose products interact with the ion channels in the membranes of heart muscle cells, resulting in changes in electrical conduction between the cells and a prolonged time interval between heartbeats. Its symptoms depend on the genes that mutated and its severity correlates with the number of mutated genes.

TABLE 14.1

GMP Herbal Medicines for a 12-Year-Old Child with Romano-Ward Syndrome

Romano-Ward syndrome (OrphaCode: 101016)

A disease with a prevalence of ~4 in 10,000

Disease-causing germline mutation(s): triadin (*TRDN* / Entrez: 10345) at 6q22.31

Disease-causing germline mutation(s) (loss of function): potassium voltage-gated channel subfamily H member 2 (*KCNH2* / Entrez: 3757) at 7q36.1

Disease-causing germline mutation(s) (loss of function): potassium voltage-gated channel subfamily Q member 1 (*KCNQ1* / Entrez: 3784) at 11p15.5-p15.4

Disease-causing germline mutation(s) (gain of function): caveolin 3 (*CAV3* / Entrez: 859) at 3p25.3

Disease-causing germline mutation(s) (loss of function): ankyrin 2 (*ANK2* / Entrez: 287) at 4q25-q26

Disease-causing germline mutation(s) (loss of function): potassium voltage-gated channel subfamily E regulatory subunit 1 (*KCNE1* / Entrez: 3753) at 21q22.12

Disease-causing germline mutation(s) (loss of function): potassium voltage-gated channel subfamily E regulatory subunit 2 (*KCNE2* / Entrez: 9992) at 21q22.11

(Continued)

DOI: 10.1201/9781032726625-14

TABLE 14.1 *(Continued)*

GMP Herbal Medicines for a 12-Year-Old Child with Romano-Ward Syndrome

Disease-causing germline mutation(s) (gain of function): sodium voltage-gated channel alpha subunit 5 (*SCN5A* / Entrez: 6331) at 3p22.2

Disease-causing germline mutation(s) (loss of function): A-kinase anchoring protein 9 (*AKAP9* / Entrez: 10142) at 7q21.2

Disease-causing germline mutation(s) (gain of function): sodium voltage-gated channel beta subunit 4 (*SCN4B* / Entrez: 6330) at 11q23.3

Disease-causing germline mutation(s) (gain of function): syntrophin alpha 1 (*SNTA1* / Entrez: 6640) at 20q11.21

Disease-causing germline mutation(s) (loss of function): potassium inwardly rectifying channel subfamily J member 5 (*KCNJ5* / Entrez: 3762) at 11q24.3

Modifying germline mutation: nitric oxide synthase 1 adaptor protein (*NOS1AP* / Entrez: 9722) at 1q23.3

Disease-causing germline mutation(s): calmodulin 1 (*CALM1* / Entrez: 801) at 14q32.11

Disease-causing germline mutation(s): calmodulin 2 (*CALM2* / Entrez: 805) at 2p21

Disease-causing germline mutation(s) (loss of function): sodium voltage-gated channel alpha subunit 10 (*SCN10A* / Entrez: 6336) at 3p22.2

Disease-causing germline mutation(s) (loss of function): T-box transcription factor 5 (*TBX5* / Entrez: 6910) at 12q24.21

Disease-causing germline mutation(s): calcium voltage-gated channel subunit alpha1 C (*CACNA1C* / Entrez: 775) at 12p13.33

Disease-causing germline mutation(s): calmodulin 3 (*CALM3* / Entrez: 808) at 19q13.32

Autosomal dominant, Autosomal recessive

Prolonged QTc interval

Syncope, Sinus bradycardia, Abnormal T-wave

Seizure, Sudden cardiac death, Torsades de pointes, Ventricular arrhythmia, Abnormal autonomic nervous system physiology, Abnormal cardiac exercise stress test

All ages

Syncope (D013575):

Shēngmàiyǐn 5g + xuèfǔzhúyūtāng 5g + sānqī 1g + dānshēn 1g.

Shēngmàiyǐn 5g + bǔzhōngyìqìtāng 5g + xuèfǔzhúyūtāng 4-0g + dānshēn 1-0g + yùjīn 1-0g + xiāngfù 1-0g + yìmǔcǎo 1-0g.

Shēngmàiyǐn 5g + zhìgāncǎotāng 5g + língguìshùgāntāng 5-0g + zīshèntōngěrtāng 5-0g + yǎngxīntāng 5-0g.

Shēngmàiyǐn 5g + zhìgāncǎotāng 5-3g + bǔzhōngyìqìtāng 5-0g + chuānqī 1-0g + dānshēn 1-0g.

Zhìgāncǎo 5g + fùzǐ 4-2g + dǎngshēn 2-0g + gānjiāng 0g.

Zhìgāncǎo 5g + dǎngshēn 5-2g + bànxià 3-1g + hòupò 3-1g + chuānqī 2-0g + shēngjiāng 0g + dàhuáng 0g.

Zhìgāncǎo 5g + dǎngshēn 5-4g + hòupò 5-2g + bànxià 3-2g + gānjiāng 0g + dàhuáng 0g.

Seizure (345.9), Torsades de pointes (D016171) [Long QT syndrome (426.82)]:

Cháihújiālónggǔmǔlìtāng 5g + wēndǎntāng 5g + shíchāngpú 1g + yuǎnzhì 1g + tiānmá 1-0g + gōuténg 1-0g + yùjīn 1-0g.

Cháihújiālónggǔmǔlìtāng 5g + gāncǎoxiǎomàidàzǎotāng 4-2g + yuǎnzhì 1g + shíchāngpú 1-0g + gōuténg 1-0g + fúshén 1-0g + tiānmá 1-0g.

Tiānwángbǔxīndān 5g + cháihújiālónggǔmǔlìtāng 5-0g + bǔyánghuánwǔtāng 5-0g + tiānmá 1-0g + shíchāngpú 1-0g + yuǎnzhì 1-0g.

Tiānwángbǔxīndān 5g + yìgānsǎn 5g + shíchāngpú 1g + mǔlì 1g + yuǎnzhì 1g.

Xuánshēn 5g + dìhuáng 5g + màiméndōng 5g + hòupò 5-1g + zhǐshí 5-0g + dàhuáng 1-0g + hòupò 0g.

Huángqí 5g + chìsháo 1g + fángfēng 1g + dàhuáng 0g.

Gāncǎo 5g + báizhǐ 5g + shārén 5g + huángqín 5g + dàhuáng 0g.

Báizhǐ 5g + zhìgāncǎo 4g + shārén 4g + huángqín 4g + dàhuáng 0g.

Shēngmàiyǐn, translated to "pulse generating drink," was introduced in Sections 2.39, 2.55, 3.20, and 6.15 to be cardio- and neuroprotective. Active compounds from Xuánshēn (cf. Section 1.3) were shown in hypertensive rats to prevent ventricular remodeling (Zhang et al., 2016), the persistency of which leads to heart failure. Tiānwángbǔxīndān, comprising Xuánshēn and Màiméndōng, was introduced in Section 3.15 for cardiac dysrhythmias. Adjunctive use of Dānshēn, Huángqí, Dàhuáng, Fùzǐ, Zhìgāncǎotāng, Xuèfǔzhúyūtāng, Tiānwángbǔxīndān, or Shēngmàiyǐn was found to improve the survival of patients with ischemic heart disease in a cohort study (Hung et al., 2022).

14.2 PLACENTAL INSUFFICIENCY

Placental insufficiency, or uteroplacental vascular insufficiency, is insufficient oxygen and nutrient supply to the fetus through the placenta during pregnancy, leading to fetal hypoxemia and fetal growth restriction that can be diagnosed by Doppler ultrasounds for fetal blood flow or by a decelerated fetal heart rate. Disturbances in the blood flow to the placenta cause placental insufficiency. Maternal preeclampsia, advanced maternal age, smoking, alcoholism, and drug use during pregnancy are risk factors.

TABLE 14.2

GMP Herbal Medicines for a 40-Year-Old Woman with Placental Insufficiency

Placental insufficiency (OrphaCode: 439167)

A clinical syndrome with a prevalence of ~3 in 10,000

Not applicable

Abnormality of the placenta

Intrauterine growth retardation, Small for gestational age, Proportionate short stature, Small placenta, Abnormal umbilical cord blood vessels, Hypoxemia

Autism, Autistic behavior, Systemic lupus erythematosus, Antiphospholipid antibody positivity, Neurodevelopmental abnormality

Insulin resistance, Abnormal heart morphology, Abnormal lung morphology, Spontaneous abortion, Maternal hypertension, Cerebral palsy, Eclampsia, Preeclampsia

Adult

Hypoxemia (D000860):

Sìnìtāng 5g + bànxià 1g + rénshēn 1-0g + shēngjiāng 1-0g + guìzhī 1-0g + xìxīn 1-0g + dàhuáng 0g.

Sìnìtāng 5g + guìzhī 2g + máhuáng 1g + xìxīn 1g + dàhuáng 0g.

Lǐzhōngtāng 5g + bànxià 1g + shārén 1g + fúlíng 1g + dàhuáng 0g.

Gānjiāng 5g + bànxià 4-2g + rénshēn 4-0g + dàhuáng 0g.

Autism (299.0), Systemic lupus erythematosus (710.0):

Tiānwángbǔxīndān 5g + jiāwèixiāoyáosǎn 5g + gāncǎoxiǎomàidàzǎotāng 5g + cháihújiālónggǔmǔlìtāng 5-0g.

Jiāwèixiāoyáosǎn 5g + zhībódìhuángwán 5g + gāncǎoxiǎomàidàzǎotāng 5-0g + cháihújiālónggǔmǔlìtāng 5-0g + nǚzhēnzǐ 1-0g + hànliáncǎo 1-0g.

Gāncǎoxiǎomàidàzǎotāng 5-4g + cháihújiālónggǔmǔlìtāng 5-4g + zhībódìhuángwán 5-0g + yuǎnzhì 2-1g + shíchāngpú 2-0g + dānshēn 2-0g + yèjiāoténg 1-0g + fúshén 1-0g + suānzǎorén 1-0g + zhúrú 1-0g + gōuténg 1-0g.

Tiānwángbǔxīndān 5g + zhībódìhuángwán 5g + cháihújiālónggǔmǔlìtāng 5g + shíchāngpú 1g + yuǎnzhì 1g + suānzǎorén 1g.

Báizhú 5g + fùzǐ 5g + cháihú 5g + báisháo 4g + fúlíng 4g + tiānhuā 2g + dǎngshēn 2g + guìzhī 2g + huángqín 2g + wǔwèizǐ 2-0g + xìxīn 2-0g + shēngjiāng 2-0g + gāncǎo 1g + mǔlì 1g + gānjiāng 1g + dàhuáng 1-0g.

Huángqín 5g + báizhú 5-3g + shārén 3-2g + gāncǎo 3-0g + tiānhuā 2-1g + xìxīn 1-0g + dàhuáng 0g.

Běishāshēn 5g + yùzhú 5g + hòupò 5g + zhǐshí 5g + dàhuáng 1g.

Abnormal heart morphology (746.9), Cerebral palsy (343.0, 343.3, 343.2):

Jiāwèixiāoyáosǎn 5g + dāngguīsháoyàosǎn 5g + dānshēn 1g + xiāngfù 1g + yìmǔcǎo 1g + yuǎnzhì 1-0g + zélán 1-0g + yùjīn 1-0g.

Tiānwángbǔxīndān 5g + jiāwèixiāoyáosǎn 5g + yèjiāoténg 1g + dānshēn 1-0g + mǔlì 1-0g + huángliánshàngqīngwán 1-0g + yùjīn 1-0g + ējiāo 1-0g + yínyánghuò 1-0g + mázǐrénwán 1-0g.

Dāngguīsìnìtāng 5g + shēngjiāng 1g + wúzhūyú 1g.

Rénshēnyǎngróngtāng 5g + zuǒguīwán 5g + dùzhòng 1g + yínyánghuò 1g + tùsīzǐ 1g.

Rénshēnyǎngróngtāng 5g + jiāwèixiāoyáosǎn 5g + tiānmá 1g + niúxī 1g + yìmǔcǎo 1g + zélán 1g.

Bànxià 5g + dāngguī 5g + gāncǎo 3g + báisháo 3g + chìsháo 3g + guìzhī 3g + huángbò 3g + acupuncture.

Bànxià 5g + ējiāo 5g + zǐcǎo 5g + dǎngshēn 5g + fùzǐ 3g + gānjiāng 3g.

Báizhú 5g + fùzǐ 5g + cháihú 5g + báisháo 4g + fúlíng 4g + tiānhuā 2g + dǎngshēn 2g + guìzhī 2g + huángqín 2g + wúzhūyú 2-0g + shēngjiāng 2-0g + gāncǎo 1g + mǔlì 1g + gānjiāng 1g + huánglián 1-0g.

Dàzǎo 5g + dānshēn 5g + gāncǎo 5g + báisháo 5g + bǎihé 5g + xìngrén 5g + fúxiāomài 5g + fúshén 5g + chénpí 5g + màiméndōng 5g + suānzǎorén 5g.

Sìnìtāng was introduced in Sections 1.46 and 1.70 for heart diseases. Sìnìtāng was also shown to ameliorate interrelated lung injury in septic mice (Wang et al., 2020). Heart and lung diseases are common causes of hypoxemia. Dāngguīsháoyàosǎn (cf. Section 3.22) has been a popular formula in gynecologic and obstetric TCM (Lee et al., 2016). It is used today for disorders of menstruation and other abnormal bleeding from the female genital tract (Wang, 2019). Zǐcǎo (Radix Arnebiae) "cools Blood, enlivens Blood, removes toxins, promotes eruptions" and was shown to attenuate atrial injury in rats with atrial fibrillation (Zhou et al., 2020).

14.3 BRUGADA SYNDROME

Brugada syndrome is a subtype of irregular heartbeat called idiopathic ventricular fibrillation, Brugada type. Brugada syndrome was first described and associated with mutations of the *SCN5A* gene that encodes sodium ion channels of heart muscle cells. Today, inherited or *de novo* defects in many other ions transport genes are associated with Brugada syndrome, which manifests a fast heartbeat during sleep or at rest.

Zhìgāncǎo (cf. Sections 1.11, 1.25, 1.68, and 2.55), making up Zhìgāncǎotāng (cf. Section 14.1), invigorates Qi and restores the pulse (Zhang et al., 2018). Xuèfǔzhúyūtāng, translated to "blood-mansion stasis-dispersing decoction," benefits the cardiovascular system (cf. Sections 1.70, 2.45,

---

TABLE 14.3
GMP Herbal Medicines for a 19-Year-Old Man with Brugada Syndrome

Brugada syndrome (OrphaCode: 130)

A disease with a prevalence of ~2 in 10,000

Candidate gene tested: hyperpolarization activated cyclic nucleotide gated potassium channel 4 (*HCN4* / Entrez: 10021) at 15q24.1

Candidate gene tested: ATP binding cassette subfamily C member 9 (*ABCC9* / Entrez: 10060) at 12p12.1

Candidate gene tested: calcium voltage-gated channel auxiliary subunit beta 2 (*CACNB2* / Entrez: 783) at 10p12

Disease-causing germline mutation(s): calcium voltage-gated channel subunit alpha1 C (*CACNA1C* / Entrez: 775) at 12p13.33

Candidate gene tested: calcium voltage-gated channel auxiliary subunit alpha2delta 1 (*CACNA2D1* / Entrez: 781) at 7q21.11

Candidate gene tested: potassium voltage-gated channel subfamily E regulatory subunit 3 (*KCNE3* / Entrez: 10008) at 11q13.4

Candidate gene tested: glycerol-3-phosphate dehydrogenase 1 like (*GPD1L* / Entrez: 23171) at 3p22.3

Candidate gene tested: potassium voltage-gated channel subfamily D member 3 (*KCND3* / Entrez: 3752) at 1p13.2

Candidate gene tested: sodium voltage-gated channel beta subunit 3 (*SCN3B* / Entrez: 55800) at 11q24.1

Candidate gene tested: transient receptor potential cation channel subfamily M member 4 (*TRPM4* / Entrez: 54795) at 19q13.33

Candidate gene tested: sodium voltage-gated channel alpha subunit 10 (*SCN10A* / Entrez: 6336) at 3p22.2

Disease-causing germline mutation(s): sarcolemma associated protein (*SLMAP* / Entrez: 7871) at 3p14.3

Candidate gene tested: sodium voltage-gated channel beta subunit 1 (*SCN1B* / Entrez: 6324) at 19q13.11

Candidate gene tested: A-kinase anchoring protein 9 (*AKAP9* / Entrez: 10142) at 7q21.2

Candidate gene tested: potassium voltage-gated channel subfamily E regulatory subunit 5 (*KCNE5* / Entrez: 23630) at Xq23

Candidate gene tested: RAN guanine nucleotide release factor (*RANGRF* / Entrez: 29098) at 17p13.1

Disease-causing germline mutation(s): sodium voltage-gated channel alpha subunit 5 (*SCN5A* / Entrez: 6331) at 3p22.2

Disease-causing germline mutation(s): sodium channel epithelial 1 subunit alpha (*SCNN1A* / HGNC:10599) at 12p13

Disease-causing germline mutation(s): semaphorin 3A (*SEMA3A* / Entrez: 10371) at 7q21.11

Disease-causing germline mutation(s): sodium voltage-gated channel beta subunit 2 (*SCN2B* / Entrez: 6327) at 11q23.3

Candidate gene tested: potassium inwardly rectifying channel subfamily J member 8 (*KCNJ8* / Entrez: 3764) at 12p12.1

Candidate gene tested: plakophilin 2 (*PKP2* / Entrez: 5318) at 12p11.21

Autosomal dominant, Not applicable

Right bundle branch block, ST segment elevation, Syncope, Cardiac arrest

Tachycardia, Ventricular fibrillation, Paroxysmal ventricular tachycardia, Supraventricular tachycardia, Sick sinus syndrome, First-degree atrioventricular block

Childhood, Adult

(Continued)

TABLE 14.3 *(Continued)*
GMP Herbal Medicines for a 19-Year-Old Man with Brugada Syndrome

Syncope (D013575), Cardiac arrest (427.5):

Shēngmàiyǐn 5g + zhìgāncǎotāng 5g + xuèfǔzhúyūtāng 5-0g.	Zhìgāncǎo 5g + fùzǐ 5-3g + dǎngshēn 5-0g + gānjiāng 1-0g.
Shēngmàiyǐn 5g + zhìgāncǎotāng 5g + bǔzhōngyìqìtāng 5-0g + dānshēn 2-1g + chuānqí 1-0g + yùjīn 1-0g.	

Tachycardia (D013610) [Tachycardia, unspecified (785.0)]:

Tiānwángbǔxīndān 5g + jiāwèixiāoyáosǎn 5g.	Zhìgāncǎo 5g + jiégěng 5g + xuánshēn 3g + mǔlì 3g + bèimǔ 3g + liánqiáo 3g + zhīzǐ 2-0g + shānzhīzǐ 1-0g.
Zhìgāncǎotāng 5g + tiānwángbǔxīndān 5-0g + shēngmàiyǐn 4-0g + dānshēn 1-0g + yùjīn 1-0g.	Zhìgāncǎo 5g + gānjiāng 5g + fùzǐ 3g + rénshēn 3-0g + gǒuqǐzǐ 3-0g + júhuā 3-0g.
	Fùzǐ 5g + báizhú 3g + cháihú 3g + báisháo 2g + fúlíng 2g + tiānhuā 2g + dǎngshēn 2g + guìzhī 1g + huángqín 1g + gāncǎo 1g + mǔlì 1g + gānjiāng 1g.
	Huángqí 5g + zhìgāncǎo 3g + dāngguī 2-0g + wǔwèizǐ 1g.

and 14.1). Jiégěng, introduced in Sections 2.57, 8.11, and 12.2 for respiratory symptoms, is used for chest pain, too (Wang, 2020).

14.4 FAMILIAL ISOLATED DILATED CARDIOMYOPATHY

Dilated cardiomyopathy (DCM) occurs when the muscles of at least one heart chamber become thinned and weakened. When DCM is the only atypical cardiac manifestation in the patient, it is called *isolated DCM*. When DCM is found in two or more first-degree relatives in a family, it is

TABLE 14.4
GMP Herbal Medicines for a 40-Year-Old Adult with Familial Isolated Dilated Cardiomyopathy

Familial isolated dilated cardiomyopathy (OrphaCode: 154)

A disease with a prevalence of ~2 in 10,000

Disease-causing germline mutation(s): TATA-box binding protein associated factor, RNA polymerase I subunit A (*TAF1A* / Entrez: 9015) at 1q41

Disease-causing germline mutation(s): myosin binding protein C3 (*MYBPC3* / Entrez: 4607) at 11p11.2

Disease-causing germline mutation(s): phosphopantothenoylcysteine synthetase (*PPCS* / Entrez: 79717) at 1p34.2

Disease-causing germline mutation(s): cyclase associated actin cytoskeleton regulatory protein 2 (*CAP2* / Entrez: 10486) at 6p22.3

Disease-causing germline mutation(s): ATP binding cassette subfamily C member 9 (*ABCC9* / Entrez: 10060) at 12p12.1

Disease-causing germline mutation(s): actin alpha cardiac muscle 1 (*ACTC1* / Entrez: 70) at 15q14

Disease-causing germline mutation(s): presenilin 1 (*PSEN1* / Entrez: 5663) at 14q24.2

Disease-causing germline mutation(s): presenilin 2 (*PSEN2* / Entrez: 5664) at 1q42.13

Disease-causing germline mutation(s) (gain of function): sodium voltage-gated channel alpha subunit 5 (*SCN5A* / Entrez: 6331) at 3p22.2

Disease-causing germline mutation(s): succinate dehydrogenase complex flavoprotein subunit A (*SDHA* / Entrez: 6389) at 5p15.33

Disease-causing germline mutation(s): sarcoglycan delta (*SGCD* / Entrez: 6444) at 5q33.2-q33.3

Disease-causing germline mutation(s): tafazzin, phospholipid-lysophospholipid transacylase (*TAFAZZIN* / Entrez: 6901) at Xq28

Disease-causing germline mutation(s): titin-cap (*TCAP* / Entrez: 8557) at 17q12

Disease-causing germline mutation(s): troponin I3, cardiac type (*TNNI3* / Entrez: 7137) at 19q13.42

Disease-causing germline mutation(s): troponin T2, cardiac type (*TNNT2* / Entrez: 7139) at 1q32.1

(Continued)

TABLE 14.4 *(Continued)*

GMP Herbal Medicines for a 40-Year-Old Adult with Familial Isolated Dilated Cardiomyopathy

Disease-causing germline mutation(s): tropomyosin 1 (*TPM1* / Entrez: 7168) at 15q22.2

Disease-causing germline mutation(s): titin (*TTN* / Entrez: 7273) at 2q31.2

Disease-causing germline mutation(s): crystallin alpha B (*CRYAB* / Entrez: 1410) at 11q23.1

Disease-causing germline mutation(s): cysteine and glycine rich protein 3 (*CSRP3* / Entrez: 8048) at 11p15.1

Disease-causing germline mutation(s): desmin (*DES* / Entrez: 1674) at 2q35

Disease-causing germline mutation(s): dystrophin (*DMD* / Entrez: 1756) at Xp21.2-p21.1

Disease-causing germline mutation(s): desmoglein 2 (*DSG2* / Entrez: 1829) at 18q12.1

Disease-causing germline mutation(s): fukutin (*FKTN* / Entrez: 2218) at 9q31.2

Disease-causing germline mutation(s): LIM domain binding 3 (*LDB3* / Entrez: 11155) at 10q23.2

Disease-causing germline mutation(s) (loss of function): dolichol kinase (*DOLK* / Entrez: 22845) at 9q34.11

Disease-causing germline mutation(s): myosin heavy chain 6 (*MYH6* / Entrez: 4624) at 14q11.2

Disease-causing germline mutation(s): myosin heavy chain 7 (*MYH7* / Entrez: 4625) at 14q11.2

Disease-causing germline mutation(s): Raf-1 proto-oncogene, serine/threonine kinase (*RAF1* / Entrez: 5894) at 3p25.2

Disease-causing germline mutation(s): thymopoietin (*TMPO* / Entrez: 7112) at 12q23.1

Disease-causing germline mutation(s): troponin C1, slow skeletal and cardiac type (*TNNC1* / Entrez: 7134) at 3p21.1

Disease-causing germline mutation(s): vinculin (*VCL* / Entrez: 7414) at 10q22.2

Disease-causing germline mutation(s): actinin alpha 2 (*ACTN2* / Entrez: 88) at 1q43

Disease-causing germline mutation(s): four and a half LIM domains 2 (*FHL2* / Entrez: 2274) at 2q12.2

Disease-causing germline mutation(s): phospholamban (*PLN* / Entrez: 5350) at 6q22.31

Disease-causing germline mutation(s): BAG cochaperone 3 (*BAG3* / Entrez: 9531) at 10q26.11

Disease-causing germline mutation(s): RNA binding motif protein 20 (*RBM20* / Entrez: 282996) at 10q25.2

Disease-causing germline mutation(s) (loss of function): nexilin F-actin binding protein (*NEXN* / Entrez: 91624) at 1p31.1

Disease-causing germline mutation(s) (loss of function): thioredoxin reductase 2 (*TXNRD2* / Entrez: 10587) at 22q11.21

Disease-causing germline mutation(s): GATA zinc finger domain containing 1 (*GATAD1* / Entrez: 57798) at 7q21.2

Disease-causing germline mutation(s): myopalladin (*MYPN* / Entrez: 84665) at 10q21.3

Disease-causing germline mutation(s): laminin subunit alpha 4 (*LAMA4* / Entrez: 3910) at 6q21

Disease-causing germline mutation(s): PR/SET domain 16 (*PRDM16* / Entrez: 63976) at 1p36.32

Disease-causing germline mutation(s): ankyrin repeat domain 1 (*ANKRD1* / Entrez: 27063) at 10q23.31

Disease-causing germline mutation(s): lamin A/C (*LMNA* / Entrez: 4000) at 1q22

Disease-causing germline mutation(s): desmoplakin (*DSP* / Entrez: 1832) at 6p24.3

Disease-causing germline mutation(s) (loss of function): heart and neural crest derivatives expressed 2 (*HAND2* / Entrez: 9464) at 4q34.1

Disease-causing germline mutation(s) (loss of function): BAG cochaperone 5 (*BAG5* / Entrez: 9529) at 14q32.33

Autosomal dominant, Autosomal recessive, Mitochondrial inheritance, X-linked recessive

Dilated cardiomyopathy

Sensorineural hearing impairment, Palmoplantar keratoderma, Abnormality of neutrophils, Myopathy, Elevated circulating creatine kinase concentration, EMG abnormality, Lipoatrophy

All ages

Sensorineural hearing impairment (389.1), Myopathy (359.9):

Xiǎocháihútāng 5g + língguìshùgāntāng 5g + shíchāngpú 1g + yuǎnzhì 1g + qīnghāo 1-0g + jiégěng 1-0g + héyè 1-0g + tiānmá 1-0g + mǔlì 1-0g.

Lóngdǎnxiègāntāng 5g + língguìshùgāntāng 2g.

Yínqiàosǎn 5g + jiégěng 3g + qīngzàojiùfèitāng 2g + cāngěrsǎn 2g + shēngmàiyǐn 1g + shíhúsuī 1g + yúxīngcǎo 1g.

Liùwèidìhuángwán 5g + yìqìcōngmíngtāng 5g + shíchāngpú 1g + cháihú 1g + yuǎnzhì 1g.

Huángbò 5g + shārén 4-3g + guībǎn 3-0g + zhìgāncǎo 2-0g + gāncǎo 2-0g + fùzǐ 2-0g.

Shúdìhuáng 5g + báizhú 4-3g + fùzǐ 4-0g + fúlíng 3-2g + báisháo 3-0g + qiànshí 3-0g + yìyǐrén 3-0g + báijièzǐ 2g + dǎngshēn 2g + shānzhūyú 2-0g + wǔwèizǐ 2-0g + dùzhòng 2-0g + guìzhī 2-0g + yìzhìrén 1-0g + júhóng 1-0g + gāncǎo 1-0g + shēngjiāng 1-0g + máhuáng 1-0g + huánglián 0g + shārén 0g.

Shānzhūyú 5g + shānyào 5g + chuānxiōng 5g + bājǐtiān 5g + niúxī 5g + ròucōngróng 5g + dùzhòng 5g + fángjǐ 5g + zhìgāncǎo 5g + fùzǐ 5g + gǒuqǐzǐ 5g + fúlíng 5g + xìxīn 5g + tùsīzǐ 5g + dāngguī 5g.

Báizhǐ 5g + zhìgāncǎo 5-3g + shārén 5-3g + huángqín 5-3g + tiānhuā 2-0g + máhuáng 1-0g + dàhuáng 0g.

called *familial DCM*. Familial isolated DCM is caused by mutations in the genes that instruct the production of proteins essential for heart muscle contraction.

Guībǎn (Carapax et Plastrum Testudinis) "nourishes yin, suppresses overactive yang" and is used today for neuralgia, neuritis, radiculitis, and sleep disturbances (Wang, 2020). Liver diseases and hearing loss are associated (Chen et al., 2017; Deutsch et al., 1998; Jung, 2023; Koff et al., 1973). The association is established in TCM through the gallbladder meridian, which connects the liver and the ear (cf. Section 1.3). We therefore see liver-benefiting formulas such as Xiǎocháihútāng and Lóngdǎnxièmgāntāng for hearing impairment in Table 14.4. Indeed, Lóngdǎnxièmgāntāng, combined with antibiotics, was found to be more effective than treatment with antibiotics alone for acute otitis media in a systematic review of randomized controlled trials (Son et al., 2017).

14.5 CATECHOLAMINERGIC POLYMORPHIC VENTRICULAR TACHYCARDIA

Catecholaminergic polymorphic ventricular tachycardia (CPVT), also known as bidirectional ventricular tachycardia induced by catecholamine, is the occurrence of abnormally accelerated heart rhythms during physical activities or emotional stress. CPVT is caused by gene mutations that disrupt the regulation of calcium concentrations in heart muscle cells during heartbeats.

TABLE 14.5

GMP Herbal Medicines for a 30-Year-Old Adult with Catecholaminergic Polymorphic Ventricular Tachycardia

Catecholaminergic polymorphic ventricular tachycardia (OrphaCode: 3286)

A disease with a prevalence of ~1 in 10,000

Disease-causing germline mutation(s): calsequestrin 2 (*CASQ2* / Entrez: 845) at 1p13.1

Disease-causing germline mutation(s): triadin (*TRDN* / Entrez: 10345) at 6q22.31

Disease-causing germline mutation(s): ryanodine receptor 2 (*RYR2* / Entrez: 6262) at 1q43

Disease-causing germline mutation(s): calmodulin 1 (*CALM1* / Entrez: 801) at 14q32.11

Candidate gene tested: calmodulin 2 (*CALM2* / Entrez: 805) at 2p21

Candidate gene tested: calmodulin 3 (*CALM3* / Entrez: 808) at 19q13.32

Disease-causing germline mutation(s): trans-2,3-enoyl-CoA reductase like (*TECRL* / Entrez: 253017) at 4q13.1

Autosomal dominant, Autosomal recessive

Ventricular tachycardia

Vertigo

Syncope, Sudden cardiac death

Childhood, Adolescent, Adult

Ventricular tachycardia (D017180) [Paroxysmal ventricular tachycardia (427.1)]:

Shēngmàiyǐn 5g + zhìgāncǎotāng 5g + xuèfǔzhúyūtāng 4-0g + dānshēn 1g + yùjīn 1g + bózǐrén 1-0g + yuǎnzhì 1-0g.

Zhìgāncǎotāng 5g + cháixiàntāng 5g + géxiàzhúyūtāng 5g + wēilíngxiān 2g + màiméndōng 2g.

Dǎngshēn 5g + zhìgāncǎo 5-4g + fùzǐ 5-4g + fúlíng 5-4g + gānjiāng 5-1g.

Huángqí 5g + zhīmǔ 2g + shēngmá 1g + jiégěng 1g + cháihú 1g.

Báizhú 5g + zhìgāncǎo 5g + fúlíng 5g + dǎngshēn 5g + shārén 4g + bànxià 2g + fùzǐ 2g + gānjiāng 2g.

Màiméndōng 5g + rénshēn 2g + niúxī 2g + báizhú 2g + fùzǐ 2g + wǔwèizǐ 1g.

Vertigo (386.2):

Bànxiàbáizhútiānmátāng 5g + língguìshùgāntāng 5g + chuānxiōng 1-0g.

Língguìshùgāntāng 5g + zhēnwǔtāng 5g + bànxiàbáizhútiānmátāng 5-0g.

Wǔlíngsǎn 5g + cāngzhú 2-1g + cāngěrzǐ 2-1g + gōuténg 2-1g + fùfāngdānshēnpiàn 2-1g.

Rénshēn 5g + bànxià 5g + gānjiāng 5-3g + chuānxiōng 5-0g + guālóurén 5-0g + mànjīngzǐ 5-0g + dàhuáng 0g.

Zéxiè 5g + báizhú 3-2g.

Báizhú 5g + fùzǐ 5g + cháihú 5g + báisháo 4g + fúlíng 4g + tiānhuā 2g + dǎngshēn 2g + guìzhī 2g + huángqín 2g + gāncǎo 1g + mǔlì 1g + gānjiāng 1g.

(Continued)

TABLE 14.5 *(Continued)*
GMP Herbal Medicines for a 30-Year-Old Adult with Catecholaminergic Polymorphic Ventricular Tachycardia

Syncope (D013575):

Shēngmàiyǐn 5g + xuèfǔzhúyūtāng 5g + jìshēngshènqìwán 5g + bànxiàxièxīntāng 2-0g + xiāngshāliùjūnzǐtāng 2-0g + dānshēn 1g + yùjīn 1-0g.
Shēngmàiyǐn 5g + zhìgāncǎotāng 5g + dānshēn 2g + xiāngfù 2g + yùjīn 2g.
Shēngmàiyǐn 5g + bǔzhōngyìqìtāng 5g + dānshēn 1g + shíchāngpú 1g + yuǎnzhì 1g.

Zhìgāncǎo 5g + fùzǐ 4-2g + dǎngshēn 4-0g + dàhuáng 0g + gānjiāng 0g.

Cháixiàntāng was introduced in Sections 3.28 and 5.11 for chest symptoms. Géxiàzhúyūtāng "activates circulation, dissolves stasis, moves Qi, stops pain" and is used today for essential hypertension and angina pectoris (Wang, 2019). Rénshēn was introduced in Sections 2.33, 2.49, and 5.20 for hearing. Bànxiàbáizhútiānmátāng "dries dampness, transforms phlegm, normalizes the Liver, calms Wind" and is used today for vertiginous syndromes and other disorders of the vestibular system (Wang, 2019).

14.6 INCESSANT INFANT VENTRICULAR TACHYCARDIA

Incessant infant ventricular tachycardia is the presence of ventricular tachycardia for more than 10% of a day in infants. The cause of incessant infant ventricular tachycardia is unknown but benign overgrowth of the mature, differentiated cells of the heart muscle is suggested.

Guālóurén was introduced in Section 5.11 for coughs and chest pain. Yùjīn (Radix Curcumae) was reviewed and summarized to be antitumor, hepatoprotective, anti-inflammatory, analgesic, antithrombosis, and nervous system affecting (Ao et al., 2022). It is used alone, or with

---

TABLE 14.6
GMP Herbal Medicines for a Two-Year-Old Child with Incessant Infant Ventricular Tachycardia

Incessant infant ventricular tachycardia (OrphaCode: 45453)

A disease with a prevalence of ~5 in 100,000

Not applicable

Ventricular tachycardia

Congestive heart failure, Cardiac arrest, Prolonged QRS complex, Bundle branch block, Abnormal P wave

Prenatal movement abnormality, Supraventricular tachycardia, Histiocytoid cardiomyopathy, Cardiac rhabdomyoma

Wolff-Parkinson-White syndrome

Infancy, Childhood

Ventricular tachycardia (D017180) [Paroxysmal ventricular tachycardia (427.1)]:

Zhìgāncǎotāng 5g + língguìshùgāntāng 5g + yǎngxīntāng 5g.
Zhìgāncǎotāng 5g + bǔzhōngyìqìtāng 5g.
Zhìgāncǎotāng 5g + shēngmàiyǐn 5-4g.
Tiānwángbǔxīndān 5g + zhìgāncǎotāng 5g + dānshēn 1g.

Zhǐqiào 5g + jílí 5-0g + chántuì 5-0g.
Chántuì 5g + jílí 2g.
Jílí 5g + júhóng 4g + chántuì 4g.

Bundle branch block (D002037) [Bundle branch block, other and unspecified (426.5)]:

Shēngmàiyǐn 5g + bǔzhōngyìqìtāng 5-0g.
Zhìgāncǎotāng 5g + dānshēn 1-0g.
Xiǎojiànzhōngtāng 5g + shēnlíngbáizhúsǎn 5g + gāncǎo 0g.

Zhìgāncǎo 5g + hòupò 5-0g + zhǐshí 5-0g + dàhuáng 0g.
Gāncǎo 5g + báizhǐ 5g + shārén 5-0g + huángqín 5-0g + fúlíng 5-0g + dǎngshēn 5-0g + dàhuáng 0g.

(Continued)

TABLE 14.6 *(Continued)*
GMP Herbal Medicines for a Two-Year-Old Child with Incessant Infant Ventricular Tachycardia

Supraventricular tachycardia (D013617) [Paroxysmal supraventricular tachycardia (427.0)]:

Tiānwángbǔxīndān 5g + zhìgāncǎotāng 5g + dānshēn 2-0g.	Dānshēn 5g + hónghuā 5g + táorén 5g + guālóurén 5g + xièbái 5g + yùjīn 5-0g.
Zhìgāncǎotāng 5g + dānshēn 2-1g + fúlíng 1-0g.	Dānshēn 5g + gāncǎo 5g + báisháo 5g + xìngrén 5g + fúlíng 5g + chénpí 5g + shíhú 5-0g + guālóurén 5-0g + báizhú 5-0g + màiméndōng 5-0g + huángqí 5-0g + dǎngshēn 5-0g.
	Báizhǐ 5g + gāncǎo 4g + shārén 4g + huángqín 4g + tiānhuā 3g + dàhuáng 1g.

Wolff-Parkinson-White syndrome (426.7):	
Yǎngxīntāng 5g + bǔzhōngyìqìtāng 2-0g.	
Zhēnwǔtāng 5g + wǔwèizǐ 1g + gānjiāng 1g + xìxīn 1g.	Gāncǎo 5g + báizhú 5g + fúlíng 5g + chénpí 5g + màiyá 5g + dǎngshēn 5g + huángqí 5-0g + gānjiāng 1-0g.
Xiǎojiànzhōngtāng 5g + bǔzhōngyìqìtāng 5g.	Zhìgāncǎo 5g + hòupò 3g + zhǐshí 3g + dàhuáng 0g.

Guālóurén, for chest pain (Wang, 2020). Yǎngxīntāng was introduced in Section 11.11 for cardiac dysrhythmias. We note that the doses of TCM prescriptions to infants are usually less and that the strategies of TCM for infants focus also on improving the digestion and thus growth of the baby.

REFERENCES

Ao, M., Li, X., Liao, Y., Zhang, C., Fan, S., Hu, C., Chen, Z., & Yu, L. (2022). Curcumae Radix: A review of its botany, traditional uses, phytochemistry, pharmacology and toxicology. *Journal of Pharmacy and Pharmacology*, 74(6), 779–792. https://doi.org/10.1093/jpp/rgab126

Chen, H., Chung, C., Wang, C., Lin, J., Chang, W., Lin, F., Tsao, C., Wu, Y., & Chien, W. (2017). Increased risk of sudden sensorineural hearing loss in patients with hepatitis virus infection. *PloS One*, 12(4), e0175266. https://doi.org/10.1371/journal.pone.0175266

Deutsch, E. S., Bartling, V., Lawenda, B. D., Schwegler, J., Falkenstein, K., & Dunn, S. P. (1998). Sensorineural hearing loss in children after liver transplantation. *Archives of Otolaryngology Head & Neck Surgery*, 124(5), 529. https://doi.org/10.1001/archotol.124.5.529

Hung, I., Chung, C., Hu, W., Liao, Y., Hsu, C. Y., Chiang, J., & Hung, Y. (2022). Chinese herbal medicine as an adjunctive therapy improves the survival rate of patients with ischemic heart disease: A nationwide population-based cohort study. *Evidence-Based Complementary and Alternative Medicine*, 2022, 1–10. https://doi.org/10.1155/2022/5596829

Jung, D. J. (2023). Association between fatty liver disease and hearing impairment in Korean adults: A retrospective cross-sectional study. *Journal of Yeungnam Medical Science*, 40(4), 402–411. https://doi.org/10.12701/jyms.2023.00304

Koff, R. S., Oliai, A., & Sparks, R. (1973). Sensori-neural hearing loss in alcoholic cirrhosis. *Digestion*, 8(3), 248–253. https://doi.org/10.1159/000197320

Lee, H. W., Jun, J. H., Kil, K., Ko, B., Lee, C. H., & Lee, M. S. (2016). Herbal medicine (Danggui Shaoyao San) for treating primary dysmenorrhea: A systematic review and meta-analysis of randomized controlled trials. *Maturitas*, 85, 19–26. https://doi.org/10.1016/j.maturitas.2015.11.013

Son, M. J., Kim, Y. E., Song, Y., & Kim, Y. H. (2017). Herbal medicines for treating acute otitis media: A systematic review of randomised controlled trials. *Complementary Therapies in Medicine*, 35, 133–139. https://doi.org/10.1016/j.ctim.2017.11.001

Wang, S.-C. (2019). Therapeutic classes of CHEG formulas. In S.-C. Wang (Ed.), *Clinical herbal prescriptions: Principles and practices of herbal formulations from deep learning health insurance herbal prescription big data* (pp. 16–89). World Scientific Publishing. https://doi.org/10.1142/11211

Wang, S.-C. (2020). Modern therapeutic uses of CHEG herbs and herb pairs. In S.-C. Wang (Ed.), *Veterinary herbal pharmacopoeia* (pp. 35–233). Nova Science Publishers. https://doi.org/10.52305/GHTR1903

Wang, W., Chen, Q., Yang, X., Wu, J., & Huang, F. (2020). Sini decoction ameliorates interrelated lung injury in septic mice by modulating the composition of gut microbiota. *Microbial Pathogenesis*, *140*, 103956. https://doi.org/10.1016/j.micpath.2019.103956

Zhang, C. C., Gu, W., Xian, W., Li, Y. M., Chen, C. X., & Huang, X. (2016). Active components from Radix Scrophulariae inhibits the ventricular remodeling induced by hypertension in rats. *SpringerPlus*, *5*(1). https://doi.org/10.1186/s40064-016-1985-z

Zhang, Y., Wang, M., Yang, J., & Li, X. (2018). The effects of the honey-roasting process on the pharmacokinetics of the six active compounds of licorice. *Evidence-Based Complementary and Alternative Medicine*, *2018*, 1–9. https://doi.org/10.1155/2018/5731276

Zhou, Q., Chen, B., Chen, X., Wang, Y., Ji, J., Kizaibek, M., Wang, X., Li-Xing, W., Hu, Z., Gao, X., Wu, N., Huang, D., Xu, X., Lü, W., Cai, X., Yang, Y., Ye, J., Wei, Q., Shen, J., & Cao, P. (2020). *Arnebiae Radix* prevents atrial fibrillation in rats by ameliorating atrial remodeling and cardiac function. *Journal of Ethnopharmacology*, *248*, 112317. https://doi.org/10.1016/j.jep.2019.112317

15 GMP Herbal Medicine for Rare Hepatic Diseases

Hepatic diseases are diseases of the liver. Liver diseases can be caused by viral infections, alcohol abuse, medication, toxic poisoning, and gene mutations. Many of the rare hepatic diseases of this chapter are multigenic/multifactorial.

The GMP single herbs and multi-herb formulas that are frequently discussed for the signs and symptoms of the rare hepatic diseases of this chapter are Rhubarb Root and Rhizome (Dàhuáng), Licorice Root (Gāncǎo), Salvia Root (Dānshēn), Virgate Wormwood Herb (Yīnchén), Scutellaria Root (Huángqín), Processed Licorice Root (Zhìgāncǎo), Cardamon Seed (Shārén), Dahurian Angelica Root (Báizhǐ), Ophiopogon Tuber (Màiméndōng), Red Peony Root (Chìsháo), Figwort Root (Xuánshēn), Virgate Wormwood and Five Ingredient Powder with Poria (Yīnchénwǔlíngsǎn), Minor Bupleurum Decoction (Xiǎocháihútāng), Five Ingredient Formula with Poria (Wǔlíngsǎn), Six Ingredient Pill with Rehmannia (Liùwèidìhuángwán), Free and Easy Wanderer Plus (Augmented Rambling Powder; Jiāwèixiāoyáosǎn), Tangkuei and Tribulus Decoction (Dāngguīyǐnzǐ), Wind Reducing Formula (Xiāofēngsǎn), Ginseng, Poria and Atractylodes Powder (Shēnlíngbáizhúsǎn), Gentiana Draining the Liver Decoction (Lóngdǎnxiègāntāng), Bupleurum Dredging the Liver Decoction (Cháihúshūgāntāng), and Calm the Stomach Powder (Píngwèisǎn).

In traditional Chinese medicine, the liver delivers bile, disperses Qi, stores blood, and also governs emotions.

15.1 AUTOIMMUNE HEPATITIS

Autoimmune hepatitis is a chronic condition where the immune system attacks one's own liver, causing inflammation and damage of the liver. The exact cause of autoimmune hepatitis is unknown; however, viruses and medications are two known factors that can trigger the autoimmune reaction to the liver.

Tǔfúlíng (cf. Section 8.8) "neutralizes toxins, removes dampness" and was summarized to be antioxidant, anti-inflammatory, immunomodulatory, hypouricemic, and hepatoprotective (Liang et al., 2019). Dìfūzǐ (Fructus Kochiae) "clears heat, helps draining, stops itching" and was shown to be anti-allergic and anti-pruritogenic in rats (Matsuda et al., 1997). Tǔfúlíng, Báixiānpí (cf. Section 9.1), and Dìfūzǐ are commonly used for skin conditions today (Wang, 2020). Dāngguīniántòngtāng is used

---

TABLE 15.1

GMP Herbal Medicines for a Seven-Year-Old Girl with Autoimmune Hepatitis

Autoimmune hepatitis (OrphaCode: 2137)

A disease with a prevalence of ~2 in 10,000

Not applicable

Increased circulating IgG level, Increased antibody level in blood

Elevated hepatic transaminase, Smooth muscle antibody positivity, Antineutrophil antibody positivity, Antinuclear antibody positivity, Liver kidney microsome type 1 antibody positivity, Anti-liver cytosolic antigen type 1 antibody positivity

Depression, Abdominal pain, Arthralgia, Chronic fatigue, Spider hemangioma

Glomerulonephritis, Anxiety, Jaundice, Vitiligo, Arthritis, Cirrhosis, Ascites, Splenomegaly, Inflammation of the large intestine, Gastrointestinal hemorrhage, Increased total bilirubin, Diffuse hepatic steatosis, Sclerosing cholangitis, Ulcerative colitis, Thyroiditis, Acute hepatitis

Childhood, Adolescent, Adult, Elderly

(Continued)

DOI: 10.1201/9781032726625-15

TABLE 15.1 *(Continued)*

GMP Herbal Medicines for a Seven-Year-Old Girl with Autoimmune Hepatitis

Increased antibody level in blood (D006942):

Dāngguīyǐnzǐ 5g + xiāofēngsǎn 4-0g + báixiānpí 1g + jīnyínhuā 1-0g + liánqiáo 1-0g + dìfūzǐ 1-0g + mǔdānpí 1-0g + chìsháo 1-0g.

Dāngguīniántòngtāng 5g + xiāofēngsǎn 2g + zhēnrénhuómìngyǐnqùchuānshānjiǎ 2g.

Dāngguīniántòngtāng 5g + sháoyàogāncǎotāng 4-0g + niúxī 1g + yánhúsuǒ 1-0g + dānshēn 1-0g + gāncǎo 0g + acupuncture.

Tǔfúlíng 5g + báixiānpí 5-4g + shéchuángzǐ 5-4g + dìfūzǐ 5-4g + dìhuáng 5-0g + mǔdānpí 5-0g + chìsháo 5-0g + kǔshēngēn 5-0g + dāngguī 5-0g + cāngěrzǐ 5-0g + bìxiè 4-0g + huáshí 4-0g + dàhuáng 2-0g + tōngcǎo 2-0g + zéxiè 2-0g + yìyǐrén 2-0g.

Tǔfúlíng 5g + gāncǎo 5g + báixiānpí 5g + jīnyínhuā 5g + dàhuáng 0g.

Báixiānpí 5g + dìhuáng 5g + mǔdānpí 5g + chìsháo 5g + jīnyínhuā 5g + liánqiáo 5g + zǐcǎogēn 5g + niúbàngzǐ 4g + xìngrén 4g + júhuā 4g + chántuì 4g + gāncǎo 2g.

Jīnyínhuā 5g + xuánshēn 4g + zhìgāncǎo 4g + dāngguī 4g + dàhuáng 0g.

Yìyǐrén 5g + gāncǎo 2g + báizhǐ 2g + shārén 2g + dàhuáng 1g.

Elevated hepatic transaminase (573.9):

Xiǎocháihútāng 5g + liùwèidìhuángwán 5g + xiāngshāliùjūnzǐtāng 5-0g.

Xiǎocháihútāng 5g + liùwèidìhuángwán 5g + shēnlíngbáizhúsǎn 5-0g.

Xiǎocháihútāng 5g + xiāngshāliùjūnzǐtāng 5-0g + píngwèisǎn 5-0g + shānzhā 2-0g + shénqū 2-0g + màiyá 2-0g.

Xiǎocháihútāng 5g + bǎohéwán 5g.

Xiǎocháihútāng 5g + sìjūnzǐtāng 5g.

Cháihúshūgāntāng 5g + bǔzhōngyìqìtāng 5g + gāncǎo 0g.

Lóngdǎnxiègāntāng 5g.

Huángqín 5g + báizhǐ 4g + zhìgāncǎo 3-2g + shārén 3-2g + tiānhuā 2-0g + dàhuáng 0g.

Huángqín 5g + báizhǐ 4g + shārén 2g + gāncǎo 2-1g + tiānhuā 1-0g + dàhuáng 0g.

Gāncǎo 5g + báizhǐ 5g + shārén 5g + dàhuáng 0g.

Abdominal pain (D015746), Arthralgia (D018771):

Wǔlíngsǎn 5g + píngwèisǎn 5-0g + gāncǎo 1-0g + báisháo 1-0g + tiáowèichéngqìtāng 1-0g + huángqín 1-0g + dàhuáng 0g.

Lǐzhōngtāng 5g + bǔzhōngyìqìtāng 5g + qīngyānlìgétāng 3g + tiānwángbǔxīndān 3-0g + xīnyísǎn 3-0g + fángfēng 2g + zhǐqiào 2g + jiégěng 2g + gānjiāng 2g.

Lǐzhōngtāng 5g + bànxià 1g + shārén 1g + fúlíng 1g + dàhuáng 0g.

Xuánshēn 5g + dìhuáng 5g + màiméndōng 5g + hòupò 5-1g + zhǐshí 5-1g + gāncǎo 1-0g + dàhuáng 1-0g.

Jaundice (D007565), Vitiligo (709.01), Ulcerative colitis (556, 556.5), Thyroiditis (245):

Liùwèidìhuángwán 5g + dānshēn 1g + gāncǎo 1g + hànliáncǎo 1g + chìsháo 1g + hónghuā 1g + bǔgǔzhǐ 1g + jílí 1g + cháihú 1-0g + táorén 1-0g + báizhǐ 1-0g + héshǒuwū 1-0g + nǔzhēnzǐ 1-0g + yèjiāoténg 1-0g + jīxuèténg 1-0g + dāngguī 1-0g + cǎojuémíng 1-0g.

Jiāwèixiāoyáosǎn 5g + zhībódìhuángwán 5g + dānshēn 1g + xiānhècǎo 1g + dìyú 1g + huáihuā 1g.

Báizhǐ 5g + zhìgāncǎo 5-2g + shārén 5-2g + dàhuáng 0g.

Báizhǐ 5g + gāncǎo 3-2g + shārén 3-2g + dàhuáng 0g.

Xuánshēn 5g + dìhuáng 5g + màiméndōng 5g + hòupò 2-1g + zhǐshí 1g + dàhuáng 1-0g.

today for rheumatoid arthritis and other inflammatory polyarthropathies (Wang, 2019). Autoimmune disorders such as rheumatoid arthritis and lupus manifest high levels of antibodies in the blood.

15.2 PRIMARY BILIARY CHOLANGITIS

Primary biliary cholangitis, also known as Hanot syndrome, is a slow and progressive condition in which one's immune system mistakenly attacks the liver's small bile ducts, causing small bile duct inflammation and damage. If the bile ducts are destroyed, buildup of bile in the liver can damage

TABLE 15.2

GMP Herbal Medicines for a 13-Year-Old Girl with Primary Biliary Cholangitis

Primary biliary cholangitis (OrphaCode: 186)

A disease with a prevalence of ~2 in 10,000

Major susceptibility factor: interleukin 12 receptor subunit beta 1 (*IL12RB1* / Entrez: 3594) at 19p13.11

Major susceptibility factor: Spi-B transcription factor (*SPIB* / Entrez: 6689) at 19q13.33

Major susceptibility factor: interleukin 12A (*IL12A* / Entrez: 3592) at 3q25.33

Major susceptibility factor: interferon regulatory factor 5 (*IRF5* / Entrez: 3663) at 7q32.1

Major susceptibility factor: transportin 3 (*TNPO3* / Entrez: 23534) at 7q32.1

Major susceptibility factor: membrane metalloendopeptidase like 1 (*MMEL1* / Entrez: 79258) at 1p36.32

Major susceptibility factor: POU class 2 homeobox associating factor 1 (*POU2AF1* / Entrez: 5450) at 11q23.1

Major susceptibility factor: TNF superfamily member 15 (*TNFSF15* / Entrez: 9966) at 9q32

Multigenic/multifactorial, Unknown

Hyperpigmentation of the skin, Cirrhosis, Biliary cirrhosis, Conjugated hyperbilirubinemia, Dermatographic urticaria
Jaundice, Pruritus, Orthostatic hypotension, Hepatic fibrosis, Hepatic failure, Hepatocellular carcinoma, Portal
hypertension, Recurrent fungal infections, Autoimmunity, Abnormal circulating lipid concentration, Elevated alkaline
phosphatase, Antinuclear antibody positivity, Increased circulating IgM level, Abnormality of the intrahepatic bile duct,
Onychomycosis, Abnormality of the thyroid gland

Osteoporosis, Excessive daytime somnolence, Ascites, Sleep disturbance, Celiac disease, Hypoalbuminemia, Increased
circulating IgA level, Abdominal distention, Hepatitis, Fatigue

Adolescent, Adult, Elderly

Biliary cirrhosis (571.6):

Liùwèidìhuángwán 5g + cháihúshūgāntāng 5g + dānshēn 1g.

Liùwèidìhuángwán 5g + jiāwèixiāoyáosǎn 5g + nǚzhēnzǐ 1-0g + dānshēn
1-0g + hànliáncǎo 1-0g + tùsīzǐ 1-0g.

Xiǎojiànzhōngtāng 5g + bǔzhōngyìqìtāng 4g + shānzhā 1g + shénqū 1g +
màiyá 1g + jīnèijīn 1g.

Cháihúshūgāntāng 5g + wēndǎntāng 5g + shānzhā 1g + dānshēn 1g +
yùjīn 1g.

Cháihúshūgāntāng 5g + gānlùxiāodúdān 4g + dānshēn 1g + yīnchén 1g +
púgōngyīng 1g.

Xiǎocháihútāng 5g + liùwèidìhuángwán 5g.

Yīnchén 5g + shānzhīzǐ 4g + dàhuáng
1g + huǒmárén 1g.

Yīnchén 5g + dānshēn 3g + bǎnlángēn
3g + hónghuā 3-0g + shānzhīzǐ 2g +
chēqiánzǐ 2g + huángbò 2g + yùjīn 2g.

Dìhuáng 5g + mǔdānpí 5g + chìsháo
5g + hónghuā 5g + guìzhī 5g + táorén
5g + huángbò 5g + dāngguī 5g.

Jaundice (D007565), Pruritus (D011537), Portal hypertension (572.3), Abnormality of the thyroid gland (246.9):

Jiāwèixiāoyáosǎn 5g + zhībódìhuángwán 5-4g + nǚzhēnzǐ 1g + gǒuqǐzǐ
1g + huángqí 1g + màiméndōng 1-0g + wǔwèizǐ 1-0g + dānshēn 1-0g +
huángbò 0g.

Jiāwèixiāoyáosǎn 5g + xiāngshāliùjūnzǐtāng 5g + dānshēn 1g + shénqū 1g +
liánqiáo 1g + yùjīn 1g.

Jiāwèixiāoyáosǎn 5g + yīnchénwǔlíngsǎn 5g + dānshēn 2-1g + huángshuǐqié
2-1g + hǔzhàng 2-0g + yùjīn 2-0g + wǔwèizǐ 1-0g.

Yīnchénwǔlíngsǎn 5g + huángliánjiědútāng 2g + jīnyínhuā 1g + púgōngyīng
1g + yùjīn 1g.

Yīnchénwǔlíngsǎn 5g + huòxiāngzhèngqìsǎn 5g + sānqī 1g + dānshēn 1g +
chìsháo 1g + hónghuā 1g.

Xuánshēn 5g + mǔlì 5g + bèimǔ 5g +
zhìgāncǎo 5g + jiégěng 5g + liánqiáo
5-4g + shānzhīzǐ 2-0g + xìngrén 2-0g +
zhīzǐ 2-0g.

Gāncǎo 5g + báizhǐ 5g + tiānhuā 3g +
shārén 3g + huángqín 3g + dàhuáng 0g.

Xuánshēn 5g + dìhuáng 5g +
màiméndōng 5g + hòupò 5-1g + zhǐshí
5-1g + dàhuáng 1-0g.

Osteoporosis (733.0), Celiac disease (579.0), Fatigue (D005221):

Shēnlíngbáizhúsǎn 5g + bǔzhōngyìqìtāng 5g.

Shēnlíngbáizhúsǎn 5g + shānzhā 2-1g + shénqū 2-1g + màiyá 2-1g + jīnèijīn
1-0g + shārén 1-0g + wūméi 1-0g.

Zuǒguīwán 5g + shēnlíngbáizhúsǎn 5g + shānzhā 1g + shénqū 1g +
màiyá 1g.

Shānyào 5g + huáihuā 5-2g + cāngzhú
5-0g + jīxuèténg 5-0g.

Mǔdānpí 5g + huáihuā 5g + cāngzhú
5-0g.

Xiānhècǎo 5g + huáihuā 5g + cāngzhú
5-0g + mǔdānpí 5-0g.

Bànzhīlián 5g + huáihuā 5g + cāngzhú 2g.

the liver. Primary biliary cholangitis was reported to occur in families and variant genes associated with the condition have been identified.

Yīnchén was introduced in Sections 1.57 and 4.21 to be hepatoprotective. Shānyào (cf. Sections 1.62 and 3.4) was shown to inhibit bone loss in rats with ovariectomy-induced osteopenia (Zhang et al., 2014). Huáihuā was introduced in Sections 12.7 and 13.7 for digestive conditions such as neoplasm of the gastrointestinal tract. Furthermore, Fructus Sophorae was reviewed to be antiosteoporosis (Shi et al., 2023). Shēnlíngbáizhúsăn (cf. Sections 1.5, 2.23, and 2.26) "replenishes Qi, strengthens the Spleen, harmonizes the Stomach, helps infiltrate" and was shown in the human fetal osteoblast cell line to prevent osteoporosis by inhibiting cell apoptosis and promoting cell proliferation (Liang et al., 2022).

15.3   ACUTE LIVER FAILURE

Acute liver failure is loss of liver function after the first signs in patients who have no previous liver diseases. Causes of acute liver failure include hepatitis A or B, alcohol overconsumption, medication overdose, toxins, and idiosyncratic reaction to medication.

TABLE 15.3

GMP Herbal Medicines for a 35-Year-Old Adult with Acute Liver Failure

Acute liver failure (OrphaCode: 90062)

A clinical syndrome with a prevalence of ~2 in 10,000

Not applicable

Jaundice, Hepatocellular necrosis, Elevated hepatic transaminase, Hepatitis

Agitation, Adrenal insufficiency, Bruising susceptibility, Confusion, Slurred speech, Mood changes, Thrombocytopenia, Hypoglycemia, Hyperammonemia, Vomiting, Diarrhea, Nausea, Drowsiness, Hepatic necrosis, Hepatic periportal necrosis, Hypotension, Abnormal pattern of respiration, Functional respiratory abnormality, Reduced coagulation factor V activity, Abnormality of the coagulation cascade, Prolonged prothrombin time, Reduced factor VII activity, Reduced factor X activity, Increased factor VIII activity

Depression, Skin rash, Seizure, Ataxia, Coma, Encephalopathy, Abnormal bleeding, Acute kidney injury, Acidosis, Fever, Alkalosis, Intracranial hemorrhage, Cerebral edema, Gastrointestinal hemorrhage, Incoordination, Increased intracranial pressure, Deep venous thrombosis, Hyperventilation, Pain insensitivity, Hypocapnia, Shock, Euphoria

Jaundice (D007565), Elevated hepatic transaminase (573.9):

Lóngdǎnxiègāntāng 5g + jiāwèixiāoyáosǎn 4-0g + huángliánjiědútāng 4-0g + yīnchén 1g + huángshuǐqié 1-0g + dàhuáng 0g.	Hǔzhàng 5g + nǚzhēnzǐ 3-2g + tiānhuā 3-2g + shíhú 3-2g + hànliáncǎo 3-2g + shāshēn 3-2g + zhìgāncǎo 3-2g + gǒuqǐzǐ 3-1g + chuānliànzǐ 2-1g + màiméndōng 2-1g + júhuā 2-1g + huángjīng 2-1g + héshǒuwū 2-0g.
Yīnchénwǔlíngsǎn 5g + lóngdǎnxiègāntāng 5g + bǎnlángēn 1g + jīnyínhuā 1g + yīnchén 1g.	Shānzhīzǐ 5g + yīnchén 5g + shānzhā 3g + dàhuáng 2g + dàfùpí 2g + hǎipiāoxiāo 2g.
	Yīnchén 5g + liánqiáo 5g + dàhuáng 3g + bànxià 3g + zhúrú 3g + fángfēng 3g + jīnyínhuā 3g + zhǐqiào 3g + jiégěng 3g + cháihú 3g + jīngjiè 3g + zhīzǐ 3g + huángqín 3g + bòhé 3g.

Bruising susceptibility (D004438), Confusion (D003221), Thrombocytopenia (287.5), Hypoglycemia (251.2), Vomiting (D014839), Diarrhea (D003967), Nausea (D009325), Abnormality of the coagulation cascade (286):

Wǔlíngsǎn 5g + gāncǎo 1g.	Gāncǎo 5g + báizhǐ 5g + shārén 5-3g + huángqín 5-0g + guālóugēn 3-0g + tiānhuā 2-0g + huánglián 1-0g + dàhuáng 1-0g.
Gāncǎo 5g + báizhú 5g + fúlíng 5g + gānjiāng 5g + dǎngshēn 5g + xiǎochéngqìtāng 5g.	
Gāncǎo 5g + báizhú 5g + fúlíng 5g + gānjiāng 5g + dǎngshēn 5g + dǐdāngtāng 5-2g.	Gāncǎo 5g + xìngrén 5g + jiégěng 5g + tiānméndōng 3g + dìgǔpí 3g + sāngbáipí 3g + màiméndōng 3g + huángqín 3g.
Gāncǎo 5g + báizhú 5g + fúlíng 5g + gānjiāng 5g + mázǐrénwán 5-2g + dàhuáng 0g.	Gāncǎo 5g + yúxīngcǎo 5-0g + tǔfúlíng 4g + báijiāngcán 4g + dìlóng 4g + fángfēng 4g + jiégěng 4g + jīngjiè 4g + bòhé 4g + púgōngyīng 4-0g.
Gāncǎo 5g + báizhú 5g + fúlíng 5g + gānjiāng 5g + tiáowèichéngqìtāng 5-1g + fùzǐ 3-0g.	

(Continued)

TABLE 15.3 *(Continued)*
GMP Herbal Medicines for a 35-Year-Old Adult with Acute Liver Failure

Skin rash (782.1), Seizure (345.9), Ataxia (D002524), Coma (D003128), Encephalopathy (348.30, 348.9), Fever (D005334), Incoordination (D001259), Hyperventilation (D006985), Hypocapnia (D016857):

Xiǎofēngsǎn 5g + dāngguīyǐnzǐ 5-0g + tǔfúlíng 1-0g + báixiānpí 1-0g + dìfūzǐ 1-0g + mǔdānpí 1-0g + chìsháo 1-0g + jílì 1-0g.

Xiǎofēngsǎn 5g + tǔfúlíng 1g + báixiānpí 1g + dìfūzǐ 1g + chìsháo 1g + jīngjiè 1g + yìyǐrén 1g.

Dāngguīyǐnzǐ 5g + xiāofēngsǎn 3g + tǔfúlíng 1g + báixiānpí 1g + dìfūzǐ 1g + liánqiáo 1g + jīnchán 1-0g + chìsháo 1-0g + jīnyínhuā 1-0g.

Huángqí 5g + chìsháo 1g + fángfēng 1g + xìxīn 0g + huánglián 0g.

Gāncǎo 5g + báizhǐ 5g + shārén 5g + huángqín 5g + tiānhuā 2g + xìxīn 2g + dàhuáng 1-0g.

Huángqín 5g + báizhǐ 2g + zhìgāncǎo 2g + shārén 2g + tiānhuā 1g + dàhuáng 0g.

Huángqín 5g + báizhǐ 2g + gāncǎo 2g + shārén 2g + tiānhuā 1g + xìxīn 1-0g + dàhuáng 1-0g + acupuncture.

Hǔzhàng was introduced in Section 4.32 for jaundice. Xiǎochéngqìtāng, containing Dàhuáng (cf. Sections 2.17, 8.4, and 11.8), is used for functional digestive disorders (Wang, 2019). Yúxīngcǎo (cf. Section 4.22) was shown to ameliorate hyperlipidemia-induced liver and heart impairments in hyperlipidemic mice via reduced hepatic and cardiac oxidative stress (Cao et al., 2020).

15.4 PRIMARY SCLEROSING CHOLANGITIS

Primary sclerosing cholangitis (PSC) is inflammation and scarring of the bile ducts, which carry bile from the liver to the gallbladder and small intestine. Narrowing and blockage of the ducts result in buildup of bile in the liver, damaging the liver. The cause of PSC is unknown; however, as PSC usually affects people with inflammatory bowel disease, PSC is thought to be an autoimmune disease.

Sāngbáipí (cf. Section 3.34) was shown to ameliorate hepatic injury and insulin resistance in rats with type 2 diabetes associated with nonalcoholic fatty liver disease (Ma et al., 2018). Cháihúshūgāntāng "relaxes the Liver, regulates Qi" and is used today for chronic liver disease and cirrhosis (Wang, 2019). Dàzǎo (cf. Sections 2.8 and 9.10) is used today for dyspepsia and anemia

TABLE 15.4
GMP Herbal Medicines for a 40-Year-Old Man with Primary Sclerosing Cholangitis

Primary sclerosing cholangitis (OrphaCode: 171)

A disease with a prevalence of ~8 in 100,000

Disease-causing germline mutation(s): semaphorin 4D (*SEMA4D* / Entrez: 10507) at 9q22.2

Major susceptibility factor: G protein-coupled receptor 35 (*GPR35* / Entrez: 2859) at 2q37.3

Major susceptibility factor: macrophage stimulating 1 (*MST1* / Entrez: 4485) at 3p21.31

Major susceptibility factor: transcription factor 4 (*TCF4* / Entrez: 6925) at 18q21.2

Multigenic/multifactorial

Cholestasis, Autoimmunity, Abnormal biliary tract morphology

Cirrhosis, Hepatic fibrosis, Portal hypertension, Hepatosplenomegaly, Ascites, Splenomegaly, Weight loss, Fever, Hepatomegaly, Elevated hepatic transaminase, Elevated alkaline phosphatase of hepatic origin, Spider hemangioma, Abnormal large intestine physiology, Dilated superficial abdominal veins, Ulcerative colitis, Palmar telangiectasia

Renal insufficiency, Depression, Osteopenia, Osteoporosis, Jaundice, Pruritus, Cholelithiasis, Hepatocellular carcinoma, Congestive heart failure, Pancreatitis, Abdominal pain, Pleural effusion, Celiac disease, Hypoalbuminemia, Polyclonal elevation of IgM, Generalized amyotrophy, Low levels of vitamin A, Prolonged prothrombin time, Low levels of vitamin K, Hepatitis, Fatigue, Cholangiocarcinoma, Adenocarcinoma of the large intestine, Low levels of vitamin D, Low levels of vitamin E, Chronic hepatic failure, Thyroiditis, Type I diabetes mellitus

Childhood, Adolescent, Adult, Elderly

(Continued)

TABLE 15.4 *(Continued)*
GMP Herbal Medicines for a 40-Year-Old Man with Primary Sclerosing Cholangitis

Cholestasis (576.2):

Xiǎocháihútāng 5g + yīnchénwǔlíngsǎn 5g + píngwèisǎn 5-0g + huàshícǎo 2-0g + jīnqiáncǎo 2-0g + jīnèijīn 2-0g + yùjīn 2-0g + dānshēn 2-0g + xiāngfù 2-0g + hǔzhàng 1-0g + yīnchén 1-0g + huángshuǐqié 1-0g.

Sìnìtāng 5g + yīnchénwǔlíngsǎn 5g + chuānliànzǐ 1g + jīnqiáncǎo 1g + yùjīn 1g.

Píngwèisǎn 5g + yīnchénwǔlíngsǎn 5g + lóngdǎnxiègāntāng 5g.

Xiǎocháihútāng 5g + wǔlíngsǎn 5g + píngwèisǎn 5-0g + yīnchén 2-0g.

Cháihúshūgāntāng 5g + lóngdǎnxiègāntāng 4g + yīnchén 1g + huángshuǐqié 1g + yùjīn 1g.

Fúlíng 5g + bànxià 3g + fùzǐ 3g + xìxīn 2-1g + dàhuáng 1-0g.

Báisháo 5g + cháihú 5g + zhǐshí 5-4g + huángqín 5-4g + bànxià 4-2g + dàzǎo 2g + shēngjiāng 2g + dàhuáng 0g.

Báimáogēn 5g + chēqiánzǐ 3g + báizhú 2g + fúlíng 2g + dàzǎo 2g + dàhuáng 2g + shēngjiāng 2g + shígāo 2g + zhìgāncǎo 2g + máhuáng 2g.

Portal hypertension (572.3), Weight loss (D015431), Fever (D005334), Elevated hepatic transaminase (573.9), Ulcerative colitis (556, 556.5):

Yīnchénwǔlíngsǎn 5g + xiǎocháihútāng 5-0g + dānshēn 2-1g + wǔwèizǐ 2-0g + hǔzhàng 2-0g + huángshuǐqié 2-0g + yùjīn 2-0g.

Cháihúshūgāntāng 5g + yīnchénwǔlíngsǎn 5g + shēnlíngbáizhúsǎn 5-0g + báihuāshéshécǎo 1g + huángshuǐqié 1g + wǔwèizǐ 1-0g + hǔzhàng 1-0g.

Wǔlíngsǎn 5g + yīnchén 2g + huángqín 2g + dàhuáng 0g.

Lǐzhōngtāng 5g + dānshēn 0g + fùzǐ 0g.

Huángqí 5g + zhìgāncǎo 3-2g + dāngguī 1-0g + wǔwèizǐ 1-0g + dàhuáng 0g.

Chēqiánzǐ 5g + yīnchén 5g + dǎngshēn 5g + fùzǐ 2g + guìzhī 2g + wūméi 2g + gānjiāng 2g + xìxīn 2g + huángbò 2g + huánglián 2g + dāngguī 2g.

Chēqiánzǐ 5g + chìxiǎodòu 5-2g + liánqiáo 5-2g + sāngbáipí 5-0g + dàzǎo 2-1g + shēngjiāng 2-1g + xìngrén 2-1g + zhìgāncǎo 2-1g + yīnchén 2-0g + máhuáng 1-0g.

Yīnchén 5g + zhīzǐ 5g + huángqín 5g + huángbò 5g + dàhuáng 0g.

Renal insufficiency (586), Osteoporosis (733.0), Jaundice (D007565), Pruritus (D011537), Congestive heart failure (428, 428.0), Pancreatitis (577.0), Abdominal pain (D015746), Celiac disease (579.0), Low levels of vitamin K (269.0), Fatigue (D005221), Thyroiditis (245):

Xiǎocháihútāng 5g + wǔlíngsǎn 5g + jìshēngshènqìwán 5-0g + yīnchén 1-0g.

Xiǎocháihútāng 5g + huòxiāngzhèngqìsǎn 5g + zhìgāncǎotāng 5-0g + xiāngshāliùjūnzǐtāng 5-0g + nǚzhēnzǐ 1-0g + báizhú 1-0g + huángqí 1-0g + fúlíng 1-0g + dǎngshēn 1-0g.

Zhìgāncǎotāng 5g + xiāngshāliùjūnzǐtāng 5g + huòxiāngzhèngqìsǎn 5g + báizhú 1g + pípáyè 1g + cháihú 1g.

Wǔlíngsǎn 5g + zhībódìhuángwán 5g + huòxiāngzhèngqìsǎn 5g + mùxiāng 1g + báizhú 1g + huángqí 1g.

Zhìgāncǎotāng 5g + xuèfǔzhúyūtāng 4g + sānqī 1g + dānshēn 1g + yùjīn 1g.

Jīnyínhuā 5g + huángqí 5g + dāngguī 5g + niúxī 2g + xuánshēn 2g + gāncǎo 2g + chìsháo 2g + dǎodìwúgōng 2g.

Jīnyínhuā 5g + gāncǎo 4-3g + xuánshēn 3-0g + dāngguī 3-0g + shārén 2-0g + dàhuáng 1-0g + huánglián 1-0g.

Báizhú 5g + dāngguī 5g + dǎngshēn 5g + ròuguì 2g + fángfēng 2g + cháihú 2g + wǔlíngzhī 2g + mǔdānpí 2g + chìsháo 2g + hónghuā 2g + táorén 2g + púhuáng 2g.

Bèimǔ 5g + gāncǎo 4g + zhīmǔ 3g + dàhuáng 0g + huánglián 0g.

Xuánshēn 5-2g + zhìgāncǎo 5-2g + jīnyínhuā 5-0g + mǔlì 5-0g + bèimǔ 5-0g + jiégěng 5-0g + liánqiáo 4-0g + zhīzǐ 2-0g + dāngguī 2-0g + dàhuáng 1-0g.

(Wang, 2020). Jīnyínhuā is anti-inflammatory (cf. Section 3.5), anti-osteoporotic (cf. Section 9.9), and antipruritic (cf. Section 3.9).

15.5 WILSON DISEASE

Wilson disease, also known as hepatolenticular degeneration, is characterized by excessive copper in the body, including the liver and brain. Wilson disease is caused by mutations in a gene whose products transfer excessive copper to bile for elimination.

TABLE 15.5
GMP Herbal Medicines for a 13-Year-Old Adolescent with Wilson Disease

Wilson disease (OrphaCode: 905)

A disease with a prevalence of ~2 in 100,000

Disease-causing germline mutation(s) (loss of function): ATPase copper transporting beta (*ATP7B* / Entrez: 540) at 13q14.3

Autosomal recessive

Abnormality of the menstrual cycle, Depression, Aggressive behavior, Jaundice, Bruising susceptibility, Pruritus, Abnormality of the hand, Intellectual disability, Dysarthria, Arthritis, Joint swelling, Cirrhosis, Hepatic steatosis, Failure to thrive, Splenomegaly, Weight loss, Thrombocytopenia, Anemia, Hepatomegaly, Clumsiness, Difficulty walking, Bone pain, Pathologic fracture, Arthralgia, Elevated hepatic transaminase, Back pain, Increased body weight, Acute hepatic failure, Proximal muscle weakness in lower limbs, Hepatitis, Hypersexuality, Kayser-Fleischer ring, Acute hepatitisChildhood, Adolescent, Adult, Elderly

Jaundice (D007565), Bruising susceptibility (D004438), Pruritus (D011537), Intellectual disability (D008607), Dysarthria (D004401), Hepatic steatosis (571.0), Weight loss (D015431), Thrombocytopenia (287.5), Anemia (285.9), Difficulty walking (D051346), Arthralgia (D018771), Elevated hepatic transaminase (573.9), Back pain (D001416), Increased body weight (D015430):

Yīnchénwǔlíngsǎn 5g + lóngdǎnxiègāntāng 5g + dàqīngyè 2g + jīnyínhuā 2g.	Yīnchén 5g + báizhú 3g + dìhuáng 3g + zhǐqiào 3g + huángqín 3g + mǔdānpí 3-2g + zéxiè 3-2g + fùzǐ 3-0g + jīnyínhuā 3-0g.
Yīnchénwǔlíngsǎn 5g + guīpítāng 5g + xiānhècǎo 2-0g + dàqīngyè 2-0g + jīnyínhuā 2-0g + jīxuèténg 2-0g.	Hǔzhàng 5g + nǚzhēnzǐ 2g + tiānhuā 2g + héshǒuwū 2g + hànliáncǎo 2g + shāshēn 2g + gǒuqǐzǐ 2g + huángjīng 2g + chuānliànzǐ 1g + zhìgāncǎo 1g + màiméndōng 1g + júhuā 1g.
	Báizhú 5g + báisháo 5g + yīnchén 5g + dǎngshēn 5g + dàzǎo 2g + shānyào 2g + zhìgāncǎo 2g + guìzhī 2g + gānjiāng 2g + dāngguī 2g + fùzǐ 1g.

Yīnchén and Yīnchénwǔlíngsǎn benefit the liver. Guīpítāng was introduced in Sections 1.2 and 4.19 for anemia and general symptoms. Guīpítāng with two extra herbs was shown to significantly improve both the behavioral and psychological symptoms of dementia and positive emotions in patients with Alzheimer's disease (Nogami et al., 2023). Processed Héshǒuwū (cf. Section 8.8) was summarized to be antiaging, immunomodulating, hepatoprotective, anticancer, and anti-inflammatory (Li et al., 2020).

15.6 BUDD-CHIARI SYNDROME

Budd-Chiari syndrome is characterized by narrowing and obstruction of the hepatic veins that drain the liver. Budd-Chiari syndrome can be caused by conditions that induce the blood to clot in the blood vessel or by compression of the vein by a tumor.

TABLE 15.6
GMP Herbal Medicines for a 30-Year-Old Adult with Budd-Chiari Syndrome

Budd-Chiari syndrome (OrphaCode: 131)

A disease with a prevalence of ~1 in 100,000

Candidate gene tested: coagulation factor V (*F5* / Entrez: 2153) at 1q24.2

Candidate gene tested: Janus kinase 2 (*JAK2* / Entrez: 3717) at 9p24.1

Disease-causing somatic mutation(s): calreticulin (*CALR* / Entrez: 811) at 19p13.13

Multigenic/multifactorial

Portal hypertension, Ascites, Splenomegaly

Cirrhosis, Fever, Abdominal pain, Esophageal varix, Hepatomegaly, Elevated hepatic transaminase

Jaundice, Cholecystitis, Weight loss, Malabsorption, Gastrointestinal hemorrhage, Peritonitis, Intestinal obstruction, Gastrointestinal infarctions, Acute hepatic failure

All ages

(Continued)

TABLE 15.6 *(Continued)*

GMP Herbal Medicines for a 30-Year-Old Adult with Budd-Chiari Syndrome

Portal hypertension (572.3), Ascites (D001201) [Ascites (789.5)]:

Wǔlíngsǎn 5g + xiǎocháihútāng 5-0g + yīnchén 2-1g + zhīzǐ 2-0g + chēqiánzǐ 1-0g + huángqín 1-0g + dàhuáng 0g.

Jiāwèixiāoyáosǎn 5g + yīnchénwǔlíngsǎn 5g + dānshēn 1g + niúxī 1g + chēqiánzǐ 1g + yùjīn 1g.

Huángqí 5g + báimáogēn 2g + chēqiánzǐ 2g + yùjīn 2g + sīguāluò 2-0g + jīnyínhuā 1g + dāngguī 1-0g.

Báimáogēn 5g + chìxiǎodòu 5g + chēqiánzǐ 5g + yìmǔcǎo 5-4g + dāngguī 2g + dàhuáng 0g.

Cirrhosis (D008103) [Cirrhosis of liver without mention of alcohol (571.5)], Fever (D005334), Abdominal pain (D015746), Elevated hepatic transaminase (573.9):

Yīnchénwǔlíngsǎn 5g + jiāwèixiāoyáosǎn 5-0g + dānshēn 2-1g + wǔwèizǐ 2-0g + yùjīn 2-0g + chìsháo 1-0g + hǔzhàng 1-0g + huángshuǐqié 1-0g.

Dàcháihútāng 5g + yīnchénwǔlíngsǎn 5g + dānshēn 1g + hǔzhàng 1g + huángshuǐqié 1g.

Dānshēn 5g + báizhú 5g + fúlíng 5g + dǎngshēn 5g + mǔdānpí 5g + báisháo 5-0g + báihuāshéshécǎo 5-0g + ējiāo 5-0g + cháihú 5-0g + huángqín 5-0g + jīnyínhuā 5-0g + táorén 5-0g + chénpí 5-0g + biējiǎ 5-0g.

Cháihú 5g + tiānhuā 2g + chìxiǎodòu 2g + guìzhī 2g + huángqín 2g + dàzǎo 1g + shēngjiāng 1g + xìngrén 1g + zhìgāncǎo 1g + mǔlì 1g + sāngbáipí 1g + gānjiāng 1g + liánqiáo 1g + máhuáng 1g.

Yīnchén 5g + bànzhīlián 2g + báizhú 2g + mǔdānpí 2g + hòupò 2g + zhǐqiào 2g + huángqín 2g + zéxiè 2g.

Dàzǎo 5g + dānshēn 5g + gāncǎo 5g + báisháo 5g + bǎihé 5g + mǔdānpí 5g + fúxiǎomài 5g + fúshén 5g + suānzǎorén 5g.

Jaundice (D007565), Cholecystitis (575.10), Weight loss (D015431), Intestinal obstruction (560.9):

Dàcháihútāng 5g + yīnchénhāotāng 5-0g + jīnqiáncǎo 1-0g + yīnchén 1-0g + yùjīn 1-0g + huǒmárén 0g.

Yīnchénwǔlíngsǎn 5g + huòxiāngzhèngqìsǎn 5g + yèjiāoténg 3g + hǎipiāoxiāo 3g + bózǐrén 2g + chìsháo 2g + cāngzhú 2g.

Wǔlíngsǎn 5g + yīnchén 1g + dàhuáng 0g.

Yīnchén 5g + shānzhīzǐ 4g + dàhuáng 2g + huǒmárén 1-0g.

Yīnchén 5g + fùzǐ 4-3g + xìxīn 4-2g + bànxià 4-0g + dàhuáng 1g.

Báimáogēn (cf. Sections 1.66, 3.11, and 12.3) was reviewed and summarized to be immuno-modulatory, antibacterial, antitumor, anti-inflammatory, and hepatoprotective (Jung & Shin, 2021). Yīnchénhāotāng "clears heat, helps draining, eliminates jaundice" and is used today for chronic liver disease and cirrhosis (Wang, 2019). Shānzhīzǐ (cf. Section 1.39) was shown to protect against intrahepatic cholestasis in rats by regulating bile acid enterohepatic circulation (Qin et al., 2024). Dàcháihútāng is used for acute liver diseases, while Xiǎocháihútāng is used for chronic liver diseases (cf. Section 5.1).

REFERENCES

Cao, K., Lv, W., Liu, X., Fan, Y., Wang, K., Feng, Z., Liu, J., Zang, W., Liu, X., & Liu, J. (2020). *Herba houttuyniae* extract benefits hyperlipidemic mice via activation of the AMPK/PGC-1α/Nrf2 Cascade. *Nutrients*, *12*(1), 164. https://doi.org/10.3390/nu12010164

Jung, Y., & Shin, D. (2021). *Imperata cylindrica*: A review of phytochemistry, pharmacology, and industrial applications. *Molecules*, *26*(5), 1454. https://doi.org/10.3390/molecules26051454

Li, D., Yang, M., & Zuo, Z. (2020). Overview of pharmacokinetics and liver toxicities of Radix polygoni multiflori. *Toxins*, *12*(11), 729. https://doi.org/10.3390/toxins12110729

Liang, G., Nie, Y., Chang, Y., Zeng, S., Liang, C., Zheng, X., Xiao, D., Zhan, S., & Zheng, Q. (2019). Protective effects of *Rhizoma smilacis glabrae* extracts on potassium oxonate- and monosodium urate-induced hyperuricemia and gout in mice. *Phytomedicine*, *59*, 152772. https://doi.org/10.1016/j.phymed.2018.11.032

Liang, J., Bao, A., Ma, H., Dong, W., Li, W., Wu, X., Li, H., Hou, H., Chen, Y., Fu, J., & Shao, C. (2022). Prevention of polycystic ovary syndrome and postmenopausal osteoporosis by inhibiting apoptosis with Shenling Baizhu powder compound. *PeerJ, 10*, e13939. https://doi.org/10.7717/peerj.13939

Ma, L., Yuan, Y., Zhao, M., Zhou, X., Jehangir, T., Wang, F., Xi, Y., & Bu, S. (2018). Mori Cortex extract ameliorates nonalcoholic fatty liver disease (NAFLD) and insulin resistance in high-fat-diet/streptozotocin-induced type 2 diabetes in rats. *Zhongguo Tianran Yaowu/Chinese Journal of Natural Medicines, 16*(6), 411–417. https://doi.org/10.1016/s1875-5364(18)30074-8

Matsuda, H., Dai, Y., Ido, Y., Yoshikawa, M., & Kubo, M. (1997). Studies on Kochiae Fructus IV. Anti-allergic effects of 70% ethanol extract and its component, momordin Ic from dried fruits of *Kochia scoparia* L. *Biological & Pharmaceutical Bulletin, 20*(11), 1165–1170. https://doi.org/10.1248/bpb.20.1165

Nogami, T., Iwasaki, K., Kimura, H., Higashi, T., Arai, M., Butler, J. P., Fujii, M., & Sasaki, H. (2023). Traditional Chinese medicine Jia Wei Gui Pi Tang improves behavioural and psychological symptoms of dementia and favourable positive emotions in patients. *Psychogeriatrics, 23*(3), 503–511. https://doi.org/10.1111/psyg.12962

Qin, S., Tian, J., Zhao, Y., Wang, L., Wang, J., Liu, S., Meng, J., Wang, F., Liu, C., Han, J., Pan, C., Zhang, Y., Yi, Y., Li, C., Liu, M., & Liang, A. (2024). Gardenia extract protects against intrahepatic cholestasis by regulating bile acid enterohepatic circulation. *Journal of Ethnopharmacology, 319*, 117083. https://doi.org/10.1016/j.jep.2023.117083

Shi, P., Liao, J., Duan, T., Wu, Q., Huang, X., Pei, X., & Wang, C. (2023). Chemical composition and pharmacological properties of *Flos sophorae immaturus*, *Flos sophorae* and *Fructus sophorae*: A review. *Journal of Future Foods, 3*(4), 330–339. https://doi.org/10.1016/j.jfutfo.2023.03.004

Wang, S.-C. (2019). Therapeutic classes of CHEG formulas. In S.-C. Wang (Ed.), *Clinical herbal prescriptions: Principles and practices of herbal formulations from deep learning health insurance herbal prescription big data* (pp. 16–89). World Scientific Publishing. https://doi.org/10.1142/11211

Wang, S.-C. (2020). Modern therapeutic uses of CHEG herbs and herb pairs. In S.-C. Wang (Ed.), *Veterinary herbal pharmacopoeia* (pp. 35–233). Nova Science Publishers. https://doi.org/10.52305/GHTR1903

Zhang, Z., Xiang, L., Dong, B., Fu, X., Wang, W., Li, Y., Liu, H., Pan, J., Li, Y., Xiao, G. G., & Ju, D. (2014). Treatment with *Rhizoma Dioscoreae* extract has protective effect on osteopenia in ovariectomized rats. *The Scientific World Journal, 2014*, 1–12. https://doi.org/10.1155/2014/645975

16 GMP Herbal Medicine for Rare Renal Diseases

Renal diseases are diseases of the kidney. Causes of kidney diseases include hypertension, diabetes, medications, lead poisoning, and genetics. Many of the rare renal diseases of this chapter are inherited but adult onset.

The GMP single herbs and multi-herb formulas that are commonly discussed for the signs and symptoms of the rare renal diseases are Imperata Rhizome (Báimáogēn), Aconite Accessory Root (Fùzǐ), Plantain Seed (Chēqiánzǐ), Poria (Fúlíng), Rhubarb Root and Rhizome (Dàhuáng), Achyranthes Root (Niúxī), Salvia Root (Dānshēn), Scutellaria Root (Huángqín), Cat's Whiskers (Huàshícǎo), Codonopsis Root (Dǎngshēn), White Atractylodis (Báizhú), Chinese Motherwort Herb (Yìmǔcǎo), Dried Ginger Rhizome (Gānjiāng), Asian Moneywort Herb (Jīnqiáncǎo), Achyranthes and Plantago Formula (Jìshēngshènqìwán), Polyporus Decoction (Zhūlíngtāng), Gardenia and Hoelen Formula (Wǔlínsǎn), Gastrodia and Uncaria Drink (Tiānmágōuténgyǐn), True Warrior Decoction (Zhēnwǔtāng), Drive Out Stasis from the Mansion of Blood Decoction (Xuèfǔzhúyūtāng), Angelica Pubescens and Taxillus Decoction (Dúhuójìshēngtāng), Tokoro Decoction (Bìxièfēnqīngyǐn), Five Ingredient Formula with Poria (Wǔlíngsǎn), Prepared Licorice Decoction (Zhìgāncǎotāng), Lotus Seed Decoction (Qīngxīnliánzǐyǐn), and Relax the Channels and Invigorate the Blood Decoction (Shūjīnghuóxuètāng).

The kidney in traditional Chinese medicine stores congenital and acquired essences for growth, development, and reproduction. It also regulates water metabolism and produces marrow. Declining and depletion of the kidney essence determine aging and death.

16.1 AUTOSOMAL DOMINANT POLYCYSTIC KIDNEY DISEASE

Autosomal dominant polycystic kidney disease, or autosomal dominant PKD, is a chronic kidney disease passed down through a parent with PKD and characterized by the formation of bilateral kidney cysts, which can cause kidney dysfunction and eventual kidney failure. Autosomal dominant PKD can also cause cysts in organs other than the kidney, including the liver, pancreas, seminal vesicles, and prostate.

TABLE 16.1

GMP Herbal Medicines for a 40-Year-Old Adult with Autosomal Dominant Polycystic Kidney Disease

Autosomal dominant polycystic kidney disease (OrphaCode: 730)

A disease with a prevalence of ~4 in 10,000

Disease-causing germline mutation(s): glucosidase II alpha subunit (*GANAB* / Entrez: 23193) at 11q12.3

Disease-causing germline mutation(s) (loss of function): ALG9 alpha-1,2-mannosyltransferase (*ALG9* / Entrez: 79796) at 11q23.1

Disease-causing germline mutation(s) (loss of function): DnaJ heat shock protein family (Hsp40) member B11 (*DNAJB11* / Entrez: 51726) at 3q27.3

Disease-causing germline mutation(s): ALG5 dolichyl-phosphate beta-glucosyltransferase (*ALG5* / Entrez: 29880) at 13q13.3

Disease-causing germline mutation(s): polycystin 1, transient receptor potential channel interacting (*PKD1* / Entrez: 5310) at 16p13.3

(Continued)

 DOI: 10.1201/9781032726625-16

TABLE 16.1 *(Continued)*

GMP Herbal Medicines for a 40-Year-Old Adult with Autosomal Dominant Polycystic Kidney Disease

Disease-causing germline mutation(s): polycystin 2, transient receptor potential cation channel (*PKD2* / Entrez: 5311) at 4q22.1

Candidate gene tested: BicC family RNA binding protein 1 (*BICC1* / Entrez: 80114) at 10q21.1

Disease-causing germline mutation(s) (loss of function): intraflagellar transport 140 (*IFT140* / Entrez: 9742) at 16p13.3 Autosomal dominant

Renal insufficiency, Renal cyst, Hepatic cysts, Elevated serum creatinine, Decreased glomerular filtration rate

Hematuria, Hypertension, Stage 5 chronic kidney disease, Pain, Abnormal urinary electrolyte concentration, Albuminuria, Chronic kidney disease

Recurrent urinary tract infections, Enlarged kidney, Nephrolithiasis, Mitral valve prolapse, Pancreatic cysts, Aortic root aneurysm, Dilatation of the cerebral artery, Polycystic liver disease, Abnormal systemic arterial morphology, Reduced sperm motility, Pyelonephritis, Arachnoid cyst

Childhood, Adolescent, Adult

Renal insufficiency (586):

Zhūlíngtāng 5g + jìshēngshènqìwán 5g + dānshēn 1-0g + niúxī 1-0g + báimáogēn 1-0g + chēqiánzǐ 1-0g + jīnqiáncǎo 1-0g + dōngkuízǐ 1-0g + wūyào 1-0g + jīnèijīn 1-0g.

Zhēnwǔtāng 5g + guīpítāng 5-0g + fùzǐ 1-0g + dānshēn 1-0g + xìxīn 1-0g + gānjiāng 1-0g + dǐdāngtāng 0g + dàhuáng 0g.

Fúlíng 5g + shānyào 4g + tiānhuā 4g + jùmài 4g + fùzǐ 2g + dàhuáng 0g.

Fúlíng 5g + fùzǐ 4-3g + dǎngshēn 4-2g + báisháo 4-0g + báizhú 4-0g + gāncǎo 2-0g + gānjiāng 1-0g.

Báimáogēn 5g + chēqiánzǐ 5g + báizhú 2g + fúlíng 2g + dàzǎo 1g + shēngjiāng 1g + shígāo 1g + zhìgāncǎo 1g + máhuáng 1g + dàhuáng 0g.

Fùzǐ 5g + gāncǎo 4g + gānjiāng 4g.

Hypertension (401-405.99), Pain (D010146), Albuminuria (D000419):

Tiānmágōuténgyǐn 5g + xuèfǔzhúyūtāng 5-0g + zhǐbódìhuángwán 5-0g + niúxī 1-0g.

Tiānmágōuténgyǐn 5g + xuèfǔzhúyūtāng 5-0g + qǐjúdìhuángwán 5-0g.

Tiānmágōuténgyǐn 5-4g + xuèfǔzhúyūtāng 5-0g + jìshēngshènqìwán 5-0g + dānshēn 1-0g + niúxī 1-0g + chìsháo 1-0g + xiàkūcǎo 1-0g + gégēn 1-0g.

Qiānghuó 5g + hòupò 5-3g + zhǐshí 5-3g + fángfēng 3-0g + huángqín 1-0g + huánglián 1-0g + dàhuáng 1-0g.

Nephrolithiasis (592), Pyelonephritis (590.80):

Wǔlínsǎn 5g + huàshícǎo 2-1g + jīnyínhuā 1-0g + huángqín 1-0g + púgōngyīng 1-0g + jīnèijīn 1-0g.

Báimáogēn 5g + chìxiǎodòu 5g + chēqiánzǐ 5g + dāngguī 3g + dàhuáng 0g.

Báimáogēn 5g + chēqiánzǐ 5-1g + jīnqiáncǎo 5-1g + niúxī 3-1g + huáshí 2-0g + dēngxīncǎo 1-0g.

Huàshícǎo 5g + chēqiáncǎo 5g + hānqiàocǎo 5g.

Jùmài (Herba Dianthi) was shown to be antinociceptive and antiedema in mice (Oh et al., 2018); it is used today for a variety of conditions ranging from respiratory, nervous, digestive, and skin, including edema (Wang, 2020). Huàshícǎo dissolves stones (cf. Section 4.27). Hānqiàocǎo (Herba Centellae), extensively used in the East, was touted as an herb that cures all (Gohil et al., 2010). It pairs with Huàshícǎo for the treatment of calculus of kidney (Wang, 2020). Jīnqiáncǎo (cf. Section 4.27) treats kidney stones and cholesterol gallstones (Xiong et al., 2015).

16.2 PRIMARY MEMBRANOPROLIFERATIVE GLOMERULONEPHRITIS

Primary membranoproliferative glomerulonephritis, or mesangiocapillary glomerulonephritis, is a type of glomerular inflammation, characterized by hypercellularity and thickening of the glomerular basement membrane, which filters wastes and fluids from the blood. Buildup of antibodies in the

TABLE 16.2

GMP Herbal Medicines for a 20-Year-Old Adult with Primary Membranoproliferative Glomerulonephritis

Primary membranoproliferative glomerulonephritis (OrphaCode: 54370)

A disease with a prevalence of ~2 in 10,000

Not applicable

Renal insufficiency, Proteinuria, Nephrotic syndrome, Hypertension, Microscopic hematuria, Glomerular subendothelial electron-dense deposits, Decreased serum complement C3, Chronic kidney disease, C3 nephritic factor positivity

Acute kidney injury, Hypoalbuminemia, Stage 5 chronic kidney disease

Adult

Renal insufficiency (586), Proteinuria (791.0), Nephrotic syndrome (581), Hypertension (401-405.99):

Zhūlíngtāng 5g + jìshēngshènqìwán 5g + dānshēn 2-0g + báimáogēn 2-0g + yìmǔcǎo 2-0g + zélán 2-0g + dōngguāzǐ 1-0g + dīngshùxiǔ 1-0g + huángqí 1-0g + dàhuáng 1-0g. Qīngxīnliánzǐyǐn 5g + zhībódìhuángwán 4g + dānshēn 1g + yìmǔcǎo 1g + dàhuáng 0g.	Fúlíng 5g + fùzǐ 4-3g + dǎngshēn 4-2g + báisháo 4-0g + báizhú 2-0g + gāncǎo 2-0g + gānjiāng 1-0g + huángqín 1-0g. Shānyào 5g + tiānhuā 5g + fùzǐ 5g + fúlíng 5g + jùmài 5g. Báimáogēn 5g + chìxiǎodòu 5g + chēqiánzǐ 4g + yìmǔcǎo 4g + dāngguī 2g + dàhuáng 0g.

membrane, due to abnormal immune response, such as autoimmune disease, cancer, and infection, causes primary membranoproliferative glomerulonephritis.

Yìmǔcǎo (Herba Leonuri) translates to "mother-benefiting herb" and is used today for disorders of menstruation and lesions in the kidney (Wang, 2020). It was also proposed to treat cardiovascular diseases (Liu et al., 2012). Zélán (Herba Lycopi), combined with Huángqí, was shown to significantly lower fasting glucose and urine albumin in diabetic rats (Fu et al., 2014). Dīngshùxiǔ (cf. Section 3.35) was demonstrated to be hypoglycemic in diabetic rats (Daisy et al., 2007).

16.3 CYSTINURIA

Cystinuria, also known as cystinuria-lysinuria syndrome, is caused by gene mutations that prevent proper reabsorption of cystine and lysine amino acids into the blood from urine. High concentrations of cystine in the urine lead to the formation of cystine stones in the kidneys, ureters, and bladder.

Chìsháo (cf. Sections 2.36 and 9.8) was shown to decrease cell viability of bladder cancer cells and reduce the bladder tumor size in mice (Lin et al., 2016). Wǔlínsǎn (cf. Sections 3.33 and 5.10),

TABLE 16.3

GMP Herbal Medicines for a 20-Year-Old Adult with Cystinuria

Cystinuria (OrphaCode: 214)

A disease with a prevalence of ~1 in 10,000

Disease-causing germline mutation(s): solute carrier family 3 member 1 (*SLC3A1* / Entrez: 6519) at 2p21

Disease-causing germline mutation(s): solute carrier family 7 member 9 (*SLC7A9* / Entrez: 11136) at 19q13.11

Autosomal recessive, Semi-dominant

Nephrolithiasis, Hematuria, Abnormality of amino acid metabolism

Renal insufficiency, Hyperuricemia

All ages

Nephrolithiasis (592):

Wǔlínsǎn 5g + huàshícǎo 2-1g + huángqín 1-0g + jīnyínhuā 1-0g + púgōngyīng 1-0g + jīnèijīn 1-0g. Bāzhèngsǎn 5g + wǔlínsǎn 5g + dǐdāngtāng 5g.	Huàshícǎo 5g + chēqiáncǎo 5g + hānqiàocǎo 5g + báijí 2-0g + xiāngfù 2-0g. Báimáogēn 5g + niúxī 2-1g + chēqiánzǐ 2-1g + jīnqiáncǎo 2-1g.

(Continued)

TABLE 16.3 *(Continued)*
GMP Herbal Medicines for a 20-Year-Old Adult with Cystinuria

Renal insufficiency (586):

Zhūlíngtāng 5g + jìshēngshènqìwán 5g + dùzhòng 1-0g + xùduàn 1-0g + dōngkuízǐ 1-0g + báimáogēn 1-0g + bìxiè 1-0g + chēqiánzǐ 1-0g + dānshēn 1-0g + niúxī 1-0g + jīnqiáncǎo 1-0g.

Wǔlíngsǎn 5g + jìshēngshènqìwán 5g.

Jìshēngshènqìwán 5g + guīpítāng 5g + dānshēn 1g.

Zhēnwǔtāng 5g + fùzǐ 1g + gānjiāng 1g + suānzǎorén 1g + tiáowèichéngqìtāng 1g.

Báimáogēn 5g + chēqiánzǐ 5g + jīnqiáncǎo 5g + niúxī 3-2g + jùmài 3-0g.

Chēqiánzǐ 5g + fúlíng 5g + shānyào 4g + tiānhuā 4g + fùzǐ 4g + jùmài 4g.

Chēqiánzǐ 5g + zhìgāncǎo 5g + niúxī 3g + chìsháo 3g + fùzǐ 3g + máhuáng 3g + huángqí 3g + dàhuáng 0g.

Dìhuáng 5g + mǔdānpí 5g + chìsháo 5g + hónghuā 5g + guìzhī 5g + táorén 5g + huángbò 5g + dāngguī 5g + dàhuáng 2g.

Fúlíng 5g + fùzǐ 4-3g + dǎngshēn 4-3g + báisháo 4-0g + gāncǎo 3-0g + báizhú 1-0g + gānjiāng 1-0g.

Fúlíng 5g + huángqí 3g + gāncǎo 2g + fùzǐ 2g + chénpí 2g + zéxiè 2g + dǎngshēn 2g + shānzhā 1g + shénqū 1g + màiyá 1g + dàhuáng 0g.

containing Chìsháo, "clears heat, cools Blood, induces urination, relieves stranguria" and is used today for cystitis (Wang, 2019). Note that herbal prescriptions for patients with the same symptoms but different ages may differ (cf. Tables 16.1 and 16.3).

16.4 ADENINE PHOSPHORIBOSYLTRANSFERASE DEFICIENCY

Adenine phosphoribosyltransferase deficiency, also called APRT deficiency or 2,8-dihydroxyadenine urolithiasis, is characterized by the recurrent formation of stones in the kidneys and urinary tract. APRT deficiency is caused by mutations in the *APRT* gene, whose products are part of the purine salvage pathway. Deficiency in purine adenine recycling leads to accumulation and crystallization of 2,8-dihydroxyadenine in urine and formation of the stone.

Bìxiè (Rhizoma Dioscoreae Septemlobae) was shown to be anti-hyperuricemic and nephroprotective in hypertensive mice (Su et al., 2014) and is used for diabetes (Wang, 2020). Bìxièfēnqīngyǐn,

TABLE 16.4
GMP Herbal Medicines for a 19-Year-Old Adult with Adenine Phosphoribosyltransferase Deficiency

Adenine phosphoribosyltransferase deficiency (OrphaCode: 976)

A disease with a prevalence of ~5 in 100,000

Disease-causing germline mutation(s) (loss of function): adenine phosphoribosyltransferase (*APRT* / Entrez: 353) at 16q24.3

Autosomal recessive

Abnormal enzyme/coenzyme activity

Renal insufficiency, Proteinuria, Nephrolithiasis, Hypertension, Acute kidney injury, Chronic kidney disease, Dysuria

Recurrent urinary tract infections, Urinary retention, Urinary hesitancy, Uric acid nephrolithiasis, Stage 5 chronic kidney disease, Atrial fibrillation, Abdominal colic, Macroscopic hematuria, Flank pain, Oliguria

Infancy, Childhood, Adolescent, Adult, Elderly

Renal insufficiency (586), Proteinuria (791.0), Nephrolithiasis (592), Hypertension (401-405.99), Dysuria (D053159):

Zhūlíngtāng 5g + jìshēngshènqìwán 5g + báimáogēn 2-1g + yìmǔcǎo 2-1g + dānshēn 2-0g + zélán 2-0g + jīxuèténg 2-0g + bìxiè 1-0g + dàhuáng 1-0g.

Bìxièfēnqīngyǐn 5g + jìshēngshènqìwán 5g + báimáogēn 1g + yìmǔcǎo 1g.

Jìshēngshènqìwán 5g + zhūlíngtāng 4-3g + huángqí 2-0g + dīngshùxiǔ 1-0g + xiānhècǎo 1-0g + báimáogēn 1-0g + bìxiè 1-0g + ǒujiē 1-0g + dàhuáng 0g.

Chìxiǎodòu 5g + chēqiánzǐ 5-2g + yìmǔcǎo 5-2g + báimáogēn 5-0g + dāngguī 3-2g + dàhuáng 0g.

Fúlíng 5g + fùzǐ 4-2g + dǎngshēn 2g + gāncǎo 2g + gānjiāng 1g.

Fúlíng 5g + jùmài 5g + shānyào 3g + tiānhuā 3g + fùzǐ 3g + dàhuáng 0g.

Fúlíng 5g + báisháo 3g + fùzǐ 3g + dǎngshēn 3g + báizhú 2g.

(Continued)

TABLE 16.4 *(Continued)*

GMP Herbal Medicines for a 19-Year-Old Adult with Adenine Phosphoribosyltransferase Deficiency

Atrial fibrillation (427.31), Abdominal colic (D003085), Flank pain (D021501), Oliguria (D009846):

Zhìgāncǎotāng 5g + yǎngxīntāng 5g.	Xièbái 5g + guālóurén 2g + bànxià 2-0g + dānshēn 1-0g +
Zhìgāncǎotāng 5g + cháixiàntāng 5g.	hónghuā 1-0g + jiàngzhēnxiāng 1-0g.
Zhìgāncǎotāng 5g + dānshēn 1-0g + wǔwèizǐ 0g +	Fùzǐ 5g + gāncǎo 5-4g + fúlíng 5-0g + gānjiāng 4-3g +
màiméndōng 0g + yùjīn 0g.	suānzǎorén 3-0g.
Cháixiàntāng 5g + fùfāngdānshēnpiàn 5g + yǎngxīntāng 5g.	Guālóurén 5g + xièbái 5-4g + bànxià 3-0g + guìzhī 3-0g +
	hòupò 2-0g + zhǐshí 2-0g.

containing Bìxiè, was introduced in Section 3.16 for nephritis and nephropathy. Xièbái "connects yang, dissolves congelation, moves Qi, conducts stagnation" and is used for palpitations (cf. Section 12.9). Fúlíng not only benefits the skin (cf. Section 7.3) but also protects the kidney (Nie et al., 2020). Yǎngxīntāng, containing Fúlíng, is used for cardiac dysrhythmias (cf. Section 11.11) as well as for neurotic disorders (Wang, 2019).

16.5 GITELMAN SYNDROME

Gitelman syndrome is an autosomal recessive trait characterized by an imbalance of potassium, magnesium, and calcium ions in the body. Gitelman syndrome is caused by mutations in a gene coding for sodium-chloride cotransporters, which are found in kidney nephrons responsible for the regulation of potassium, sodium, calcium, and pH.

TABLE 16.5

GMP Herbal Medicines for a 12-Year-Old Child with Gitelman Syndrome

Gitelman syndrome (OrphaCode: 358)

A disease with a prevalence of ~2 in 100,000

Disease-causing germline mutation(s) (loss of function): solute carrier family 12 member 3 (*SLC12A3* / HGNC:10912) at 16q13

Disease-causing germline mutation(s) (loss of function): chloride voltage-gated channel Kb (*CLCNKB* / Entrez: 1188) at 1p36.13

Autosomal recessive

Hypokalemia

Muscle weakness, Failure to thrive, Prolonged QT interval, Abdominal pain, Low-to-normal blood pressure, Hypomagnesemia

Nocturia, Proteinuria, Renal potassium wasting, Enuresis, Delayed puberty, Glucose intolerance, Insulin resistance, Nausea and vomiting, Hypocalcemia, Hypermagnesemia, Muscle spasm, Salt craving, Metabolic alkalosis

Childhood

Muscle weakness (D018908), Abdominal pain (D015746):

Dúhuójìshēngtāng 5g + shūjīnghuóxuètāng 4g + acupuncture.	Báizhú 5g + báisháo 5g + fùzǐ 5g + fúlíng 5g +
Dúhuójìshēngtāng 5g + sháoyàogāncǎotāng 4g +	dǎngshēn 5g.
shūjīnghuóxuètāng 4g + acupuncture.	Báizhú 5g + fùzǐ 5g + cháihú 5g + báisháo 4g + fúlíng
Dúhuójìshēngtāng 5g + shūjīnghuóxuètāng 4g + niúxī 1g +	4g + tiānhuā 2g + dǎngshēn 2g + guìzhī 2g + huángqín
mòyào 1g + rǔxiāng 1g + yánhúsuǒ 1g + fùzǐ 1g + guìzhī 1g +	2g + wǔwèizǐ 2-0g + xìxīn 2-0g + shēngjiāng 2-0g +
jīxuèténg 1g.	gāncǎo 1g + mǔlì 1g + gānjiāng 1g.
Dúhuójìshēngtāng 5g + dùzhòng 1g + gǔsuìbǔ 1g + xùduàn	Báizhú 5g + fúlíng 5-4g + zhìgāncǎo 3g + gānjiāng 3g +
1g + gǒujǐ 1-0g + niúxī 1-0g + acupuncture.	niúxī 3-2g + fùzǐ 3-2g + guìzhī 3-2g + dàhuáng 0g.

(Continued)

TABLE 16.5 *(Continued)*
GMP Herbal Medicines for a 12-Year-Old Child with Gitelman Syndrome

Nocturia (D053158), Proteinuria (791.0), Muscle spasm (D009120):

Wǔlíngsǎn 5g + qīngxīnliánzǐyǐn 5g + bìxièfēnqīngyǐn 5-0g.

Wǔlíngsǎn 5g + bìxièfēnqīngyǐn 5g + jìshēngshènqìwán 5g + gāncǎo 0g.

Wǔlíngsǎn 5g + jìshēngshènqìwán 5g + báimáogēn 1g + chēqiánzǐ 1g.

Liùjūnzǐtāng 5g + liùwèidìhuángwán 5g + bìxièfēnqīngyǐn 5g.

Qiànshí 5g + yìyǐrén 5g + fùpénzǐ 5-0g + báizhú 2-0g + fúlíng 1-0g + chēqiánzǐ 0g + ròuguì 0g.

Dìhuáng 5g + qínpí 5g + fúlíng 5g + huángbò 5g + zéxiè 5g + dàhuáng 0g.

Zhǐqiào 5g + jílí 5g + chántuì 5g.

Dúhuójìshēngtāng (cf. Sections 2.10 and 8.1), combined with Western medicine, was concluded to be beneficial for patients with knee osteoarthritis in a systematic review and meta-analysis of randomized clinical trials (Zhang et al., 2016). Qiànshí (Semen Euryales) "benefits the Kidney, retains semen, strengthens the Spleen, stops diarrhea, eliminates dampness, arrests leukorrhea" and is used today for urinary frequency, nephrotic syndrome, proteinuria, leukorrhea, and so on (Wang, 2020). Fùpénzǐ is used for urinary frequency and urinary incontinence (cf. Section 2.31). Qīngxīnliánzǐyǐn (cf. Section 3.11) for nephrotic syndrome in children was reviewed (Zhang et al., 2023).

REFERENCES

Daisy, P., Rayan, A., & Rajathi, D. (2007). Hypoglycemic and other related effects of *Elephantopus scaber* extracts on alloxan induced diabetic rats. *Journal of Biological Sciences*, 7(2), 433–437. https://doi.org/10.3923/jbs.2007.433.437

Fu, X., Song, B., Guo-Wei, T., & Li, J. (2014). The effects of the water-extraction of Astragali Radix and Lycopi herba on the pathway of TGF-smads-UPP in a rat model of diabetic nephropathy. *Pharmacognosy Magazine*, 10(40), 491. https://doi.org/10.4103/0973-1296.141773

Gohil, K. J., Patel, J. A., & Anuradha, G. (2010). Pharmacological review on *Centella asiatica*: A potential herbal cure-all. *Indian Journal of Pharmaceutical Sciences*, 72(5), 546. https://doi.org/10.4103/0250-474x.78519

Lin, M., Chiang, S., Li, Y., Chen, M., Chen, Y., Wu, J., & Liu, Y. (2016). Anti-tumor effect of Radix Paeoniae Rubra extract on mice bladder tumors using intravesical therapy. *Oncology Letters*, 12(2), 904–910. https://doi.org/10.3892/ol.2016.4698

Liu, X. H., Pan, L., & Zhu, Y. (2012). Active chemical compounds of traditional Chinese medicine Herba Leonuri: Implications for cardiovascular diseases. *Clinical and Experimental Pharmacology & Physiology*, 39(3), 274–282. https://doi.org/10.1111/j.1440-1681.2011.05630.x

Nie, A., Chao, Y., Zhang, X., Jia, W., Zhou, Z., & Zhu, C. (2020). Phytochemistry and pharmacological activities of *Wolfiporia cocos* (F.A. Wolf) Ryvarden & Gilb. *Frontiers in Pharmacology*, 11, 505249. https://doi.org/10.3389/fphar.2020.505249

Oh, Y., Jeong, Y. H., Cho, W., Hwang, Y., & Yeul, J. (2018). Inhibitory effects of Dianthi Herba ethanolic extract on inflammatory and nociceptive responses in murine macrophages and mouse models of abdominal writhing and ear edema. *Journal of Ethnopharmacology*, 211, 375–383. https://doi.org/10.1016/j.jep.2017.09.010

Su, J.-X., Wei, Y., Liu, M., Liu, T., Li, J., Ji, Y., & Liang, J. (2014). Anti-hyperuricemic and nephroprotective effects of *Rhizoma Dioscoreae septemlobae* extracts and its main component dioscin via regulation of mOAT1, mURAT1 and mOCT2 in hypertensive mice. *Archives of Pharmacal Research*, 37(10), 1336–1344. https://doi.org/10.1007/s12272-014-0413-6

Wang, S.-C. (2019). Therapeutic classes of CHEG formulas. In S.-C. Wang (Ed.), *Clinical herbal prescriptions: Principles and practices of herbal formulations from deep learning health insurance herbal prescription big data* (pp. 16–89). World Scientific Publishing. https://doi.org/10.1142/11211

Wang, S.-C. (2020). Modern therapeutic uses of CHEG herbs and herb pairs. In S.-C. Wang (Ed.), *Veterinary herbal pharmacopoeia* (pp. 35–233). Nova Science Publishers. https://doi.org/10.52305/GHTR1903

Xiong, Y., Wang, J.-W., & Deng, J. (2015). [Comparison between Lysimachiae Herba and Desmodii Styracifolii Herba in pharmacological activities]. *Zhongguo Zhong Yao Za Zhi*, *40*(11), 2106–2111. [Article in Chinese] https://pubmed.ncbi.nlm.nih.gov/26552164

Zhang, W., Wang, S., Zhang, R., Zhang, Y., Li, X., Lin, Y., & Wei, X. (2016). Evidence of Chinese herbal medicine Duhuo Jisheng decoction for knee osteoarthritis: A systematic review of randomised clinical trials. *BMJ Open*, *6*(1), e008973. https://doi.org/10.1136/bmjopen-2015-008973

Zhang, Y., Du, L., Liu, B., & Wang, H. (2023). Study on the progress of application of Qingxin Lianzi drink in paediatric nephrotic syndrome. *Alternative Therapies in Health and Medicine*, *29*(8), 882–891. https://pubmed.ncbi.nlm.nih.gov/37708561

17 GMP Herbal Medicine for Rare Immune Diseases

Immune diseases are diseases of the immune system which seeks and destroys harmful invaders. Causes of immune diseases include virial infections, medications, and genetics. Many rare immune diseases of this chapter are inherited.

The GMP single herbs and multi-herb formulas that are frequently prescribed for the signs and symptoms of the rare immune diseases are Licorice Root (Gāncǎo), Rhubarb Root and Rhizome (Dàhuáng), Cardamon Seed (Shārén), Dahurian Angelica Root (Báizhǐ), Scutellaria Root (Huángqín), Processed Licorice Root (Zhìgāncǎo), Virgate Wormwood Herb (Yīnchén), Ophiopogon Tuber (Màiméndōng), Bitter Apricot Kernel (Xìngrén), Five Ingredient Formula with Poria (Wǔlíngsǎn), Schizonepeta and Siler Formula (Jīngfángbàidúsǎn), Minor Bupleurum Decoction (Xiǎocháihútāng), Free and Easy Wanderer Plus (Augmented Rambling Powder; Jiāwèixiāoyáosǎn), Sweet Dew Decoction (Gānlùyǐn), Virgate Wormwood and Five Ingredient Powder with Poria (Yīnchénwǔlíngsǎn), Ephedra, Apricot Kernel, Gypsum, and Licorice Decoction (Máxìnggānshítāng), Ginseng, Poria and Atractylodes Powder (Shēnlíngbáizhúsǎn), Bupleurum Dredging the Liver Decoction (Cháihúshūgāntāng), Regulate the Stomach and Order the Qi Decoction (Tiáowèichéngqìtāng), Minor Construct the Middle Decoction (Xiǎojiànzhōngtāng), and Minor Blue Dragon Decoction (Xiǎoqīnglóngtāng).

In traditional Chinese medicine (TCM), the Qi running under the skin plays the role of immunity. In addition, TCM products that clear heat are immunosuppressing, and those that supplement Qi are immunoenhancing. TCM can thus contribute to contemporary immunomodulatory therapies (Ma et al., 2013).

17.1 T-B+ SEVERE COMBINED IMMUNODEFICIENCY DUE TO GAMMA CHAIN DEFICIENCY

T-B+ severe combined immunodeficiency due to gamma chain deficiency, or T-B+ SCID due to gamma chain deficiency, is the most common form of severe combined immunodeficiency (SCID) characterized by low mature T- and NK cell numbers and high numbers of dysfunctional B-cell. It is caused by mutations in a gene, on chromosome X, coding for the gamma chain of the IL-2 receptor. SCID is life-threatening, resulting in recurrent infection, diarrhea, and failure to thrive in newborns.

TABLE 17.1

GMP Herbal Medicines for a One-Year-Old Boy with T-B+ Severe Combined Immunodeficiency Due to Gamma Chain Deficiency

T-B+ severe combined immunodeficiency due to gamma chain deficiency (OrphaCode: 276)

A disease with a prevalence of ~5 in 100,000

Disease-causing germline mutation(s): interleukin 2 receptor subunit gamma (*IL2RG* / Entrez: 3561) at Xq13.1

X-linked recessive

Lymphopenia, Recurrent fever, Pneumonia, Decreased proportion of CD4-positive T cells, Abnormal immunoglobulin level, Decreased lymphocyte proliferation in response to mitogen, Reduced proportion of naive T cells, Reduced natural killer cell count

(Continued)

DOI: 10.1201/9781032726625-17

TABLE 17.1 *(Continued)*

GMP Herbal Medicines for a One-Year-Old Boy with T-B+ Severe Combined Immunodeficiency Due to Gamma Chain Deficiency

Skin rash, Diarrhea, Recurrent bacterial infections, Decreased circulating IgA level, Decreased circulating IgG level, Recurrent opportunistic infections, Cough, Abnormally low T-cell receptor excision circle level, Decreased proportion of CD3-positive T cells, Sepsis

Failure to thrive, Chronic mucocutaneous candidiasis, Lymph node hypoplasia, Recurrent herpes, Recurrent Haemophilus influenzae infections, Recurrent bacterial skin infections, Severe recurrent varicella, Chronic oral candidiasis, Recurrent cutaneous fungal infections, Absent tonsils

Neonatal

Lymphopenia (288.51):

Xiǎojiànzhōngtāng 5g + shēnlíngbáizhúsǎn 5-0g + shānzhā 1-0g + màiyá 1-0g + jīnèijīn 1-0g.

Shēnlíngbáizhúsǎn 5g + bǎohéwán 2-0g + shānzhā 1-0g + màiyá 1-0g + shénqū 0g.

Sìjūnzǐtāng 5g.

Xiǎojiànzhōngtāng 5g + yùpíngfēngsǎn 5-2g.

Xiāngshāliùjūnzǐtāng 5g + shānzhā 2g + shénqū 2g + màiyá 2g.

Gāncǎo 5g + báizhǐ 5-2g + shārén 5-2g + jīnyínhuā 2-0g + dàhuáng 1-0g.

Xuánshēn 5g + dìhuáng 5g + màiméndōng 5g + hòupò 2-1g + zhǐshí 2-1g + dàhuáng 1-0g.

Zhìgāncǎo 5g + shārén 5g + báizhǐ 3g + dàhuáng 1g.

Skin rash (782.1), Diarrhea (D003967), Cough (D003371):

Xiāofēngsǎn 5g + jīngfángbàidúsǎn 5-0g + báixiānpí 1-0g + dìfūzǐ 1-0g.

Jīngfángbàidúsǎn 5g + jīnyínhuā 1g + liánqiáo 1g.

Gānlùxiāodúdān 5g + jīngfángbàidúsǎn 5g + gāncǎo 0g.

Wǔlíngsǎn 5g.

Báizhǐ 5g + gāncǎo 4g + shārén 4-3g + huángqín 4-0g + guālóugēn 2-0g + tiānhuā 1-0g + dàhuáng 0g.

Gāncǎo 5g + báizhǐ 5g + shārén 5g + huángqín 5-0g + jīnyínhuā 2-0g + dàhuáng 1-0g.

A compound in Gāncǎo (cf. Section 1.1) was shown to enhance significantly a specific antibody and cellular immune response against ovalbumin in mice (Sun & Pan, 2006). The immune regulating effect of Xuánshēn (cf. Sections 8.7 and 8.16) was demonstrated through the synergistic "yin-nourishing" effect of its compounds on yin-deficient mice (Gong et al., 2020). The term jiànzhōng in Xiǎojiànzhōngtāng (cf. Sections 5.23 and 9.9) is meant to enhance the functions and activities of the organs inside the body. Xiāofēngsǎn (cf. Section 1.23) is used today for eczema and urticaria (Wang, 2019).

17.2 AUTOSOMAL DOMINANT HYPER-IgE SYNDROME

Autosomal dominant hyper-IgE syndrome is also known as Buckley syndrome, Job syndrome, or STAT3 deficiency. It is a multisystem immunodeficiency disorder, characterized by elevated levels of immunoglobulin E in the serum, which affects the connective tissues, lungs, and skeleton. It is caused by mutations in a gene involved in the STAT3 pathway, resulting in reduced protection against bacterial and fungal infections and in other abnormal immune responses.

TABLE 17.2

GMP Herbal Medicines for a One-Year-Old Baby with Autosomal Dominant Hyper-IgE Syndrome

Autosomal dominant hyper-IgE syndrome (OrphaCode: 2314)

A disease with a prevalence of ~5 in 100,000

Disease-causing germline mutation(s): signal transducer and activator of transcription 3 (*STAT3* / Entrez: 6774) at 17q21.2

Autosomal dominant

(Continued)

TABLE 17.2 *(Continued)*
GMP Herbal Medicines for a One-Year-Old Baby with Autosomal Dominant Hyper-IgE Syndrome

Eczema, Skin rash, Pruritus, Recurrent respiratory infections, Recurrent infections, Increased circulating total IgE level, Generalized abnormality of skin, Atelectasis, Skin ulcer

Abnormality of the dentition, Cleft palate, Gingivitis, Abnormality of the face, Chronic otitis media, Wide nasal bridge, Deeply set eye, Delayed eruption of teeth, Osteopenia, Abnormality of the hair, Paronychia, Eosinophilia, Scoliosis, Recurrent fractures, Joint hyperflexibility, Dystrophic fingernails, Prominent forehead, Cough, Papule

Craniosynostosis, Fever, Dilatation, Lymphoma, Osteomyelitis, Cellulitis, Skin vesicle

Neonatal, Infancy

Skin rash (782.1), Pruritus (D011537):	
Jīngfángbàidúsǎn 5g + dìfūzǐ 2-0g + shéchuángzǐ 2-0g + huánglián 2-0g + jílí 2-0g + jīnchán 1-0g + wǔbèizǐ 0g.	Gāncǎo 5g + jīnyínhuā 5g + liánqiáo 5g.
Xiāofēngsǎn 5g + báixiānpí 1g + dìfūzǐ 1g + jílí 1g.	Jīnyínhuā 5g + gāncǎo 4-2g + báizhǐ 4-0g + shārén 4-0g + dàhuáng 0g.
	Báizhǐ 5g + gāncǎo 5-3g + shārén 5-3g + huángqín 2-0g + guālóugēn 2-0g + dàhuáng 1-0g.
Cleft palate (749.0), Gingivitis (523.0, 523.1), Deeply set eye (376.5), Eosinophilia (288.3), Cough (D003371):	
Gānlùyǐn 5g + zhībódìhuángwán 5-0g + qīngwèisǎn 5-0g + dǎochìsǎn 5-0g.	Huángqín 5g + báizhǐ 4g + zhìgāncǎo 3-2g + shārén 3-2g + tiānhuā 2g + xìxīn 1-0g + dàhuáng 1-0g.
Gānlùyǐn 5g + bǎohéwán 5-0g + xiāngshāliùjūnzǐtāng 5-0g + màiyá 2-0g + jīnèijīn 2-0g + xuánshēn 1-0g + mǔdānpí 1-0g + jīnyínhuā 1-0g + liánqiáo 1-0g + gāncǎo 1-0g.	Huángqín 5g + báizhǐ 4g + tiānhuā 3g + gāncǎo 3g + shārén 3g + dàhuáng 0g.
Dǎochìsǎn 5g + gāncǎo 0g.	Zhìgāncǎo 5g + shārén 5g + dàhuáng 0g.
Gānlùyǐn 5g + xīnyíqīngfèitāng 5g.	Zhǐqiào 5g + jílí 2g.
	Júhuā 5g + jílí 3-0g + zhǐqiào 2-0g.
Fever (D005334), Dilatation (442.9):	
Wǔlíngsǎn 5g + gāncǎo 1-0g + báisháo 1-0g + tiáowèichéngqìtāng 1-0g + dàhuáng 0g.	Gāncǎo 5g + báizhǐ 5-4g + shārén 5-3g + huángqín 5-0g + dàhuáng 0g.
Xiǎojiànzhōngtāng 5g + gāncǎo 1g + dàhuáng 0g.	
Máxìnggānshítāng 5g + dàzǎo 2g + tínglìzǐ 2g + dàhuáng 0g.	
Guìzhītāng 5g + gāncǎo 2g + tiáowèichéngqìtāng 1g + dàhuáng 0g.	

Jīnyínhuā was introduced in Sections 3.5 and 3.9 to be immune regulating and inflammation suppressing. Dǎochìsǎn was formulated to treat "heat in the Heart meridian and the Small Intestine meridian," which can give rise to sores on the mouth and tongue. Its modern uses include diseases of the urinary system and oral soft tissues (cf. Section 3.19). Huángqín was summarized in Section 2.1 to be antibacterial and antiviral. Wǔlíngsǎn (cf. Section 10.5) improves body fluid metabolism.

17.3 COMMON VARIABLE IMMUNODEFICIENCY

Common variable immunodeficiency, also known as primary antibody deficiency or primary hypogammaglobulinemia, is characterized by low counts of IgG, IgM, and IgA antibodies in the circulation and thus recurrent infections. The cause of the majority of common variable immunodeficiency cases is unknown and mutations in many genes altogether are believed to contribute to the failure of antibody production.

Shúdìhuáng was introduced in Section 2.36 to supplement "body essence and marrow," which enhance one's immunity (Luo et al., 2020). The herb was indeed shown to enhance growth performance, immune response, and bacterial resistance in fish (Wu et al., 2019). Tiānméndōng was introduced in Sections 1.71 and 8.10 for coughs. Dìgǔpí (Cortex Lycii) "cools Blood, relieves (bone) steaming, cleanses the Lung, clears heat" and is used today for both skin and respiratory conditions (Wang, 2020). Huángshuǐqié (Herba Solani Incani) "pacifies the Liver, neutralizes pathogens,

TABLE 17.3
GMP Herbal Medicines for a 35-Year-Old Adult with Common Variable Immunodeficiency

Common variable immunodeficiency (OrphaCode: 1572)

A disease with a prevalence of ~5 in 100,000

Disease-causing germline mutation(s): CD19 molecule (*CD19* / Entrez: 930) at 16p11.2

Disease-causing germline mutation(s): inducible T cell costimulator (*ICOS* / Entrez: 29851) at 2q33.2

Disease-causing germline mutation(s): complement C3d receptor 2 (*CR2* / Entrez: 1380) at 1q32.2

Disease-causing germline mutation(s): TNF receptor superfamily member 13C (*TNFRSF13C* / Entrez: 115650) at 22q13.2

Disease-causing germline mutation(s): membrane spanning 4-domains A1 (*MS4A1* / Entrez: 931) at 11q12.2

Disease-causing germline mutation(s): CD81 molecule (*CD81* / Entrez: 975) at 11p15.5

Disease-causing germline mutation(s): protein kinase C delta (*PRKCD* / Entrez: 5580) at 3p21.1

Disease-causing germline mutation(s) (loss of function): TNF superfamily member 12 (*TNFSF12* / Entrez: 8742) at 17p13.1

Disease-causing germline mutation(s) (gain of function): TNF superfamily member 12 (*TNFSF12* / Entrez: 8742) at 17p13.1

Disease-causing germline mutation(s): nuclear factor kappa B subunit 1 (*NFKB1* / Entrez: 4790) at 4q24

Disease-causing germline mutation(s): nuclear factor kappa B subunit 2 (*NFKB2* / Entrez: 4791) at 10q24.32

Disease-causing germline mutation(s) (gain of function): interferon regulatory factor 2 binding protein 2 (*IRF2BP2* / Entrez: 359948) at 1q42.3

Disease-causing germline mutation(s): TNF receptor superfamily member 13B (*TNFRSF13B* / Entrez: 23495) at 17p11.2

Autosomal dominant, Autosomal recessive, Not applicable

Brachycephaly, Otitis media, Chronic otitis media, Lymphopenia, Autoimmune thrombocytopenia, Pneumonia, Recurrent respiratory infections, Immunodeficiency, Recurrent bronchitis, Decreased antibody level in blood

Purpura, Abnormality of the liver, Splenomegaly, Hemolytic anemia, Anal atresia, Bronchiectasis, Lymphadenopathy, Elevated hepatic transaminase

Failure to thrive in infancy, Restrictive ventilatory defect, Emphysema, Vasculitis, Lymphoma, Arthralgia, Posterior pharyngeal cleft, Gastrointestinal stroma tumor

All ages

Otitis media (382.9), Lymphopenia (288.51), Autoimmune thrombocytopenia (287.31), Immunodeficiency (279.3):

Yínqiàosăn 5g + lóngdănxiègāntāng 5-0g + xuánshēn 1-0g + dìhuáng 1-0g + màiméndōng 1-0g + dàhuáng 1-0g.

Yìqìcōngmíngtāng 5g + bŭzhōngyìqìtāng 4g + dānshēn 1g + shíchāngpú 1g + yuănzhì 1g.

Línggùishùgāntāng 5g + huángqí 2g + dānggūi 1g + dàhuáng 0g.

Liùwèidìhuángwán 5g + línggùishùgāntāng 5g + gūipítāng 5g + xiānhècăo 1g.

Rénshēnyăngróngtāng 5g + gūipítāng 5-0g + jiāwèixiāoyáosăn 5-0g + zhībódìhuángwán 5-0g.

Shúdìhuáng 5g + báizhú 4g + fùzĭ 4g + báisháo 3g + fúlíng 3g + báijièzĭ 2g + dăngshēn 2g + shēngjiāng 1g + máhuáng 1g + dàhuáng 1-0g + gāncăo 1-0g + huánglián 0g.

Huángqí 5g + dìhuáng 4g + dānggūi 4g + shúdìhuáng 4g + huángqín 2g + huángbò 2g + huánglián 2g.

Gāncăo 5g + báizhĭ 5g + shārén 5g + huángqín 5g + dàhuáng 1g.

Bànxià 5g + ējiāo 5g + zĭcăo 5g + dăngshēn 5g + fùzĭ 3g + gānjiāng 3g.

Purpura (D011693), Abnormality of the liver (573.9), Bronchiectasis (494):

Jiāwèixiāoyáosăn 5g + xuèfŭzhúyūtāng 5g + dānshēn 1g + wŭwèizĭ 1g + màiméndōng 1g.

Jiāwèixiāoyáosăn 5g + cháihúshūgāntāng 5g + yīnchénwŭlíngsăn 5-0g + dānshēn 1-0g + yīnchén 1-0g + yùjīn 1-0g + huángshuĭqié 1-0g.

Yīnchénwŭlíngsăn 5g + xiăocháihútāng 4g + máxìnggānshítāng 3g + fángfēng 1g + cāngĕrzĭ 1g.

Yīnchénwŭlíngsăn 5g + jiāwèixiāoyáosăn 4g + máxìnggānshítāng 3g + huángqí 1g + fángfēng 1g + cāngĕrzĭ 1g.

Cháihúshūgāntāng 5g + gānlùxiāodúdān 4g + yīnchénwŭlíngsăn 4g + hŭzhàng 1g + huángshuĭqié 1g.

Xiăocháihútāng 5g + yīnchénwŭlíngsăn 5g + jiāwèixiāoyáosăn 5-0g + wŭwèizĭ 1-0g + hŭzhàng 1-0g + huángshuĭqié 1-0g.

Wŭwèizĭ 5g + bànxià 5g + zhìgāncăo 5g + cháihú 5g + gānjiāng 5g + huángqín 5g + dàhuáng 1-0g.

Dānshēn 5g + gāncăo 5g + xìngrén 5g + zhīmŭ 5g + jīnyínhuā 5g + qiánhú 5g + huángqín 5g.

Băibù 5g + zĭwăn 5g + báiqián 4g + xìngrén 4g + jiégĕng 4g + jīngjiè 4g + máhuáng 4g + kuăndōnghuā 4g + gāncăo 2g + chénpí 2g.

Tiānméndōng 5g + dìgŭpí 5g + xìngrén 5g + zhìgāncăo 5g + jiégĕng 5g + sāngbáipí 5g + màiméndōng 5g + huángqín 5g.

Gāncăo 5g + chuānqí 3g + báijiāngcán 3g + xìngrén 3g + fángfēng 3g + jiégĕng 3g + jīngjiè 3g + bòhé 3g + niúbàngzĭ 2g.

Gāncăo 5g + wŭwèizĭ 4g + jiégĕng 4g + fúlíng 4g + xìxīn 1g + gānjiāng 0g.

(Continued)

TABLE 17.3 *(Continued)*

GMP Herbal Medicines for a 35-Year-Old Adult with Common Variable Immunodeficiency

Emphysema (492.8), Arthralgia (D018771):

Xiǎoqīnglóngtāng 5g + xìngrén 1-0g + hòupò 1-0g + fúlíng 1-0g.

Máxìnggānshítāng 5g + tínglìzǐ 2-0g + dàzǎo 1-0g + dàhuáng 0g.

Zhēnwǔtāng 5g + wǔwèizǐ 0g + bànxià 0g + gānjiāng 0g + xìxīn 0g.

Gāncǎo 5g + máhuáng 2g + yínyánghuò 2g + shúdìhuáng 2g.

Gāncǎo 5g + báizhú 5g + bǎihé 5g + xìngrén 5g + bèimǔ 5g + fúlíng 5g + dǎngshēn 5g.

Dàzǎo 5g + gāncǎo 5g + xìngrén 5g + jiégěng 5g + kuǎndōnghuā 5g + zǐwǎn 5g + tínglìzǐ 5g + máhuáng 4g + wǔwèizǐ 2g + xìxīn 1g + gānjiāng 1g.

Guālóurén 5g + tiānméndōng 3g + xìngrén 3g + bèimǔ 3g + sāngbáipí 3g + màiméndōng 3g + zhīmǔ 2g + zǐwǎn 2g + huángqín 2g + júhóng 2g + gāncǎo 2g + zhǐqiào 2g + jiégěng 2g.

Wǔwèizǐ 5g + gāncǎo 5g + xìngrén 5g + fùzǐ 5g + gānjiāng 5g + xìxīn 5g.

---

scatters wind, stops pain" and is used for skin and malignant neoplasms of the liver and lungs (Wang, 2020). Kuǎndōnghuā (Flos Farfarae) "moistens the Lung, stops coughing, dissolves phlegm" and is used today mainly for coughs and bronchitis (Wang, 2020). Wǔwèizǐ was introduced in Sections 7.10, 12.2, and 12.10 for respiratory conditions.

17.4 GRAFT VERSUS HOST DISEASE

Graft versus host disease (GVH) is a multisystem disorder that occurs when, after a bone marrow or stem cell transplantation, the T cells in the donor's tissue recognize the recipient's cells as foreign and thus attack the recipient's organs. GVH is acute when symptoms occur within 100 days after the transplantation.

Shíhú (cf. Section 4.15) is used today for functional disorders of the intestines (Wang, 2020). Héshǒuwū (cf. Sections 8.8 and 15.5) was shown to attenuate nonalcoholic fatty liver disease in zebrafish (Yu et al., 2020) and its modern uses include benign essential hypertension and alcoholic fatty liver (Wang, 2020). Tōngcǎo (Medulla Tetrapanacis) was shown to alleviate inflammation and infection in a murine macrophage cell line (Kwok et al., 2023) and is used for pruritis, dyspepsia, and neuralgia (Wang, 2020). Hǔzhàng (cf. Section 4.32) pairs with Shāshēn (cf. Section 10.2) for the treatment of alcoholic fatty liver (Wang, 2020), while Yīnchén (cf. Sections 1.57 and 4.21) combines with Tōngcǎo for chronic hepatitis (Wang, 2020).

TABLE 17.4

GMP Herbal Medicines for a 56-Year-Old Adult with Graft Versus Host Disease

Graft versus host disease (OrphaCode: 39812)

A disease with a prevalence of ~5 in 100,000

Not applicable

Inflammatory abnormality of the skin

Oral ulcer, Diarrhea, Recurrent infections, Elevated hepatic transaminase, Stomatitis, Maculopapular exanthema, Skin erosion, Chronic hepatitis

Irritability, Jaundice, Arthritis, Hepatosplenomegaly, Tachycardia, Vomiting, Nausea, Abdominal pain, Pneumonia, Pulmonary infiltrates, Hyperbilirubinemia, Limited elbow movement, Elevated alkaline phosphatase, Skeletal muscle atrophy, Gastrointestinal inflammation, Limited shoulder movement, Hemophagocytosis, Recurrent gastroenteritis, Cutaneous sclerotic plaque, Lichenoid skin lesion, Scaling skin, Inflammatory abnormality of the eye, Fasciitis, Myositis, Acute hepatitis

All ages

(Continued)

TABLE 17.4 *(Continued)*

GMP Herbal Medicines for a 56-Year-Old Adult with Graft Versus Host Disease

Diarrhea (D003967), Elevated hepatic transaminase (573.9), Chronic hepatitis (570, 571.4, 571.41):

Xiǎocháihútāng 5g + jiāwèixiāoyáosǎn 5g + shēnlíngbáizhúsǎn 5g + shānzhā 1g + dānshēn 1g + xiàkūcǎo 1g.

Xiǎocháihútāng 5g + xiāngshāliùjūnzǐtāng 5g + huòxiāngzhèngqìsǎn 5g.

Wǔlíngsǎn 5g + píngwèisǎn 5g + cháihúshūgāntāng 5g + yīnchén 1g.

Xiǎocháihútāng 5g + wǔlíngsǎn 5g + píngwèisǎn 5-0g + yīnchén 2-0g + zhīzǐ 2-0g + púgōngyīng 1-0g.

Jiāwèixiāoyáosǎn 5g + yīnchénwǔlíngsǎn 5g + wǔwèizǐ 1g + hǔzhàng 1g + yīnchén 1g + huángshuǐqié 1g.

Hǔzhàng 5g + nǔzhēnzǐ 3-2g + tiānhuā 3-2g + shíhú 3-2g + hànliáncǎo 3-2g + shāshēn 3-2g + zhìgāncǎo 3-2g + chuānliànzǐ 2-1g + gǒuqǐzǐ 2-1g + màiméndōng 2-1g + júhuā 2-1g + huángjīng 2-1g + héshǒuwū 2-0g.

Yīnchén 5g + báimáogēn 2g + chēqiánzǐ 2g + chìxiǎodòu 2g + dàzǎo 1g + shēngjiāng 1g + xìngrén 1g + zhìgāncǎo 1g + sāngbáipí 1g + liánqiáo 1g + máhuáng 0g.

Shúdìhuáng 5g + báizhú 4g + fùzǐ 4g + báisháo 3g + fúlíng 3g + báijièzǐ 2g + dǎngshēn 2g + gāncǎo 1g + shēngjiāng 1g + máhuáng 1g + huánglián 0g.

Jaundice (D007565), Vomiting (D014839), Nausea (D009325), Abdominal pain (D015746), Skeletal muscle atrophy (D009133), Fasciitis (729.4):

Wǔlíngsǎn 5g + shūjīnghuóxuètāng 5g + dāngguīniántòngtāng 5-0g + yánhúsuǒ 1-0g + acupuncture.

Wǔlíngsǎn 5g + báisháo 1-0g + yīnchén 1-0g + huángqín 1-0g + guìzhī 1-0g.

Yīnchénwǔlíngsǎn 5g + huòxiāngzhèngqìsǎn 5g + yèjiāoténg 3g + hǎipiāoxiāo 3g + bózǐrén 2g + chántuì 2g + chìsháo 2-0g + cāngzhú 2-0g.

Yīnchén 5g + shānzhīzǐ 4-0g + dàhuáng 2-0g + tōngcǎo 1-0g + huǒmárén 1-0g.

Tiānméndōng 5g + gāncǎo 5g + dìgǔpí 5g + jiégěng 5g + sāngbáipí 5g + màiméndōng 5g + xìngrén 4g + huángqín 2g.

Fùzǐ 5g + fúlíng 5g + báisháo 3g + dǎngshēn 3g + báizhú 2g.

Gāncǎo 5g + chìsháo 5g + zhīmǔ 5g + fùzǐ 5g + máhuáng 5g + huángbò 5g + huángqí 5g.

REFERENCES

Gong, P., He, Y., Qi, J., Chai, C., & Yu, B. (2020). Synergistic nourishing 'Yin' effect of iridoid and phenylpropanoid glycosides from Radix Scrophulariae in vivo and in vitro. *Journal of Ethnopharmacology*, *246*, 112209. https://doi.org/10.1016/j.jep.2019.112209

Kwok, C. T., Chow, W. N., Cheung, K., Zhang, X., Mok, D. K. W., Kwan, Y. W., Chan, G., Leung, G. P., Cheung, K. W., Lee, S. M., Wang, N., Li, J., & Seto, S. W. (2023). *Medulla Tetrapanacis* water extract alleviates inflammation and infection by regulating macrophage polarization through MAPK signaling pathway. *Inflammopharmacology*, *32*, 393–404. https://doi.org/10.1007/s10787-023-01266-1

Luo, C., Qin, S., Liang, P., Ling, W., & Zhao, C. (2020). Advances in modern research on pharmacological effects of *Radix Rehmanniae*. *AIP Conference Proceedings*, *2252*, 020034. https://doi.org/10.1063/5.0020348

Ma, H., Deng, Y., Tian, Z., & Lian, Z. (2013). Traditional Chinese medicine and immune regulation. *Clinical Reviews in Allergy & Immunology*, *44*(3), 229–241. https://doi.org/10.1007/s12016-012-8332-0

Sun, H., & Pan, H. (2006). Immunological adjuvant effect of *Glycyrrhiza uralensis* saponins on the immune responses to ovalbumin in mice. *Vaccine*, *24*(11), 1914–1920. https://doi.org/10.1016/j.vaccine.2005.10.040

Wang, S.-C. (2019). Therapeutic classes of CHEG formulas. In S.-C. Wang (Ed.), *Clinical herbal prescriptions: Principles and practices of herbal formulations from deep learning health insurance herbal prescription big data* (pp. 16–89). World Scientific Publishing. https://doi.org/10.1142/11211

Wang, S.-C. (2020). Modern therapeutic uses of CHEG herbs and herb pairs. In S.-C. Wang (Ed.), *Veterinary herbal pharmacopoeia* (pp. 35–233). Nova Science Publishers. https://doi.org/10.52305/GHTR1903

Wu, C. Y., Shan, J., Feng, J., Wang, J., Qin, C., Nie, G., & Ding, C. (2019). Effects of dietary *Radix Rehmanniae Preparata* polysaccharides on the growth performance, immune response and disease resistance of *Luciobarbus capito*. *Fish & Shellfish Immunology*, *89*, 641–646. https://doi.org/10.1016/j.fsi.2019.04.027

Yu, L., Gong, L., Wang, C., Hu, N., Tang, Y., Li, Z., Dai, X., & Li, Y. (2020). Radix Polygoni Multiflori and its main component emodin attenuate non-alcoholic fatty liver disease in zebrafish by regulation of AMPK signaling pathway. *Drug Design, Development and Therapy*, *Volume 14*, 1493–1506. https://doi.org/10.2147/dddt.s243893

18 GMP Herbal Medicine for Rare Disorders Due to Toxic Effects

Poisoning can be categorized according to the affected organ systems. Neurotoxic poisons attack the central and peripheral nervous systems, making moving and breathing difficult. Hemotoxic poisons destroy red blood cells and change blood clotting, causing anemia and bleeding. Immunotoxic agents interfere with the innate and adaptive immune systems, causing immune suppression, hypersensitivity, or autoimmunity. Genotoxic substances damage DNA, increasing the risk of cancer development. The rare disorders of this chapter are due to heavy metal and snake venom toxicities.

The GMP single herbs and multi-herb formulas that are frequently used for the signs and symptoms of the rare disorders due to toxic effects are Rhubarb Root and Rhizome (Dàhuáng), Licorice Root (Gāncǎo), Immature Bitter Orange (Zhǐshí), Magnolia Bark (Hòupò), Poria (Fúlíng), Cardamon Seed (Shārén), Dahurian Angelica Root (Báizhǐ), Notopterygium Root (Qiānghuó), Donkey Hide Glue (Ējiāo), White Atractylodis (Báizhú), Scutellaria Root (Huángqín), Chinese Angelica Root (female Ginseng; Dāngguī), Blighted Wheat (Fúxiǎomài), Tonify the Middle and Augment the Qi Decoction (Bǔzhōngyìqìtāng), Gastrodia and Uncaria Drink (Tiānmágōuténgyǐn), Jade Windscreen Powder (Yùpíngfēngsǎn), Tangkuei and Tribulus Decoction (Dāngguīyǐnzǐ), Earth Restoring Decoction (Guīpítāng), Regulate the Middle Decoction (Lǐzhōngtāng), Uncaria Formula (Gōuténgsǎn), Schizonepeta and Siler Formula (Jīngfángbàidúsǎn), Minor Construct the Middle Decoction (Xiǎojiànzhōngtāng), Preserve Harmony Pill (Bǎohéwán), Clear the Throat and Enable the Diaphragm Decoction (Qīngyānlìgétāng), and Wind Reducing Formula (Xiāofēngsǎn).

18.1 MERCURY POISONING

Mercury poisoning, also called hydrargyria or mercurialism, is exposure to mercury, which is a neurotoxic and immunotoxic heavy metal. In developed parts of the world, the major route of mercury poisoning is through the consumption of fish and shellfish that have gathered high levels of methylmercury in their bodies through the food chain. Pregnant women are advised to minimize

---

TABLE 18.1

GMP Herbal Medicines for a 24-Year-Old Adult with Mercury Poisoning

Mercury poisoning (OrphaCode: 330021)

A disease with a prevalence of ~5 in 100,000

Not applicable

Hypertension, Seizure, Confusion, Dystonia, Tremor, Tachycardia, Acute kidney injury, Nausea, Anorexia, Dyspnea, Respiratory distress, Abnormal cerebral white matter morphology, Episodic vomiting, Episodic abdominal pain, Hypotension, Respiratory failure, Hypokalemia, Generalized muscle weakness, Interstitial pneumonitis, Loss of consciousness, Insomnia

All ages

Hypertension (401-405.99), Seizure (345.9), Confusion (D003221), Dystonia (D004421), Tremor (D014202), Nausea (D009325), Anorexia (D000855), Respiratory distress (D004417), Loss of consciousness (D014474):

Tiānmágōuténgyǐn 5g + gōuténgsǎn 5-0g + dānshēn 1-0g + báisháo 1-0g + xiàkūcǎo 1-0g + huángqín 1-0g + niúxī 1-0g + gōuténg 1-0g + chuānqī 1-0g.	Qiānghuó 5g + hòupò 5-3g + zhǐshí 5-3g + fángfēng 5-0g + huángqín 2-0g + huánglián 2-0g + dàhuáng 1-0g.
Dāngguīsìnìtāng 5g + shēngjiāng 1g + wúzhūyú 1g + fùzǐ 1g.	Hòupò 5g + zhǐshí 5g + dàhuáng 1g + huǒmárén 1g.

DOI: 10.1201/9781032726625-18

seafood ingestion as the fetus is developing its central nervous system. In other areas of the world, mining workers have a high risk of exposing to mercury.

Qiānghuó was introduced in Sections 2.14 and 4.10 for hypertension. Gōuténg (cf. Section 2.43) was reviewed and summarized to have such pharmacological effects as antihypertension, antiinflammation, anticancer, antioxidation, antivirus, anti-epilepsy, antidepression, anti-ischemic brain injury, neuroprotection, anti-Alzheimer's disease, anti-Parkinson's disease, and antiasthma (Zhang et al., 2023). Both Tiānmágōuténgyǐn and Gōuténgsǎn contain Gōuténg and are used today for essential hypertension (cf. Sections 1.4, 3.21, and 3.30).

18.2 SNAKEBITE ENVENOMATION

Snakebite envenomation is injection of poisonous secretion of a venomous snake into a person's body through a bite by the snake. Snake's venom consists of up to a hundred toxins, which can be neurotoxic, hemotoxic, and cytotoxic. There are about 600 species of venomous snakes worldwide, including vipers and cobras. Farmers, hunters, and hikers are at a high risk of snakebite envenomation.

Púgōngyīng (Herba Taraxaci) was shown to increase the frequency of urination in humans (Clare et al., 2009); it is used for digestive and skin conditions (Wang, 2020). Láifúzǐ (Semen Raphani) "digests food, removes stagnation, lowers rising Qi, dissolves phlegm" and is used for noninfectious gastroenteritis and colitis, flatulence, eructation, gas pain, and coughs (Wang, 2020). Huòxiāng was introduced in Section 3.14 to dry dampness. Fúxiǎomài was introduced in Section 4.7 for the

---

TABLE 18.2

GMP Herbal Medicines for a 35-Year-Old Adult with Snakebite Envenomation

Snakebite envenomation (OrphaCode: 449285)

A disease with a prevalence of ~5 in 100,000

Not applicable

Edema

Erythema, Localized skin lesion, Pain, Ecchymosis

Abnormality of the nervous system, Stroke, Tachycardia, Thrombocytopenia, Abnormal bleeding, Abnormality of coagulation, Vomiting, Intracranial hemorrhage, Cerebral ischemia, Rhabdomyolysis, Paralysis, Muscle fiber necrosis, Pseudobulbar paralysis, Speech articulation difficulties, Hypofibrinogenemia

All ages

Edema (D004487):

Lǐzhōngtāng 5g + bànxià 2-1g + shārén 2-1g + fúlíng 2-1g + dàhuáng 0g.

Lǐzhōngtāng 5g + bǔzhōngyìqìtāng 5g + qīngyānlìgétāng 3g + qínjiāobiējiǎsǎn 3-0g + xiǎojiànzhōngtāng 3-0g + báizhǐ 2g + fángfēng 2g + zhǐqiào 2g + jiégěng 2g + gānjiāng 2g.

Lǐzhōngtāng 5g + bǔzhōngyìqìtāng 5g + liùwèidìhuángwán 3g + qīngyānlìgétāng 3g + fángfēng 2g + zhǐqiào 2g + jiégěng 2g + gānjiāng 2g.

Báizhú 5g + báidòukòu 5g + fúlíng 5g + shíchāngpú 4g + hòupò 4g + zhǐqiào 4g + púgōngyīng 4-0g + láifúzǐ 4-0g.

Báizhú 5g + fúlíng 5g + huòxiāng 5-0g + zhǐshí 4g + shénqū 4g + shānzhā 4-0g + chénpí 4-0g + xiāngfù 4-0g + mùxiāng 4-0g + cháihú 4-0g + púgōngyīng 4-0g + shēngmá 2-0g + báizhǐ 2-0g.

Erythema (D005483), Pain (D010146):

Yùpíngfēngsǎn 5g + bǔzhōngyìqìtāng 5g + mǔlì 1-0g + fúxiǎomài 1-0g + máhuánggēn 1-0g + wǔwèizǐ 1-0g + wūméi 1-0g.

Yùpíngfēngsǎn 5g + bǔzhōngyìqìtāng 5-2g + língguìshùgāntāng 5-0g + xīnyí 2-0g + cāngěrzǐ 2-0g.

Yùpíngfēngsǎn 5g + guìzhītāng 5g + bǔzhōngyìqìtāng 5-0g + cāngěrsǎn 5-0g.

Fúxiǎomài 5g + dàzǎo 2g + gāncǎo 2g + báisháo 2-1g + bǎihé 2-0g + ējiāo 2-0g + bózǐrén 2-0g + fúshén 2-0g + huángqín 2-0g + suānzǎorén 2-0g + gānjiāng 2-0g.

Fúxiǎomài 5g + báisháo 4g + dìhuáng 4g + mǔlì 4g + màiméndōng 4g + zhìgāncǎo 2g + ējiāo 2g + guībǎn 2g + biējiǎ 2g + wǔwèizǐ 1g + huǒmárén 1g.

Fúxiǎomài 5g + dìhuáng 3g + mǔlì 2g + huángqín 2g + huángbò 2g + huángqí 2g + huánglián 2g + dāngguī 2g + shúdìhuáng 2g.

(Continued)

TABLE 18.2 *(Continued)*

GMP Herbal Medicines for a 35-Year-Old Adult with Snakebite Envenomation

Thrombocytopenia (287.5), Abnormality of coagulation (286), Vomiting (D014839), Paralysis (D010243), Pseudobulbar paralysis (335.23):

Bǔzhōngyìqìtāng 5g + guīpítāng 5g + nǔzhēnzǐ 1-0g + xiānhècǎo 1-0g + hànliáncǎo 1-0g + báimáogēn 1-0g + ējiāo 1-0g.

Guīpítāng 5g + bǔzhōngyìqìtāng 3g + xiānhècǎo 1g + dìyú 1-0g.

Shíquándàbǔtāng 5g + guīpítāng 5g + dānshēn 1g + jīxuèténg 1g.

Ējiāo 5g + dāngguī 5-3g + dǎngshēn 5-0g + chuānxiōng 2-0g + gāncǎo 2-0g + dàzǎo 2-0g + shēngjiāng 2-0g + gānjiāng 2-0g + shēngmá 1-0g + cháihú 1-0g + dàhuáng 1-0g.

Shúdìhuáng 5g + báizhú 4g + fùzǐ 4g + báisháo 3g + fúlíng 3g + báijièzǐ 2g + dǎngshēn 2g + gāncǎo 1g + shēngjiāng 1g + máhuáng 1g + dàhuáng 0g.

treatment of erythema. Yùpíngfēngsǎn was shown to ameliorate recurrent allergic inflammation of atopic dermatitis in mice (Zheng et al., 2019).

18.3 LEAD POISONING

Lead poisoning, also called plumbism or saturnism, is a buildup of lead in the body. Lead is a neurotoxic, hemotoxic, immunotoxic, and genotoxic agent. It can be found in paint, leaded gasoline, toys, water pipes, pottery, and cosmetics. Children under the age of 6 are at a high risk of lead poisoning because of their hand-to-mouth behaviors.

Shānzhā (cf. Section 8.8) helps digestion and is used for metabolic and digestive conditions such as hypercholesterolemia and gas pain (Wang, 2020). Mázǐrénwán treats constipation in Section 4.25. Liánqiáo was summarized to be anti-inflammatory, antibacterial, antiviral, antioxidant, and neuroprotective (Dong et al., 2017) and is used today mainly for skin conditions (cf. Section 1.28). Dāngguīyǐnzǐ (cf. Section 3.28) has been used to treat various skin diseases associated with a TCM pattern of blood deficiency and wind dryness (Su et al., 2023). The prescriptions in the table are seen to address the immune, neural, and/or hematologic symptoms of patients with lead poisoning.

TABLE 18.3

GMP Herbal Medicines for a Four-Year-Old Child with Lead Poisoning

Lead poisoning (OrphaCode: 330015)

A disease with a prevalence of ~2 in 100,000

Not applicable

Hypertension, Vomiting, Nausea, Constipation, Abdominal pain, Anorexia, Abdominal distention, Fatigue

Renal tubular dysfunction, Delayed eruption of teeth, Behavioral abnormality, Depression, Skin rash, Specific learning disability, Small for gestational age, Premature birth, Anemia, Headache, Memory impairment, Distal muscle weakness, Abnormality of the immune system, Spontaneous abortion, Imbalanced hemoglobin synthesis, Decreased pulmonary function, Poor fine motor coordination, Poor gross motor coordination, Attention deficit hyperactivity disorder, Impairment of activities of daily living, Abdominal cramps, Abnormality of vitamin D metabolism, Low levels of vitamin D, Cognitive impairment, Preeclampsia, Insomnia

All ages

Hypertension (401-405.99), Vomiting (D014839), Nausea (D009325), Constipation (564.0), Abdominal pain (D015746), Anorexia (D000855), Fatigue (D005221):

Bǎohéwán 5g + shānzhā 2-1g + wūméi 2-0g + gāncǎo 1-0g.

Xiǎojiànzhōngtāng 5g + shānzhā 1-0g + wūméi 1-0g + xiǎochéngqìtāng 0g.

Wǔlíngsǎn 5g + shānzhā 1-0g + gāncǎo 1-0g.

Gōuténgsǎn 5g + mázǐrénwán 2g + gāncǎo 1g.

Qiānghuó 5g + hòupò 5g + zhǐshí 5g + dàhuáng 1-0g.

Xuánshēn 5g + dìhuáng 5g + màiméndōng 5g + hòupò 3-0g + zhǐshí 3-0g + dàhuáng 0g.

(Continued)

TABLE 18.3 *(Continued)*

GMP Herbal Medicines for a Four-Year-Old Child with Lead Poisoning

Skin rash (782.1), Anemia (285.9), Headache (D006261), Memory impairment (D008569):

Xiāofēngsǎn 5g + dāngguīyǐnzǐ 5g + báixiānpí 2-1g + dìfūzǐ 2-1g + mǔdānpí 1-0g.

Jīngfángbàidúsǎn 5g + dāngguīyǐnzǐ 5-0g + báixiānpí 2-0g + dìfūzǐ 2-0g + gāncǎo 2-0g + chìsháo 1-0g + zǐcǎo 1-0g.

Jīngfángbàidúsǎn 5g + bǔzhōngyìqìtāng 5g + báixiānpí 1g + dìfūzǐ 1g + chántuì 1g.

Xiǎojiànzhōngtāng 5g + huángqí 1g + dānggui 0g.

Gāncǎo 5g + báizhǐ 5g + shārén 5g + liánqiáo 5-0g + dàhuáng 1-0g.

Báizhǐ 5g + zhìgāncǎo 5g + shārén 5g + huángqín 5g + dàhuáng 1g.

Báizhǐ 5g + huángqín 5-0g + gāncǎo 4-2g + shārén 4-2g + tiānhuā 2-0g + guālóugēn 2-0g + dàhuáng 1-0g.

REFERENCES

Clare, B., Conroy, R., & Spelman, K. (2009). The diuretic effect in human subjects of an extract of *Taraxacum officinale* folium over a single day. *Journal of Alternative and Complementary Medicine*, 15(8), 929–934. https://doi.org/10.1089/acm.2008.0152

Dong, Z., Lu, X., Tong, X., Dong, Y., Tang, L., & Liu, M. (2017). *Forsythiae Fructus*: A review on its phytochemistry, quality control, pharmacology and pharmacokinetics. *Molecules*, 22(9), 1466. https://doi.org/10.3390/molecules22091466

Su, J., Li, M., Teng, Y., Zhao, H., & Li, C. (2023). Textual research classic decoction Danggui Yinzi by ancient and modern literatures. *International Journal of Traditional Chinese Medicine*, (6), 129–135. https://pesquisa.bvsalud.org/portal/resource/en;/wpr-989604

Wang, S.-C. (2020). Modern therapeutic uses of CHEG herbs and herb pairs. In S.-C. Wang (Ed.), *Veterinary herbal pharmacopoeia* (pp. 35–233). Nova Science Publishers. https://doi.org/10.52305/GHTR1903

Zhang, Z., Li, Y., Wu, G., Li, Y., Zhang, D., & Wang, R. (2023). A comprehensive review of phytochemistry, pharmacology and clinical applications of Uncariae Ramulus Cum Uncis. *Arabian Journal of Chemistry*, 16(5), 104638. https://doi.org/10.1016/j.arabjc.2023.104638

Zheng, J., Wang, X., Tao, Y., Wang, Y., Yu, X., Liu, H., Ji, L., Bao, K., Wang, C., Jia, Z., & Hong, M. (2019). Yu-Ping-Feng-San ameliorates recurrent allergic inflammation of atopic dermatitis by repairing tight junction defects of the epithelial barrier. *Phytomedicine*, 54, 214–223. https://doi.org/10.1016/j.phymed.2018.09.190

19 GMP Herbal Medicine for Rare Gynecologic or Obstetric, Otorhinolaryngologic, Infertility, Odontologic, and Urogenital Diseases

Gynecologic diseases affect women's reproductive system. Obstetric diseases affect the health of women during pregnancy, childbirth, and postpartum period. Otorhinolaryngologic diseases are diseases of the ear, nose, throat, and related parts of the head and neck. Infertility is a condition in males or females with which a pregnancy is not achieved after one year of regular and unprotected sex. Odontologic diseases affect the teeth and their surrounding tissues. Urogenital diseases are diseases of the genitals and the urinary tract including the kidneys, ureters, bladder, and urethra. Among the rare diseases of this chapter, the rare gynecologic or obstetric are acquired and adult onset; the rare otorhinolaryngologic and rare odontologic diseases are inherited and early onset.

The GMP herbs and GMP formulas that are most frequently used for rare gynecologic or obstetric diseases are Salvia Root (Dānshēn), Chinese Motherwort Herb (Yìmǔcǎo), White Peony Root (Báisháo), Cyperus Rhizome (Xiāngfù), Astragalus Root (Huángqí), Cuscuta (Chinese Dodder Seed; Tùsīzǐ), Bitter Orange (Zhǐqiào), White Atractylodis (Báizhú), Schisandra Berry (Wǔwèizǐ), Chinese Angelica Root (female Ginseng; Dānguī), Black Jujube (Dàzǎo), Asiatic Cornelian Cherry Fruit (Shānzhūyú), Ginger Rhizome (Shēngjiāng), Free and Easy Wanderer Plus (Augmented Rambling Powder; Jiāwèixiāoyáosǎn), Gastrodia and Uncaria Drink (Tiānmágōuténgyǐn), Tangkuei and Peony Formula (Dāngguīsháoyàosǎn), Tangkuei and Gelatin Combination (Xiōngguījiāoàitāng), Virgate Wormwood and Five Ingredient Powder with Poria (Yīnchénwǔlíngsǎn), Tonify the Middle and Augment the Qi Decoction (Bǔzhōngyìqìtāng), Tokoro Decoction (Bìxièfēnqīngyǐn), Minor Bupleurum Decoction (Xiǎocháihútāng), Earth Restoring Decoction (Guīpítāng), Anemarrhena, Phellodendron, and Rehmannia Pill (Zhībódìhuángwán), and Warm the Menses Decoction (Wēnjīngtāng).

The GMP herbs and GMP formulas that are most frequently used for rare otorhinolaryngologic diseases are Rhubarb Root and Rhizome (Dàhuáng), Fritillaria Bulb (Bèimǔ), Figwort Root (Xuánshēn), Oyster Shell (Mǔlì), Licorice Root (Gāncǎo), Cardamon Seed (Shārén), Sweetflag Rhizome (Shíchāngpú), Chinese Senega Root (Yuǎnzhì), Prunella Spike (Xiàkūcǎo), Dahurian Angelica Root (Báizhǐ), Forsythia Fruit (Liánqiào), Tonify Yang and Restore Five Decoction (Bǔyánghuánwǔtāng), Poria, Cinnamon, Atractylodis and Licorice Decoction (Língguìshùgāntāng), Prepared Licorice Decoction (Zhìgāncǎotāng), Six Ingredient Pill with Rehmannia (Liùwèidìhuángwán), Ginseng, Astragalus and Pueraria Combination (Yìqìcōngmíngtāng), True Man's Decoction to Revitalize Life (Zhēnrénhuómìngyǐn), Disperse the Swelling and Break the Hardness Decoction (Sǎnzhǒngkuìjiāntāng), Minor Bupleurum Decoction (Xiǎocháihútāng), and Minor Construct the Middle Decoction (Xiǎojiànzhōngtāng). In addition, acupuncture is also frequently prescribed for the signs and symptoms of rare otorhinolaryngologic diseases.

DOI: 10.1201/9781032726625-19

The GMP herbs and GMP formulas that are most frequently used for rare infertility are Horny Goat Weed (Yínyánghuò), Cistanche Herb (Ròucōngróng), Cuscuta (Chinese Dodder Seed; Tùsīzǐ), Morinda Root (Bājǐtiān), Fleshy Stem of Cynomorium (Suǒyáng), Goji Berry (Chinese Wolfberry; Gǒuqǐzǐ), Chinese Raspberry (Fùpénzǐ), Plantain Seed (Chēqiánzǐ), Chinese Angelica Root (female Ginseng; Dāngguī), Asiatic Cornelian Cherry Fruit (Shānzhūyú), Schisandra Berry (Wǔwèizǐ), Cnidium Fruit (Shéchuángzǐ), Youth Return Formula (Huánshǎodān), Restore the Right Kidney Pill (Yòuguīwán), Lotus Stamen Formula (Jīnsuǒgùjīngwán), Restore the Left Kidney Pill (Zuǒguīwán), and Six Ingredient Pill with Rehmannia (Liùwèidìhuángwán).

The GMP herbs and GMP formulas that are most frequently used for rare odontologic diseases are Indigo Woad Leaf (Dàqīngyè), Licorice Root (Gāncǎo), Scutellaria Root (Huángqín), Chameleon Plant (Yúxīngcǎo), Hedyotis Herb (Báihuāshéshécǎo), Patrinia (Bàijiàngcǎo), Dandelion (Púgōngyīng), Trichosanthes Root (Tiānhuā), Figwort Root (Xuánshēn), Dendrobium Stem (Shíhú), Jade Woman Decoction (Yùnǚjiān), Sweet Dew Decoction (Gānlùyǐn), and Coptis and Rehmannia Formula (Clear the Stomach Powder; Qīngwèisǎn).

Finally, the GMP herbs and GMP formulas that are most frequently used for rare urogenital diseases are Poria (Fúlíng), Plantain Seed (Chēqiánzǐ), Codonopsis Root (Dǎngshēn), Aconite Accessory Root (Fùzǐ), Licorice Root (Gāncǎo), Rhubarb Root and Rhizome (Dàhuáng), Rehmannia Root (Dìhuáng), Dried Ginger Rhizome (Gānjiāng), Amur Cork Tree Bark (Huángbò), Achyranthes Root (Niúxī), Ash Bark (Qínpí), Water Plantain Rhizome (Zéxiè), Five Ingredient Formula with Poria (Wǔlíngsǎn), Guide out the Red Powder (Dǎochìsǎn), Gentiana Draining the Liver Decoction (Lóngdǎnxiègāntāng), Gardenia and Hoelen Formula (Wǔlínsǎn), and Polyporus Decoction (Zhūlíngtāng).

19.1   PREECLAMPSIA

Preeclampsia is a condition that develops in pregnant women in their second half of pregnancy. It is characterized by high blood pressure and high protein concentrations in the urine of pregnant women with preeclampsia. The exact cause of preeclampsia is uncertain, although it is believed to be related to problems with the placenta. Diabetes, hypertension, kidney disease before pregnancy, and autoimmune disorder increase the risk of developing preeclampsia.

Zhǐqiào (cf. Section 3.3), combined with Sāngyè (Folium Mori), was shown to prevent damage to blood vessels induced by diabetes in rats (Park et al., 2007). Both Shēngjiāng (Rhizoma Zingiberis Recens) and Gānjiāng (Rhizoma Zingiberis) improve digestion. However, Shēngjiāng is considered more dispersing and Gānjiāng is warmer. Compounds extracted from Yèjiāoténg (cf. Section 2.35) were shown to improve the sleeping of mice (Li et al., 2007). Hǎipiāoxiāo (cf. Section 4.23), a marine animal medicine in TCM, "tastes salty, stops bleeding, kills pain" and is used for gastric ulcer (Wang, 2020).

TABLE 19.1

GMP Herbal Medicines for a 38-Year-Old Woman with Preeclampsia

Preeclampsia (OrphaCode: 275555)

A disease with a prevalence of ~4 in 10,000

Major susceptibility factor: fms related receptor tyrosine kinase 1 (*FLT1* / Entrez: 2321) at 13q12.3

Major susceptibility factor: storkhead box 1 (*STOX1* / Entrez: 219736) at 10q22.1

Major susceptibility factor: corin, serine peptidase (*CORIN* / Entrez: 10699) at 4p12

Not applicable

Proteinuria, Hypertension, Elevated systolic blood pressure, Elevated diastolic blood pressure, Abnormality of the placenta

Abnormality of the kidney, Abnormality of vision, Abnormality of the nervous system, Intrauterine growth retardation, Small for gestational age, Abdominal pain, Headache, Elevated hepatic transaminase, Abnormality of the hepatic vasculature, Increased body mass index

Adult

(Continued)

TABLE 19.1 *(Continued)*

GMP Herbal Medicines for a 38-Year-Old Woman with Preeclampsia

Proteinuria (791.0), Hypertension (401-405.99):

Tiānmágōuténgyǐn 5g + bìxièfēnqīngyǐn 5-4g + zhībódìhuángwán 5-0g + dānshēn 1-0g + chēqiánzǐ 1-0g.

Bìxièfēnqīngyǐn 5g + tiānmágōuténgyǐn 5-4g + liùwèidìhuángwán 5-0g + dānshēn 1-0g + sāngjìshēng 1-0g + yìmǔcǎo 1-0g + zélán 1-0g.

Tiānmágōuténgyǐn 5g + jìshēngshènqìwán 5g + dānshēn 1g + mǔlì 1g + gégēn 1g.

Tiānmágōuténgyǐn 5g + zhūlíngtāng 4g + báimáogēn 1g + chēqiánzǐ 1g.

Tiānmágōuténgyǐn 5g + zhībódìhuángwán 5g + qīngxīnliánzǐyǐn 5-0g + jiāwèixiāoyáosǎn 4-0g + xuánshēn 1-0g + xiàkūcǎo 1-0g.

Zhǐqiào 5g + sāngbáipí 5g + jílí 5g + chántuì 5g.

Zhǐqiào 5g + júhuā 5-0g + jílí 5-0g + chántuì 5-0g.

Abdominal pain (D015746), Headache (D006261), Elevated hepatic transaminase (573.9):

Xiǎocháihútāng 5g + yīnchénwǔlíngsǎn 5g + dānshēn 1g + wǔwèizǐ 1-0g + bǎnlángēn 1-0g + hǔzhàng 1-0g + huángshuǐqié 1-0g.

Yīnchénwǔlíngsǎn 5g + huòxiāngzhèngqìsǎn 5g + yèjiāoténg 3g + hǎipiāoxiāo 3g + bózírén 2g + cāngzhú 2g.

Jiāwèixiāoyáosǎn 5g + cháihúshūgāntāng 5-0g + guìzhīfúlíngwán 5-0g + yīnchénwǔlíngsǎn 5-0g + dānshēn 1g + xiāngfù 1-0g + yìmǔcǎo 1-0g + yùjīn 1-0g + wǔwèizǐ 1-0g + hǔzhàng 1-0g + huángshuǐqié 1-0g + zélán 1-0g.

Cháihúshūgāntāng 5g + yīnchénwǔlíngsǎn 5g + hǔzhàng 1g + huángshuǐqié 1g.

Gāncǎo 5g + báizhǐ 5g + shārén 5g + huángqín 5g + dàhuáng 0g.

Báizhú 5g + fúlíng 5g + dǎngshēn 5g + xiǎohuíxiāng 4g + bànxià 4g + zhìgāncǎo 2g + gānjiāng 2-0g + fùzǐ 1g.

Báizhú 5g + báisháo 5g + báibiǎndòu 5g + fúlíng 5g + huángqí 5g + dàzǎo 2g + shēngjiāng 2g + zhìgāncǎo 2-0g.

Cháihú 5g + huángqín 5g + bànxià 4g + shēngjiāng 4g + báisháo 4g + zhǐshí 4g + dàhuáng 0g.

Báisháo 5g + cháihú 5g + huángqín 5g + dàzǎo 4g + bànxià 4g + shēngjiāng 4g + zhǐshí 4g + dàhuáng 0g.

Huángqí 5g + gāncǎo 5-2g + báizhú 5-2g + báisháo 5-2g + báibiǎndòu 5-2g + fúlíng 5-2g + dàzǎo 2-1g + shēngjiāng 2-1g.

19.2 ASHERMAN SYNDROME

Asherman syndrome is scarring of the uterine walls after surgical scraping and cleaning of the uterine wall tissues in miscarriage or abortion. Chronic inflammation of the endometrium from genital tuberculosis infection can also cause scars in the uterus and cervix, and so can surgical removal of uterine leiomyomas.

Guìzhī (cf. Sections 2.30 and 8.14) was summarized to be antibacterial, anti-inflammatory, antiviral, antitumor, antipyretic, analgesic, antidiabetic, and antiplatelet aggregation (Liu et al., 2019) and is used for rhinitis, headaches, and so on (Wang, 2020). Táorén (Semen Persicae) "enlivens Blood, dissolves stasis, moistens bowels, passes stools" and is used today for endometriosis and leiomyoma of the uterus (Wang, 2020). Shānzhūyú (cf. Section 2.18) was shown to improve the ovarian function in natural aging mice (Wang et al., 2019). Tùsīzǐ (cf. Section 10.10) was demonstrated to restore the levels of testosterone

TABLE 19.2

GMP Herbal Medicines for a 30-Year-Old Woman with Asherman Syndrome

Asherman syndrome (OrphaCode: 137686)

A disease with a prevalence of ~4 in 10,000

Not applicable

Abnormality of the menstrual cycle, Decreased fertility in females, Oligomenorrhea

Infertility, Secondary amenorrhea, Episodic abdominal pain, Spontaneous abortion, Dysmenorrhea, Metrorrhagia

Adult

(Continued)

TABLE 19.2 *(Continued)*
GMP Herbal Medicines for a 30-Year-Old Woman with Asherman Syndrome

Oligomenorrhea (D009839) [Scanty or infrequent menstruation (626.1)]:

Jiāwèixiāoyáosăn 5g + wēnjīngtāng 5g + dānshēn 1g + xiāngfù 1g + yìmŭcăo 1g + zélán 1-0g + yùjīn 1-0g.	Zhìgāncăo 5g + guìzhī 5g + táorén 5g + zhǐqiào 5-3g + dàhuáng 1-0g + hónghuā 1-0g.
Jiāwèixiāoyáosăn 5g + dāngguīsháoyàosăn 5g + dānshēn 1g + yìmŭcăo 1g + xiāngfù 1-0g + zélán 1-0g.	Shānzhūyú 5g + shānyào 5g + báisháo 5g + gŏuqǐzǐ 5g + tùsīzǐ 5g + huángqí 5g + shúdìhuáng 5g + dǎngshēn 5g + báizhú 5-0g + dāngguī 5-0g + bǎihé 5-0g + ējiāo 5-0g + suānzǎorén 5-0g + zhìgāncăo 3-0g.
Xiāoyáosăn 5g + guìzhīfúlíngwán 4g + dānshēn 2g + niúxī 2g + zélán 2g + wŭlíngzhī 1g + púhuáng 1g.	Dānggui 5g + shēngjiāng 2g + ējiāo 2g.
Liùwèidìhuángwán 5g + sìwùtāng 5g + bājítiān 1g + yínyánghuò 1g + tùsīzǐ 1g.	Shānyào 5g + báisháo 5g + dìhuáng 5g + dāngguī 5g + xiānmáo 3g + dùzhòng 3g + sāngjìshēng 3g + guālóugēn 3g + fúlíng 3g + yínyánghuò 3g + tùsīzǐ 3g + huángqín 3g + huángjīng 3g.
Táohóngsìwùtāng 5g + dāngguīsháoyàosăn 5g + xiāngfù 1g + yìmŭcăo 1g + zélán 1g.	

Dysmenorrhea (D004412), Metrorrhagia (D008796) [Metrorrhagia (626.6)]:

Xiōngguījiāoàitāng 5g + dāngguīsháoyàosăn 5g + xiānhècăo 1g + xiāngfù 1g.	Báisháo 5g + dìhuáng 5g + mŭdānpí 5g + ējiāo 5g + dāngguī 5g + dìyú 5-0g + dàzăo 3g + niúxī 3g + xiāngfù 3g + huángbò 3g.
Xiōngguījiāoàitāng 5g + bǔzhōngyìqìtāng 5g + guīpítāng 5-0g + xiānhècăo 2-0g + yìmŭcăo 1-0g + dìyú 1-0g.	Shānzhūyú 5g + tùsīzǐ 2g + nǚzhēnzǐ 2g + hànliáncăo 2g + wǔwèizǐ 2-1g + yìmŭcăo 2-1g + guālóupí 2-1g + huángqí 2-0g + huángjīng 2-0g.
Jiāwèixiāoyáosăn 5g + dāngguīsháoyàosăn 5g + yìmŭcăo 1g + dānshēn 1-0g + yánhúsuǒ 1-0g + xiāngfù 1-0g + xiānhècăo 1-0g.	Dānggui 5g + ējiāo 3g + shēngjiāng 3g.

and androgen receptor gene and protein expression in the kidney and testicle of kidney yang deficient mice (Yang et al., 2008); it is used for lumbago and disorders of menstruation (Wang, 2020). Xiōngguījiāoàitāng (cf. Section 4.9) contains Báisháo, Dìhuáng, Ējiāo, Dānggui, and so on, and is used for disorders of menstruation and other abnormal bleeding from female genital tract (Wang, 2019).

19.3   PENDRED SYNDROME

Pendred syndrome, also known as goiter-deafness syndrome, is a genetic disease characterized by bilateral hearing loss and an enlarged thyroid gland. Pendred syndrome is caused by mutations in genes that express in the cochlea and thyroid to transport negatively charged ions including chloride and iodide across cell membranes.

TABLE 19.3
GMP Herbal Medicines for a One-Year-Old Infant with Pendred Syndrome

Pendred syndrome (OrphaCode: 705)

A malformation syndrome with a prevalence of ~7 in 100,000

Disease-causing germline mutation(s): solute carrier family 26 member 4 (*SLC26A4* / Entrez: 5172) at 7q22.3

Disease-causing germline mutation(s): potassium inwardly rectifying channel subfamily J member 10 (*KCNJ10* / Entrez: 3766) at 1q23.2

Disease-causing germline mutation(s): forkhead box I1 (*FOXI1* / Entrez: 2299) at 5q35.1

Autosomal recessive

Abnormality of the inner ear, Sensorineural hearing impairment, Hypoplasia of the cochlea, Enlarged vestibular aqueduct

Hypothyroidism, Goiter

Nephropathy, Hyperparathyroidism, Intellectual disability, Ataxia, Respiratory insufficiency, Neurological speech impairment, Vertigo, Tracheal stenosis, Thyroid carcinoma

Neonatal, Infancy

(Continued)

TABLE 19.3 *(Continued)*

GMP Herbal Medicines for a One-Year-Old Infant with Pendred Syndrome

Sensorineural hearing impairment (389.1):

Xiǎojiànzhōngtāng 5g + língguìshùgāntāng 5-0g + shíchāngpú 1-0g + héyè 1-0g + yuǎnzhì 1-0g.

Xiǎojiànzhōngtāng 5g + yùpíngfēngsǎn 5-0g + gāncǎo 1-0g + huángqí 0g.

Xìngsūyǐnyòukē 5g + xīnyíqīngfèitāng 5g + yínqiàosǎn 5-0g.

Féiérbāzhēngāo 5g + shēnlíngbáizhúsǎn 5g.

Jīngjièliánqiáotāng 5g + shíchāngpú 1g + yuǎnzhì 1g + gāncǎo 1g.

Zhìgāncǎo 5g + shārén 5-0g + báizhǐ 4-0g + xìxīn 1-0g + dàhuáng 1-0g.

Sīguāluò 5g + júhuā 5-0g + júhóng 5-0g + zhǐqiào 4-0g.

Yùzhú 5g + shāshēn 5g + hòupò 5g + zhǐshí 5g + xuánshēn 2g + dìhuáng 2g + màiméndōng 2g + dàhuáng 1g.

Gāncǎo 5g + shārén 5g + dàhuáng 1g.

Hypothyroidism (244.9), Goiter (240.9):

Sǎnzhǒngkuìjiāntāng 5g + èrchéntāng 2-0g + xiàkūcǎo 2-0g + xuánshēn 1-0g + mǔlì 1-0g + bèimǔ 1-0g + jiégěng 1-0g.

Zhēnrénhuómìngyǐn 5g + xiǎocháihútāng 5-0g + sǎnzhǒngkuìjiāntāng 5-0g + xiàkūcǎo 2g + bèimǔ 2-1g + xuánshēn 2-0g + mǔlì 2-0g.

Gāncǎo 5-3g + báizhǐ 5-2g + shārén 5-2g + huángqín 5-0g + dàhuáng 1-0g.

Báizhǐ 5g + zhìgāncǎo 4g + shārén 4g + dàhuáng 0g.

Hyperparathyroidism (252.0), Intellectual disability (D008607), Ataxia (D002524), Neurological speech impairment (D013064), Vertigo (386.2), Thyroid carcinoma (193):

Zhìgāncǎotāng 5g + bèimǔ 1g + xuánshēn 1-0g + mǔlì 1-0g + xiàkūcǎo 1-0g + liánqiáo 1-0g + hǎizǎo 1-0g + dàhuáng 0g.

Língguìshùgāntāng 5g + bànxià 2g + xuánshēn 2-0g + mǔlì 2-0g + bèimǔ 2-0g + xiàkūcǎo 2-0g + fùzǐ 2-0g + shārén 2-0g + dàhuáng 1-0g.

Èrchéntāng 5g + mǔlì 1g + bèimǔ 1g + xiàkūcǎo 1g + xuánshēn 1g.

Zhìgāncǎo 5g + jiégěng 5g + bèimǔ 5-3g + liánqiáo 5-2g + xuánshēn 5-2g + mǔlì 5-2g + shānzhīzǐ 3-2g + dàhuáng 1-0g.

Gāncǎo 5g + xuánshēn 4-2g + mǔlì 4-2g + bèimǔ 4-2g + jiégěng 4-2g + liánqiáo 2g + shānzhīzǐ 2-0g + zhīzǐ 1-0g + dàhuáng 1-0g.

Bèimǔ 5g + zhìgāncǎo 5g + jiégěng 5g + xuánshēn 3g + mǔlì 3g + liánqiáo 3g + shānzhīzǐ 2-0g + dàhuáng 1-0g.

Báizhú 5g + fùzǐ 5g + cháihú 5g + báisháo 4g + fúlíng 4g + tiānhuā 2g + dǎngshēn 2g + wǔwèizǐ 2g + guìzhī 2g + xìxīn 2g + huángqín 2g + gāncǎo 1g + mǔlì 1g + gānjiāng 1g.

Zhìgāncǎo "benefits Qi and Blood." Xiǎojiànzhōngtāng "replenishes interior deficiency." Féiérbāzhēngāo "benefits Qi and the Spleen." They are all supposed to strengthen the affected baby's constitution. Zhìgāncǎotāng, Zhēnrénhuómìngyǐn, Xiàkūcǎo, Xuánshēn, Bèimǔ, and Mǔlì were the most commonly prescribed GMP herbal extract granules to hyperthyroidism patients in Taiwan (Chang et al., 2022). Jīngjièliánqiáotāng (cf. Section 3.11) is used for chronic sinusitis (Wang, 2019), which is associated with sensorineural hearing loss (Lin et al., 2019). Sǎnzhǒngkuìjiāntāng is used today for tumors and goiters (cf. Sections 4.11 and 8.7).

19.4 FULL NF2-RELATED SCHWANNOMATOSIS

Full NF2-related schwannomatosis, also known as nonmosaic neurofibromatosis type 2, is a benign nerve sheath tumor of the nerves that transmit signals between the inner ear and the brain. Mutations in the *NF2* gene, which regulates a tumor suppressor, cause full NF2-related schwannomatosis.

Dàndòuchǐ (Semen Sojae Praeparatum) was shown to alter depression-like behaviors in chronic, unpredictable mild stress rats through the microbiota-gut-brain axis (Chen et al., 2021); it is used for gastrojejunal ulcer and sleep disturbances (Wang, 2020). Jiānghuáng (Rhizoma Curcumae Longae) was summarized to be antitumor, anti-inflammatory, antioxidant, neuroprotective, antibacterial, and hypolipidemic (Liu et al., 2022) and is used for a multitude of conditions including functional disorders of the intestines, monoplegia, and myalgia (Wang, 2020).

TABLE 19.4

GMP Herbal Medicines for a 13-Year-Old Adolescent with Full NF2-Related Schwannomatosis

Full NF2-related schwannomatosis (OrphaCode: 637)

A disease with a prevalence of ~2 in 100,000

Disease-causing germline mutation(s): NF2, moesin-ezrin-radixin like (MERLIN) tumor suppressor (*NF2* / Entrez: 4771) at 22q12.2

Autosomal dominant

Neuroma

Sensorineural hearing impairment, Abnormality of the eye, Myelopathy, Meningioma, Reduced visual acuity, Posterior subcapsular cataract, Bilateral vestibular Schwannoma, Peripheral Schwannoma, Spinal cord tumor, Intracranial meningioma, Hyperesthesia

Hydrocephalus, Tinnitus, Visual loss, Abnormality of the optic nerve, Blindness, Amblyopia, Diplopia, Sensory neuropathy, Hyperpigmentation of the skin, Seizure, Dysarthria, Hemiparesis, Polyneuropathy, Abnormal cerebellum morphology, Dysphagia, Postural instability, Unsteady gait, Memory impairment, Brain stem compression, Ependymoma, Sensory impairment, Cranial nerve paralysis, Neoplasm of the skin, Foot dorsiflexor weakness, Retinal hamartoma, Mononeuropathy, Facial palsy, Wrist drop, Spinal meningioma, Epiretinal membrane, Cortical cataract

All ages

Sensorineural hearing impairment (389.1), Abnormality of the eye (379.90), Myelopathy (336.9), Bilateral vestibular Schwannoma (237.72), Spinal cord tumor (192.2), Hyperesthesia (D006941):

Liùwèidìhuángwán 5g + yìqìcōngmíngtāng 5-0g + bǔyánghuánwǔtāng 5-0g + shíchāngpú 1-0g + gǒuqǐzǐ 1-0g + yuǎnzhì 1-0g + báijiāngcán 1-0g + acupuncture.

Jīngjièliánqiáotāng 5g + báijiāngcán 1g + hángjú 1g + xiàkūcǎo 1g + chántuì 1g + acupuncture.

Qǐjúdìhuángwán 5g + zīshènmíngmùtāng 5g + bǔyánghuánwǔtāng 5g + acupuncture.

Yìqìcōngmíngtāng 5g + bǔzhōngyìqìtāng 5g + shíchāngpú 1g + acupuncture.

Dàhuáng 5g + gāncǎo 5g + báizhǐ 5g + shārén 5g + huángqín 5g + acupuncture.

Huángbò 5g + shārén 4-2g + dìhuáng 3-1g + bǎihé 3-1g + dàndòuchǐ 3-1g + shānzhīzǐ 3-0g + gāncǎo 2-1g + chìsháo 2-1g + ējiāo 2-1g + huángqín 2-1g + jiānghuáng 2-1g + jiāngcán 2-1g + zhīzǐ 2-0g + chántuì 2-0g + yùjīn 2-0g + huánglián 0g + dàhuáng 0g.

Hydrocephalus (331.4, 331.3), Tinnitus (D014012), Blindness (D001766), Amblyopia (368.01, 368.00), Diplopia (D004172), Seizure (345.9), Dysarthria (D004401), Hemiparesis (D010291), Polyneuropathy (357.82), Unsteady gait (D020233), Memory impairment (D008569), Sensory impairment (D006987), Cranial nerve paralysis (352.9), Mononeuropathy (355.9, 354.5), Epiretinal membrane (362.56):

Bǔyánghuánwǔtāng 5g + tiānmá 1g + shíchāngpú 1g + yuǎnzhì 1g + acupuncture.

Bǔyánghuánwǔtāng 5g + língguìshùgāntāng 5-3g + shíchāngpú 1g + yuǎnzhì 1g + dānshēn 1-0g + acupuncture.

Bǔyánghuánwǔtāng 5-4g + tōngqiàohuóxuètāng 5-4g + shíchāngpú 1g + yuǎnzhì 1g + sānqī 1-0g + acupuncture.

Qǐjúdìhuángwán 5g + língguìshùgāntāng 5g + tiānmá 1g + shíchāngpú 1g + yuǎnzhì 1g.

Língguìshùgāntāng 5g + tiānmá 1g + shíchāngpú 1g + yuǎnzhì 1g + acupuncture.

Tiānmá 5g + chìsháo 5g + júhuā 5g + mànjīngzǐ 5g + zéxiè 5g + gōuténg 5g + dàhuáng 4g + chuānxiōng 2g + báizhǐ 2g + hónghuā 2g + táorén 2g.

Tiānmá 5g + dìhuáng 5g + dìlóng 5g + zhǐshí 5g + shénqū 5g + huángqí 5g + fúlíng 5-0g + bèimǔ 5-0g + yìyǐrén 5-0g + shíchāngpú 3g + yuǎnzhì 3g.

Júhuā 5g + mànjīngzǐ 5g + bòhé 5g + chìsháo 5-4g + shēngmá 4-2g + chuānxiōng 4-0g + guànzhòng 4-0g + xīnyí 2-0g + dàhuáng 2-0g.

Jiāngcán (cf. Section 12.5) or Báijiāngcán (Bombyx Batryticatus) are used for unspecified vertiginous syndromes and labyrinthine disorders, migraine, facial nerve disorder, and neuralgia (Wang, 2020). Dìlóng (cf. Sections 1.22, 1.69, and 12.10) was reviewed to be antifibrotic, anticoagulant, antithrombotic, antibacterial, antitussive, and anti-asthmatic (Xu et al., 2022) and is used for essential hypertension, cardiac dysrhythmia, and peripheral enthesopathies (Wang, 2020). Bòhé (cf. Section 2.43) was shown to attenuate neuroinflammation in murine microglial cells (Park et al., 2022).

19.5 PARTIAL CHROMOSOME Y DELETION

Partial chromosome Y deletion, also called male sterility due to chromosome Y deletion, is missing genes on the Y chromosome. Since many genes on the Y are responsible for spermatogenesis, men with partial chromosome Y deletion can produce normal, reduced, or zero amounts of sperm depending on which segment of the Y chromosome is missing.

Bājǐtiān was introduced in Sections 1.58 and 2.19 for male infertility. Ròucōngróng (cf. Section 1.58) is antioxidant, neuroprotective, and antiaging and used for chronic renal disease, impotence, female infertility, morbid leukorrhea, profuse metrorrhagia, and senile constipation (Li et al., 2016; Wang, 2020). Yínyánghuò (Herba Epimedii) is anti-osteoporotic (Wang et al., 2015)

TABLE 19.5

GMP Herbal Medicines for a 32-Year-Old Man with Partial Chromosome Y Deletion

Partial chromosome Y deletion (OrphaCode: 1646)

A malformation syndrome with a prevalence of ~2 in 10,000

Role: the phenotype of azoospermia factor 1 (*AZF1* / HGNC:908) at Yq11

Role: the phenotype of ubiquitin specific peptidase 9 Y-linked (*USP9Y* / Entrez: 8287) at Yq11.221

Candidate gene tested: deleted in azoospermia 1 (*DAZ1* / Entrez: 1617) at Yq11.223

Candidate gene tested: deleted in azoospermia 2 (*DAZ2* / Entrez: 57055) at Yq11.223

Candidate gene tested: deleted in azoospermia 3 (*DAZ3* / Entrez: 57054) at Yq11.23

Candidate gene tested: deleted in azoospermia 4 (*DAZ4* / Entrez: 57135) at Yq11.23

Candidate gene tested: DEAD-box helicase 3 Y-linked (*DDX3Y* / Entrez: 8653) at Yq11.221

Candidate gene tested: RNA binding motif protein Y-linked family 1 member A1 (*RBMY1A1* / Entrez: 5940) at Yq11.223

Modifying germline mutation: testis specific protein Y-linked 1 (*TSPY1* / Entrez: 7258) at Yp11.2

Not applicable, Y-linked

Male infertility, Abnormal spermatogenesis, Decreased testicular size, Non-obstructive azoospermia

Oligospermia

Cryptorchidism

Adult

Male infertility (606):

Yòuguīwán 5g + zuǒguīwán 5g + bājǐtiān 1g + ròucōngróng 1g + yínyánghuò 1g + tùsīzǐ 1g.

Yòuguīwán 5g + huánshǎodān 5g + bājǐtiān 1g + ròucōngróng 1g + yínyánghuò 1g + suǒyáng 1-0g + tùsīzǐ 1-0g.

Jīnsuǒgùjīngwán 5g + huánshǎodān 5g + yínyánghuò 1g + bājǐtiān 1-0g + ròucōngróng 1-0g + suǒyáng 1-0g + tùsīzǐ 1-0g + bǔgǔzhǐ 1-0g + shéchuángzǐ 1-0g.

Bāwèidìhuángwán 5g + bājǐtiān 1g + ròucōngróng 1g + yínyánghuò 1g + tùsīzǐ 1g.

Zuǒguīwán 5g + huánshǎodān 5g + ròucōngróng 1g + yínyánghuò 1g + tùsīzǐ 1g + suǒyáng 1g.

Oligospermia (606.1):

Liùwèidìhuángwán 5g + huánshǎodān 5g + bājǐtiān 1g + tùsīzǐ 1g + ròucōngróng 1-0g + yínyánghuò 1-0g + suǒyáng 1-0g + fùpénzǐ 1-0g.

Yòuguīwán 5g + huánshǎodān 5g + ròucōngróng 1g + yínyánghuò 1g + bājǐtiān 1-0g + suǒyáng 1-0g.

Zuǒguīwán 5g + huánshǎodān 5g + wūwèizǐ 1g + chēqiánzǐ 1g + gǒuqǐzǐ 1g + tùsīzǐ 1g + fùpénzǐ 1g.

Qǐbǎoměirándān 5g + huánshǎodān 5g + bājǐtiān 1g + ròucōngróng 1g + yínyánghuò 1g + suǒyáng 1g.

Liùwèidìhuángwán 5g + bājǐtiān 1g + ròucōngróng 1g + yínyánghuò 1g + tùsīzǐ 1g.

Bājǐtiān 5g + yínyánghuò 5g + bǔgǔzhǐ 5g + ròucōngróng 5-0g + suǒyáng 5-0g + tùsīzǐ 5-0g + dùzhòng 5-0g.

Bājǐtiān 5g + zhīmǔ 5g + yínyánghuò 5g + tùsīzǐ 5g + huángbò 5g + dāngguī 5g + suǒyáng 5g.

Yìzhìxiāng 5g + yínyánghuò 1g + tùsīzǐ 1g + bǔgǔzhǐ 1g + gāncǎo 0g.

Tùsīzǐ 5g + wūwèizǐ 2g + chēqiánzǐ 2g + gǒuqǐzǐ 2g + shānzhūyú 2-0g.

Shānzhūyú 5g + shānyào 5g + bājǐtiān 5g + gǒuqǐzǐ 5g + yínyánghuò 5g + tùsīzǐ 5g + dāngguī 5g + shúdìhuáng 5g + chénpí 5-0g + fùpénzǐ 5-0g + ròucōngróng 5-0g + chēqiánzǐ 5-0g.

Gǒuqǐzǐ 5g + tùsīzǐ 5g + fùpénzǐ 3g + chēqiánzǐ 2g + wūwèizǐ 1g.

Yìzhìxiāng 5g + gǒuqǐzǐ 1g + tùsīzǐ 1g + fùpénzǐ 1g + huángqí 1-0g + dāngguī 1-0g + yínyánghuò 1-0g + shāyuànzǐ 1-0g + chēqiánzǐ 1-0g.

Héshǒuwū 5g + chēqiánzǐ 5g + gǒuqǐzǐ 5g + yínyánghuò 5g + tùsīzǐ 5g + fùpénzǐ 5g.

(Continued)

TABLE 19.5 *(Continued)*
GMP Herbal Medicines for a 32-Year-Old Man with Partial Chromosome Y Deletion

Cryptorchidism (752.51):

Yòuguīwán 5g + ròucōngróng 1g + yínyánghuò 1g + suǒyáng 1g + bājǐtiān 1-0g + shéchuángzǐ 1-0g.

Zuǒguīwán 5g + bājǐtiān 1g + ròucōngróng 1g + yínyánghuò 1g + suǒyáng 1-0g + tùsīzǐ 1-0g.

Huánshǎodān 5g + jīnsuǒgùjīngwán 5-0g + yòuguīwán 5-0g + bājǐtiān 1g + ròucōngróng 1g + yínyánghuò 1g + suǒyáng 1-0g + shéchuángzǐ 1-0g.

Tùsīzǐ 5g + wǔwèizǐ 3-1g + gǒuqǐzǐ 3-0g + yínyánghuò 3-0g + bǔgǔzhī 3-0g + shānzhūyú 2-0g + ròucōngróng 2-0g + shéchuángzǐ 2-0g + shúdìhuáng 2-0g + ròuguì 1-0g.

Yínyánghuò 5g + shéchuángzǐ 5-0g + ròucōngróng 3-0g + tùsīzǐ 3-0g + wǔwèizǐ 2-0g + yuǎnzhì 2-0g.

Zhīmǔ 5g + huángbò 5g + ròuguì 2g.

and used for impotence of organic origin, disorders of male genital organs, and osteoporosis (Wang, 2020). Suǒyáng (Herba Cynomorii) was shown to increase mitochondrial ATP generation and glutathione-dependent antioxidant response in embryonic rat cardiomyocytes (Chen et al., 2014) and is used today for impotence of organic origin, among other urinary and gynecologic conditions (Wang, 2020). Huánshǎodān (cf. Section 1.30) "replenishes Qi/Blood, nourishes yin, benefits the Kidney" and is used for neurotic disorders (Wang, 2019). Shéchuángzǐ (Fructus Cnidii) "kills worms, relieves itching, warms the Kidney, and enhances yang." It has traditionally been used for the relief of genital itching and is used today for leukorrhea and eczema (Wang, 2020). Jīnsuǒgùjīngwán "replenishes the Kidney, retains semen" and is used today for neurotic disorders, and nephritis and nephropathy (Wang, 2019).

19.6   DENTINOGENESIS IMPERFECTA

Dentinogenesis imperfecta, also known as dentinogenesis imperfecta without osteogenesis imperfecta (DGI without OI) or opalescent teeth without osteogenesis imperfecta, is a genetic disorder affecting the development of dentin, which is the bone-like substance making up

TABLE 19.6
GMP Herbal Medicines for a Six-Year-Old Child with Dentinogenesis Imperfecta

Dentinogenesis imperfecta (OrphaCode: 49042)

A disease with a prevalence of ~1 in 10,000

Disease-causing germline mutation(s): dentin sialophosphoprotein (*DSPP* / Entrez: 1834) at 4q22.1

Autosomal dominant

Obliteration of the pulp chamber, Abnormality of the dental root

Grayish enamel, Shell teeth, Joint hypermobility, Generalized hypoplasia of dental enamel, Yellow-brown discoloration of the teeth, Abnormality of the dental pulp, Abnormality of dentin, Hypocalcification of dental enamel, Fragile teeth

Bruising susceptibility, Selective tooth agenesis, Finger joint hypermobility, Persistence of primary teeth, Short dental roots, Hyperextensibility at elbow, Knee joint hypermobility

Childhood

Bruising susceptibility (D004438):

Yùnǔjiān 5g + gānlùyǐn 5g + qīngwèisǎn 5-0g.

Yùnǔjiān 5g + gānlùyǐn 5g + mázǐrénwán 2-0g + tiānhuā 1-0g + xuánshēn 1-0g + shíhú 1-0g.

Yùnǔjiān 5g + gānlùyǐn 5g + zhúyèshígāotāng 5-0g + tiānhuā 1-0g.

Yùnǔjiān 5g + xiāofēngsǎn 5g + jīngfángbàidúsǎn 5g.

Yùnǔjiān 5g + qīngwèisǎn 5g + jīnyínhuā 1-0g + liánqiáo 1-0g + xuánshēn 1-0g.

Dàqīngyè 5g + yúxīngcǎo 5g + huángqín 5g + báihuāshéshécǎo 5-0g + bàijiàngcǎo 5-0g + púgōngyīng 5-0g + bǎnlángēn 5-0g + gāncǎo 2g + hǎipiāoxiāo 2-0g + acupuncture.

Dàqīngyè 5g + gāncǎo 5g + bǎibù 5g + yúxīngcǎo 5g + máhuáng 5g + huángqín 5g + cāngěrzǐ 5g.

most of the teeth. DGI without OI is caused by mutations in the gene whose products are components of dentin.

Dàqīngyè was introduced in Section 9.12 for skin conditions. Bàijiàngcǎo (Herba Patriniae) "clears heat, neutralizes pathogens, eliminates carbuncles, drains pus, resolves stasis, stops pain" and is used for nasopharyngitis and pruritic disorder (Wang, 2020). Cāngěrzǐ (Fructus Xanthii (stir-baked)) "dispels Wind, eliminates dampness, opens orifices, stops pain" and is used for rhinitis and eczema (Wang, 2020). Yùnǚjiān is used for eczema and gingival and periodontal diseases (cf. Sections 1.51 and 5.17).

19.7 INTERSTITIAL CYSTITIS

Interstitial cystitis, also called painful bladder syndrome, is a chronic condition characterized by recurring pain, pressure, and discomfort in the pelvic floor region including the bladder. Although the pelvic symptoms resemble those with an infection, interstitial cystitis is not caused by an infection. The exact cause of interstitial cystitis is unknown; however, mast cells are believed to play a role.

TABLE 19.7

GMP Herbal Medicines for a 45-Year-Old Woman with Interstitial Cystitis

Interstitial cystitis (OrphaCode: 37202)

A disease with a prevalence of ~3 in 10,000

Unknown

Pollakisuria, Urinary bladder inflammation, Functional abnormality of the bladder, Urinary urgency, Abnormality of the bladder, Nocturia, Abnormality of the labia, Abnormality of the genital system, Abnormality of the menstrual cycle, Abnormality of the urethra, Pain, Dyspareunia

Abnormality of the vagina

All ages

Urinary bladder inflammation (595), Nocturia (D053158), Pain (D010146):

Wǔlíngsǎn 5g + wǔlínsǎn 5g + dǎochìsǎn 5-0g.	Fúlíng 5g + fùzǐ 4-3g + dǎngshēn 3g + báisháo 3-0g + gāncǎo 3-0g + báizhú 2-0g + gānjiāng 2-0g.
Wǔlíngsǎn 5g + dǎochìsǎn 5-4g + jìshēngshènqìwán 5-0g + niúxī 1-0g + chēqiánzǐ 1-0g.	Chìxiǎodòu 5g + dānggui 5-2g + chēqiánzǐ 5-0g + yìmǔcǎo 5-0g.
Wǔlíngsǎn 5g + lóngdǎnxiègāntāng 5g + wǔlínsǎn 5-0g.	Gāncǎo 5g + báizhǐ 5g + shārén 5g + dàhuáng 0g.
Zhūlíngtāng 5g + jiāwèixiāoyáosǎn 4-0g + niúxī 1g + chēqiánzǐ 1g + báimáogēn 1-0g + jīnqiáncǎo 1-0g.	Dìhuáng 5g + qínpí 5g + fúlíng 5g + huángbò 5g + zéxiè 5g + dàhuáng 1-0g.

Fúlíng (cf. Sections 7.3 and 16.4) relieves skin and urinary conditions by "removing dampness and promoting urination." Dìhuáng (cf. Sections 1.55 and 6.16) is used for diabetes and urinary frequency (Wang, 2020). Note that Wǔlíngsǎn, Wǔlínsǎn, Zhūlíngtāng, and Jiāwèixiāoyáosǎn contain Fúlíng, while Dǎochìsǎn and Lóngdǎnxiègāntāng contain Dìhuáng. Moreover, Zéxiè (cf. Section 3.2) composes Wǔlíngsǎn, Zhūlíngtāng, and Lóngdǎnxiègāntāng.

REFERENCES

Chang, C. T., Wu, S., Lai, Y., Hung, Y., Hsu, C. Y., Chen, H., Chu, C., Cheng, J., Hu, W., & Kuo, C. (2022). The utilization of Chinese herbal products for hyperthyroidism in National Health Insurance System (NHIRD) of Taiwan: A population-based study. *Evidence-Based Complementary and Alternative Medicine*, *2022*, 1–11. https://doi.org/10.1155/2022/5500604

Chen, J., Wong, H. S., & Ko, K. M. (2014). Ursolic acid-enriched Herba cynomorii extract induces mitochondrial uncoupling and glutathione redox cycling through mitochondrial reactive oxygen species generation: Protection against menadione cytotoxicity in H9C2 cells. *Molecules*, *19*(2), 1576–1591. https://doi.org/10.3390/molecules19021576

Chen, Y., Xiao, N., Chen, Y., Chen, X., Zhong, C., Cheng, Y., Du, B., & Li, P. (2021). Semen Sojae Praeparatum alters depression-like behaviors in chronic unpredictable mild stress rats via intestinal microbiota. *Food Research International, 150*, 110808. https://doi.org/10.1016/j.foodres.2021.110808

Li, Z., Lin, H., Gu, L., Gao, J., & Tzeng, C. (2016). Herba cistanche (Rou Cong-Rong): One of the best pharmaceutical gifts of traditional Chinese medicine. *Frontiers in Pharmacology, 7.* https://doi.org/10.3389/fphar.2016.00041

Li, Z.-X., Yang, Z.-P., Shi, B.-X., Che, H.-L., Chen, Y., Xiao, W., Zhu, X.-J., & He, J.-G. (2007). Study on slumber improving with *Caulis polygoni* multiflori in mice. *Food Science, 28*(4), 327–331. https://www.spkx.net.cn/EN/abstract/abstract20518.shtml

Lin, X., Shan, X., Shen, L., Shu, B., Wang, Y., & Xiao, W. (2019). Is sensorineural hearing loss related to chronic rhinosinusitis caused by outer hair cell injury? *Medical Science Monitor, 25*, 627–636. https://doi.org/10.12659/msm.912382

Liu, J., Zhang, Q., Li, R., Wei, S., Huang, C., Gao, Y., & Pu, X. (2019). The traditional uses, phytochemistry, pharmacology and toxicology of *Cinnamomi ramulus*: A review. *Journal of Pharmacy and Pharmacology, 72*(3), 319–342. https://doi.org/10.1111/jphp.13189

Liu, S. T., Zheng, S. W., Hou, A. J., Zhang, J. X., Wang, S., Wang, X. J., Yu, H., & Yang, L. (2022). A review: The phytochemistry, pharmacology, and pharmacokinetics of *Curcumae Longae Rhizoma* (Turmeric). *World Journal of Traditional Chinese Medicine, 8*(4), 463–490. https://journals.lww.com/wtcm/fulltext/2022/08040/a_review__the_phytochemistry,_pharmacology,_and.1.aspx

Park, J.-S., Park, C.-H., Jun, C.-Y., Choi, Y.-K., Hwang, G.-S., & Kim, D.-W. (2007). The anti-diabetes and vasoelasticity effects of *Mori Folium* and *Aurantii Fructus* in streptozotocin induced type II diabetes mellitus model. *The Journal of Internal Korean Medicine, 28*(3), 544–559. https://www.jikm.or.kr/journal/view.php?number=1249

Park, Y. J., Yang, H. J., Li, W., Oh, Y., & Go, Y. (2022). Menthae herba attenuates neuroinflammation by regulating CREB/NRF2/HO-1 pathway in BV2 microglial cells. *Antioxidants, 11*(4), 649. https://doi.org/10.3390/antiox11040649

Wang, L., Yu, L., Guo, Y., Ma, R., Fu, M., Niu, J., S, G., & Zhang, D. (2015). *Herba Epimedii*: An ancient Chinese herbal medicine in the prevention and treatment of osteoporosis. *Current Pharmaceutical Design, 22*(3), 328–349. https://doi.org/10.2174/1381612822666151112145907

Wang, S.-C. (2019). Therapeutic classes of CHEG formulas. In S.-C. Wang (Ed.), *Clinical herbal prescriptions: Principles and practices of herbal formulations from deep learning health insurance herbal prescription big data* (pp. 16–89). World Scientific Publishing. https://doi.org/10.1142/11211

Wang, S.-C. (2020). Modern therapeutic uses of CHEG herbs and herb pairs. In S.-C. Wang (Ed.), *Veterinary herbal pharmacopoeia* (pp. 35–233). Nova Science Publishers. https://doi.org/10.52305/GHTR1903

Wang, Y., Wu, J., Yu, L., & Xu, Q. (2019). Polysaccharides of *Fructus corni* improve ovarian function in mice with aging-associated perimenopause symptoms. *Evidence-Based Complementary and Alternative Medicine, 2019*, 1–8. https://doi.org/10.1155/2019/2089586

Xu, T., Liu, X., Wang, S., Kong, H., Yu, X., Liu, C., Song, H., Gao, P., & Zhang, X. (2022). Effect of *Pheretima aspergillum* on reducing fibrosis: A systematic review and meta-analysis. *Frontiers in Pharmacology, 13*. https://doi.org/10.3389/fphar.2022.1039553

Yang, J.-X., Wang, Y., Yu, B., & Guo, J. (2008). The total flavones from *Semen cuscutae* reverse the reduction of testosterone level and the expression of androgen receptor gene in kidney-yang deficient mice. *Journal of Ethnopharmacology, 119*(1), 166–171. https://doi.org/10.1016/j.jep.2008.06.027

Index